Soft Tissue Surgery in Exotic Animals

Editors

JOSÉ ROSAS-NAVARRO
CARLO PAOLETTI

VETERINARY CLINICS OF NORTH AMERICA: EXOTIC ANIMAL PRACTICE

www.vetexotic.theclinics.com

Consulting Editor
JÖRG MAYER

September 2026 • Volume 29 • Number 3

ELSEVIER

1818 Market Street • Suite 3323 • Philadelphia, Pennsylvania, 19103-2899
http://www.vetexotic.theclinics.com

VETERINARY CLINICS OF NORTH AMERICA: EXOTIC ANIMAL PRACTICE Volume 29, Number 3
September 2026 ISSN 1094-9194, ISBN-13: 978-0-443-47316-6

Editor: Stacy Eastman
Developmental Editor: Niharika Saxena

Publishing Office: *Veterinary Clinics of North America: Exotic Animal Practice* (ISSN 1094-9194) is published in January, May, and September by Elsevier Inc., 1818 Market Street, Philadelphia, PA 19103, United States. Periodicals postage paid at New York, NY and additional mailing offices. USA POSTMASTER: Send address changes to *Veterinary Clinics of North America: Exotic Animal Practice*, Elsevier Customer Service Department, 3251 Riverport Lane, Maryland Heights, MO 63043, USA. Subscription prices are $314.00 per year for US individuals, $100.00 per year for US students and residents, $366.00 per year for Canadian individuals, $381.00 per year for international individuals, $100.00 per year Canadian students/residents, and $165.00 per year for international students/residents. For institutional access pricing please contact Customer Service via the contact information below. To receive student/resident rate, orders must be accompanied by name of affiliated institution, date of term, and the *signature* of program/residency coordinator on institution letterhead. Orders will be billed at individual rate until proof of status is received. Foreign air speed delivery is included in all *Clinics* subscription prices. All prices are subject to change without notice. Orders, claims, and journal inquiries: Please visit our Support Hub page https://service.elsevier.com for assistance.

Reprints. For copies of 100 or more of articles in this publication, please contact the Commercial Reprints Department, Elsevier Inc., 360 Park Avenue South, New York, New York 10010-1710. Tel.: 212-633-3874; Fax: 212-633-3820; E-mail: reprints@elsevier.com.

Veterinary Clinics of North America: Exotic Animal Practice is covered in *MEDLINE/PubMed (Index Medicus).*

Contributors

CONSULTING EDITOR

JÖRG MAYER, Dr med vet, Msc
Diplomate, American Board of Veterinary Practitioners (Exotic Companion Mammals); Diplomate, European College of Zoological Medicine (Small Mammals); Diplomate, American College of Zoological Medicine; Professor of Zoological Medicine, Department of Small Animal Medicine and Surgery, University of Georgia College of Veterinary Medicine, Athens, Georgia, USA

EDITORS

JOSÉ ROSAS-NAVARRO, DVM
Diplomate of the European College of Zoological Medicine (Small Mammals); Postgraduate University Diploma in Microsurgical Techniques (Faculty of Medicine, Sorbonne University, Paris); Head, the Exotic Animal Department, Centre Hospitalier Vétérinaire AniCura-ADVETIA, Vélizy-Villacoublay, France

CARLO PAOLETTI, DVM
Diplomate of the European College of Zoological Medicine (Small Mammals); Postgraduate University Diploma in Microsurgical Techniques (Faculty of Medicine, Sorbonne University, Paris); Exotic Animal Department, Centre Hospitalier Vétérinaire AniCura-ADVETIA, Vélizy-Villacoublay, France

AUTHORS

PANAGIOTIS AZMANIS, DVM, PhD
Diplomate of the European College of Zoological Medicine (Avian), Diplomate of Zoo and Wildlife Medicine (RCVS); Avian and Wildlife Veterinarian, Dubai Falcon Hospital, Wadi Al Safa Wildlife Center, Dubai, United Arab Emirates

CÉCILE BERNHARD, DVM
Diplomate of the European College of Zoological Medicine (Small Mammals); Veterinarian, Veterinary Clinic l'Arche Des NAC, Pontoise, France

DANIEL CALVO CARRASCO, LV CertAVP(ZM), MRCVS
Diplomate of the European College of Zoological Medicine (Avian); Assistant Vice President of Veterinary Healthcare and Scientific Programmes, Bird Paradise, Mandai Wildlife Group, Singapore

MATHILDE CHARRASSE, DVM
Exotic Animal Department, Centre Hospitalier Vétérinaire AniCura-ADVETIA, Vélizy-Villacoublay, France

LUCILE CHASSANG, DVM
Diplomate of the European College of Zoological Medicine (Small Mammals); Clinician, Eläinsairaala Evidensia Tammisto Animal Hospital, Vantaa, Finland

CIRO COCOCCETTA, DMV
Diplomate of the European College of Zoological Medicine (Avian); Veterinary Specialist, Centre Hospitalier Vétérinaire (CHV) Saint-Martin, Allonzier-la-Caille, France

ISABELLE DESPREZ, DVM
Diplomate of the European College of Zoological Medicine (Small Mammals), Diplomate of the American Board of Veterinary Practitioners (Exotic Companion Mammal); Associate Professor, Department of Small Animal Clinical Sciences, Western College of Veterinary Medicine, Saskatoon, Saskatoon, Canada

NICOLA DI GIROLAMO, DVM, PhD
Diplomate of the European College of Zoological Medicine(Herp); Diplomate of the American College of Zoological Medicine; Diplomate of the American College of Veterinary Preventive Medicine; Associate Professor of Exotic Pet Medicine, Department of Clinical Sciences, College of Veterinary Medicine, Cornell University, Ithaca, New York, USA

SHEYLA DOMINGUEZ, DVM
Diplomate of the European College of Zoological Medicine (Small Mammal); Veterinary Specialist, Department of Exotic Animal, ExoVet Exotic Veterinary Hospital, Ngau Tau Kok, Hong Kong

DARIO D'OVIDIO, DVM, MS, SpecPACS, PhD
Diplomate of the European College of Zoological Medicine (Small Mammals); Head of Avian and Exotic Pet Service, Clinica Veterinaria Malpensa, Samarate, Referral Veterinarian for Exotic Pets, Naples, Italy

LUCAS FLENGHI, DMV
Diplomate of the European College of Zoological Medicine (Small Mammals); Exotic Animal Veterinarian in Private Practice, Exotic ClinicSevetys, Nandy, France

MIKEL SABATER GONZÁLEZ, LV, MRCVS, CertZooMed
Diplomate of the European College of Zoological Medicine (Avian); Veterinary Specialist, Exoticsvet, Valencia, Spain

AURE-ELINE GRILLOT, DVM
Diplomate of the European College of Veterinary Ophthalmologists; Veterinary Ophthalmologist, Department of Ophthalmology, AniCura–ADVETIA Veterinary Hospital, Vélizy-Villacoublay, France

DAVID GUILLIER, DVM
Diplomate of the European College of Zoological Medicine (Small Mammal); Head, Exotic Pet Service, Clinique Vétérinaire Ric et Rac, Le Cannet, France

MINH HUYNH, DVM, MRCVS
Diplomate of the European College of Zoological Medicine (Avian); Diplomate of the American College of Zoological Medicine; Head, Department of Exotic Pet Medicine, Clinique vétérinaire Sevetys Crozatier, Paris, France

LUCIANA MANDRIOLI, DVM, PhD
EBVS© Specialist, Diplomate of the European College of Aquatic Animal Health (ECAAH); Associate Professor, Department of Veterinary Medical Sciences, Alma Mater Studiorum, University of Bologna, Bologna, Italy

EMMA MONGE, DVM
Diplomate of the European College of Zoological Medicine (Small Mammals); Veterinarian, Department of Zoological Medicine, New Companion Animals (NAC) clinic, Ecole Nationale Vétérinaire de Toulouse-INRAE, UMR IHAP VIRAL, France

GIANPIERO NIEDDU, DVM
Chief Veterinarian, Aquarium and Civic Hydrobiological Station, Milan, Italy

CLÉMENT PAILLUSSEAU, DVM
Diplomate of the European College of Zoological Medicine (Herpetology); Veterinary Specialist, Veterinary Clinic SpéNAC, Paris, France

CARLO PAOLETTI, DVM
Diplomate of the European College of Zoological Medicine (Small Mammals); Postgraduate University Diploma in Microsurgical Techniques (Faculty of Medicine, Sorbonne University, Paris); Exotic Animal Department, Centre Hospitalier Vétérinaire AniCura-ADVETIA, Vélizy-Villacoublay, France

MARÍA LUISA PÉREZ ORRICO, LICVET, MRCVS, CES OPHTALMOLOGIE VETERINAIRE
Veterinary Ophthalmologist, Head of the Ophthalmology Service, Hospital Veterinario, Universidad Católica de Valencia, Specialist Clinician, Exoticsvet, Valencia, Spain

ALBERT PHOURATSAMAY, DVM
Diplomate of the European College of Zoological Medicine (Small Mammals); Veterinarian, Department of Exotic Pet Medicine, Nacology Veterinary Clinic, Sevetys Crozatier Veterinary Clinic, Paris; Veterinary Surgeon, Department of Exotic Animal Department, Centre Hospitalier Vétérinaire AniCura-ADVETIA, Vélizy-Villacoublay, France

CHARLY PIGNON, DVM
Diplomate of the European College of Zoological Medicine (Small Mammals); Head, Exotics Medicine Service, Ecole Nationale Vétérinaire d'Alfort, Maisons-Alfort, France

PAUL RAYMOND, DMV
Diplomate of the European College of Zoological Medicine (Small Mammals); Veterinary Specialist, Exotic Medicine Service, Sevetys Clinic, Paris, France

JOSÉ ROSAS-NAVARRO, DVM
Diplomate of the European College of Zoological Medicine (Small Mammals); Postgraduate University Diploma in Microsurgical Techniques (Faculty of Medicine, Sorbonne University, Paris); Head, the Exotic Animal Department, Centre Hospitalier Vétérinaire AniCura-ADVETIA, Vélizy-Villacoublay, France

DIEGO ROSSETTI, DVM
Diplomate of the European College of Veterinary Surgeons; Head, Department of Surgery, Centre Hospitalier Vétérinaire AniCura-ADVETIA, Vélizy-Villacoublay, France

VICENTE SOLER, DVM
Diplomate of the European College of Zoological Medicine (Small Mammal); Veterinary Specialist, Department of Exotic Animal, Tai Wai Small Animal and Exotic Hospital, New Territories, Hong Kong

ALESSANDRO VETERE, DVM, PhD, MSc
Diplomate of the European College of Zoological Medicine (Herpetology); Researcher, Department of Veterinary Science, University of Parma, Parma, Italy

LAURA VILALTA, DVM, PhD
Diplomate of the European College of Zoological Medicine (Small Mammal); Veterinary Specialist, Department of Exotic Animal, Hospital Veterinari Canis, Girona, Spain

LAËTITIA VOLAIT-ROSSET, DVM, MVS
Diplomate of the European College of Zoological Medicine (Small Mammal), Diplomate of the American Board of Veterinary Practitioners (Exotic Companion Mammal); Senior Lecturer in Rabbit, Exotics & Wildlife Medicine and Surgery, Royal (Dick) School of Veterinary Studies, Midlothian, United Kingdom

GRAHAM ZOLLER, DMV
IPSAV (Zoologic Medicine), Diplomate of the European College of Zoological Medicine (Avian); Head, Department of Exotic Pet, OnlyVet Veterinary Hospital Center, Saint-Priest, France

Contents

VETERINARY CLINICS OF NORTH AMERICA: EXOTIC ANIMAL PRACTICE

FORTHCOMING ISSUES

January 2027
Toxicology
Lisa A. Murphy and Peter M. DiGeronimo, *Editors*

September 2027
Alternative Therapy
Tara Harrison, *Editor*

RECENT ISSUES

May 2026
Recent Advances in Exotic Animal Oncology
Shangzhe Xie and Michelle Sutherland, *Editors*

January 2026
Updates in Internal Medicine
Alyssa Scagnelli, *Editor*

September 2025
Oral Cavity Disorders in Exotic Animals
Vladimír Jekl, *Editor*

SERIES OF RELATED INTEREST

Veterinary Clinics: Small Animal Practice
https://www.vetsmall.theclinics.com/
Advances in Small Animal Care
https://www.advancesinsmallanimalcare.com

Preface
Soft Tissue Surgery in Exotic Animals

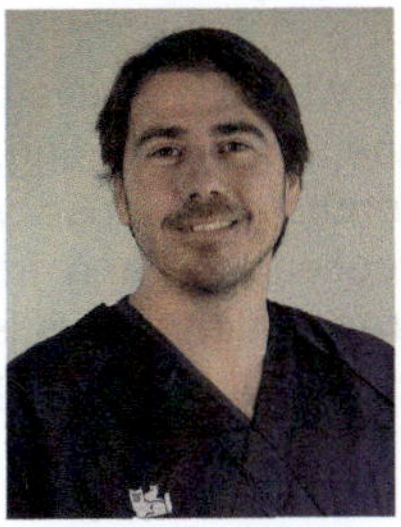

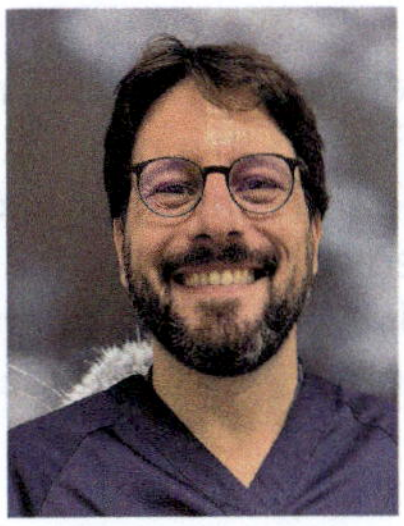

José Rosas-Navarro, DVM   Carlo Paoletti, DVM
Editors

For this long-awaited issue of *Veterinary Clinics of North America: Exotic Animal Practice* on *Soft Tissue Surgery in Exotic Animals*, we have brought together internationally recognized authors with well-established expertise and strong clinical and scientific backgrounds. This selection reflects our commitment to providing readers with authoritative, up-to-date, and clinically relevant content in a rapidly evolving field.

This issue addresses the principal classes of exotic animal patients of clinical interest that are fish, amphibians, reptiles, birds, and small mammals, following a logical and clinically oriented structure. Particular emphasis has been placed on recent literature and current advances. Readers seeking foundational concepts or historical perspectives are referred to the previous *Veterinary Clinics of North America: Exotic Animal Practice* issue on soft tissue surgery published in 2016.

The veterinary literature on exotic animal surgery remains, in some areas, incomplete or affected by inconsistencies. To help overcome these limitations, contributors were encouraged to explore and critically assess relevant nonveterinary scientific sources where appropriate, fostering a more comprehensive and reliable understanding of anatomy, surgical principles, and outcomes. In recent years, surgery in exotic species has progressed considerably, driven by growing clinical interest in these patients and by the expanding expertise of colleagues worldwide, whose work continues to refine and broaden current knowledge.

Surgical challenges in exotic species are substantially greater than those encountered in traditional carnivore surgery. These difficulties arise from the remarkable diversity of species, their distinctive anatomic and physiologic characteristics, and the often very small size of many patients. Consequently, surgical procedures must strictly adhere to the principles of sound surgical practice and be supported by advanced anesthetic and analgesic management, as well as a detailed, species-specific understanding of anatomy and physiology.

Vet Clin Exot Anim 29 (2026) xiii–xiv
https://doi.org/10.1016/j.cvex.2026.04.006
1094-9194/26/© 2026 Published by Elsevier Inc.
vetexotic.theclinics.com

For the most advanced and minimally invasive procedures, the use of state-of-the-art technologies, such as endoscopic approaches and microsurgical techniques, including the operating microscope, is essential. We strongly encourage readers to pursue dedicated training programs and advanced courses to develop the theoretic knowledge and practical skills required in this highly demanding and fascinating discipline. This issue is further enriched by supplementary video material, which complements the existing iconography and provides enhanced visual guidance for the surgical techniques presented.

We wish to express our sincere gratitude to our families, from whom we have taken valuable time to devote ourselves to this project. Their patience, understanding, and unwavering support were fundamental throughout these months of intense work. We also warmly thank our dedicated team, as well as the colleagues and friends who supported us and patiently endured us during the long preparation of this issue. Their encouragement, collaboration, and friendship were invaluable in bringing this project to completion.

DISCLOSURES

The guest editors declare that they have no commercial or financial relationships that could be construed as a potential conflict of interest. No external funding was received in support of this work.

José Rosas-Navarro, DVM
AniCura–ADVETIA Veterinary Hospital
Exotics Department
9 Av. Louis Breguet
Vélizy-Villacoublay 78140, France

Carlo Paoletti, DVM
AniCura–ADVETIA Veterinary Hospital
Exotics Department
9 Av. Louis Breguet
Vélizy-Villacoublay 78140, France

E-mail addresses:
jose.rosas.vet@gmail.com (J. Rosas-Navarro)
carlovet@gmail.com (C. Paoletti)

Soft Tissue Surgery in Fish

Gianpiero Nieddu, DVM[a,*], Luciana Mandrioli, DVM, PhD[b,c]

KEYWORDS

- Bony fish surgery • Celomatic surgery • Elasmobranch surgery • Fishes

KEY POINTS

- Soft tissue surgery in fish has become increasingly feasible and effective allowing safe removal of masses and repair of trauma with acceptable morbidity and mortality.
- Evidence of nociception and pain in fish supports the routine inclusion of perioperative analgesia and structured postoperative management (water quality, mucus protection, and nutritional support) to improve welfare and recovery outcomes.
- A One Health approach is crucial in fish surgery, linking antibiotic stewardship, zoonotic risk management, and environmental biosecurity, and requiring coordinated work between veterinarians, environmental scientists, and public health professionals.
- The field still suffers from a lack of standardization and robust data; there is a need for minimally invasive techniques, consensus guidelines, multicenter registries, and dedicated training programs to transform fish surgery into a fully evidence-based, ethically grounded discipline.

Video content accompanies this article at http://www.vetexotic.theclinics.com.

INTRODUCTION

Soft tissue surgery in fish is a rapidly developing discipline,[1] driven by growing interest in several contexts.[2,3] Traditionally, surgeries in fish were considered impractical due to anatomic, physiologic, and environmental constraints.[4] However, advances in anesthetic techniques, microsurgical instrumentation, and perioperative care have progressively enabled veterinarians to undertake complex procedures in teleosts and elasmobranchs with acceptable morbidity and mortality rates.[5,6] The applications of soft tissue surgery are numerous and vary according to the context: ornamental (koi, goldfish, cichlids, and other species of high economic and emotional value),[7] aquaculture (in fish production, surgery is less frequent, but may involve breeding animals of high genetic value),[8] zoological-conservative (in public aquariums and research centers, interventions are carried out on rare elasmobranchs and teleosts,

[a] Aquarium and Civic Hydrobiological Station, Viale Gadio 2, 20100, Milan, Italy; [b] Department of Veterinary Medical Sciences, Alma Mater Studiorum, University of Bologna, Ozzano Emilia, Via Tolara di Sopra 50, 40064, Bologna, Italy; [c] Diplomate of the European College of Aquatic Animal Health (ECAAH)
* Corresponding author.
E-mail address: gianpieronieddu@gmail.com

Vet Clin Exot Anim 29 (2026) 449–468
https://doi.org/10.1016/j.cvex.2026.04.001 vetexotic.theclinics.com

Abbreviation	
STS	soft tissue sarcoma

to ensure the individual well-being and survival of precious specimens),[9] research (includes procedures for sensor and telemetry implantation, tissue biopsies, or sampling for toxicologic and physiologic studies).[10,11]

This scientific review builds upon the previous edition prepared for the Veterinary Clinics of North America (Sladky KK & Clarke EO, 2016), which serves as an essential supplement to the current edition.

PRESURGICAL PREPARATION

A comprehensive clinical evaluation (Video 1), including diagnostic imaging and laboratory tests, is necessary in presurgical planning.[4] X-rays are useful for detecting masses, swim bladder abnormalities, and skeletal structures (**Fig. 1**). Ultrasonography provides a real-time assessment of soft tissue masses, reproductive organs, and celomatic fluid[12] (**Figs. 2** and **3**). Endoscopy can also be used for direct visualization and biopsy of internal tissues, especially in larger species.[13] Unlike terrestrial species, the external signs of disease in fish may initially be nonspecific or not noticeable, and the disease often becomes manifest only in advanced stages[14] (**Fig. 4**).

SURGICAL PREPARATION

Environmental control: because fish are ectothermic and depend on water for respiration and homeostasis, environmental parameters must be tightly controlled before, during, and after surgery.[15] The temperature should be kept within the species' preferred range to prevent metabolic stress. Sudden changes can induce shock. Dissolved oxygen must be close to saturation and ammonia, nitrites and other water quality parameters must be monitored and kept within safe limits (**Fig. 5**).[4]

Sedation and manipulation: minimizing stress during initial handling is essential.[16] Before induction of anesthesia, fish may be lightly sedated (eg, with low-dose MS-222 or eugenol) to facilitate restraint with the net.[17] Physical restraint should be gentle, using soft nets or wet towels to avoid mucus loss and skin abrasions.[18]

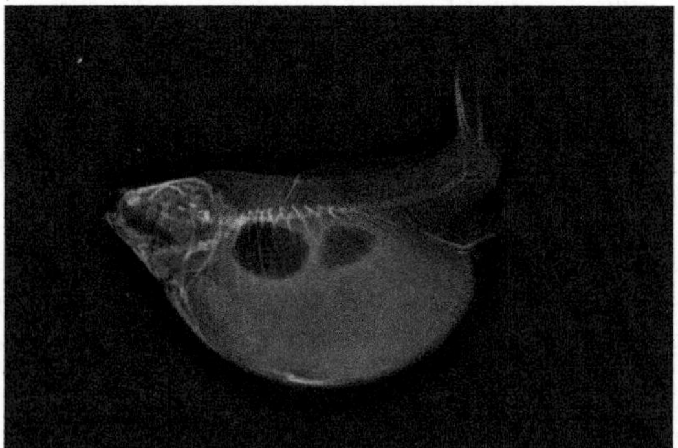

Fig. 1. The X-ray examination performed with the patient under sedation (50 mg/L of methanesulfonate tricaine) revealed a significant accumulation of fluid within the celomatic cavity. (Image Courtesy of Dr Nieddu.)

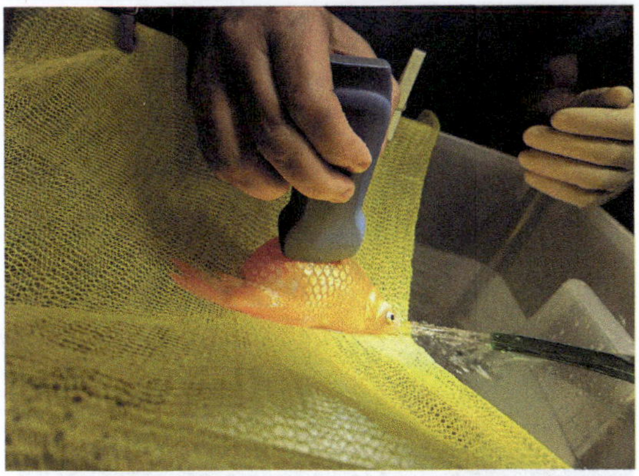

Fig. 2. Ultrasound examination with the patient under sedation was performed in addition to the radiological study. (Image Courtesy of Dr Nieddu.)

Skin preparation and asepsis: the preparation of a sterile surgical field in an aquatic organism is complex.[19] The skin can be appropriately prepared with disinfectants such as diluted povidone iodine (0.5%–1%) or chlorhexidine (0.05%), which can be applied and rinsed before incision, taking care to protect the gills from exposure.[5] The fish should be placed on a moistened and disinfected surface, and irrigation with water should be continuous to avoid overdrying of the fish body exposed to air.[4]

Anesthesia and Analgesia

Proper anesthesia is obviously a key component.[18] It must provide adequate immobility, analgesia and muscle relaxation while maintaining cardiorespiratory function and minimizing recovery time.[20] Analgesia is increasingly recognized as an essential component of perioperative care due to the increasing evidence of nociception and pain perception in fish (**Table 1**).[18,21]

Most fish are anesthetized by immersion in water containing dissolved anesthetic agents.[20] Tricaine methanesulfonate, probably remains the most widely used drug.[22]

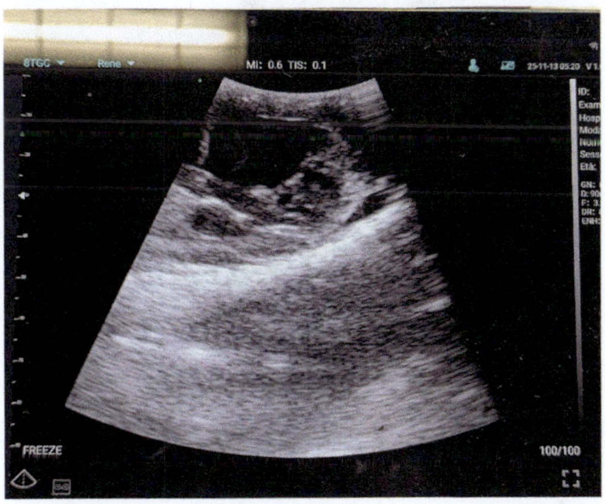

Fig. 3. Ultrasound confirmed the fluid in the celomic cavity and revealed the presence of echogenic structures (consistent with ovarian tissue) that were not detected by X-rays. (Image Courtesy of Dr Nieddu.)

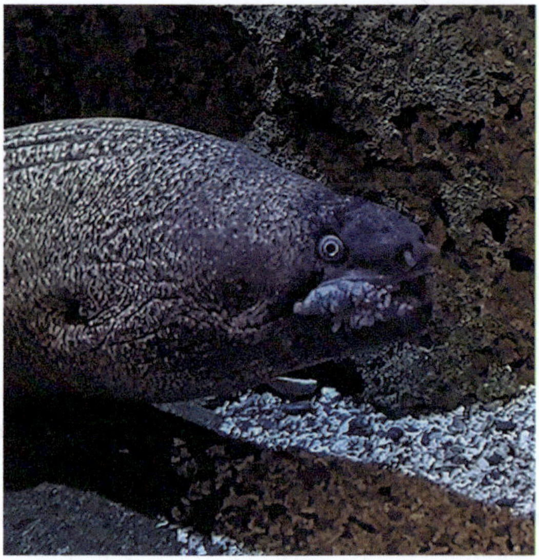

Fig. 4. A Mediterranean moray eel (*Muraena helena*) affected by a condition known as oral stomatopapillomatosis. This condition should be preferably treated by a surgical approach. Since papillomatosis can reach esophagus and stomach, it would be advisable to add a CT scan or MRI to evaluate the level of its extent. (Image Courtesy of Dr Nieddu.)

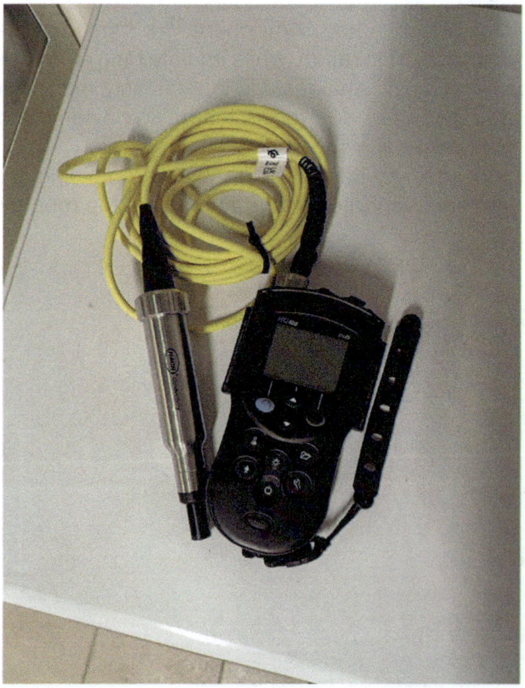

Fig. 5. A probe can be useful for accurately determining certain parameters during patient sedation. pH, temperature, salinity, and so on must be monitored. (Image Courtesy of Dr Nieddu.)

Table 1
Analgesic drugs

Category	Molecule (Drug)	Dose	Administration Route	Efficacy/Indications	Safety Notes
Non-steroidal anti-inflammatory drugs	Meloxicam	0.2–1.0 mg/kg every 24–48 h	Intramuscular or intracelomic injection	Reduces inflammation, mild to moderate analgesia	Use with caution in compromised fish
Non-steroidal anti-inflammatory drugs	Carprofen	2–4 mg/kg	Intramuscular or intracelomic injection	Limited data available	Generally safe, but limited data
Opioids	Butorphanol	0.2–0.4 mg/kg	Intramuscular or intracelomic injection	Moderate to severe analgesia, behavioral improvement	May depress respiration at high doses
Opioids	Buprenorphine	0.01–0.05 mg/kg	Intramuscular or intracelomic injection	Experimental evidence of behavioral improvement	Monitor respiratory function
Opioids	Morphine	variable	Not specified	Variable efficacy, prolonged recovery in some species	Can cause respiratory depression, slow recovery
Local anesthetics	Lidocaine	2–4 mg/kg	Incisional infiltration	Local analgesia before closure	Local use, toxic risk if systemic
Local anesthetics	Bupivacaine	1–2 mg/kg	Incisional infiltration	Local analgesia before closure	Local use, avoid excessive doses

Typical induction doses range from 50 to 150 mg/L, and it is always necessary to monitor the pH of the water due to its tendency to acidify.[23] The use of baking soda may be necessary to buffer this tendency.[24] Eugenol is effective at lower costs and provides good induction and recovery.[25] Benzocaine, alfaxalone and 2-phenoxyethanol are also used, particularly in Europe.[26]

Injectable anesthetics are useful for prolonged or invasive procedures and in large individuals where immersion is not practical.[26] Drugs include ketamine, propofol, and alfaxalone, often combined with sedatives (dexmedetomidine, diazepam) or opioids (butorphanol, buprenorphine).[27] These drugs require species-specific dosing and close monitoring due to the variable pharmacokinetics in ectotherms.[28]

Different molecules[29] and different doses can be used to achieve a specific anesthetic plan (**Table 2**).[30–32]

The stages of induction and awakening of anesthesia in fish are well described by veterinary protocols and can be summarized in recognizable sequences depending on the depth of anesthesia and the response to stimuli.[20,33]

Anesthesia Induction

Light sedation: slowing of movements, reduced reactivity to external stimuli, swimming still coordinated.

Deep sedation: slowed movements, partial loss of balance, and reduced response to tactile stimuli.

Surgical anesthesia: loss of the balance reflex (the fish lies on the bottom), absence of response to stimuli, shallow and regular breathing, abolition of reflexes (such as dorsal fin reflex and operculum).

Table 2
Main anesthetic drugs in fish

Anesthetic Drugs	Recommended Dosage	Notes
Tricaine methanesulfonate (MS-222)	50–150 mg/L for anesthesia	Dose varies according to the species; buffer with baking soda; Effective in most freshwater and marine species
Clove oil (eugenol)	20–40 mg/L for anesthesia, 2–4 mg/L for sedation	Widely used in aquaculture
Benzocaine	30–100 mg/L for anesthesia	Mainly for ornamental fish
2-phenoxyethanol	200–400 mg/L for anesthesia	Suitable for ornamental fish, quick effect but short
Propofol	5–10 mg/L for anesthesia	Limited use, especially in research approach
Xylazine (use in combination)	1–2 mg/kg IM	Sometimes with other agents for deep interventions
Compound	**Recommended Dosage**	**Notes**
	Alternative and Innovative Compounds:	
Alfaxalone	2–10 mg/L immersion	anesthetic, administered by immersion
Butorphanol	0.4 mg/kg IM	Used for analgesia in combination with alphaxalone
Thiopental sodium	Variable dosage	Injectable barbiturate (Pentothal Sodium)
Ketamine	50–100 mg/L immersion, 10–30 mg/kg injection IM	Used primarily in combination with other agents for surgical anesthesia

Overdose: respiratory arrest, risk of serious injury or death; attention to concentration, and time of exposure should be avoided (Video 2).[34]

Planning the Surgical Approach: Positioning and Stabilization

Careful planning of the surgical approach minimizes tissue trauma, operative time, and can improve postoperative outcomes.[4]

The fish should be positioned to allow optimal access to the surgical site while maintaining gill irrigation and avoiding compression of the gills or viscera.[16] Common positions include dorsal decubitus (for ventral celiotomy), lateral decubitus (for flank access), and ventral decubitus (for dorsal or cranial procedures).[35]

From this point onwards, it is necessary to keep the gills constantly oxygenated to ensure breathing and maintain the desired level of anesthesia.[5] This is typically accomplished by using a recirculating irrigation system that delivers water with the dissolved anesthetic to the gills via a tube or catheter in the mouth. The amount of water supplied to the gills should be carefully adjusted according to the size of the fish (Video 3).[28] Respiratory support is also necessary in the case of injectable anesthesia when the respiratory rate tends to decrease, to maintain an adequate level of blood oxygenation.

Instrumentation

Surgical instruments should be appropriately sized for the patient.

Minimally invasive approaches should be preferred whenever possible, endoscopic approaches can reduce surgical trauma, improve visualization, and shorten recovery time.[10] These techniques remain experimental in fish, but are increasingly reported, especially in large elasmobranchs or sturgeons.[9,36] Preoperative imaging should guide incision planning to avoid unnecessary dissections.[12,37–39]

COMMON SOFT TISSUE SURGICAL PROCEDURES

Removal of Celomatic Masses

Celomatic masses can be of more often neoplastic[40] and less often inflammatory or dysplastic origin; they are relatively common in ornamental and research fishes in captivity.[41]

The surgical approach to a fish with a gonadal neoplasm is often preceded by an instrumental diagnosis (usually ultrasound) following clinical examination that reveals abnormal and sometimes asymmetric abdominal distension.[42,43] Ultrasound, in addition to detecting abnormalities in the coelomic cavity, often allows visualization of pathologic effusion, which can arise from multiple underlying conditions, including organ dysfunction.[43] Once the fish is adequately sedated and positioned dorsoventrally, a midline incision is made to provide proper access to the coelomic cavity. At this stage, aspiration of the fluid present may be necessary to improve visualization of the organs.

Unfortunately, diagnosis of these conditions is often delayed, and neoplasia may already have infiltrated surrounding organs when presenting for surgery.[44] In such cases, surgery can aim to remove as much of the mass as possible, even if not completely. After excision, the surgical wound could be closed in one or 2 layers using absorbable material (generally Polyglactin 910). This avoids the need to resedate the fish to remove sutures once the surgical site is healed (**Fig. 6**).[45–47]

During surgery, if sedation is achieved with tricaine methanesulfonate, it is necessary to continuously monitor pH due to the acidifying effect of the anesthetic on the water.[41] At the end of surgery, the fish is transferred to a recovery container with

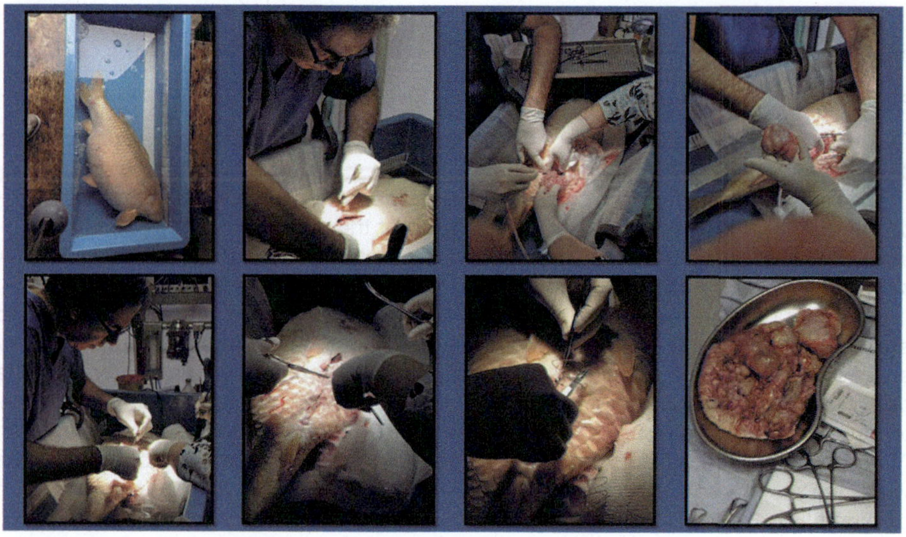

Fig. 6. Removal of celomatic masse. (Image Courtesy of Dr Nieddu.)

water of the same chemical characteristics as its original habitat.[48] Anti-inflammatory drugs may be administered before full recovery to accelerate postoperative improvement.[49,50]

Resumption of normal functions occurs gradually: first an increase in respiratory rate, then attempts to regain proper swimming posture, and finally swimming stability. At this stage, the patient should be placed in a container large enough to allow comfortable swimming and effective observation for several days.[25] Some fish may require the presence of conspecifics to restore a *social* environment that relieves postoperative stress, calms the patient, and speeds up recovery (Video 4).

Not Neoplastic Reproductive Surgery

It has high relevance in the percentage of surgical treatments.[38] Surgical interventions on the reproductive system in fish are performed for therapeutic, management or research purposes.[48] These surgeries are often technically challenging due to the fragility and high vascularization of the gonadal tissue.[51]

Proximity to the main vessels requires careful dissection.[10]

In teleosts, the reproductive system includes paired elongated gonads, efferent ducts, and a genital papilla, with gonads suspended dorsally in the coelomic cavity and often joined caudally. Teleosts show wide reproductive diversity, but ovaries are mainly cystovarian (oocytes into an ovarian lumen continuous with the oviduct) or gymnovarian (eggs first into the coelom), without a true uterine analog; the basic germinal units are the ovarian follicle and testicular spermatocyst.[52]

In elasmobranchs, gonads are associated with the cranial epigonal organ; males have paired testes, whereas females typically have a right ovary in sharks, a left ovary in rays, and paired ovaries in skates and chimaeras, with paired oviducts and uteri opening through a common ostium. Internal fertilization is universal, mediated by paired claspers in males, and sperm is stored in oviducal glands; reproductive modes span oviparity, aplacental viviparity, and placental viviparity, reflecting extensive diversification of chondrichthyan reproductive anatomy and strategies.[51]

Oophorectomy/Orchiectomy

Access is usually via a ventral celiotomy (preferably performed using a radiosurgical/electrosurgical or laser scalpel) to minimize disruption of other organs. After isolating the gonad, the vessels are tied with a thin, absorbable suture or hemoclips. The gonad is then gently removed. In some cases, only a partial gonadectomy is performed to remove the pathologic tissue while preserving endocrine function. Excessive traction should be avoided to avoid tearing and bleeding (**Fig. 7**A–D).[51]

Dystocia occurs in oviparous fish when mature oocytes are not expelled, often due to triggering environmental factors (unsuitable environmental conditions or unsuitable environmental enrichment), anatomic obstruction or poor conditions that affect spawning. Conservative treatments include environmental modification, hormonal induction (gonadotropin releasing hormone analogues, human chorionic gonadotropin) and manual pressure under anesthesia. If these fail, surgical removal of the retained eggs via ventral celiotomy is indicated. Care must be taken to avoid breaking the eggs, which can cause a serious celomitis.

Repair of Cutaneous Traumatic Injuries

Traumatic wounds, lacerations, and bite injuries are common in captive fish, especially in densely populated systems or among aggressive species.[45] Surgical repair is indicated when wounds are deep, extensive, or unlikely to heal by secondary intention. The wound margins must be managed to remove necrotic tissue and promote vascularization. The edges of the skin are sutured with absorbable materials so that no subsequent sedation is required for their removal.[5]

Excision of Cutaneous and Subcutaneous Masses

Some goldfish (*Carassius auratus*) varieties have distinctive head conformations characterized by the growth of tissue known as *wen*. In high-quality fish, the wen is usually well developed and symmetric, but in some cases, it may grow abnormally, covering the eyes and impairing vision and the quality of life.[53] In these situations, reduction of the wen is necessary and various surgical techniques are available, including the use of a surgical laser.[54] The fish, sedated with tricaine methanesulfonate or for example, phenoxyethanol, can be manipulated appropriately for a rapid procedure, and the surgical laser produces a precise tissue incision, reducing the need for suturing,

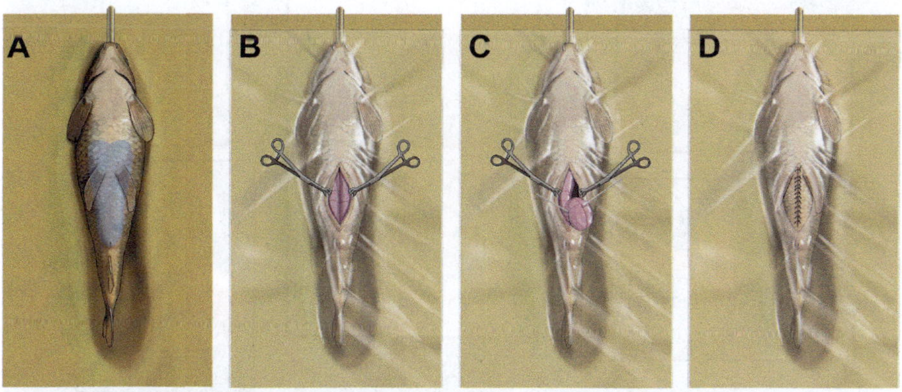

Fig. 7. (*A–D*) koi carp (*Cyprinus carpio*), ventral frontal view. (surgical approach for ovariectomy). ((c)Digital Illustration (2025) by Cristian Rovea (@corporevivi).)

minimizing tissue bleeding, and decreasing the risk of infection at the treated sites.[54] Once awakened, the fish can immediately be returned to the community tank, where, having regained optimal visual capacity, it resumes normal routines (**Fig. 8**).

Goldfish are frequently affected by cutaneous masses. They often affect the skin and fins, present as single or even multiple masses and are histologically consistent with tumors that were variably named as neurofibroma, fibrosarcoma, schwannoma, peripheral nerve sheath tumors, and nerve sheath tumors[55–60] (see the benchmark publication of Schlumberger, 1953).[61] About their histologic classification, these tumors can be listed under the more general category of cutaneous soft tissue sarcoma (STSs). In the absence of standardized histologic criteria in fish species, the authors of this article encourage a collaboration among professionals and between diagnostic laboratories and suggest the use of the broader term of cutaneous STSs. Very often these cutaneous masses can be surgically treated using a surgical laser (Videos 5–7).

In some cases, masses to be removed may be of viral origin.[62,63] Lesions from lymphocystivirus (LCDV) can impair certain bodily functions if they develop in critical areas. Lesions near the mouth may obstruct or hinder mouth opening, reducing the ability to grasp food and compromising the fish's health. In these cases, as well, the use of a surgical laser allows for rapid removal of the mass, minimizing the risk of bleeding and postoperative infections.[64] The fish, sedated with tricaine methanesulfonate or clove oil, can be properly handled for quick excision. Given the lesion's location, placement of a tube to facilitate gill oxygenation can be difficult (**Figs. 9** and **10**).

LESS COMMON SOFT TISSUES PROCEDURES

Gastrointestinal Surgery

It is highly dependent on the fish species with which it is working. Occasionally, surgical interventions on the gastrointestinal tract are necessary for the removal of foreign bodies (fishhooks, plastic material, bottom material, and so on), intussusception, among others.[38,65]

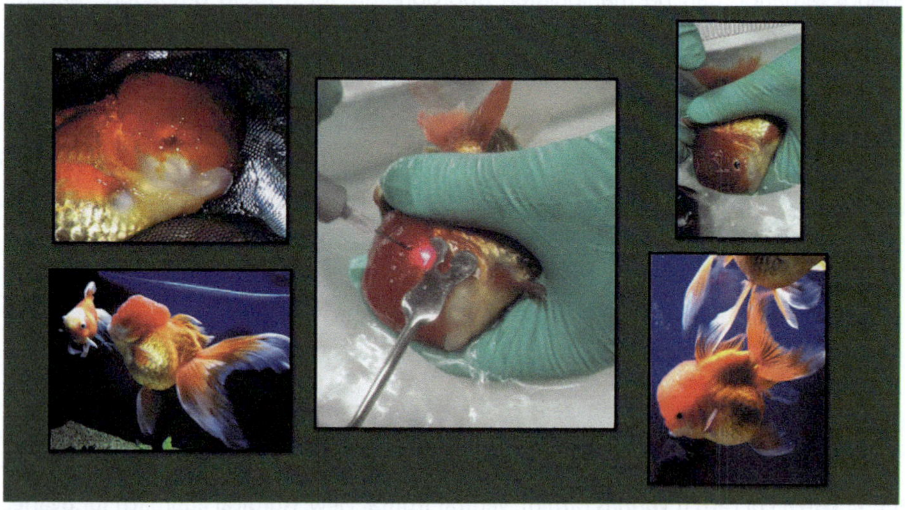

Fig. 8. Excision of cutaneous and subcutaneous masses of goldfish *Carassius auratus*.

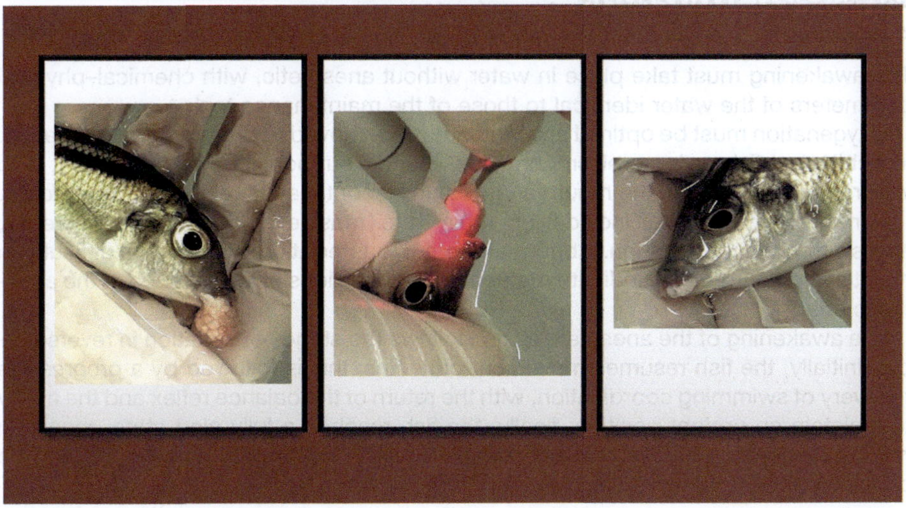

Fig. 9. Laser-assisted excision of an LCDV-related oral mass in a sedated fish (*Mylochromis lateristriga*); airway management and limited access noted due to lesion location. (Image Courtesy of Dr Nieddu.)

A ventral celiotomy allows exposure of the gastrointestinal tract. The intestine is gently exteriorized with moistened applicators with a cotton tip. Enterotomy or gastrotomy is performed using a thin scalpel or microscissors and the tract is sutured in 2 planes (mucosa/submucosa and seromuscular), when possible, with absorbable monofilament suture (5–0 to 7–0).[45,47] The suture should be very accurate to avoid celomatic contamination caused by intestinal contents and consequent infection.

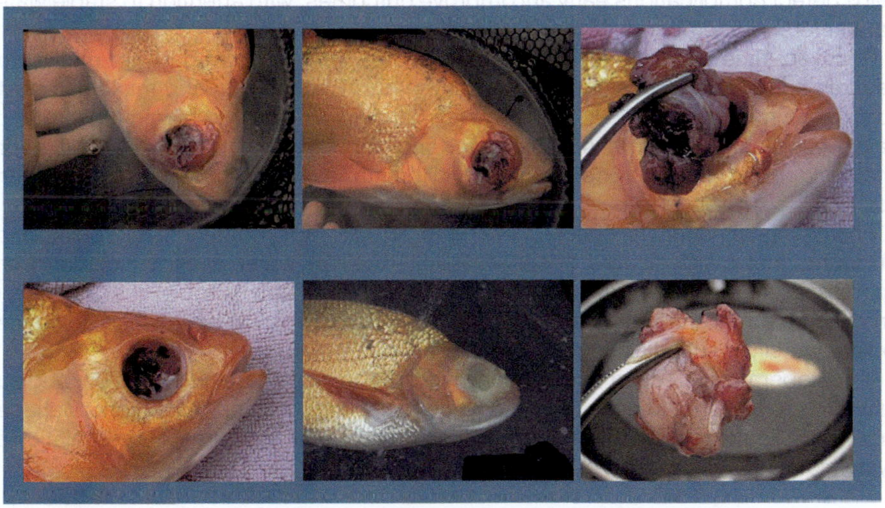

Fig. 10. Some eye conditions should be treated by surgery. During enucleation, with the patient under appropriate sedation, the eyeball is detached from the surrounding soft tissues, taking care to ligate the optic nerve and blood vessels located posteriorly to limit any bleeding. (Image Courtesy of Dr Barbé.)

POSTSURGICAL MANAGEMENT

Awakening

The awakening must take place in water without anesthetic, with chemical–physical parameters of the water identical to those of the maintenance tank.

Oxygenation must be optimal and water must be moved to promote gills ventilation. In debilitated fish or large elasmobranchs, manual support may be necessary, with water irrigation through the mouth and gills until spontaneous respiration is restored.

Parameters to monitor include: opercular rate, muscle tone, straightening reflex, and swimming coordination. Abnormalities such as erratic swimming or difficulty in maintaining posture may indicate metabolic complications or persistence of the anesthetic effect.

The awakening of the anesthetized fish follows the stages of sedation in reverse order. Initially, the fish resumes movement of its fins; this is followed by a progressive recovery of swimming coordination, with the return of the balance reflex and the ability to maintain an upright position; finally, the fish reaches a fully alert state, regaining normal responsiveness to external stimuli, baseline respiratory activity and can be considered ready for complete release.[66,67]

Supportive Therapy

It focuses on restoring osmotic balance, which is often affected by stress and trauma. Effective support includes maintaining optimal water parameters, administering fluids to larger fish, minimizing handling and density to preserve the mucus layer, and using commercial mucus protectants, for example, formulations combining aloe vera with polyvinylpyrrolidone (PVP) have been shown to enhance mucus production and wound healing in cyprinids[68] or low-dose salt baths to promote healing.[67]

Reducing stress postoperatively is essential, achieved through visual barriers, low lighting, and minimal disturbances. Nutritional support is also key: food should only resume when fish show normal alertness and interest, using highly digestible and palatable foods.[36] Continuous monitoring of water quality and the fish's behavior helps detect complications early and improve outcomes, with attention to stable water parameters and temperature (see **Fig. 9**).[28]

Recovery time varies by species and procedure, ranging from days for minor procedures up to several weeks for major surgeries.[18] Recognizing and managing postsurgical pain is important[69–71]; fish display behavioral and physiologic indicators of pain[72] such as lethargy, loss of appetite, and abnormal posture.[73,74] A multimodal analgesic approach is recommended,[75] though evidence-based guidelines are scarce.[76]

Preventing infection is critical, given the aquatic environment's microbial load. Measures include dedicated hospital tanks, excellent water quality, isolation from aggressive tankmates, and, where indicated, targeted antimicrobial therapy based on cultures rather than routine broad-spectrum use.[77] Topical agents like povidone-iodine and silver sulfadiazine may be used on skin wounds.

If postoperative infection occurs, early signs (redness, swelling, ulceration, and suture dehiscence) should prompt cytology, cultures, imaging, and bloodwork. Management may require removal of necrotic tissue, replacement of sutures, and escalation of systemic antibiotics guided by microbiological testing.

THE *ONE HEALTH* PARADIGM APPLIED TO FISH SURGERY

A *One Health* approach in fish surgery, as part of the aquaculture framework, is a systemic, transdisciplinary strategy that integrates human, animal, and environmental health to promote sustainability and global biosecurity.[78] This paradigm extends beyond traditional biomedical models by addressing how biological, environmental, and societal factors intersect to influence disease, productivity, and public health.[79,80]

In the context of fish surgery, *One Health* principles require rigorous antibiotic stewardship and careful management of zoonotic risks, given the potential for antimicrobial residues and resistant bacteria to impact both aquatic and human ecosystems.[81]

Implementing this model calls for close collaboration among veterinarians, environmental scientists, and public health professionals to ensure responsible use of therapeutics, high standards of animal welfare, and ecological protection. Embracing the *One Health* framework enables innovation, improves risk mitigation, and supports safe, sustainable aquaculture practices that underpin global food security.[81]

Development of Minimally Invasive Techniques

Endoscopic and laparoscopic techniques have the potential to reduce tissue trauma, shorten recovery time, and improve visualization of internal structures,[82] especially in large teleosts and elasmobranchs.[83] Early reports of laparoscopic gonadectomy and biopsy procedures in sturgeon and elasmobranchs demonstrate feasibility, but remain technically challenging and resource-intensive.[10]

Standardization of Surgical Techniques and Reporting of Results

The current literature on fish soft tissue surgery is dominated by case reports and anecdotal descriptions, with limited controlled trials or standardized outcome data.[84] This hampers evidence-based refinement of techniques and comparison of results between institutions.

There is a clear need to

- Consensus guidelines on surgical terminology, technique description, and reporting standards
- Creation of multicenter registries documenting surgical procedures, complications, survival rates, and long-term outcomes[85]
- Adoption of objective metrics for the evaluation of wound healing, pain and functional recovery[86]
- Integration of digital imaging and video recording to facilitate peer review and training[87,88]

Such standardization would accelerate the evolution of fish surgery from a set of individualized practices to a cohesive, evidence-based discipline.

Integration Between Welfare and Ethical Considerations

- As recognition of fish sentience increases, ethical control of invasive procedures is likely to intensify. This requires the proactive incorporation of wellness principles into surgical decision-making and experimental design.
    - Future efforts should emphasize.
- Refinement of surgical indications to ensure that interventions are justified by tangible benefits in terms of well-being or conservation.
- Development of validated welfare assessment tools for perioperative fish care.[74,89]
- Mandatory inclusion of pain mitigation protocols in institutional guidelines for animal care and use.[71,74,90]
- Incorporating welfare considerations within the scientific framework of fish surgery will support the ethical legitimacy and public acceptance of the field.[91–93]

Training, Education and Capacity Building

- There is currently a shortage of veterinarians trained in fish surgery, which limits access to advanced care and slows the spread of new techniques. Capacity building through targeted training programs is essential to support the growth of this discipline.[94,95]

SUMMARY

The field of fish soft tissue surgery is at a turning point. Advances in anesthesia, microsurgical instrumentation, and postoperative care have made complex procedures increasingly feasible, but substantial gaps in knowledge, standardization, and training remain. Addressing these challenges through coordinated research, technological innovation, and ethical management will enable the transition of fish surgery from a niche capability to a robust, evidence-based discipline. Ultimately, such advances will improve the welfare and survival outcomes of fish under human care, benefiting ornamental aquaculture, biomedical research, and conservation efforts.

CLINICS CARE POINTS

- Always buffer and monitor anesthetic solutions, adjusting pH and exposure time to avoid acidotic overdose and delayed recovery.
- Tailor multimodal anesthesia and perioperative analgesia to species, size, and procedure length, and never equate rapid recovery with absence of pain.
- Do not schedule surgery without complete water-quality data and species-specific temperature ranges, as environmental optimization often stabilizes fragile patients more than drug changes.
- Use imaging systematically to plan incision sites and approaches, minimizing unnecessary coelomic exploration and shortening operative time.
- Maintain continuous, size-adjusted gill irrigation with oxygenated, temperature-controlled water throughout air-exposed surgery.
- Protect skin and mucus with gentle handling, wet towels, and non-abrasive supports, and avoid over-zealous antisepsis that can damage gills and integument.
- Match instruments and closure materials to body size and wall thickness, favoring minimally invasive techniques and absorbable sutures when re-anesthesia for removal is high-risk.
- Anticipate advanced disease and friable tissues in coelomic and reproductive surgery, using meticulous hemostasis and clear preoperative communication about palliative versus curative intent.
- Standardize recovery in dedicated hospital tanks with identical water chemistry, optimal oxygenation, delayed feeding until full coordination, and routine mucus-supportive measures.
- Detect and treat postoperative infection early using cytology, culture, and targeted antibiotics, embedding One Health–based antimicrobial stewardship into every surgical plan.

ACKNOWLEDGMENTS

The authors would like to thank Dr Carla Iacono Isidoro, librarian (Leon Battista Alberti Central Library, Alma Mater Studiorum University of Bologna, Italy) for her valuable assistance into setting up the bibliographic research.

We would also like to thank Dr Tim Barbé for kindly providing the plate about the eye surgery, Dr Carlo Paoletti and Dr José Rosas-Navarro for kindly providing some surgery videos and Cristian Rovea for the scientific drawing.

DISCLOSURE

The authors have nothing to disclose.

SUPPLEMENTARY DATA

Supplementary data related to this article can be found online at https://doi.org/10.1016/j.cvex.2026.04.001.

REFERENCES

1. Harms CA, Lewbart GA. Surgery in fish. Vet Clin Exot Anim Pract 2000;3(3):759–74.
2. Kang G, Woo WS, Kim KH, et al. Clinical assessment of thermotherapy applications during hepatectomy and laparotomy in sturgeon (acipenser ruthenus): impact on bioparameter variations based on liver condition. Vet Sci 2023;10-(12):682.
3. da Rocha JNNM, Bastos AC, Meneguelli M, et al. Cirurgia em peixes. Res Soc Dev 2020;9(11). https://doi.org/10.33448/rsd-v9i11.9849. e2659119849.
4. Saint-Erne N. Surgery. In: The handbook of ornamental fish health and welfare. CABI Books; 2024. p. 148–57. https://doi.org/10.1079/9781789246032.0016.
5. Sladky KK, Clarke EO. Fish surgery. Vet Clin Exot Anim Pract 2016;19(1):55–76.
6. Mylniczenko ND, Burns C, Greene W, et al. Bony fish (lungfish, sturgeon, and teleosts). In: West G, Heard D, Caulkett N, editors. Zoo animal and wildlife immobilization and anesthesia. wiley; 2025. p. 225–345. https://doi.org/10.1002/9781119539278.ch8.
7. Mansur VFR, Melo N, Di Chiacchio IM, et al. Sex identification of the ornamental Amazon fish Astronotus ocellatus by videoceloscopy and gonadal biopsy. Anim Reprod Sci 2021;230:106780. https://doi.org/10.1016/j.anireprosci.2021.106780.
8. Hegna J, Scribner K, Baker E. Evaluation of optimal surgical techniques for intracoelomic transmitter implantation in age-0 lake sturgeon. Fish Res 2019;218:198–208.
9. Abraham Gabriel A, Yee-Nin ST, Adamu L, et al. Enucleation in a cownose ray (Rhinoptera bonasus). Case Rep Vet Med 2018;2018(1):5048948. https://doi.org/10.1155/2018/5048948.
10. Falahatkar B, Tolouei Gilani MH, Falahatkar S, et al. Laparoscopy, a minimally-invasive technique for sex identification in cultured great sturgeon *Huso huso*. Aquaculture 2011;321(3):273–9.
11. Tagger effects in aquatic telemetry. Short term and delayed effects of surgery in Atlantic Salmon smolts | North American Journal of Fisheries Management | Oxford Academic. Available at: https://academic.oup.com/najfm/article/44/2/262/7811729?login=false. Accessed September 22, 2025.
12. Kehoe SP, Divers SJ, Mayer J, et al. Computed tomographic and ultrasonographic diagnosis with successful excision of a lipoma in a shusui koi (Cyprinus carpio). J Am Vet Med Assoc 2020;256(12):1379–85.
13. Sladakovic I, Divers S. Surg Endosc 2021;213–32. https://doi.org/10.1002/9781119259886.ch11.

14. Cutaneous haemangiosarcoma with ovarian metastases in an aquarium-managed mirror carp (Cyprinus carpio) - rich - 2024 - veterinary record case reports - wiley online library. Available at: https://bvajournals.onlinelibrary.wiley.com/doi/10.1002/vrc2.831. Accessed October 30, 2025.
15. Flecknell P. Laboratory animal anaesthesia and analgesia, fifth edition. Elsevier; 2023. https://doi.org/10.1016/C2018-0-03009-1.
16. Surgery of Exotic Animals - Fish surgery 1 2022.
17. Guidelines on fish anesthesia analgesia and surgery – animal care & use program. Available at: https://az.research.umich.edu/animalcare/guidelines/guidelines-fish-anesthesia-analgesia-and-surgery/. Accessed August 8, 2025.
18. Anesthesia and analgesia - clinical guide to fish medicine - Wiley online library. Available at: https://onlinelibrary.wiley.com/doi/10.1002/9781119259886.ch10. Accessed September 19, 2025.
19. Vergneau-Grosset C, Cruz Benedetti IC. Fish sedation and anesthesia. Vet Clin Exot Anim Pract 2022;25(1):13–29.
20. Schroeder P, Lloyd R, McKimm R, et al. Anaesthesia of laboratory, aquaculture and ornamental fish: proceedings of the first LASA-FVS symposium. Lab Anim 2021;55(4):317–28.
21. Sneddon LU. Clinical anesthesia and analgesia in fish. J Exot Pet Med 2012; 21(1):32–43.
22. Parker-Graham CA, Lima KM, Soto E. The effect of anesthetic time and concentration on blood gases, acid-base status, and electrolytes in koi (Cyprinus carpio) anesthetized with buffered tricaine methanesulfonate (MS-222). J Zoo Wildl Med 2020;51(1):102–9.
23. Carter KM, Woodley CM, Brown RS. A review of tricaine methanesulfonate for anesthesia of fish. Rev Fish Biol Fish 2011;21(1):51–9.
24. Applegate JR, Dombrowski DS, Christian LS, et al. Tricaine methanesulfonate (MS-222) sedation and anesthesia in the purple-spined sea urchin (ARBACIA PUNCTULATA). J Zoo Wildl Med Off Publ Am Assoc Zoo Vet 2016;47(4):1025–33.
25. Narumanchi S, Perttunen S, Laine P, et al. Tricaine, eugenol and etomidate for repetitive procedural anesthesia in adult zebrafish, Danio rerio: effect on stress and behavior. Front Vet Sci 2025;12. https://doi.org/10.3389/fvets.2025.1562425.
26. Adel M, Sadegh AB, Yeganeh S, et al. Anesthetic efficacy of clove oil, propofol, 2-Phenoxyethanol, and ketamine hydrochloride on Persian sturgeon, Acipenser persicus, juveniles. J World Aquacult Soc 2016;47(6):812–9.
27. De Freitas SSLR, Fanger IS, Tsuruta SA, et al. Use of propofol associated with methadone and local blockade with lidocaine in 6 specimens of freshwater stingrays (Potamotrygon spp.). J Exot Pet Med 2025;53:28–31.
28. Grosset C, Weber IIIE. Fish Surgery 2021;46–62. https://doi.org/10.1002/9781119139614.ch5.
29. Pedrazzani AS, Neto AO. The anaesthetic effect of camphor (Cinnamomum camphora), clove (Syzygium aromaticum) and mint (Mentha arvensis) essential oils on clown anemonefish, Amphiprion ocellaris (Cuvier 1830). Aquac Res 2016; 47(3):769–76.
30. Anaesthetic efficacy of eugenol on iridescent shark, Pangasius hypophthalmus (Sauvage, 1878) in different size classes - hoseini - 2015 - aquaculture Research - wiley Online Library. Available at: https://onlinelibrary.wiley.com/doi/10.1111/are.12188. Accessed September 19, 2025.
31. Tarkhani R, Imani A, Sarvi K. Anaesthetic efficacy of eugenol on flowerhorn (Amphilophus labiatus × Amphilophus trimaculatus). Aquac Res 2016;47. https://doi.org/10.1111/are.13151.

32. Reis TS, de Araújo DB, da Paz CA, et al. Etomidate as an anesthetic in Colossoma macropomum: behavioral and electrophysiological data complement each other as a tool to assess anesthetic safety. PLoS One 2024;19(8):e0305093. https://doi.org/10.1371/journal.pone.0305093.
33. Yaşar TÖ, Yardımcı M, Yağcılar Ç. Determination of the average intraocular pressure values, optimum anesthesia dose and phenotypic characteristics in Oscar fish (Astronotus ocellatus). J Adv VetBio Sci Tech 2021;6(2):142–9.
34. Fernández-Parra R, Donnelly TM, Pignon C, et al. Immersion anesthesia with alfaxalone in a goldfish (*Carassius auratus*). J Exot Pet Med 2017;26(4):276–82.
35. Surgery and Endoscopy - Clinical Guide to Fish Medicine - Wiley Online Library. Available at: https://onlinelibrary.wiley.com/doi/abs/10.1002/9781119259886.ch11. Accessed September 22, 2025.
36. Pujol J, Lamglait B, Vanore M, et al. A post-operative Follow-Up of an endangered saltwater fish lensectomy for cataract management in a public aquarium: a case series. Vet Sci 2023;10(10):611.
37. Heniff A, Lewbart G, Applegate J. Removal of malignant melanophoroma with intramuscular invasion in a bowfin fish (Amia calva). Vet Rec Case Rep 2022; 10:e474. https://doi.org/10.1002/vrc2.474.
38. FiLik N, FiLik F. Selected Research and Dramatic Surgery Fish Cases of Incisive Complete in Fish Surgical. Bull Biotechnol. 2023;4(1):30–35. https://doi.org/10.51539/biotech.1215628.
39. Chow D, Westermeyer H, Fernando N, et al. Unilateral ventral strabismus in an aquarium Silver Arowana (Osteoglossum bicirrhosum). Vet Ophthalmol 2015; 19. https://doi.org/10.1111/vop.12320.
40. Wright SE, Pawlik M, Snyman HN, et al. Review of neoplasia in fish at a large display aquarium, 2005–2021. J Vet Diagn Invest 2024;36(3):362–7.
41. Stevens B, Sanchez-Migallon Guzman D, Phillips K, et al. Evaluation of diagnostic coelioscopy in koi (Cyprinus carpio). Am J Vet Res 2019;80:221–9.
42. Royan MR, Kanda S, Kayo D, et al. Gonadectomy and blood sampling procedures in small size teleost models. Front Endocrinol 2020;11. https://doi.org/10.1101/2020.08.30.271478.
43. Neoplasia of fish - exotic and laboratory animals. MSD veterinary manual. Available at: https://www.msdvetmanual.com/exotic-and-laboratory-animals/aquarium-fish/neoplasia-of-fish. Accessed November 7, 2025.
44. Cutaneous haemangiosarcoma with ovarian metastases in an aquarium-managed mirror carp (Cyprinus carpio) | Request PDF. Available at: https://www.researchgate.net/publication/380899734_Cutaneous_haemangiosarcoma_with_ovarian_metastases_in_an_aquarium-managed_mirror_carp_Cyprinus_carpio. Accessed October 30, 2025.
45. Boone S, Hernandez S, Camus A, et al. Evaluation of four suture materials for surgical incision closure in Siberian sturgeon. Trans Am Fish Soc 2013;142:649–59.
46. Mones AB, Harms CA, Stoskopf MK. Implications of comparative ventral body wall histology on selection of abdominal surgical approach and closure in 12 species of fish. J Fish Biol 2021;98(5):1342–8.
47. Cannizzo SA, Roe SC, Harms CA, et al. Effect of water temperature on the hydrolysis of two absorbable sutures used in fish surgery. FACETS 2017;1:44–54.
48. The handbook of ornamental fish health and welfare - Surgery 1.
49. Fredholm D, Mylniczenko N, Kukanich B. Pharmacokinetic evaluation of meloxicam after intravenous and intramuscular administration in nile tilapia (Oreochromis niloticus). J Zoo Wildl Med 2016;47:736–42.

50. Martins T, Valentim A, Pereira N, et al. Anaesthetics and analgesics used in adult fish for research: a review. Lab Anim 2019;53(4):325–41.
51. Anderson CE, Gillis JD, Miller SN, et al. Production of live offspring following unilateral (left) ovariectomized Potamotrygon rays (Potamotrygon castexi, Potamotrygon leopoldi, and Potamotrygon motoro). J Am Vet Med Assoc 2023; 261(8):1–4.
52. Osteichthyes. In: Pathology of wildlife and zoo animals. Academic Press; 2018. p. 953–1001. https://doi.org/10.1016/B978-0-12-805306-5.00039-0.
53. Surgical management and histopathology of wen overgrowth and neoplasia in four oranda goldfish (Carassius auratus) - mones - 2021 - veterinary record case reports - wiley Online Library. Available at: https://bvajournals.onlinelibrary.wiley.com/doi/abs/10.1002/vrc2.27. Accessed November 9, 2025.
54. Laparoscopic and laser techniques in fish. CABI databases. Available at: https://www.cabidigitallibrary.org/doi/pdf/10.5555/20053197540. Accessed November 7, 2025.
55. Armando F, Pigoli C, Gambini M, et al. Peripheral nerve sheath tumors resembling human atypical neurofibroma in Goldfish (Carassius auratus, linnaeus, 1758). Animals 2021;11(9):2621.
56. Duncan TE, Harkin JC. Electron microscopic studies of goldfish tumors previously termed neurofibromas ans schwannomas. Am J Pathol 1969;55(2):191–202.
57. Rezaie A, Tulaby Dezfuly Z, Peyghan R. Fibrosarcoma in a Goldfish (carassius auratus): a case report. Iran J Vet Sci Technol 2017;9(1):45–8.
58. Marino F, Germanà A, Bambir S, et al. Calretinin and S100 expression in goldfish, Carassius auratus (L.), schwannoma. J Fish Dis 2007;30:251–3.
59. Sirri R, Diana A, Scarpa F, et al. Ultrasonographic and pathologic study of schwannoma in a goldfish (Carassius auratus). Vet Clin Pathol 2015;44(4):586–91.
60. Arbuatti A, Defourny SVP, Salda LD, et al. Multifocal cutaneous peripheral nerve sheath tumors in a goldfish, *Carassius auratus* (L.). J Exot Pet Med 2021;36:84–5.
61. Schlumberger HG. Nerve sheath tumors in an isolated goldfish population. Cancer Res 1952;12(12):890–9.
62. Lymphocystis - an overview | ScienceDirect topics. Available at: https://www.sciencedirect.com/topics/veterinary-science-and-veterinary-medicine/lymphocystis. Accessed November 7, 2025.
63. FA181/FA181: lymphocystis disease in fish. Ask IFAS - powered by EDIS. Available at: https://edis.ifas.ufl.edu/publication/FA181. Accessed November 7, 2025.
64. Chung SH, Mazur E. Surgical applications of femtosecond lasers. J Biophot 2009;2(10):557–72.
65. Stratton HS, Davis R, Lewbart GA. Gastrotomy for removal of a gastric fishhook foreign body in a blue catfish (Ictalurus furcatus). Vet Rec Case Rep 2024; 12(3):e918. https://doi.org/10.1002/vrc2.918.
66. Pujol J, Jalenques M, Lair S, et al. Occurrence of germ cell neoplasia in male striped bass (MORONE SAXATILIS) under human care in a public aquarium: surgical treatment and outcome. J Zoo Wildl Med 2024;55(1):248–55.
67. Christiansen EF, Cray C, Lewbart GA, et al. Plasma protein electrophoresis and acute phase proteins in koi carp (*Cyprinus carpio*) following exploratory coeliotomy. J Exot Pet Med 2015;24(1):76–83.
68. Shivappa RB, Christian LS, Law JM, et al. Laboratory evaluation of different formulations of stress coat® for slime production in goldfish (Carassius auratus) and koi (Cyprinus carpio). PeerJ 2017;5:e3759. https://doi.org/10.7717/peerj.3759.

69. Sneddon LU. Evolution of nociception and pain: evidence from fish models. Philos Trans R Soc B Biol Sci 2019;374(1785):20190290. https://doi.org/10.1098/rstb.2019.0290.
70. Crivelaro RM, Thiesen R, Aldrovani M, et al. Behavioural and physiological effects of methadone in the perioperative period on the nile tilapia Oreochromis niloticus. J Fish Biol 2019;94(5):823–7.
71. Walters E. Defining pain and painful sentience in animals Commentary on Sneddon et al. on Sentience Denial. Anim Sentience 2018;3. https://doi.org/10.51291/2377-7478.1360.
72. Schultz S. Do opioids provide adequate analgesia for surgical coeliotomy in teleost fish? Vet Evid 2025;10. https://doi.org/10.18849/ve.v10i1.702.
73. Sneddon L, Schroeder P, Roque A, et al. Pain management in zebrafish: report from a FELASA working group. Lab Anim 2023;58. https://doi.org/10.1177/00236772231198733.
74. Causes and therapies for pain in fish: implications for aquaculture. Available at: https://www.pubtexto.com/pdf/?causes-and-therapies-for-pain-in-fish-implications-for-aquaculture. Accessed October 30, 2025.
75. Chatigny F, Creighton C, Stevens D. Updated review of fish analgesia. J Am Assoc Lab Anim Sci 2018;57:5–12.
76. Sladky K. Treatment of pain in fish. Vet Clin Exot Anim Pract 2023;26:11–26.
77. Cameron AS, Rub AMW, Sandford BP. Evaluation of healing progression at surgical incision sites and the use of antiseptics for enhancing post-operative survival in subyearling Chinook salmon (Oncorhynchus tshawytscha). PLoS One 2023;18(7):e0288056. https://doi.org/10.1371/journal.pone.0288056.
78. Bass D, Baron S, Travers MA, et al. *One health* in fish and shellfish. Bull Eur Assoc Fish Pathol 2024;45(1). https://doi.org/10.48045/001c.124752.
79. Gozlan RE, Bommarito C, Caballero-Huertas M, et al. A one-health approach to non-native species, aquaculture, and food security. Water Biol Secur 2024;3(2):100250. https://doi.org/10.1016/j.watbs.2024.100250.
80. Stentiford GD, Tyler CR, Ellis RP, et al. Defining and averting syndemic pathways in aquaculture: a major global food sector. Front Sustain Food Syst 2023;7. https://doi.org/10.3389/fsufs.2023.1281447.
81. Hailat E, Amiri M, Debnath N, et al. Strengthening the one health approach in the Eastern Mediterranean Region. Interact J Med Res 2023;12:e41190. https://doi.org/10.2196/41190.
82. Read 6 Min. Minimally invasive techniques for soft tissue surgery in small animals. Vet Pract 2024. Available at: https://www.veterinary-practice.com/article/minimally-invasive-techniques-soft-tissue-surgery-small-animals. Accessed November 11, 2025.
83. Stetter M. Minimally invasive surgical techniques in bony fish (Osteichthyes). Vet Clin Exot Anim Pract 2010;13:291–9.
84. Trotter AW, Rathjens L, Schmiegel S, et al. Short-term effects of standard procedures associated with surgical transmitter implantation on a benthic shark species requiring anaesthesia. Fish Res 2024;270:106880. https://doi.org/10.1016/j.fishres.2023.106880.
85. Acre MR, Bonjour SM, Griffin JN, et al. Long-term surgery survival, body condition effects, and incision healing of silver carp and buffalo species comparing sedation methods across seasons. Trans Am Fish Soc 2025;154(4):424–39.
86. Kuciński M, Liszewski T, Własow T, et al. Histological and transcriptomic characterization of full-thickness skin wound healing in Maraena Whitefish (Coregonus maraena Bloch, 1779). Int J Mol Sci 2025;26(17):8315.

87. Shahrezaei A, Sohani M, Taherkhani S, et al. The impact of surgical simulation and training technologies on general surgery education. BMC Med Educ 2024; 24:1297.
88. Kheriji L, Kouadri A, Mansouri M. Deep learning-based fish health monitoring and diagnosis: a review. IEEE Access 2025;13:181599–616.
89. Zion B. The use of computer vision technologies in aquaculture – a review. Comput Electron Agric 2012;88:125–32.
90. Cooke S, Wilson A, Elvidge C, et al. Ten practical realities for institutional animal care and use committees when evaluating protocols dealing with fish in the field. Rev Fish Biol Fish 2016;26. https://doi.org/10.1007/s11160-015-9413-y.
91. Sloman KA, Bouyoucos IA, Brooks EJ, et al. Ethical considerations in fish research. J Fish Biol 2019;94(4):556–77.
92. Alvarado MV, Cerdá-Reverter JM, Espigares F. A functional framework for a comprehensive study of welfare in fishes. Proc R Soc B Biol Sci 2025;292:20251833. https://doi.org/10.1098/rspb.2025.1833.
93. Bennett RH, Ellender BR, Mäkinen T, et al. Ethical considerations for field research on fishes. Koedoe 2016;58(1):1–15.
94. Khademi-Vidra A, Urbányi B, Bakos IM. Educational and training innovation opportunities in the aquaculture and fisheries sector of Hungarian secondary agricultural education. Aquac Int 2024;32(5):5437–59.
95. Wirajing MAK, Nanfosso RT. Establishing a sustainable fishing industry: the role of environmental stringency, fishery training and education infrastructure in the maritime Cameroon. Mar Policy 2025;178:106730. https://doi.org/10.1016/j.marpol.2025.106730.

Soft Tissue Surgery in Amphibians

Alessandro Vetere, DVM, PhD, MSc, DECZM (Herpetology)[a,*],
Clément Paillusseau, DVM, DECZM (Herpetology)[b]

KEYWORDS

- Amphibians • Surgery • Coeliotomy • Ovariectomy • Anatomy

KEY POINTS

- Coeliotomy is the most versatile surgical approach in amphibians, providing access for gastrointestinal, urinary, hepatic, and reproductive procedures.
- Cotton-tipped applicators provide a gentle and practical means of exerting localized pressure on small vessels, being easier to manipulate than gauze in confined fields.
- Surgical procedures involving the gastrointestinal tract in amphibians require delicate handling due to the fragility and high vascularization of the tissues.
- Adequate hydration and temperature maintenance before, during, and after surgery are critical to prevent physiologic stress and ensure successful recovery.

Video content accompanies this article at http://www.vetexotic.theclinics.com.

INTRODUCTION

There are 3 orders of amphibians: Anura, Urodela (Caudata), and Gymnophiona. The AmphibiaWeb database currently contains 8925 amphibian species (https://amphibiaweb.org; September 2025). Over the past decades, amphibians have experienced a dramatic global decline, making them the most threatened vertebrate group. Approximately 40.7% are now classified as threatened (Vulnerable, Endangered, or Critically Endangered).[1] Available knowledge on amphibian surgery is still largely based on outdated textbooks and sporadic case reports, with few systematic studies supporting current practice.[2–5] This review offers clinicians practical guidance for performing both routine and advanced surgical procedures in captive amphibians.

INCLUSION CRITERIA

The databases Google Scholar, PubMed, and Scopus were searched with the following keywords: "amphibian's surgery, soft tissue surgery, anura, caudata,

[a] Department of Veterinary Science, University of Parma, Strada del Taglio 10, 43126, Parma, Italy; [b] Veterinary Clinic SpéNAC, 100 Boulevard de la Tour-Maubourg, 75007, Paris, France
* Corresponding author.
E-mail addresses: alessandro.vetere@unipr.it; alessandro.vetere88@gmail.com

Vet Clin Exot Anim 29 (2026) 469–488
https://doi.org/10.1016/j.cvex.2026.04.007 vetexotic.theclinics.com

Abbreviation	
IM	intramuscular

urodela, gymnophiona." Only peer-reviewed articles were considered for inclusion. Articles that either did not meet this criterion or were deemed irrelevant to the review's objectives were discarded. Only amphibian species commonly maintained in captivity, including those housed in zoologic institutions, are here discussed.

SURGICAL AND PERISURGICAL CONSIDERATIONS

In amphibian medicine, the majority of surgical interventions involves soft tissues.[2–6] These include wound management through debridement and closure, collection of diagnostic biopsies, implantation of devices for pharmacologic or populations studies, and the excision of abscesses, parasitic lesions, neoplasms, or foreign bodies.[6] Coeliotomy represents a valuable approach for diagnostic exploration and is indicated in reproductive surgery as well as for the removal of gastrointestinal foreign material, retained ova, neoplastic formations, or uroliths.[2–11]

Surgical Equipment

In amphibian surgery, the choice of surgical instruments and techniques must be tailored to the patient's size and the type of procedure. For delicate interventions, ophthalmic or microsurgical instruments with fine tips such as scissors, forceps, and hemostats are preferred.[6] Skin incisions are typically performed with No. 11 or No. 15 scalpel blades, while ophthalmic knives of various sizes and angles can be particularly advantageous in smaller individuals.[2,6] Clear plastic drapes are frequently used, as they provide an aseptic field while minimizing cutaneous desiccation.[2] However, according to the authors' experience, surgical procedures are sometimes performed without the use of drapes, particularly in aquatic species. Throughout the procedure, the skin should be kept moist with dechlorinated water, delivered using syringes or infusion bags.[6] Eyelid retractors and adjustable plastic ring retractors (eg, Lone Star [Alcyon Italia S.p.A, Via Del Lavoro 10, Cherasco, Italy]) are effective for coelomic exposure.[2,6] Magnification systems and bright, cool illumination enhance precision, especially in small patients. Hemostasis in cases with limited expected hemorrhage can be achieved through electrocautery, radiosurgery, or diode laser.[2] The diode laser, although not commonly used, has been applied for the excision of cutaneous lesions and neoplasms, with anecdotal evidence suggesting reduced postoperative infections compared to sharp dissection or radiosurgery.[12] Cotton-tipped applicators provide a gentle and practical means of exerting localized pressure on small vessels, being easier to manipulate than gauze in confined fields.[6] The choice of suture material is an important consideration in all species; however, amphibians exhibit species-specific tissue responses that warrant particular attention.[2,6] Experimental work in African clawed frogs (*Xenopus laevis*) has demonstrated that, similarly to what is observed in mammals, monofilament nylon induces the lowest inflammatory response and is therefore considered the most suitable material for cutaneous closure. In contrast, chromic gut and silk provoke marked reactions and are associated with higher dehiscence rates, and their use is discouraged.[13] Absorbable materials such as polydioxanone, polyglactin 910, or poliglecaprone 25 are appropriate for internal tissues and muscle closure, although polyglactin may elicit stronger inflammatory responses.[14] Antibiotic-impregnated sutures may provide additional protection against bacterial contamination, especially in gastrointestinal, urinary bladder, and skin procedures.[2,6] Tapered swaged needles are generally less traumatic than cutting needles.

Surgical glues or cyanoacrylate tissue adhesives may serve as an alternative or adjunct for skin closure, offering a watertight seal and antimicrobial activity, particularly against gram-positive bacteria.[15–17]

Preoperative Management

Maintaining physiologic homeostasis in amphibian patients before, during, and after surgery is essential for a successful outcome. Environmental temperature should be continuously monitored and maintained within the species' preferred optimal range, as hypothermia is neither a safe nor acceptable method for restraint or analgesia.[10,11] Preoperative management includes ensuring adequate hydration, typically achieved by soaking the animal in shallow, dechlorinated water for about 1 hour before surgery. Proper hydration should be maintained throughout and after the procedure[2,6] (**Table 1**). Antibiotic and analgesic needs must be carefully assessed and administered when indicated.[3] Handling should be as atraumatic as possible; amphibians can be gently restrained by wrapping them in a moistened paper towel.[2] The use of powder-free, moistened gloves (or powdered gloves thoroughly rinsed with sterile saline) is strongly recommended to avoid microbial or chemical contamination and to protect handlers from cutaneous secretions. Special attention should be given to material selection, as certain substances such as latex can be toxic, particularly for larval stages.[18,19] Presurgical fasting is generally unnecessary, as amphibians maintain a tightly closed larynx even under anesthesia, minimizing aspiration risk. However, in large frogs and toads, withholding food for 24 to 48 hours before anesthesia may facilitate visualization during coelomic surgery and reduce gastrointestinal complications associated with decreased metabolic activity.[2,6,10,11] Preparation of the surgical site should be minimal to preserve the natural antimicrobial barrier provided by cutaneous secretions.[20,21] Gentle cleaning of the incision area with sterile cotton-tipped applicators moistened with sterile saline, or with a diluted 2% povidone-iodine solution in saline, is generally sufficient.[2,4,6] Caution applies to facultative neotenic species within Ambystomatidae, Plethodontidae, and Salamandridae, as iodophor-containing disinfectants can be absorbed transcutaneously and may induce metamorphosis in species capable of completing this process.[6] Care is warranted when using chlorhexidine, as exposure to 0.75% chlorhexidine in African clawed frogs (*Xenopus laevis*) has been associated with epidermal degeneration and necrosis.[22]

Anesthesia, Analgesia, and Postoperative Care

Safe anesthesia in amphibians requires species-specific protocols including preanesthetic evaluation, drug and route selection, continuous monitoring, and controlled recovery (**Fig. 1**).[10] Immersion anesthesia exploits the highly vascularized skin and is most commonly achieved with buffered tricaine methanesulfonate (MS-222; 0.2–5 g/L, pH 7.0–7.5),[10,23] clove oil (300–450 mg/L),[10] or benzocaine (0.01%–0.03%).[10,24] MS-222 remains the preferred agent when buffered, as acidic solutions can damage the skin and alter uptake.[10] Topical isoflurane acts rapidly but may irritate if overdosed; a gel mixture with water and lubricant has also been described.[11]

Parenteral anesthesia (intramuscular [IM], intracoelomic, or dorsal lymph sac) can be obtained with ketamine (20–40 mg/kg IM) or propofol (25–35 mg/kg IC), though both may cause respiratory or cardiac depression.[25] Inhalant isoflurane (5% induction, 1%–3% maintenance) is suitable for larger, intubated species.[10,26] α_2-agonists such as medetomidine (0.15 mg/kg) rarely induce anesthesia alone but enhance dissociatives.[10] Alfaxalone provides consistent sedation via intramuscular, subcutaneous, or immersion routes but does not reliably achieve surgical anesthesia.[11,27] As it lacks intrinsic analgesia, adjunctive systemic or local agents are required.

Table 1
Rehydration fluids commonly used in amphibians[6]

Solutions	Composition (in a Liter of Distilled Water)	pH (T°C)	Osmolarity (mmol/L)	Indication
Ringer lactate (amphibian)	6.6 g NaCl 0.15 g KCl 0.15 g $CaCl_2$ 0.2 g $NaHCO_3$	7.99 (21.7)	229	*Isotonic* Maintenance rehydration
Ringer lactate (mammal)	/	6.5 (21)	273	*Isotonic*
Holtfreter's solution	3.46 g NaCl 0.05 g KCl 0.1 g $CaCl_2$ 0.2 g $NaHCO_3$	8.06 (22)	122	*Hypotonic* External parasite control Initial rehydration
Steinberg's solution	3.4 g NaCl 0.05 g KCl 0.05 g $CaCl_2$ 0.205 g $MgSO_4$ 0.56 g $C_4H_{11}NO_3$	6.97 (21.9)	130	*Hypotonic* External parasite control Initial rehydration
Whitaker-Wright's solution	113 g NaCl 1.7 g KCl 4.2 g $CaCl_2$ 8.6 g $MgSO_4$	7.3 (20.5)	3815	Storage solution
Whitaker-Wright's 10%	/	7.17 (21.3)	357	*Hypertonic* Treatment of hydrocoeloma or edema subcutaneously (SC).
Whitaker-Wright's 5%	/	7 (21.7)	206	*Isotonic* Initial rehydration
Sodium chloride (NaCl) 0.6%	/	/	190	*Isotonic (± hypotonic)* Initial rehydration
Sodium chloride (NaCl) 0.9%	/	/	308	*Hypertonic* Treatment of hydrocoeloma or edema subcutaneously (SC)
One-third NaCl 0.9% and two-thirds glucose 5%	/	/	314	*Isotonic (± hypertonic)* Maintenance rehydration
Seven-eighths NaCl 0.9% and one-eighth distilled water	/	/	270	*Isotonic* Maintenance rehydration

From Whitaker BR, Wright KM. Amphibian soft tissue surgery. In: Divers SJ, Stahl SJ, editors. Mader's Reptile and Amphibian Medicine and Surgery. 3rd edition. St. Louis (MO): Elsevier; 2019. p. 1096–1099.[6]

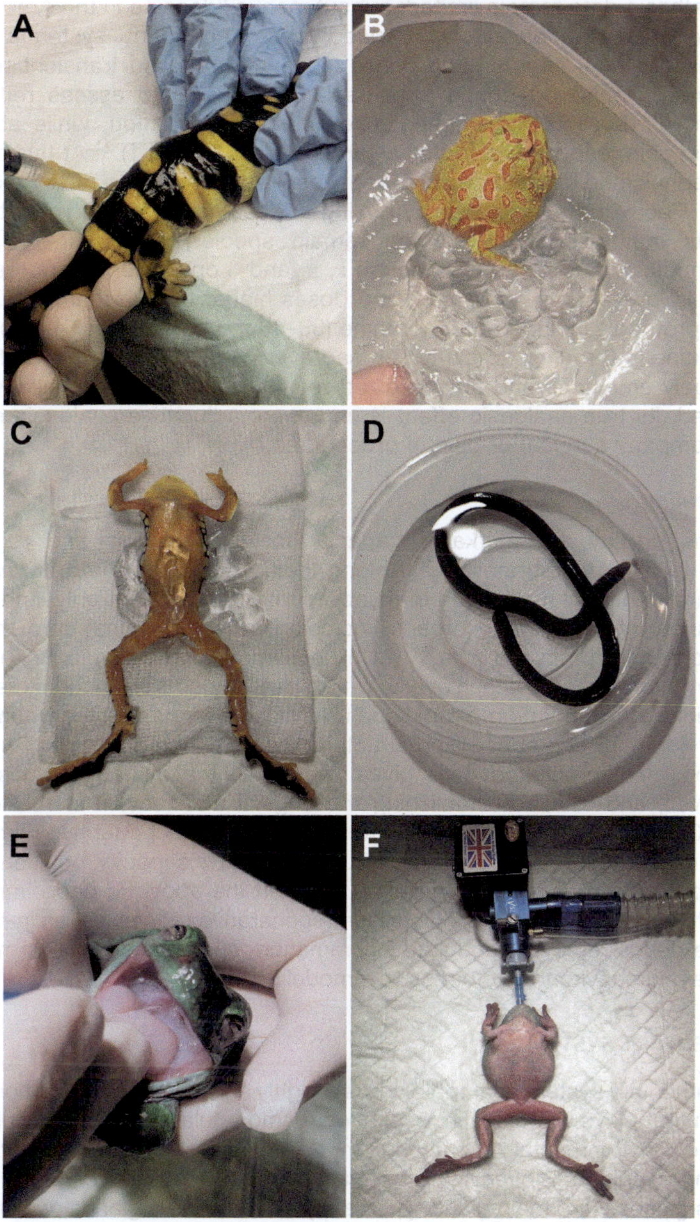

Fig. 1. (*A–F*) Various anesthetic procedures in different amphibian species. (*A*) Intrathecal injection for a cutaneous tail surgery in an Eastern tiger salamander (*Ambystoma tigrinum*). (*B*) Induction using a mixture of isoflurane and gel (1:10) in a Cranwell's horned frog (*Ceratophrys cranwelli*). (*C*) After loss of the righting reflex, the mixture is applied to the ventral skin in a fringed leaf frog (*Cruziohyla craspedopus*). (*D*) Induction with alfaxalone (5 mg/L) in a Congo caecilian (*Herpele squalostoma*). (*E* and *F*) Intubation and maintenance with isoflurane via intermittent positive pressure ventilation in a White's tree frog (*Pelodryas caerulea*). (Image Courtesy of Dr Clément Paillusseau.)

Local anesthesia data remain limited: subcutaneous lidocaine in the American bullfrog (*Lithobates catesbeianus*) produced dose-dependent systemic sedation without reliable local effects; high doses (50 mg/kg) caused transient respiratory depression.[27] Monitoring during anesthesia is essential to assess reflexes and respiration.[10,11] Loss of the righting reflex indicates sedation, while absence of corneal and pain responses denotes a surgical plane (Video 1).[11] At this depth, animals are apneic and depend on cutaneous respiration, requiring moist, oxygenated skin.[4,10,11] Recovery is facilitated by rinsing in anesthetic-free, oxygenated water; antagonists may assist reversal but remain species-dependent.[4,10] Analgesic data in amphibians are scarce. Although κ, μ, and δ opioid receptors are present, selectivity is low, effects prolonged, and doses higher than in mammals.[25,26,28–33] Reported protocols include buprenorphine (38–46 mg/kg SC every 4–6 h) and dexmedetomidine (0.6 mg/kg dorsal lymph sac every 8 h).[2,4,31] Analgesic efficacy remains largely empirical, and standardized regimens are lacking. While MS-222 is widely used, its true analgesic effect is unproven; adjunctive analgesia should always accompany surgical or painful procedures.[10,28]

Wound Healing

Amphibians display a remarkable capacity for tissue repair and regeneration compared to other vertebrates.[34–36] Among them, the axolotl (*Ambystoma mexicanum*) is an exceptional model due to its ability to regenerate not only limbs but also a wide variety of tissues and organs, including skin, tail, spinal cord, heart, and even portions of the brain and jaws.[34–36] Unlike mammals, which typically heal through scarring and fibrosis, axolotl achieve scar-free healing and full functional restoration. Following injury or amputation, a rapid epithelial closure forms over the wound, leading to the development of a specialized structure known as the blastema. This mass of proliferating, dedifferentiated cells gives rise to all the missing tissues (muscle, bone, nerves, and skin) re-establishing the original architecture of the lost structure.[34–36] Comparative data in frogs show that maturation of adaptive immunity and persistent inflammation correlate with loss of regenerative capacity, positioning immunity as a primary gatekeeper of outcome.[37] Given the above, a good immunologic health status is essential for effective tissue regenerative processes, as immune cells coordinate debris removal, modulate inflammation, and promote the formation of a permissive microenvironment for tissue remodeling.

INTEGUMENTARY SYSTEM

The integumentary system of amphibians is a highly specialized and functionally complex organ that plays vital roles in respiration, osmoregulation, thermoregulation, defense, and environmental interaction.[20,21] Amphibian skin consists of a thin, nonkeratinized epidermis overlying a well-vascularized dermis that contains numerous cutaneous glands. Two main gland types are present: mucus glands, which maintain surface moisture and facilitate cutaneous respiration, and granular (serous) glands, which secrete bioactive compounds including antimicrobial peptides, alkaloids, and toxins.[20,21] The dermis is richly supplied with capillaries, lymphatic channels, and chromatophores, contributing to gas exchange, fluid balance, and color variation. Amphibian skin also functions as a major site of water absorption, particularly in the pelvic patch region (drink patches), where specialized epithelial cells permit rapid uptake of water from the environment.[2,6] Because of its high permeability and biological activity, the integument is extremely sensitive to trauma, desiccation, and chemical exposure, posing unique challenges for surgical intervention.

Surgery of the Integument

The majority of cutaneous surgical procedures in amphibians involves tissue biopsy, management of traumatic skin lesions, excision of trematodes or cutaneous masses,[2,38–42] and placement of subcutaneous implants.[38,43] These interventions can be performed using a combination of techniques, including cryosurgery, radiosurgery, diode laser surgery, and conventional scalpel dissection, selected according to lesion type, size, and location[2,6] (**Fig. 2**). Firm abscesses and neoplastic lesions should be surgically removed with an adequate safety margin to minimize local recurrence.[2,39,40] Although no evidence-based guidelines exist regarding surgical safety margins for oncologic procedures in amphibians, principles should be extrapolated from mammalian surgical oncology.[43] When primary closure of large skin defects is not feasible, healing by second intention is generally recommended. As in reptiles, amphibian skin closure is achieved with everting sutures. Due to the frequent presence of high tension, interrupted sutures are generally preferred. Postoperative management should include topical antimicrobial therapy, such as silver sulfadiazine cream or benzalkonium chloride formulations, to prevent secondary infection and promote tissue regeneration.[2,6] Systemic antibiotic treatment is indicated in cases of extensive, contaminated, or nonhealing wounds.[6]

Coeliotomy

Coeliotomy in amphibians provides surgical access to the coelomic cavity, allowing exploration, biopsy, intervention on major internal organs such as the gastrointestinal tract,[2,7,44–46] gonads,[45,46] and urinary bladder[9] and implantation of intracoelomic devices for population studies. The animal is positioned in dorsal recumbency, and the surgical field is prepared aseptically. A single, clean paramedian ventral skin incision is preferred to minimize tissue trauma. After incising the skin and the abdominal muscles, the coelomic membrane is gently elevated and opened, with special attention to avoid

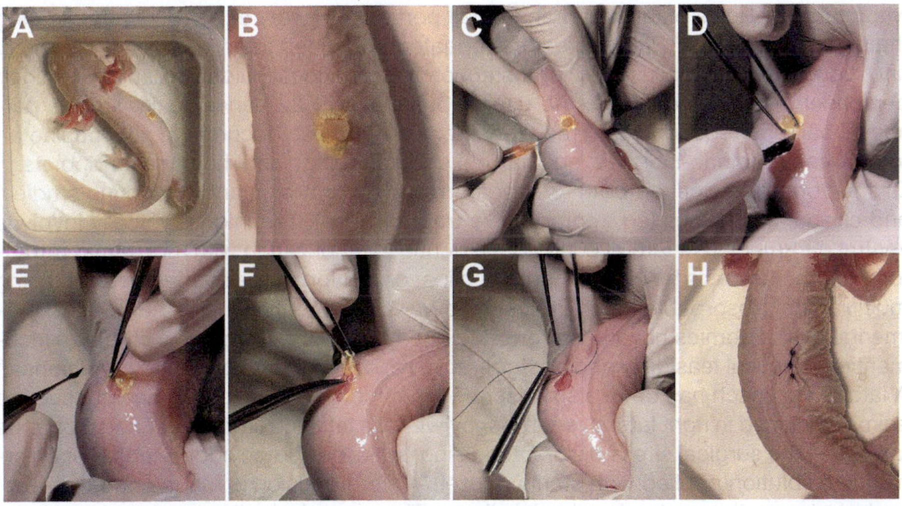

Fig. 2. (*A–H*) Surgical excision of a cutaneous fibropapilloma in an axolotl (*Ambystoma mexicanum*). (*A, B*) Preoperative views of the lesion. (*C*) Local anesthesia achieved by subcutaneous infiltration of lidocaine. (*D–F*) Excision of the mass performed using a keratome blade and fine scissors. (*G, H*) Closure of the surgical site in a single layer with interrupted U-stitches. (Image Courtesy of Dr Clément Paillusseau.)

damaging the lungs, distended bladder, gastrointestinal tract, lymph hearts, or the midventral vein.[2,6] Seasonal variations or differences in nutritional status may influence visualization, as large fat bodies or ovarian follicles can obscure deeper structures.[2]

Throughout the procedure, all exposed tissues must be kept moist using sterile saline or dechlorinated water to prevent desiccation.[6] Retractors such as eyelid retractors are useful for maintaining gentle exposure of the coelomic cavity.[7] Closure is typically performed in 2 layers: a simple continuous suture for the coelomic wall and musculature, followed by interrupted everting sutures or tissue adhesive for the skin.[2,6,11] Postoperative care includes thermal and hydration support, topical antimicrobials, and close monitoring for signs of dehiscence or infection.[2,6]

REPRODUCTIVE SYSTEM

The amphibian reproductive system varies widely among taxa but generally consists of paired gonads positioned dorsally within the coelomic cavity, cranial to the kidneys.[15,47,48] In males, the smooth, ovoid testes lie adjacent to the mesonephric kidneys; sperm pass through the efferent ducts into the Wolffian (archinephric) ducts, which also perform excretory functions before entering the cloaca.[47,48] In females, the large, lobulated ovaries can fill much of the coelomic cavity during the breeding season.[47] Each ovary is suspended by a mesovarium and connected to the cloaca via thick, glandular oviducts responsible for ovum transport, coating, and jelly deposition.[47] Some species possess a functional or rudimentary cloacal sphincter that aids reproductive control.[47] The high vascularity and fragility of gonadal tissues, and their proximity to renal and gastrointestinal organs, complicate surgeries such as ovariectomy, oocyte collection, and castration.[47,48]

Reproductive Surgery

Surgical collection of oocytes is routinely performed in laboratory anurans (especially in African clawed frogs [*Xenopus laevis*]) via coeliotomy under appropriate anesthesia, with mature follicles exteriorized and small portions of ovary excised without ligating the pedicle.[2,14,15,48,49] Procedures are repeated at defined intervals to limit morbidity and reduce total animal use.[15,48,49] Institutional and national guidelines specify trained personnel, aseptic technique, the use of buffered MS-222 anesthesia, limited per-animal harvest frequency, and recovery monitoring; these documents also outline alternatives (hormone-induced egg laying and stripping) and humane endpoints.[48] Ovariectomy is described both for research (oocyte provision and endocrine studies) and clinical indications (eg, reproductive tract disease). Technique typically involves ventral paramedian or lateral coeliotomy, gentle exteriorization with moistened retractors, and hemostasis by bipolar cautery, clips, or ligation of the ovarian pedicle (using multifilament absorbable suture); closure is performed routinely[2,14,15] (**Fig. 3**). Experimental ovariectomies have been reported in anurans for morphologic studies, documenting practical feasibility and postoperative recovery under controlled conditions.[14] A lateral approach has been also described in caudates.[50] Following anesthesia, the animal is placed in right lateral recumbency with the left hind limb positioned along the tail base. The surgical site is disinfected using either diluted povidone-iodine or chlorhexidine solution applied with sterile gauze. A lateral incision is made caudal to midbody, between the pectoral and pelvic limbs. The muscular wall is gently elevated and incised to enter the coelomic cavity, which is then retracted to expose the ovary. Hemostasis is achieved by cauterizing adjacent vessels with electrocautery or a diode laser. Closure of the coelomic wall is performed routinely. Reported complications of ovariectomy in amphibians include infection, wound dehiscence, and ovarian

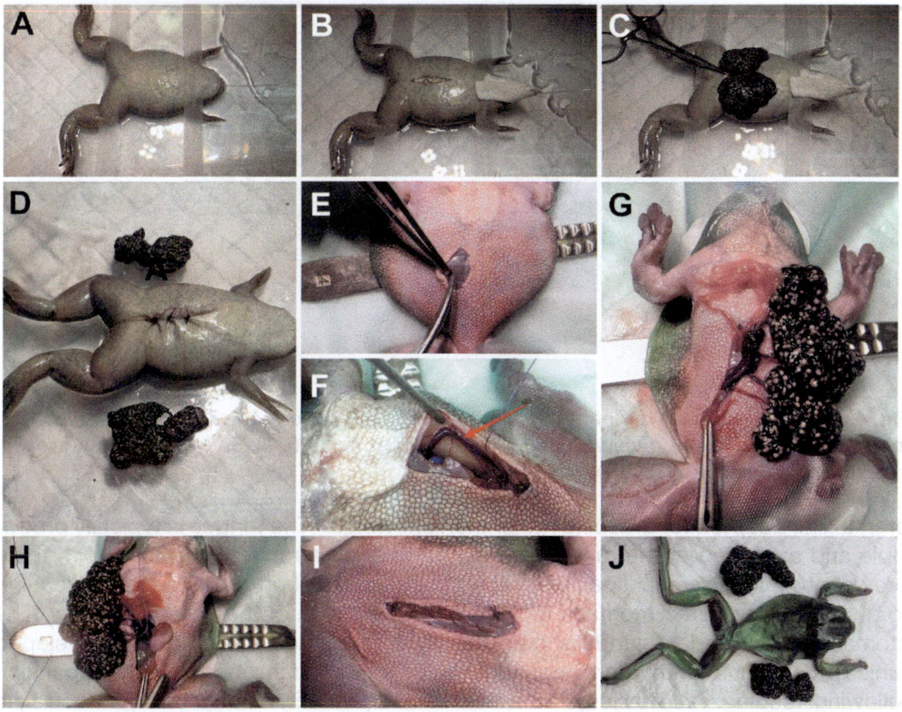

Fig. 3. (*A–J*) Ovariectomy from ventral approach in an African clawed frog (*Xenopus laevis*). (*A, B*) The animal is positioned in dorsal recumbency, and a longitudinal cutaneous incision is made. (*C, D*) Following muscular incision, the ovaries are gently exteriorized excised. The same procedure is performed in a White's tree frog (*Pelodryas caerulea*). (*E, F*) After incision of the skin and abdominal muscles, the ventral abdominal vein is identified (*red arrow*). (*G, H*) The ovaries are exteriorized, and a ligature is placed around the ovarian vessels before transection. (*I*) View of the coelomic wall closure. (*J*) Postoperative aspect showing the ovary-to-body size ratio. (Image Courtesy of Dr Clément Paillusseau.)

remnancy (personal experience, C.P.; **Fig. 4**). Castration in amphibians is primarily indicated for clinical management of testicular disease (including neoplasia, orchitis, or torsion), for the treatment of hormonally driven reproductive disorders, or for research purposes.[2] It follow the same surgical principles as ovariectomy, employing a ventral or paramedian coeliotomy to access the intracoelomic testes located cranial to the kidneys.[2] Following careful identification of the gonads, vascular control is achieved using fine absorbable multifilament ligatures or overlapping microclips to minimize the risk of hemorrhage, while the deferent ducts may be transected or cauterized to ensure sterility.[2] The coelomic wall and integument are routinely closed to promote optimal healing and minimize the risk of infection.

DIGESTIVE SYSTEM

The amphibian digestive system exhibits structural simplicity compared to that of amniotes, but shows functional specialization across species with different feeding ecologies.[44] The oral cavity is wide and lined with a stratified epithelium; many anurans possess keratinized dental ridges or pedicellate teeth attached to the maxilla and

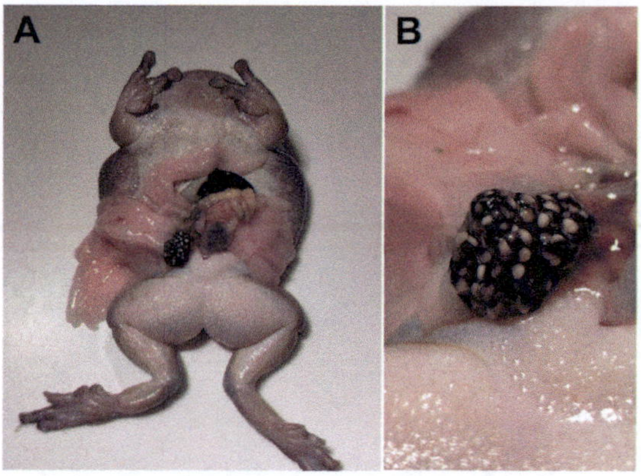

Fig. 4. (*A, B*) (*A*) Ovarian remnant in a White's tree frog (*Pelodryas caerulea*) observed during necropsy. (*B*) Close-up view. Same individual as in **Fig. 3** (*E–J*), 5 years after the procedure. (Image Courtesy of Dr Clément Paillusseau.)

premaxilla, adapted for grasping rather than chewing.[51] The tongue is typically protrusible and anchored at the mandibular symphysis, an arrangement that allows rapid prey capture in terrestrial species.[44] The esophagus is short and distensible, leading to a single-chambered stomach located on the left side of the coelomic cavity. The stomach wall includes glandular mucosa, a thin submucosa, and a well-developed tunica muscularis, with prominent rugal folds that permit considerable expansion following feeding.[2,44] The large intestine serves primarily for water and electrolyte resorption before material passes into the cloaca, which is divided into the coprodeum, urodeum, and proctodeum. The liver is proportionally large and bilobed (anura and urodela), with a gallbladder that empties via the bile duct into the proximal small intestine. The pancreas is a diffuse organ located between the stomach and duodenum and contributes to both digestive and endocrine functions.[2,51]

Gastrotomy and Enterotomy

In anurans and urodela, the stomach is positioned on the left side of the coelomic cavity and is composed of a glandular mucosa, a thin submucosa, and a well-developed tunica muscularis. The transition between the stomach and the small intestine occurs at the pyloric region, similar to mammals.[44] However, the amphibian small intestine is structurally simpler, characterized by fewer mucosal folds and villi, and shows minimal regional differentiation, making it difficult to distinguish discrete segments such as duodenum, jejunum, and ileum.[44] Gastrotomy and enterotomy are relatively uncommon procedures in amphibian medicine, typically performed only in cases of gastrointestinal obstruction, foreign body ingestion (**Fig. 5**), or focal disease where less invasive approaches are not feasible.[2,51,52] In one case of a Budgett's frog (*Lepidobatrachus laevis*), a gastrotomy was performed to remove ingested gravel that caused gastric impaction. A paramedian ventral coeliotomy allowed access to the stomach, which was incised, the foreign bodies removed, and the incision closed in 2 layers with absorbable suture material, resulting in uneventful recovery.[53] Similarly, a case of intestinal obstruction in an Argentine horned frog (*Ceratophrys ornata*) required coeliotomy and enterotomy for removal of substrate material causing complete gastrointestinal blockage. The intestine was closed using a single-layer inverting pattern with monofilament absorbable suture, and the animal recovered well after assisted feeding and postoperative hydration.[54] Surgical procedures involving the gastrointestinal tract in amphibians require delicate handling due to the

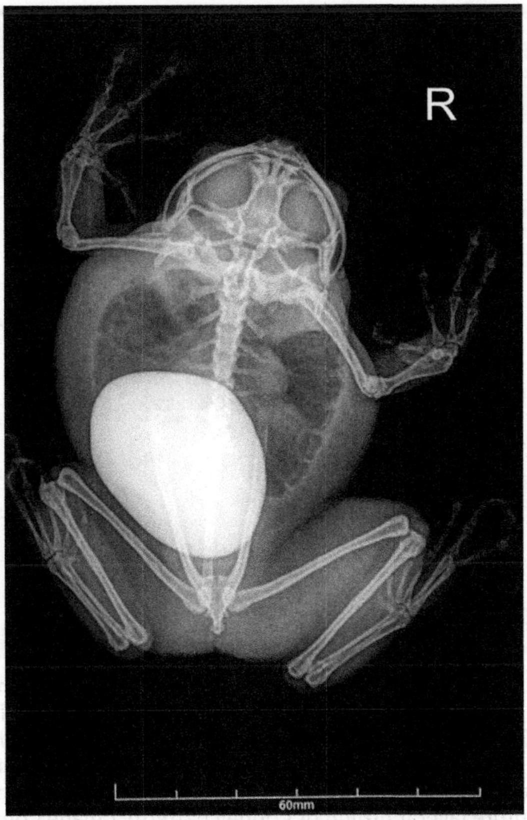

Fig. 5. Dorsoventral radiograph. Large gastric foreign body (stone) in an Australian green treefrog (*Pelodryas caerulea*). (Image Courtesy of Dr Carlo Paoletti.)

fragility and high vascularization of the tissues. The stomach and intestines are highly reactive to desiccation and manipulation, necessitating constant irrigation with isotonic saline during surgery.[2,6,51,52] Gastrotomy (**Figs. 6** and **7**) and enterotomy (**Fig. 8**) should be performed using fine instruments under magnification, with atraumatic handling to prevent tearing of the thin serosal layer.[2,6] Stay sutures placed in the gastric wall facilitate manipulation and exposure of the stomach. The incision is performed similarly to that in mammals through the antimesenteric border, and closure can be achieved with 1 or 2 layers of fine monofilament absorbable suture material. In smaller patients, a single inverting pattern is preferable to reduce the risk of gastric stenosis.[6] Postsurgical care includes maintaining optimal hydration and temperature, as gastrointestinal motility and healing are strongly influenced by environmental and physiologic homeostasis.

Prolapses

Prolapse of cloacal or rectal tissue is a common presentation in amphibians and is often associated with nematode infestation or hypocalcemia. After reduction (facilitated by applying a hyperosmotic solution to the prolapsed organ), the tissue can be lubricated with a water-soluble agent and gently repositioned into the cloaca using a moistened cotton-tipped applicator.[6] Closure of the cloacal opening with a purse-string suture for 2 to 3 days is recommended, and the animal should remain fasted until the suture is removed[6,11] (**Fig. 9** *Courtesy of* Dr Clément Paillusseau).

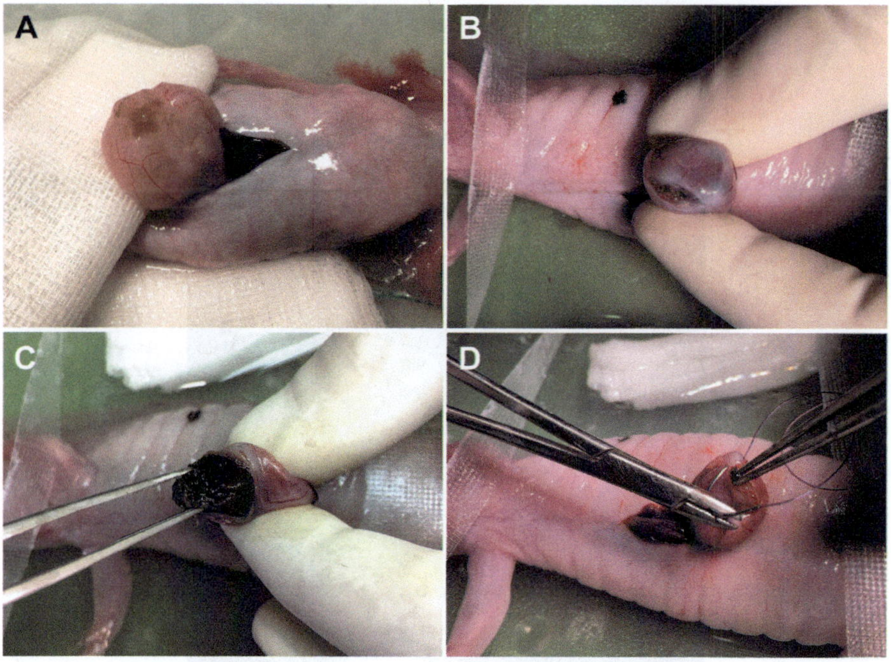

Fig. 6. (*A–D*) Gastrotomy from ventral approach in an axolotl (*Ambystoma mexicanum*). (*A*) Following aseptic preparation, the stomach is carefully exteriorized and isolated with moistened gauze swabs. (*B*) An incision is made along the antimesenteric border of the organ. (*C*) The foreign body is carefully extracted, taking care to avoid contamination of the coelomic cavity. (*D*) The stomach is then closed in 2 layers: a simple continuous monofilament suture, a second inverting suture layer (Cushing or Connell pattern). (Image Courtesy of Dr Clément Paillusseau.)

Surgery of the Hepatobiliary System

Hepatobiliary surgery in amphibians remains confined to experimental research, with current recommendations extrapolated from general amphibian soft tissue surgical principles and laboratory models rather than clinical cases.[2,45,51] The amphibian liver is highly vascularized and enclosed in a thin, friable capsule that predisposes to tearing and hemorrhage during manipulation.[45] Both open and endoscopic approaches have been described for diagnostic and research purposes, primarily in *Xenopus laevis* models.[16] Access is achieved through a ventral or paramedian coeliotomy under general anesthesia, maintaining constant tissue hydration and minimal traction to prevent capsule rupture.[2] Small peripheral wedge biopsies are the preferred diagnostic method, with hemostasis obtained using cotton-tipped applicators, bipolar cautery, or diode laser. Monofilament absorbable sutures are recommended if closure is required.[2,14] Partial hepatectomy has been experimentally performed in *Xenopus laevis*, confirming the technical feasibility of hepatic resection and demonstrating subsequent hepatic and endocrine responses, including compensatory hypertrophy of remaining lobes.[45] Reports of biliary surgery in amphibians are exceedingly limited, with no peer-reviewed clinical documentation; intraoperative bile aspiration or decompression of a distended gallbladder has only been mentioned as technically possible during exploratory coeliotomy.[2] In numerous anuran species, the gallbladder is located near the right hepatic lobe without direct attachment.

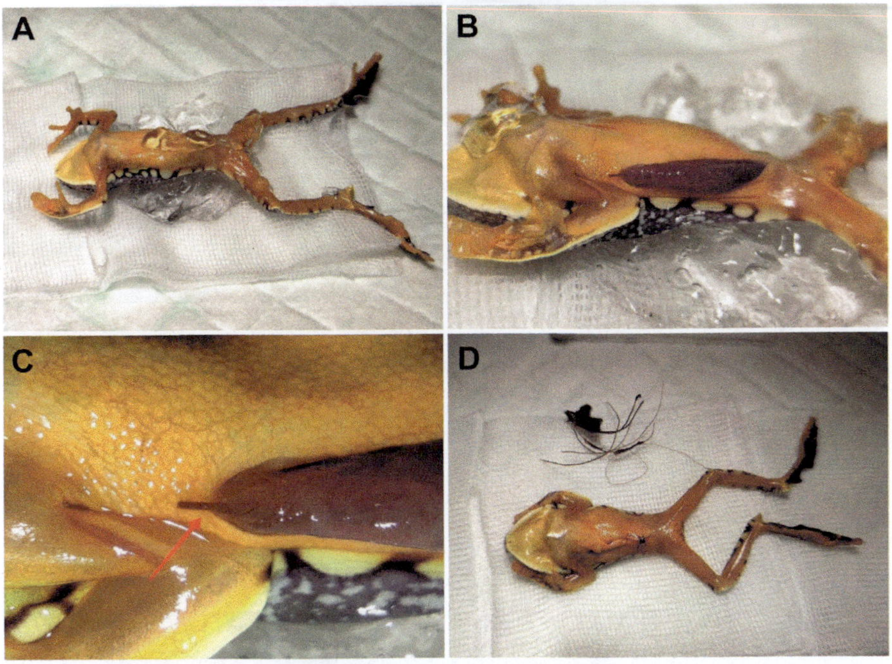

Fig. 7. (*A–D*) Coeliotomy and gastrotomy in a fringed leaf frog (*Cruziohyla craspedopus*) suffering from perforating digestive foreign body. (*A, B*) Following anesthesia, standard aseptic preparation, and coeliotomy, the stomach is carefully exteriorized. (*C*) The perforating foreign body is clearly visible (*red arrow*) and a conventional gastrotomy is performed (*D*) Postoperative aspect after coelomic closure using interrupted sutures. (Image Courtesy of Dr Clément Paillusseau.)

Cholecystectomy is readily achieved by ligating the main bile duct prior to transection (personal experience, C.P.; **Fig. 10**).

URINARY SYSTEM

The amphibian urinary system comprises paired mesonephric kidneys located dorsocaudally in the coelomic cavity. Kidneys are paired, elongated, and dorsally positioned in the caudal coelomic cavity; they are typically mesonephric in adults, consisting of nephrons adapted for both vascular and coelomic filtration. Nitrogenous waste products vary by ecology (ammonia in aquatic species, urea or uric acid in more terrestrial forms).[14,15] Each kidney drains through an archinephric (ureteral) duct that empties into the dorsolateral cloaca. The urinary bladder, thin-walled and often bilobed, serves as a major water reservoir and participates in osmoregulation.[5–10]

Cystotomy

Urogenital surgical procedures in amphibians are rarely reported but have been successfully described in selected cases, primarily involving cystotomy.[2,6,9,14] The most detailed documentation concerns waxy monkey frogs (*Phyllomedusa sauvagii*), a species predisposed to ammonium urate urolithiasis due to its uricotelic physiology and susceptibility to dehydration in captivity (**Fig. 11**).[9] Affected animals may present with coelomic distension, lethargy, and dysuria. Diagnostic imaging, especially ultrasonography, confirms the presence of radiopaque calculi within the urinary bladder.[9]

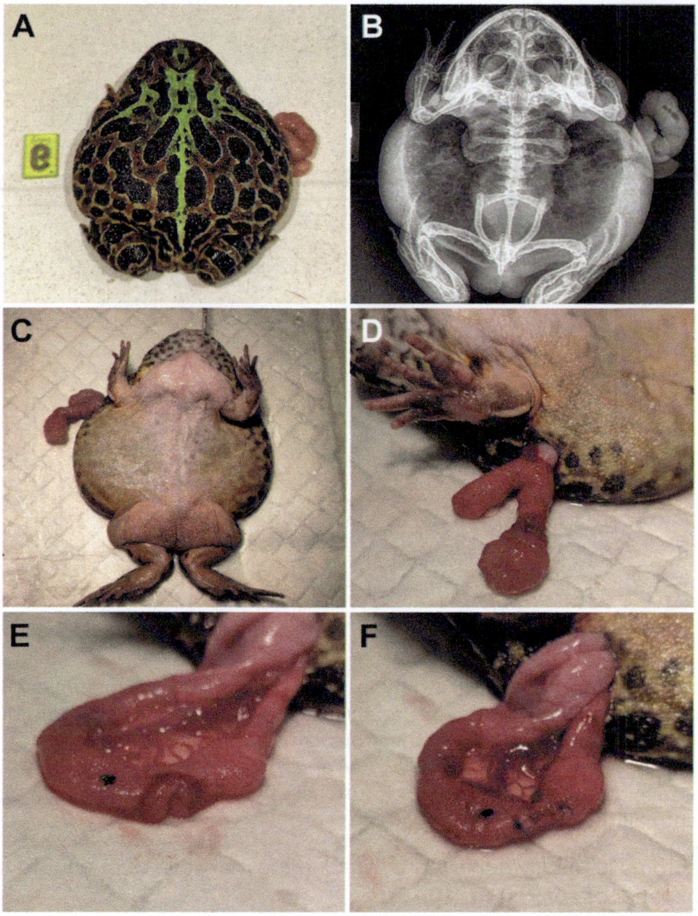

Fig. 8. (*A–F*) Surgical management of an atypical evisceration in an Ornate horned frog (*Ceratophrys ornata*). (*A*) Preoperative view showing the herniated organ. (*B*) Whole body radiographs revealing the coelomic breach. (*C*) The frog positioned in dorsal recumbency for surgery. (*D*) Close-up view of the double mucosal eversion. (*E*) Reintroduction of the everted mucosa. (*F*) Digestive wall defect closed routinely. (Image Courtesy of Dr Clément Paillusseau.)

Surgical intervention is performed via a ventral paramedian coeliotomy, with careful exteriorization of the bladder to prevent contamination of the coelomic cavity (since asymptomatic bacteriuria is a common finding in amphibians).[6,14] The ventral bladder wall is longitudinally incised using a fine, n.11 or n.15 scalpel blade, the calculi are removed, and the bladder is closed in a single or double layer using fine (eg, 6/0 or 7/0) monofilament absorbable suture (eg, poliglecaprone 25).[2] The coelomic incision is then closed routinely. Partial or total cystectomy has been mentioned as a potential option for animals with severe bladder necrosis, chronic prolapse or neoplasia; however, documented clinical cases remain extremely limited.[14] Anatomically, amphibians can tolerate the loss of the urinary bladder since both ureters open directly into the cloaca, allowing continued urine excretion.[52] Postoperative care includes maintaining optimal hydration and temperature, antibiotic therapy when indicated, environmental and dietary correction (to minimize the recurrence of urate calculi).[14]

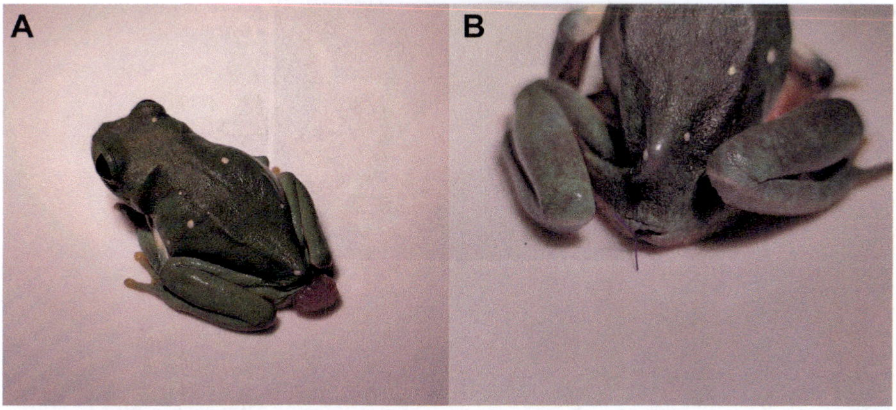

Fig. 9. (*A, B*) (*A*) Cloacal prolapse in a Mexican leaf frog (*Agalychnis dacnicolor*). (*B*) The same individual after surgical reduction and placement of purse-string suture. (Image Courtesy of Dr Clément Paillusseau.)

Nephrectomy

Nephrectomy in amphibians is documented predominantly in the experimental and biomedical literature, where African clawed frogs (*Xenopus laevis*) is used to study renal development, injury, and regeneration.[55] In larval *Xenopus laevis*, researchers have performed unilateral partial nephrectomy via microlaparotomy to remove defined

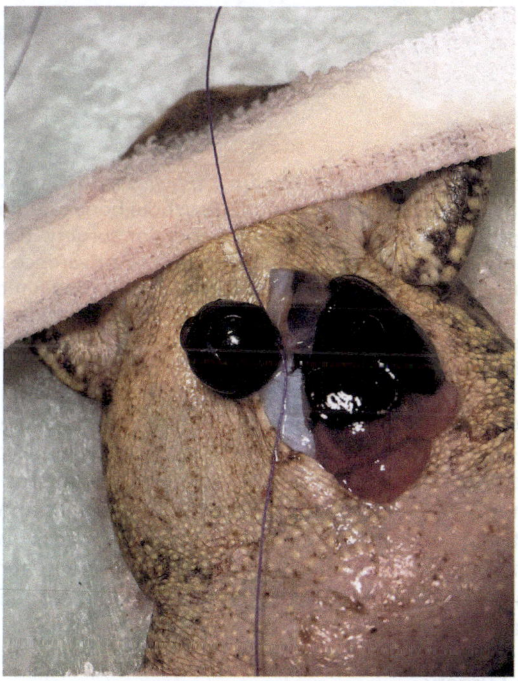

Fig. 10. Cholecystectomy in southern toad (*Anaxyrus terrestris*) suffering from bacterial cholecystitis. Cholecystectomy is readily achieved by ligating the main bile duct prior to transection. (Image Courtesy of Dr Clément Paillusseau.)

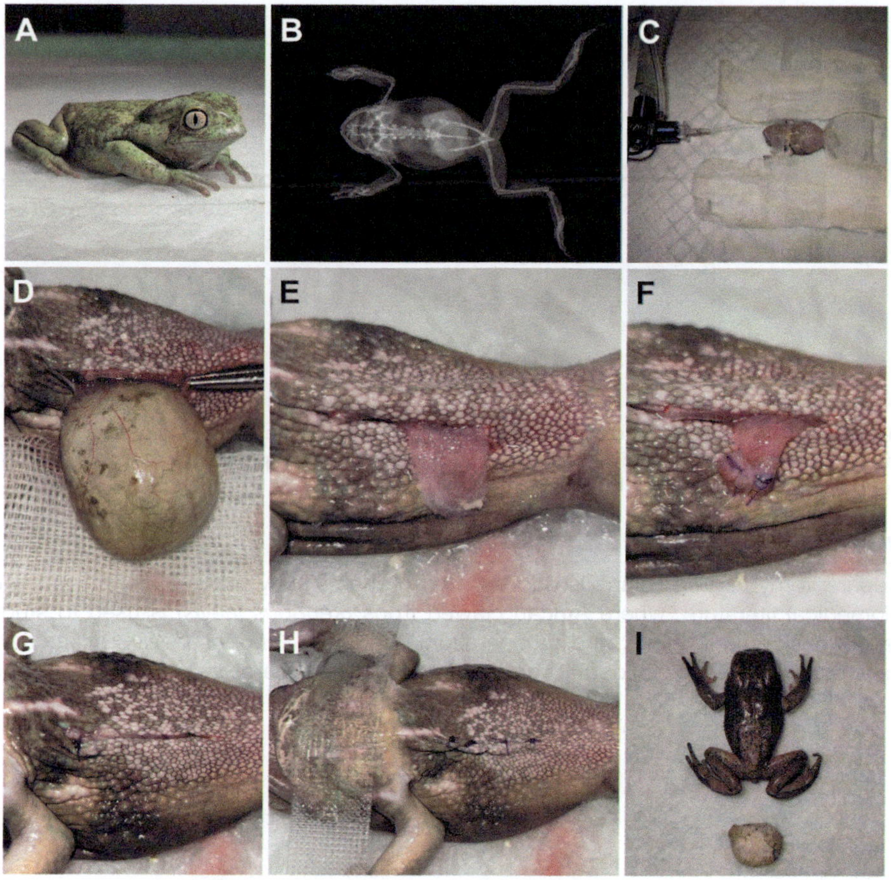

Fig. 11. (*A–I*) Cystotomy in a waxy monkey frog (*Phyllomedusa sauvagii*). (*A*) Individual before the surgery, showing coelomic distension. (*B*) Whole body radiographs revealing urolithiasis. (*C*) The frog positioned in dorsal recumbency for surgery. (*D*) After conventional coeliotomy, the urinary bladder is gently exteriorized. (*E*) Appearance of the bladder after removal of the calculi. (*F*) Suture of the urinary bladder wall using a monofilament. (*G*) Suturing of the coelomic wall using a continuous pattern with multifilament. (*H*) Skin closure using interrupted sutures with monofilament. (*I*) Postoperative aspect showing the calculi-to-body size ratio. (Image Courtesy of Dr Clément Paillusseau.)

segments of the pronephros and subsequently assess structural and functional regeneration. Under MS-222 anesthesia (~0.04%), a small lateral incision was made near the gill flap, the skin was reflected, and the dorsolateral pronephros was exposed. Using fine forceps under stereomicroscopy, a unilateral partial nephrectomy was performed by selectively excising proximal tubule segments while sparing the pronephric duct and glomus.[55] Larvae were capable of regenerating functional proximal tubules within approximately 3 weeks postresection, as confirmed by histology and functional assays.[55]

Minimally Invasive Surgery

Minimally invasive surgery is increasingly applied in amphibians, with updated protocols and indications recently reviewed.[14] Endoscopic techniques, comparable to those in other vertebrates, are used for organ biopsy, sex determination, and removal of gastrointestinal foreign bodies, as well as for procedures such as endoscopic orchiectomy in large anurans.[2,14,16] Celioscopy is typically performed in intubated amphibians positioned in dorsal recumbency, using a 3 mm paramedian incision in the midcoelomic region for telescope introduction after coelomic entry and insufflation.[2,14,16] Carbon dioxide insufflation (0.5–2.0 mm Hg; $\leq$0.5 L/min) provides adequate visualization.[2,16] A second portal, created under endoscopic view and guided by transillumination, allows insertion of atraumatic graspers. During endoscopic orchiectomy, the gonad is grasped and its vessels coagulated with a diode laser before removal.[14,16] A paramedian approach offers optimal visualization of the heart, liver, urinary bladder, and gastrointestinal tract, while a lateral entry facilitates access to gonads, adrenals, and kidneys.[2,15,16] After exploration, the coelom deflates spontaneously, and the incision is closed in a single layer with 1 or 2 interrupted sutures before recovery in a warm, oxygenated bath.[16]

CLINICS CARE POINTS

- Amphibian skin is highly permeable and sensitive; excessive surgical preparation or inappropriate disinfectants may damage the integument and impair healing.
- Monofilament suture materials are preferred for skin closure because they induce less inflammation and lower dehiscence rates.
- Continuous irrigation with sterile saline or dechlorinated water is necessary during surgery to prevent tissue desiccation.
- Amphibians possess remarkable regenerative abilities, but persistent inflammation and poor immune status may impair tissue regeneration and wound healing.
- Gastrointestinal tissues are extremely fragile and highly vascularized; atraumatic handling and magnification are recommended during gastrotomy or enterotomy.
- Gastrointestinal tissues are extremely fragile and highly vascularized; atraumatic handling and magnification are recommended during gastrotomy or enterotomy.
- Coeliotomy should be performed carefully to avoid damage to lungs, urinary bladder, lymph hearts, and major abdominal vessels.
- Minimally invasive techniques such as celioscopy provide effective diagnostic and surgical access while reducing tissue trauma and postoperative recovery time.

DISCLOSURE

The authors have nothing to disclose.

SUPPLEMENTARY DATA

Supplementary data to this article can be found online at https://doi.org/10.1016/j.cvex.2026.04.007.

REFERENCES

1. Luedtke JA, Chanson J, Neam K, et al. Ongoing declines for the world's amphibians in the face of emerging threats. Nature 2023;622(7982):308–14.
2. Chai N. Surgery in amphibians. Vet Clin North Am Exot Anim Pract 2016;19(1):77–95.
3. Wright KM. Surgical techniques. In: Wright KM, Whitaker BR, editors. Amphibian medicine and captive husbandry. Malabar (FL): Krieger; 2001. p. 274–83.

4. Wright KM. Surgery of amphibians. Vet Clin North Am Exot Anim Pract 2000;3(3): 753–8.
5. Divers SJ, Stahl SJ, editors. Mader's reptile and amphibian medicine and surgery. 3rd edition. St Louis (MO): Elsevier; 2018.
6. Whitaker BR, Wright KM. Amphibian soft tissue surgery. In: Divers SJ, Stahl SJ, editors. Mader's reptile and amphibian medicine and surgery. 3rd edition. St Louis (MO): Elsevier; 2019. p. 1096–9.
7. Sailler A, Chai N, Huberdeau P, et al. Surgical management of a digestive tract hernia in a wild marsh frog (*Pelophylax ridibundus*). J Herpetol Med Surg 2021;31(4):292–5.
8. Boss C, Plummer CE. Ophthalmology of amphibia: caecilians, salamanders, frogs, toads, and relatives. In: Montiani-Ferreira F, Moore BA, Ben-Shlomo G, editors. Wild and Exotic Animal Ophthalmology1. Cham: Springer; 2022. p. 121–41.
9. Archibald KE, Minter LJ, Dombrowski DS, et al. Cystic urolithiasis in captive waxy monkey frogs (*Phyllomedusa sauvagii*). J Zoo Wildl Med 2015;46(1):105–12.
10. Mitchell MA. Anesthetic considerations for amphibians. J Exot Pet Med 2009; 18(1):40–9.
11. DiGeronimo PM, Balko JA. Sedation and anesthesia of amphibians. Vet Clin North Am Exot Anim Pract 2022;25(1):31–47.
12. Modesto F, Nicolier A, Hurtrel C, et al. Excisional biopsy and radiotherapy for management of an olfactory neuroblastoma in an axolotl (*Ambystoma mexicanum*). J Am Vet Med Assoc 2022;260(4):436–41.
13. Tuttle AD, Law MJ, Harms CA, et al. Evaluation of reactions to five suture materials in the skin of the African clawed frog (*Xenopus laevis*). J Am Assoc Lab Anim Sci 2006;45(6):22–6.
14. Vergneau-Grosset C, Weber ES 3rd. Amphibian surgery. In: Surgery of exotic animals. 2021. p. 63–73.
15. Gentz EJ. Medicine and surgery of amphibians. ILAR J 2007;48(3):255–9.
16. Chai N. Endoscopy in amphibians. Vet Clin North Am Exot Anim Pract 2015;18(3): 479–91.
17. Waller SC, Anderson DW, Kane BJ, et al. In vitro assessment of microbial barrier properties of cyanoacrylate adhesives. Surg Infect 2019;20(6):449–52.
18. Alford R. Guidelines for the safe use of disposable gloves with amphibian larvae. Herpetol Rev 2009;40:16–8.
19. Gutleb AC, Bronkhorst M, van den Berg JH, et al. Latex laboratory gloves: an unexpected pitfall in amphibian toxicity assays. Environ Toxicol Pharmacol 2001; 10(3):119–21.
20. Rollins-Smith LA, Reinert LK, O'Leary CJ, et al. Antimicrobial peptide defenses in amphibian skin. Integr Comp Biol 2005;45(1):137–42.
21. Ladram A, Nicolas P. Antimicrobial peptides from frog skin: biodiversity and therapeutic promises. Front Biosci (Landmark Ed) 2016;21:4461–74.
22. Philips BH, Crim MJ, Hankenson FC, et al. Evaluation of presurgical skin preparation agents in African clawed frogs (*Xenopus laevis*). J Am Assoc Lab Anim Sci 2015;54(6):788–98.
23. Downes H. Tricaine anesthesia in amphibia: a review. Bull Assoc Reptil Amphib Vet 1995;5(2):11–6.
24. Crook AC, Whiteman HH. Evaluation of MS-222 and benzocaine for metamorphic and paedomorphic tiger salamanders (*Ambystoma tigrinum nebulosum*). Am Midl Nat 2006;155(2):417–22.

25. Yaw TJ, Mans C, Martinelli L, et al. Comparison of two injectable anesthetic combinations in blue poison dart frogs (*Dendrobates tinctorius azureus*). J Zoo Wildl Med 2020;50(4):868–73.
26. Smith JM, Stump KC. Isoflurane anesthesia in the African clawed frog (*Xenopus laevis*). Contemp Top Lab Anim Sci 2000;39(6):39–42.
27. Williams CJ, Alstrup AKO, Bertelsen MF, et al. Pronounced systemic effects of subcutaneous lidocaine in bullfrogs (*Lithobates catesbeianus*). Comp Biochem Physiol Mol Integr Physiol 2017;209:41–6.
28. Stevens CW. Analgesia in amphibians: preclinical studies and clinical applications. Vet Clin North Am Exot Anim Pract 2011;14(1):33–48.
29. Machin KL. Amphibian pain and analgesia. J Zoo Wildl Med 1999;30:2–10.
30. Duncan A. Reptile and amphibian analgesia. In: Fowler ME, Miller RE, editors. Fowler's zoo and wild animal medicine current therapy, vol. 7. St Louis (MO): Elsevier; 2011. p. 247–53.
31. Stevens CW. Opioid research in amphibians: an alternative pain model yielding insights on the evolution of opioid receptors. Brain Res Rev 2004;46:204–15.
32. Brenner GM, Klopp AJ, Deason LL, et al. Analgesic potency of alpha-adrenergic agents after systemic administration in amphibians. J Pharmacol Exp Therapeut 1994;270:540–5.
33. Stevens CW, Brenner GM. Spinal administration of adrenergic agents produces analgesia in amphibians. Eur J Pharmacol 1996;316(2–3):205–10.
34. Kawasumi A, Sagawa N, Hayashi S, et al. Wound healing in mammals and amphibians: toward limb regeneration in mammals. In: New perspectives in regeneration. 2012. p. 33–49.
35. Vieira WA, Wells KM, McCusker CD. Advancements to the axolotl model for regeneration and aging. Gerontology 2020;66(3):212–22.
36. Polikarpova A, Ellinghaus A, Schmidt-Bleek O, et al. The specialist in regeneration—the axolotl—a suitable model to study bone healing? npj Regen Med 2022;7(1):35.
37. Godwin JW, Rosenthal N. Scar-free wound healing and regeneration in amphibians: immunological influences on regenerative success. Differentiation 2014;87-(1–2):66–75.
38. Hardman RH, Cox S, Reinsch SD, et al. Efficacy of subcutaneous implants to provide continuous plasma terbinafine in hellbenders (*Cryptobranchus alleganiensis*). J Zoo Wildl Med 2021;52(1):300–5.
39. Sigirci BD, Alabas B, Halac B, et al. An abscess caused by *Corynebacterium pseudotuberculosis* in a Budgett's frog (*Lepidobatrachus laevis*). J Exot Pet Med 2019;31:57–60.
40. Poll CP. Wound management in amphibians: etiology and treatment of cutaneous lesions. J Exot Pet Med 2009;18(1):20–35.
41. Fischer D, Lorenz N, Heuser W, et al. Abscesses associated with a *Brucella inopinata*–like bacterium in a big-eyed tree frog (*Leptopelis vermiculatus*). J Zoo Wildl Med 2012;43(3):625–8.
42. Wiley M, Wu J, Dawson B. Comparison of two treatments for nematode infections in the túngara frog (*Engystomops pustulosus*). J Herpetol Med Surg 2009; 19(1):21–2.
43. Dobson JM. Significant advances in veterinary oncology—60 years on. J Small Anim Pract 2019;60(12):711–22.
44. Clayton LA. Amphibian gastroenterology. Vet Clin North Am Exot Anim Pract 2005;8(2):227–45.

45. Fritsch HAR, Pehlemann FW, Faltz H. Effect of partial hepatectomy on the interrenal tissues of *Xenopus laevis*. Cell Tissue Res 1977;179(2):197–209.
46. Chai N. Reproductive medicine in amphibians. Vet Clin North Am Exot Anim Pract 2017;20(2):307–25.
47. Méndez-Tepepa M, Morales-Cruz C, García-Nieto E, et al. A review of the reproductive system in anuran amphibians. Zool Lett 2023;9(1):3.
48. Ogielska M, Augustyńska R, Kotusz A, et al. A stockpile of ova in the grass frog *Rana temporaria* is a persisting feature of the ovary. Anat Rec 2013;296(1):144–58.
49. Newman K, Woodland HR. Isolation of *Xenopus* oocytes. Cold Spring Harb Protoc 2018;2018(1). pdb.prot097550.
50. Calatayud NE, Chai N, Gardner NR, et al. Reproductive techniques for ovarian monitoring and control in amphibians. J Vis Exp 2016;107:e53649.
51. Whitaker BR, Wright KM. Clinical techniques. In: Wright KM, editor. Amphibian medicine and captive husbandry. Malabar (FL): Krieger; 2001. p. 89–122.
52. Hadfield CA, Whitaker BR. Amphibian emergency medicine and care. Semin Avian Exotic Pet Med 2005;14(2):79–89.
53. Messonnier S. Foreign body removal by gastrotomy in a Budgett's frog (*Lepidobatrachus laevis*). Proc Assoc Reptil Amphib Vet 1997;30.
54. Miles S. Treating gastrointestinal obstruction in an Argentine horned frog (*Ceratophrys ornata*): coeliotomy, enterotomy and substrate impaction removal. Vet Times; 2017.
55. Caine ST, McLaughlin KA. Regeneration of functional pronephric proximal tubules after partial nephrectomy in *Xenopus laevis*. Dev Dyn 2013;242(3):219–29.

Soft Tissue Surgery in Reptiles

Clément Paillusseau, DVM, DECZM (Herpetology)[a,*],
Alessandro Vetere, DVM, PhD, DECZM (Herpetology)[b]

KEYWORDS

• Surgery • Celiotomy • Reptile • Ovariectomy

KEY POINTS

- Soft tissue surgery in reptiles follows carnivore principles but must be species-adapted and use mini-invasive techniques as possible.
- Digestive, urinary, and hepatobiliary surgeries demand meticulous dissection, hemostasis, and contamination control.
- Ovariectomy and salpingectomy are frequent reproductive surgeries, with endoscopic aid in chelonians.
- In chelonians, the prefemoral approach should be preferred over the transplastral route whenever feasible, particularly for reproductive surgeries.

Video content accompanies this article at http://www.vetexotic.theclinics.com.

INTRODUCTION

Soft tissue surgery in reptiles is an essential part of reptile medicine. The general principles established in domestic carnivores (asepsis, respect for anatomic planes, careful hemostasis, and proper suture techniques) are fully applicable but must be adapted to the anatomic and physiologic particularities of reptiles.[1,2] A thorough clinical examination, together with an assessment of husbandry and nutrition, is crucial before considering surgery, as correcting these factors may prevent recurrence of certain conditions.

INCLUSION CRITERIA

The databases Google Scholar, PubMed, and Scopus were searched with the following keywords: "reptiles's surgery, soft tissue surgery, squamata, chelonia, crocodylia." Only peer-reviewed articles were considered for inclusion. Articles that either

[a] Veterinary Clinic SpéNAC, Paris, France; [b] Department of Veterinary Science, University of Parma, Parma, Italy
* Corresponding author. Veterinary Clinic SpéNAC, 100 boulevard de la tour Maubourg, 75007 Paris, France
E-mail address: paillusseauclement@gmail.com

Vet Clin Exot Anim 29 (2026) 489–516
https://doi.org/10.1016/j.cvex.2026.04.002 vetexotic.theclinics.com

Abbreviations	
Cr	cranial
IM	intramuscular
PCR	polymerase chain reaction

did not meet this criterion or were deemed irrelevant to the review's objectives were discarded.

SURGICAL AND PERISURGICAL CONSIDERATIONS

Surgical Equipment

Most reptile surgeries can be performed with a standard small carnivore surgical kit:

- Scalpel handle with blades, needle holders, Mayo, Metzenbaum or tenotomy scissors, and various hemostatic forceps (eg, mosquito). Match instrument size to patient; ophthalmic tools for precision.
- Retractors optional (Weitlaner, Lone Star®, Retractor System, CooperSurgical Inc., Trumbull, CT).
- Gauze/swabs for hemostasis.
- Vascular hemoclips: rapid, secure ligation.
- Vessel sealing devices (advanced bipolar, ultrasonic, or hybrid systems) for efficient hemostasis and dissection.
- Laser or pure radiofrequency sealing systems for coagulation and minimally invasive tissue cutting.
- Electrosurgical or radiofrequency surgical units for general cutting and coagulation.
- Cryosurgery/microsurgery useful if available.

Procedure–specific instruments are detailed in relevant sections.

As reptiles are ectothermic poikilotherms, intraoperative thermoregulation is critical. A thermostatically controlled heating pad (approximately 32°C for most species) placed beneath the patient helps prevent hypothermia–related complications.[2]

Preoperative Management

Fasting is often unnecessary but advised before gastrointestinal surgery: skip one feeding cycle (eg, 24 hours for a small lizard, 2 weeks for a large snake).[2] Generally, 24 to 96 hours empties the stomach but not the herbivore colon. Recommended durations: approximately 48 hours for lizards and chelonians, 96 hours for snakes (personal experience, C.P.). Reptiles should be warmed and hydrated within their preferred optimal temperature zone (POTZ) before anesthesia (20°C–25°C for temperate/aquatic; 25°C–35°C for tropical species); avoid surgery after hibernation.[2,3] Fluid therapy should be guided by clinical status and laboratory values (electrolytes, ionogram); routes include intracoelomic, intravenous, or intraosseous. A common protocol is fifty-fifty lactated Ringer's and 5% glucose at about 3% body weight, but osmolarity must match species physiology. Preoperative analgesia (eg, morphine 1–5 mg/kg intramuscularly [IM] or methadone 3–5 mg/kg IM q24h in most species) and antibiotic prophylaxis should be administered hours before surgery.[4,5]

Patient and Surgical Site Preparation

Patient positioning should be adapted to the species and type of surgery, aiming to optimize surgical access while ensuring safe ventilation and avoiding pressure injuries, joint hyperextension, or surgeon fatigue.[2] Antisepsis typically uses 5%

povidone–iodine or 0.05% chlorhexidine (avoid ocular/aural areas). The ventrum should be precleaned due to contamination.[2,6] Standard drapes are often impractical; adhesive drapes adhere poorly, and towel clamps may not hold on scales or delicate skin.[2] Stay sutures are effective alternatives, and transparent drapes allow continuous monitoring.[2]

Skin and Muscle Incision

Reptile skin is keratinized; incisions begin with a stab and are extended with scissors or a guarded scalpel.[6–10] In small species, skin and muscle are cut together; in larger ones, the muscle is opened separately to protect vessels. Incision orientation and tension lines matter; scalloped incisions are often needed in snakes (in order to avoid to cut the scales). Electrosurgery or radiosurgery/laser is possible but avoided when margin histology is required.[2,6]

Muscle Closure

Closure resembles that in small carnivores, using simple interrupted or continuous patterns.[7,9,10] In celiotomy, both muscle and coelomic membrane are included, with emphasis on external fascia for strength (personal experience, C.P.).[7,9] Absorbable monofilaments such as polydioxanone, poliglecaprone 25, or polyglyconate are preferred; polyglactin 910 is avoided due to inflammation.[2,11]

Skin Closure and Healing Dynamics

Because the outer layer of reptile skin contains beta-keratin and tends to invert easily, everting patterns (horizontal mattress, continuous "U") are recommended; appositional patterns often fail.[6] Monofilament sutures are generally preferred to limit capillarity and bacterial wicking, particularly in humid environments. Suitable materials include nylon or absorbable monofilaments (polydioxanone, poliglecaprone 25). Wire sutures may be used in crocodilians.[2,6,8,11] However, in reptiles, multifilament sutures may be acceptable in selected cases (personal experience, C.P.), as the skin is typically dry and the risk of wicking appears limited; additionally, rigid monofilament knot ends, especially on ventral aspects, may adhere to the substrate, causing discomfort and increasing wound contamination. Cyanoacrylate tissue glue forms a watertight barrier and shows antimicrobial properties, especially against gram-positive bacteria.[12] Experimental use in pond turtles showed good tolerance without histotoxicity, but when applied as the sole closure method, it resulted in high dehiscence rates, indicating that glue should only be used as an adjunct, not alone, particularly for wounds under tension.[13]

Healing is slower than in mammals, averaging 6 weeks for uncomplicated closures, while second-intention healing may take months.[6] Keeping patients at the upper POTZ (30°C–32°C) accelerates repair. Sutures are usually removed after 6 to 8 weeks, though in squamates, ecdysis may cause early loss or retained exuviae, which typically resolve naturally over 1 to 3 shedding cycles.[6]

Postoperative Management

Care focuses on thermoregulation, pain control, and a quiet, clean recovery environment.[2] Surgical sites must remain dry for 5 to 14 days, and brumation avoided for 3 to 6 months.[2,14] When feasible, aquatic chelonians should be maintained in shallow water that does not cover the surgical site for 10 to 14 days.[15] In strictly aquatic reptiles (eg, Trionychidae, Cheloniidae, and Acrochordidae) dry-docking may not be feasible; in such cases, surgical wounds can be protected by applying Ilex ointment (Medcon Biolab Inc, Grafton, MA), a topical barrier that becomes impervious to water and limits wound exposure during aquatic recovery.[16] Hydration and nutrition should be supported, with assisted feeding or tubes if necessary. Analgesia must be species-specific due to documented interspecies differences.[5] Recheck at 7 to 10 days for healing and at 6 to 8 weeks for suture removal.[2]

EXTRACOELOMIC SURGERIES

Skin and Subcutaneous Tissues Surgery

Aural abscess

Complete excision and debridement of the caseous pyogranuloma is required (**Fig. 1**). After intubation, the oral cavity is packed, and the patient positioned sternal or lateral. Aseptic preparation uses dilute povidone–iodine; alcohol and chlorhexidine are avoided near the eyes.[2,15]

A ventral half-moon incision or excision of the entire tympanic scale allows direct visualization. The pyogranuloma is mobilized and removed with fine curettes, avoiding injury to the columella or Eustachian tube. Samples for cytology, Gram stain, culture, polymerase chain reaction (PCR), or histopathology are collected. The cavity and Eustachian tube are flushed with sterile saline or diluted antiseptic; a soft catheter can be fixed for postoperative topical therapy.[15]

Postoperative care includes daily saline lavage for 2 to 4 weeks, local antibiotics if indicated, and analgesia for 1 to 3 days. Aquatic species should avoid water contact over the tympanic area for 10 to 14 days to keep the surgical site dry. Environmental and dietary corrections, including vitamin A supplementation if needed, help reduce recurrence. Follow-up examinations at 1 and 6 to 8 weeks are performed to monitor healing and remove the catheter.[15] Most reptiles recover quickly and can be discharged the following day.

Subcutaneous abscess and cutaneous neoplasia

Subcutaneous abscesses (**Fig. 2**) are common in captive reptiles, appearing as firm swellings. Locations vary: rostral in boids/colubrids or following trauma/bites in multiple species. Reptile abscesses are usually caseous; complete capsule excision is required, as simple drainage is ineffective.[6,17] After incision and curettage, the cavity is flushed with sterile saline. Samples are collected for cytology, culture, or histopathology. Primary closure is possible if the abscess capsule is completely removed; otherwise, second-intention healing is required. Antibiotics are used only based on culture and sensitivity results.[6,17]

Cutaneous and subcutaneous neoplasia may also occur, requiring oncologic surgical principles (**Fig. 3**).

Venom gland removal

Venom glands are specialized modifications of the labial glands, located in the upper jaw beneath the orbit, and have evolved independently across multiple snake lineages. Their size and shape vary considerably.[18] In some snake genus (eg, *Causus*, *Atractaspis*, and *Calliophis*), glands extend caudally to the cardiac level.[19,20] In lizards, venom glands are sublingual and associated with the mandible in Helodermatidae, whereas in Anguidae and Varanidae they are mandibular, with distinct anatomic features and venom compositions.[21,22]

Venom gland surgery is indicated mainly in snakes for infection or to reduce envenomation risk, not for convenience. In snakes, venom glands are typically large, enveloped by muscle fibers, with blood supply dorsomedially. Two main surgical approaches are described:

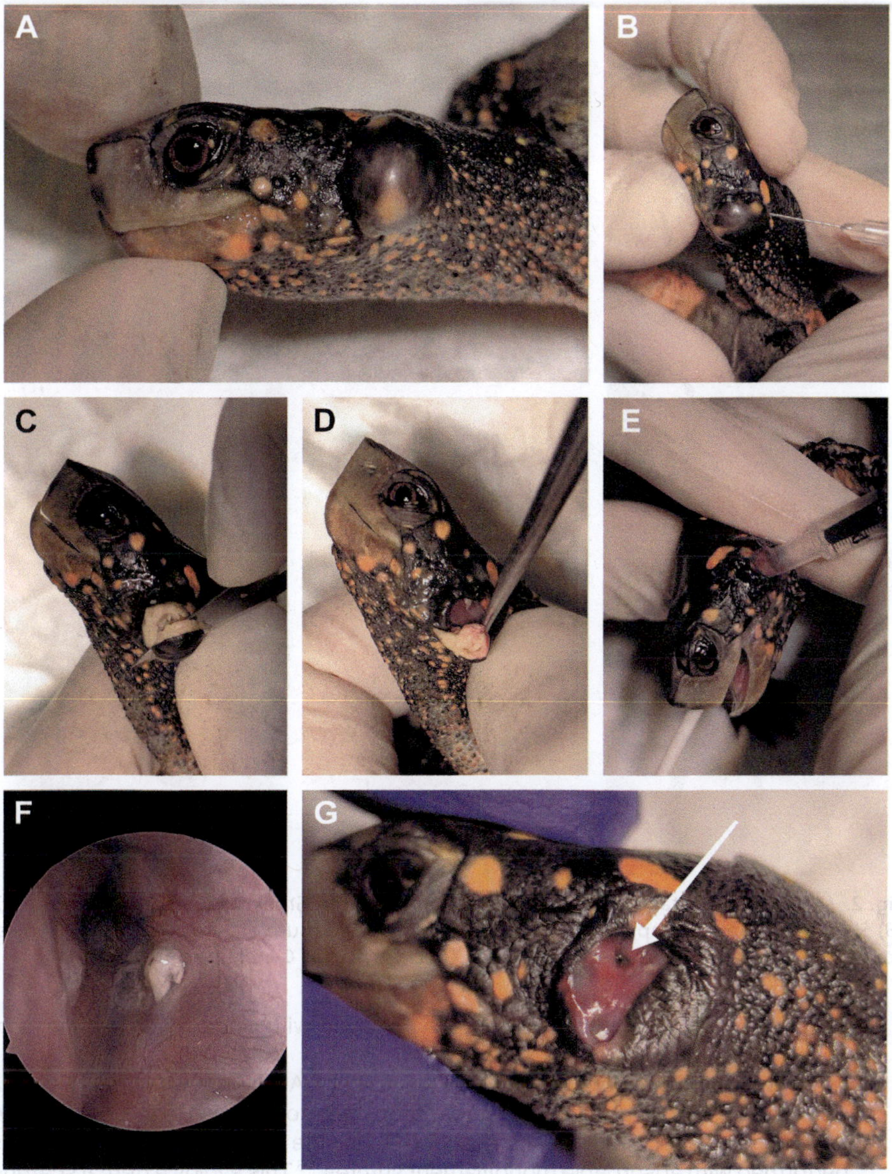

Fig. 1. (*A–G*) (*A*) Aural abscess surgery in a spotted turtle (*Clemmys guttata*). (*B, C*) Tympanic scale excision after infiltration of local anesthesia. (*D*) Pyogranuloma removal with curettes, preserving columella/Eustachian tube. (*E*) Cavity flushed with saline/antiseptic. (*F*) Endoscopic check of distal tube. (*G*) Postoperative aspect; proximal tube opening sometimes visible (*arrow*). (*Courtesy of* Dr Clément Paillusseau.)

- *Lateral approach* (**Fig. 4**): A 1 cm skin incision is made midway between the eye and upper lip. Fluorescein can be injected to visualize the duct. After fascia incision and blunt dissection, dorsomedial vessels are ligated or cauterized. The duct is cranially ligated with absorbable suture and transected; an accessory

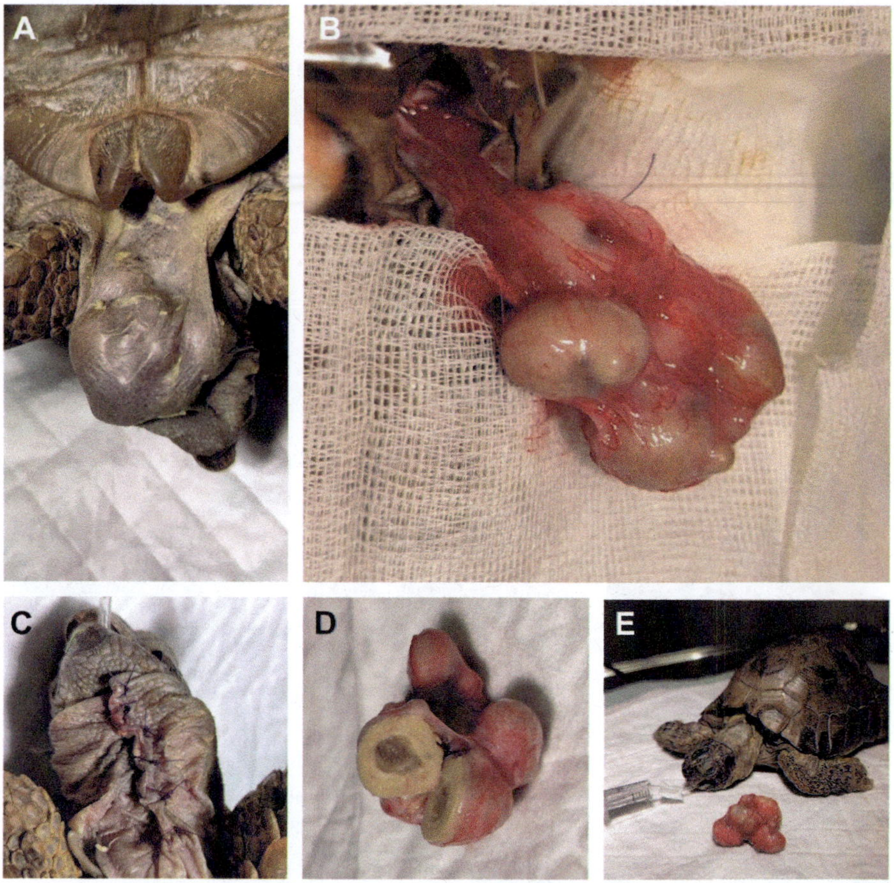

Fig. 2. (*A–E*) (*A*) Subcutaneous fungal abscess removal in a Greek tortoise (*Testudo graeca*). (*B*) Skin incision and complete capsule/pus excision. (*C*) Closure after irrigation. (*D*) Typical concentric abscess. (*E*) Postoperative aspect. (*Courtesy of* Dr Clément Paillusseau.)

gland may occur in viperids. Closure is achieved with single-layer U–sutures of absorbable material.[18]

- *Oral approach:* Fangs are immobilized (eg, tubing). A longitudinal buccal mucosa incision lateral to maxilla provides direct access to the gland and the duct. A dissection, ligation, and duct transection follow the same principles. Closure is performed with absorbable monofilament sutures.[18] This avoids external scarring but carries higher bacterial contamination risk and increases operator exposure.

Postoperative care includes minimizing handling and using absorbable sutures. Histopathology of the duct is recommended to confirm complete excision. Feeding live prey may help detect residual gland activity.

Paracloacal gland removal

Paracloacal glands are extramural exocrine glands of the distal cloaca in squamates, embedded in connective tissue and interlaced with striated muscle. Their ducts open into the distal proctodeal lumen. Secretions are important for chemical communication, including scent marking, territorial signaling, mate attraction, and species/sex

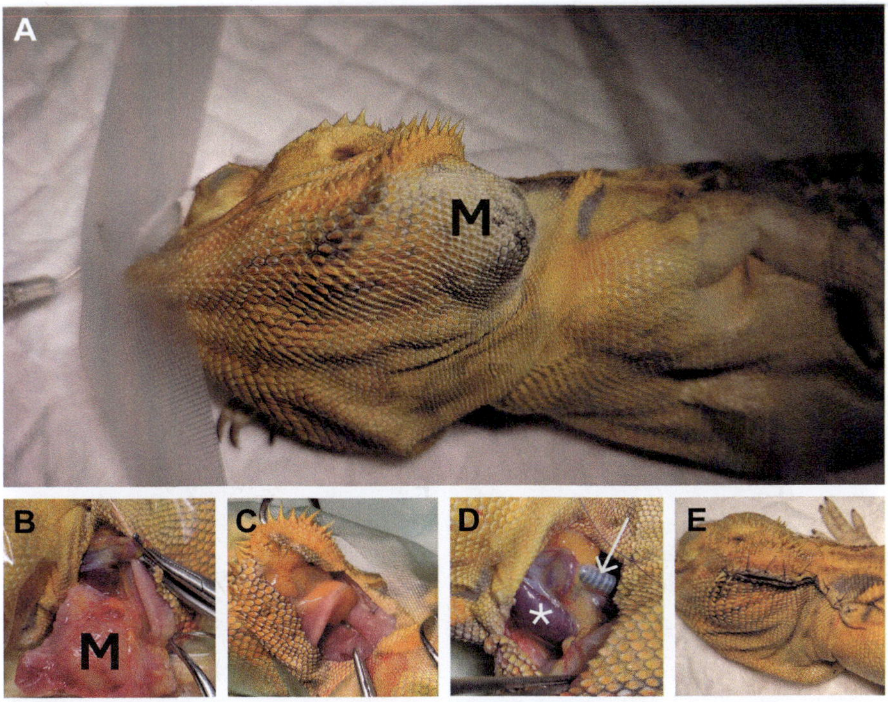

Fig. 3. (*A–E*) (*A*) Amelanotic melanoma (*M*) excision in a bearded dragon (*Pogona vitticeps*). (*B*) Intraoperative view. (*C*) Site after excision. (*D*) Oncologic margins with jugular vein (*asterisk*) and trachea (*arrow*). (*E*) Closure with U-stitches. (*Courtesy of* Dr Clément Paillusseau.)

recognition, often influenced by reproductive status.[23] Presence, epithelial type, and topography vary by species across multiple lizard and snake families.[24]

Excision of the gland (**Fig. 5**) is indicated when manual emptying fails, or in recurrent impaction, adenitis, or suspected neoplasia.[25,26]

After aseptic preparation, a skin incision is made between the first 2 lateral scale rows. The distal gland is grasped, medial adhesions dissected, and the gland remains attached only by the excretory duct. The duct is clamped, ligated, and transected; the site is flushed, and closure performed in 2 layers. Bilateral glands may be removed via the same incision or separately. Complications include gland rupture or spillage; marsupialization carries high recurrence.[25] In a series (n = 6), 90% of glands were completely excised, infections occurred in 33%, and prognosis was generally favorable with low recurrence.[26]

Urinary Tract Surgery

Renal biopsies (paracoccygian or prefemoral approaches)

In lizards with intrapelvic kidneys (eg, iguanids, geckonids, and agamids), a paracoccygeal approach is used if kidneys are not enlarged or endoscopy is unavailable (**Fig. 6**).[27,28] Patients are positioned laterally, pelvic limb retracted cranially. A 1 to 3 cm incision is made in the lateral tail groove; blunt dissection follows muscle fibers to expose the kidney. Sampling is performed with a scalpel wedge, biopsy punch, or Tru-Cut® biopsy needle, Merit Medical Systems Inc., South Jordan, UT. Hemostasis

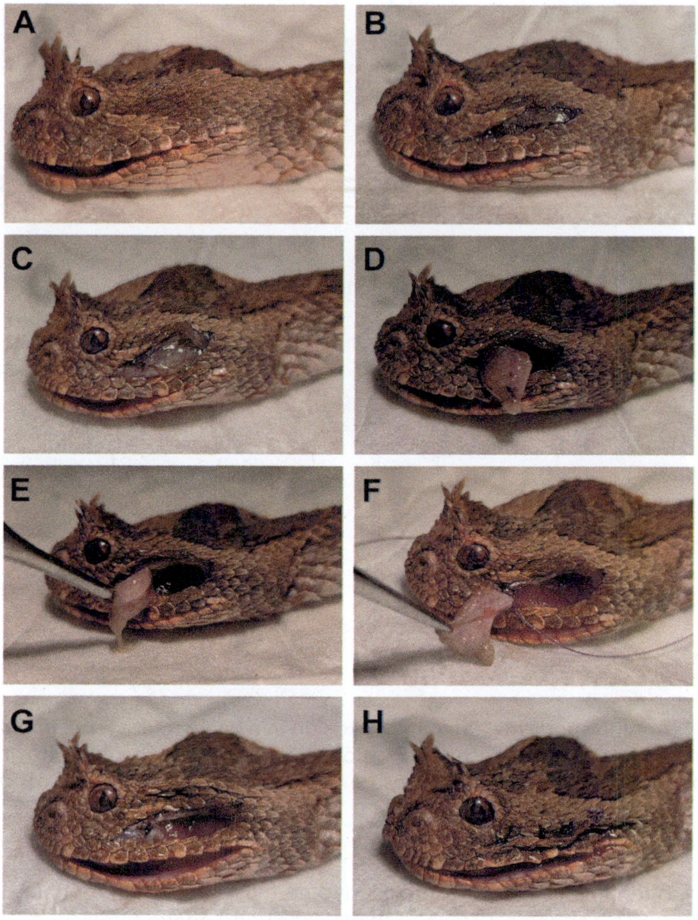

Fig. 4. (*A–H*) (*A*) Venom gland removal in a many-horned adder (*Bitis cornuta*). (*B*) Skin incision. (*C, D*) Fascia incision, blunt dissection to duct. (*E–G*) Duct ligated and transected. (*H*) Closure with absorbable U-sutures. (*Courtesy of* Dr Clément Paillusseau.)

is achieved via digital pressure, absorbable agents, or fine ligatures. Muscle and skin are closed in layers. Typically unilateral, bilateral biopsies require additional exposure.

In chelonians, renal biopsy can be performed via a prefemoral approach without celiotomy.[28] Skin incision, blunt dissection, tissue sampling, hemostasis, and layered closure follow the same principles.

Digestive Tract Surgery

Glossectomy

Glossectomy (**Fig. 7**) is indicated for trauma, necrosis, infection, neoplasia, or well-demarcated tongue lesions.[29,30] Patients are positioned sternal or lateral, with head extended; a mouth gag and oropharyngeal packing reduce aspiration risk. Partial glossectomy may use stay sutures. Circumferential epithelium incision with safety margin is followed by transection of underlying musculature. The lingual artery is controlled via ligation, electro/radiosurgery, or hemostatic agents. Tissue is excised along healthy planes, and closure is performed with fine absorbable monofilament sutures, using

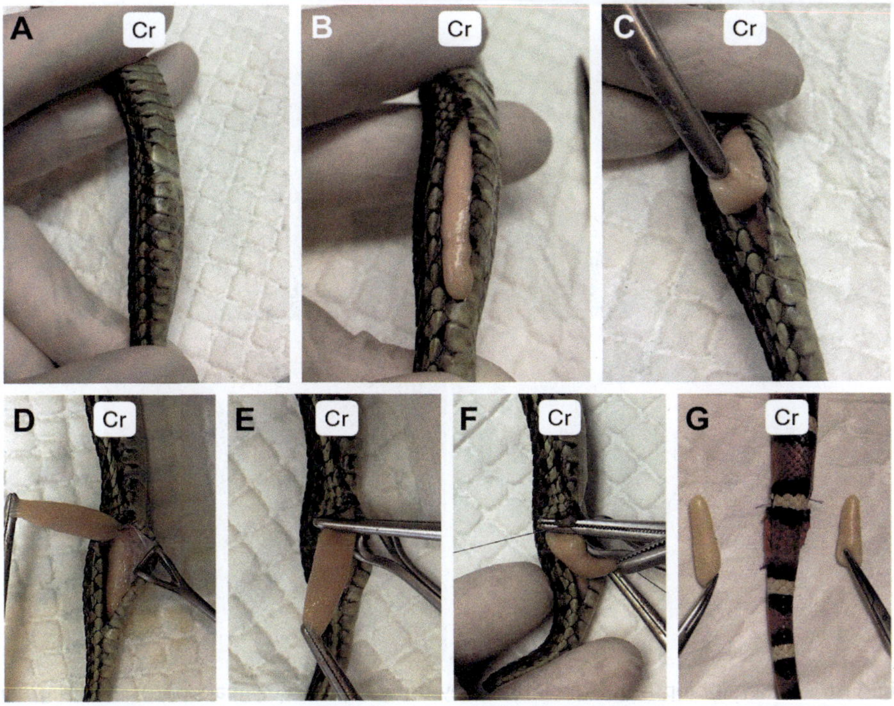

Fig. 5. (*A–G*) (*A*) Paracloacal gland excision in an Eastern ribbon snake (*Thamnophis saurita*). (*B*) Skin incision. (*C*) Distal gland grasped. (*D*) Muscular adhesions dissected. (*E, F*) Duct ligated/transected. (*G*) Two-layer closure in a Honduran milksnake (*Lampropeltis abnorma*). Cr, cranial. (*Courtesy of* Dr Clément Paillusseau.)

multiple mattress sutures if needed while preserving critical structures (eg, chameleon entoglossal process).[29,30] Nutritional support should be planned, and an esophagostomy tube may be required. Healing is usually rapid, and the patient should be monitored at 1 and 4 weeks postoperatively. A glossectomy may significantly impair key behavioral functions in squamates. Tongue flicking is essential for chemical sampling, prey detection, and orientation via the vomeronasal organ. A reduction of the tongue surface or the loss of bifurcation is, therefore, expected to decrease chemosensory efficiency and to alter foraging and exploratory strategies. Moreover, in some lizards, such as the blue-tongue skink (*Tiliqua* sp) and the green keel-bellied lizard (*Gastropholis prasina*), the tongue also serves as a visual signal in defensive or communicative displays; surgical alteration could compromise the effectiveness of these behaviors, with potential consequences on social interactions and predator deterrence.[31,32]

Esophageal tube placement

Esophagostomy tube placement (**Fig. 8**) is indicated for prolonged anorexia or when oral feeding is impossible, primarily in chelonians but applicable to all reptiles. After sedation, the left caudolateral neck is aseptically prepared, avoiding major vessels. The tube is premeasured to reach the stomach, and a small incision is made over tented esophagus using curved hemostats. The tube is guided intraluminally to the oral cavity, secured with purse-string and finger-trap sutures, and stabilized externally. Placement should be confirmed by radiography or endoscopy.[33]

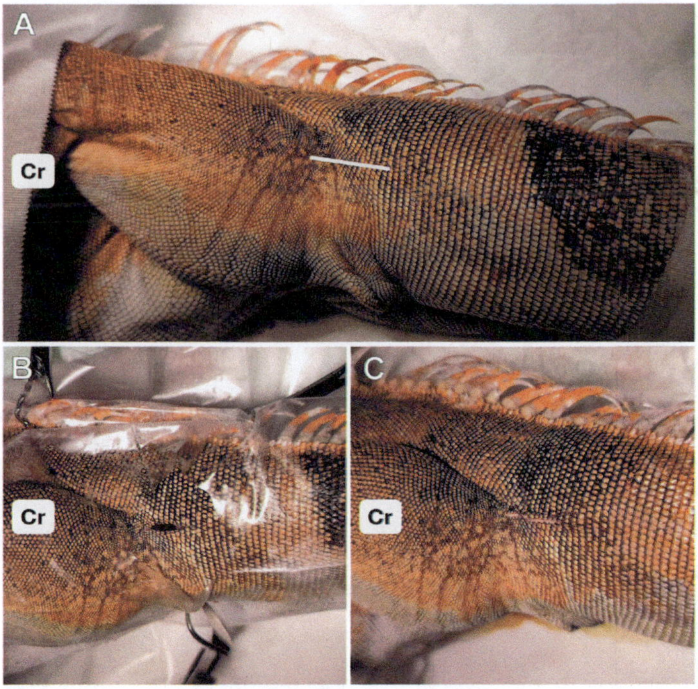

Fig. 6. (*A–C*) Renal biopsies of the left kidney using a paracoccygeal approach in a green iguana (*Iguana iguana*). (*A*) The animal is placed in right lateral recumbency, and a longitudinal incision is made along the lateral tail groove (*white line*). (*B*) Surgical site after skin incision and blunt muscle dissection. (*C*) Skin closure using interrupted monofilament sutures. Cr, cranial. (*Courtesy of* Dr Clément Paillusseau.)

Prolapsus and cloacal disease

Phallectomy (penis or hemipenis amputation). This procedure (**Fig. 9**) is indicated for prolapse of the male copulatory organ with irreversible ischemic or necrotic lesions.[34,35] In reptiles, it is relatively straightforward, as the urinary tract does not traverse the phallus. After aseptic preparation, the animal is placed in dorsal recumbency. The cloaca is everted, and a vascular clamp is applied at the penile base for temporary hemostasis. Two ligatures are placed proximal to the clamp: the most proximal is an encircling ligature completely surrounding the organ near the body wall, and the distal ligature is transfixing, passing through the penile tissue. In large chelonians, vascular clamps are often unnecessary, and ligatures can be placed directly at the base of the penis (personal experience, C.P.). The organ is transected distal to the clamp, hemostasis confirmed, and the stump repositioned into the cloaca. Closure with fine monofilament absorbable sutures may promote epithelialization and reduce irritation.[34,35]

Colonic resection–anastomosis without celiotomy. When the prolapsed mucosa is necrotic or severely damaged, segmental resection can be performed without celiotomy (**Fig. 10**).[11] After aseptic preparation, a syringe barrel is inserted into the colonic lumen and stabilized with transverse needles.[11] The distal prolapsed segment is circularly resected, and the 2 ends approximated and sutured around the barrel with simple interrupted absorbable monofilament suture. The anastomosis is reintroduced into the cloaca, with sutures inverting naturally. This reduces celiotomy trauma but carries a higher risk of postoperative dehiscence.

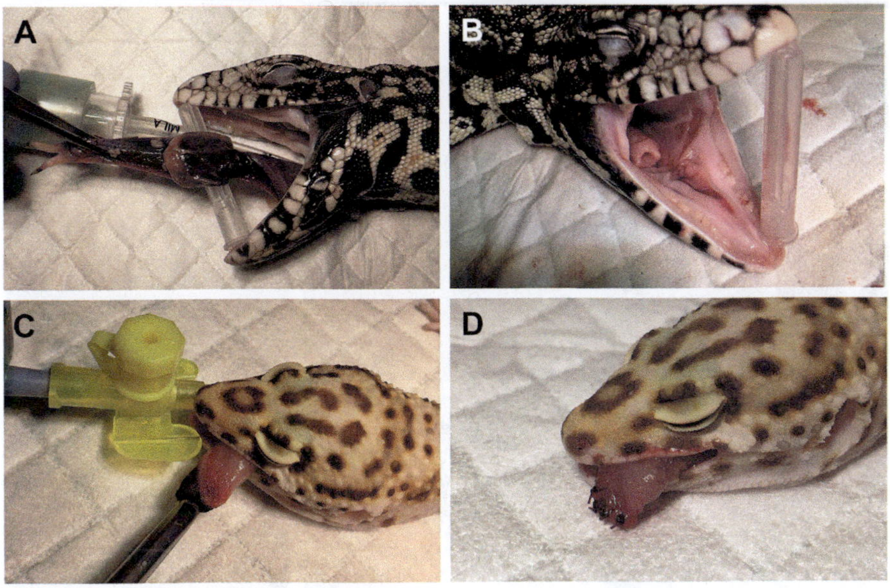

Fig. 7. (*A–D*) (*A*) Complete glossectomy in a black and white tegu (*Salvator merianae*). (*B*) Postoperative view. (*C*) Partial glossectomy in a leopard gecko (*Eublepharis macularius*). (*D*) Necrotic tip removed, sutures placed. (*Courtesy of* Dr Clément Paillusseau.)

Vascular System Surgery

Aneurysm ligature

Aneurysms mainly affect central bearded dragons (*Pogona vitticeps*), presenting as firm, sometimes pulsatile, swellings near major arteries and veins (mandible, neck, and palatine bone).[36] Infection with *Encephalitozoon pogonae* may induce vasculitis, thrombus formation, and subsequent aneurysm development.[37] In a study of 17 cases, 94% of aneurysms had ruptured, most commonly in the cranial coelomic region.[36] Histopathology revealed tunica media and adventitia degeneration with disruption of collagen and elastic fibers (100%), often with intimal thickening and thrombi (54%), dissecting hematomas (47%), vasculitis (29%), mineralization (6%), and lipid deposits (6%). These vascular alterations likely weakened vessel walls, predisposing them to rupture.[36] Preoperative evaluation includes echocardiography and abdominal ultrasonography. Surgery entails antiseptic preparation, incision, blunt dissection, proximal ligation with hemoclips or sutures, and en bloc excision. Closure uses absorbable sutures for muscle and everting mattress sutures for skin.[38] Ultrasound-guided embolization is a less-invasive alternative, reducing surgical risks and recovery time.[39]

INTRACOELOMIC SURGERIES

Celiotomy

Celiotomy in reptiles is equivalent to mammalian laparotomy, providing access to the gastrointestinal, reproductive, and urinary systems, and, due to absence of a diaphragm, the heart and lungs. Indications include exploratory surgery, ovariectomy/castration, salpingectomy/salpingotomy, gastrointestinal procedures, cystotomy, and biopsies (**Fig. 11**).[7–11]

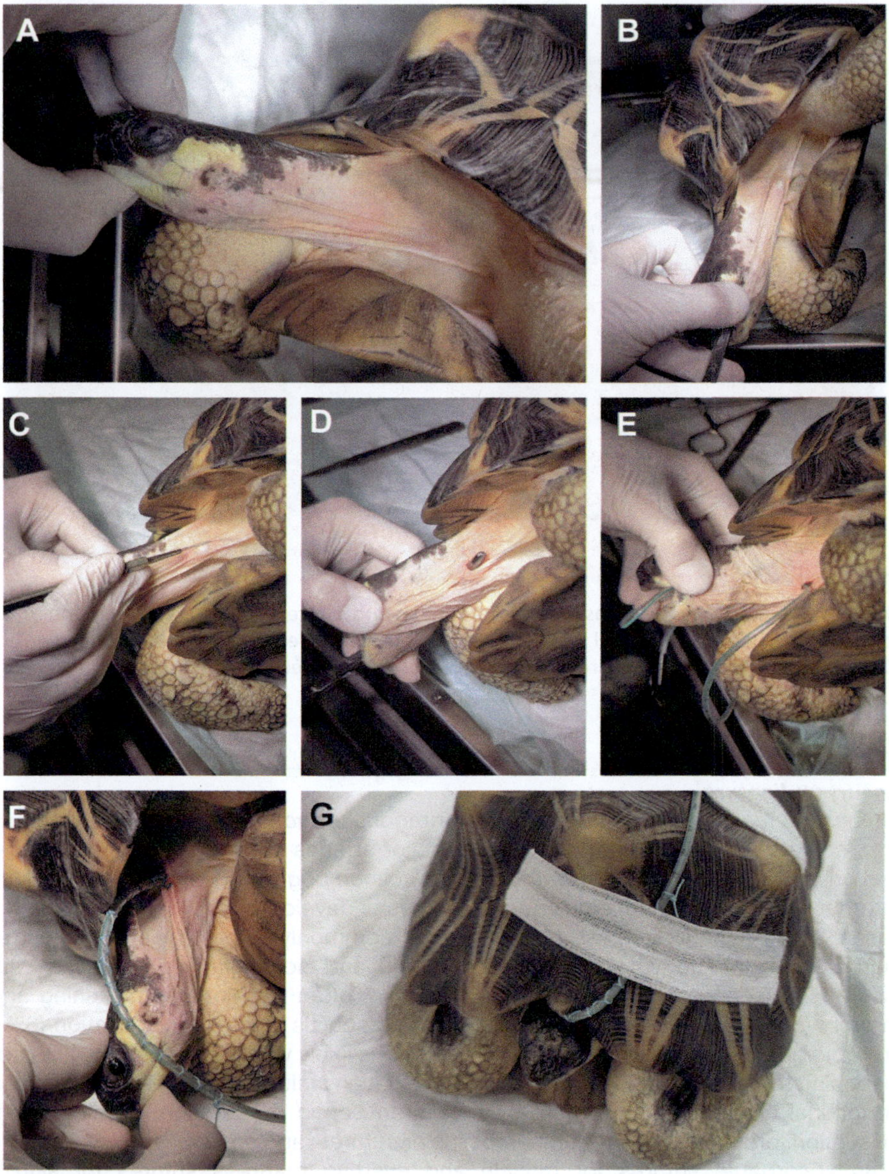

Fig. 8. (*A–G*) (*A*) Esophagostomy tube in a radiated tortoise (*Astrochelys radiata*). (*B*) Hemostats tent skin. (*C–E*) Tube passed intraluminally. (*F, G*) Secured with purse-string and finger-trap sutures. (*Courtesy of* Dr Clément Paillusseau.)

Saurians

Ventral approach

For dorsoventrally compressed lizards (eg, Agamidae, Varanidae, Gekkonidae, and Iguanidae). A midline or paramedian incision is made, sometimes incising skin and muscle together. Paramedian route avoids the ventral abdominal vein but increases

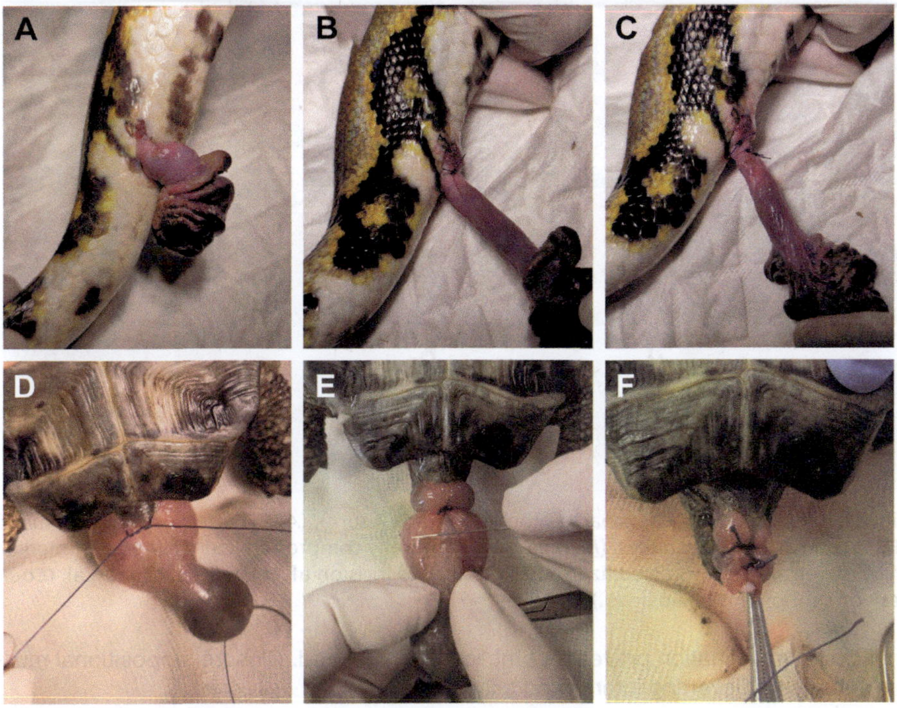

Fig. 9. (*A–F*) (*A*) Hemipenis amputation in a reticulated python (*Malayopython reticulatus*). (*B, C*) Two ligatures placed. (*D*) Same in a Greek tortoise (*Testudo graeca*). (*E, F*) Stump inspected and repositioned. (*Courtesy of* Dr Clément Paillusseau.)

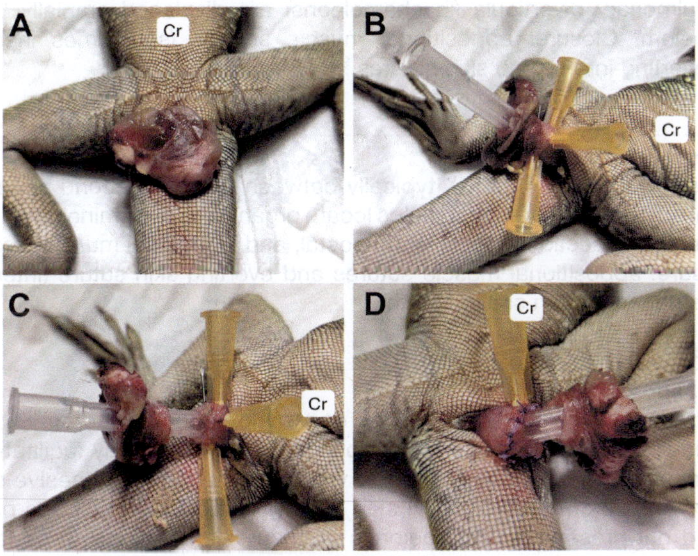

Fig. 10. (*A–D*) (*A*) Colon resection–anastomosis in a Weber's sailfin lizard (*Hydrosaurus weberi*). (*B*) Barrel placed intraluminally. (*C*) Circular resection performed. (*D*) Ends sutured around barrel (monofilament sutures are recommended). Cr, cranial. (*Courtesy of* Dr Clément Paillusseau.)

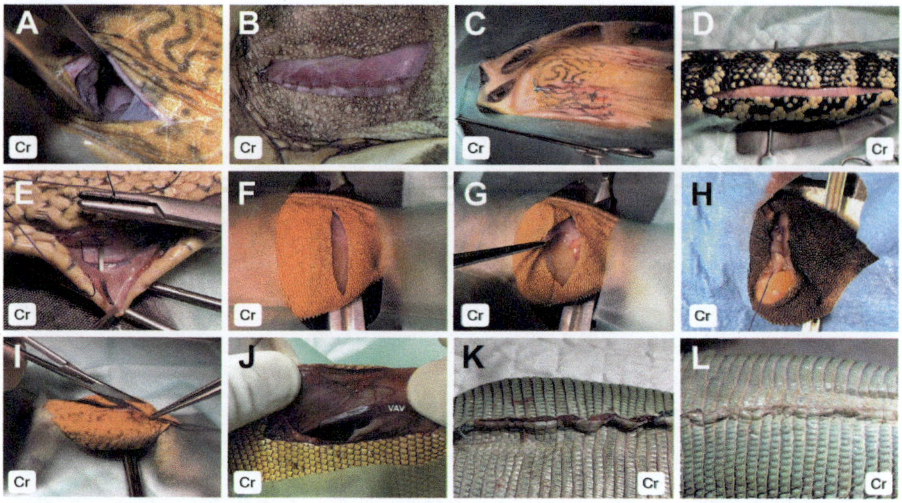

Fig. 11. (*A–L*) Celiotomy approaches (opening and closure). (*A–C*) Prefemoral in chelonians. (*D, E*) Lateroventral in snakes. (*F–H*) Lateral in laterally compressed lizards. (*I–K*) Paramedian in dorsoventrally compressed lizards. (*L*) Cutaneous incision after 6 weeks. Cr, cranial. (*Courtesy of* Dr Clément Paillusseau.)

muscle trauma; ligation prevents complications if injured. Closure: appositional muscle sutures and everting interrupted skin sutures.[9]

Lateral approach

For laterally compressed lizards (eg, Chamaeleonidae, some Agamidae). Skin incision runs perpendicular to spine along ribs; coelom entered between ribs, avoiding rib transection. Pulmonary diverticula (in chameleons) are displaced cranially to prevent pneumocoelom. Closure: appositional muscle sutures (sometimes incorporating ribs) and everting interrupted skin sutures.[9]

Ophidians

Ventrolateral approach

Skin incision over target organ(s), typically between first and second or second and third lateral scale rows. Ultrasound helps locate organs and determine optimal surgical site. Sequential dissection of axial, supracostal, and intercostal muscles exposes organs. Closure: appositional muscle sutures and everting skin suture (interrupted or continuous depending on snake length).[7]

Chelonians

Prefemoral approach

This approach is used for ovariectomy, egg removal, salpingectomy, castration, small bladder stones, and biopsies. Endoscopic assistance may facilitate the procedure. Animals are positioned laterally, with stabilization via adhesive strips and a rolled towel. A 2 cm craniocaudal skin incision exposes an adipose pad, which is retracted but preserved. The coelomic aponeurosis is incised or penetrated by advancing hemostats cranially, parallel to the table; care must be taken at this step to avoid injury to the kidneys, lungs, or urinary bladder. Closure: 2 layers—continuous suture incorporating coelomic membrane/muscle, followed by continuous or interrupted U-stitches for skin.[10]

Crocodilians

Lateral approach

Similar to saurians but complicated by multiple coelomic cavities (**Fig. 12**). Advantages include protection from body weight, avoidance of ventral osteoderms, and improved access. An optional "H"-shaped incision enhances exposure. Closure: continuous appositional muscle suture and continuous/interrupted U-stitches for skin; metallic sutures may be needed in large individuals.[8]

Digestive Tract Surgery

Surgery of the digestive tract in reptiles is indicated for obstructive foreign bodies, neoplasia, abscesses, granulomas, or volvulus. General surgical principles used in mammals apply.[1] After aseptic preparation and celiotomy, the affected segment is exteriorized and isolated with moistened swabs.[40] Because of the small size and fragility of reptilian intestines, the use of Doyen clamps are rarely feasible; instead,

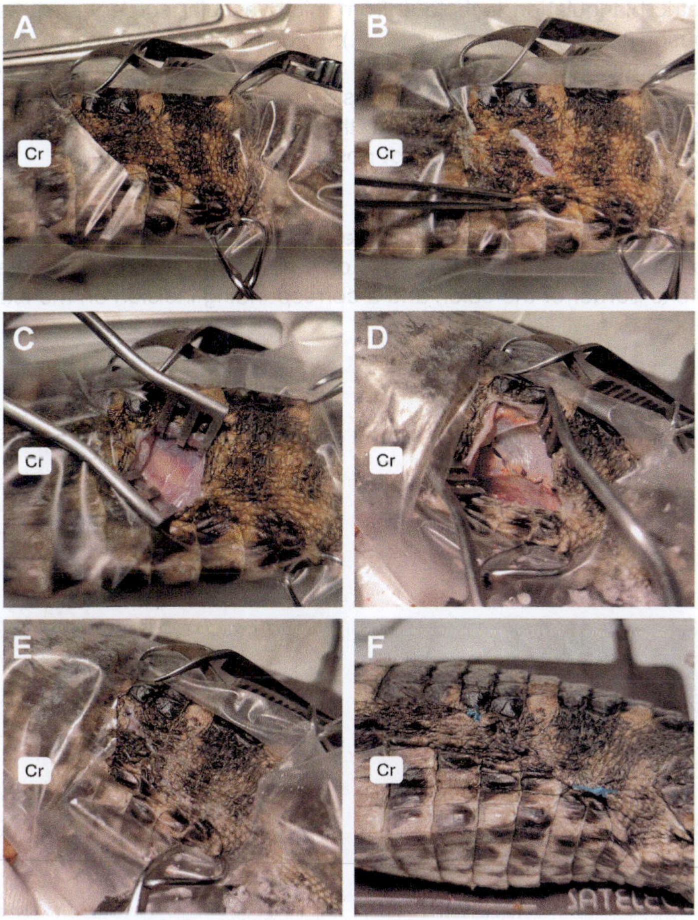

Fig. 12. (*A–F*) Lateral celiotomy in a Cuvier's dwarf caiman (*Paleosuchus palpebrosus*). (*A*) Skin incision caudal to last rib. (*B*) Avoid ventral extension. (*C*) Retractor placed. (*D*) Mesenteric sac incised, rinsed, sutured. (*E, F*) Muscle and skin closure (monofilament sutures are recommended). Cr, cranial. (*Courtesy of* Dr Clément Paillusseau.)

an assistant applies gentle digital pressure proximal and distal to the incision site to limit contamination.[40]

Opening of the digestive tract (gastrotomy, enterotomy, and colotomy)

When an incision is needed (**Fig. 13**), for example, to remove a foreign body, it is made along the antimesenteric border of the affected organ. The object is carefully extracted to avoid contamination. The organ is closed with a simple continuous or interrupted monofilament suture, rinsed outside the coelomic cavity, and new gloves and instruments are used. For gastric or colonic surgery, a second inverting layer (Cushing or Connell) may be added if stenosis risk is minimal.[40]

Resection of a portion of the digestive tract (gastrectomy, enterectomy, and colectomy)

For resection–anastomosis (**Fig. 14**), diseased segments (eg, neoplasia and necrosis) are isolated with clamps or digital pressure, mesenteric vessels ligated, and the intestine transected. Ends are approximated with simple sutures.[40] In very small patients, the symmetric biangulation technique from microvascular surgery ensures even suture distribution (personal experience, C.P.).[41] For lumen size mismatch, forceps dilation addresses minor differences, oblique transection enlarges moderate ones, and marked disparities require end-to-side or side-to-side anastomosis. After confirming watertightness, the segment is replaced, the cavity rinsed, and closed.[40] As reptiles lack an omentum, omentalization is not possible.

Colopexy (from intracoelomic approach)

This procedure secures the colon to the coelomic wall using nonabsorbable sutures.[11] After manual reduction of the prolapse, a 1 cm incision of the serosa is made along the antimesenteric border of the colon and a corresponding incision on the left coelomic

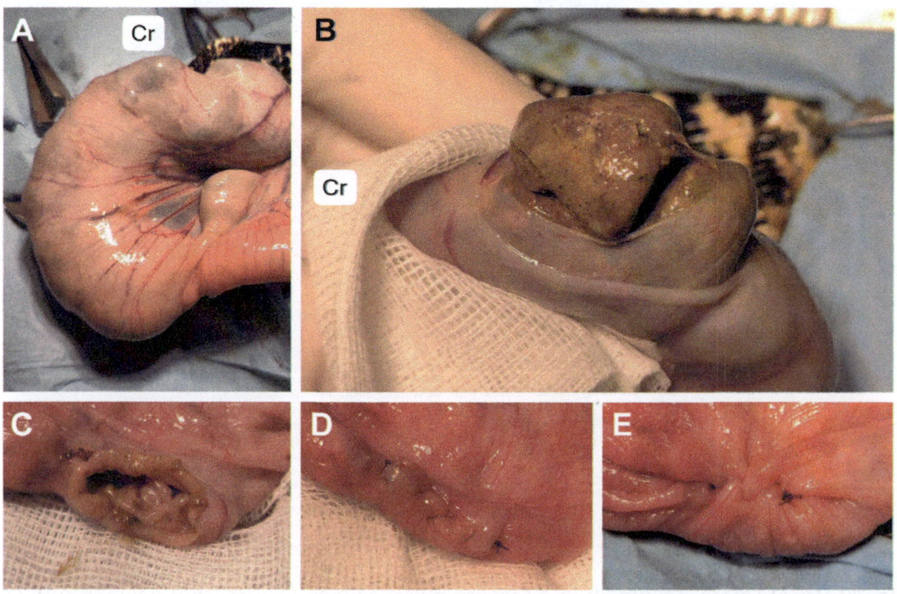

Fig. 13. (*A–E*) Colotomy in a black and white tegu (*Salvator merianae*). (*A*) Segment exteriorized. (*B*) Antimesenteric incision. (*C*) Fecaloma extracted. (*D, E*) Closure with continuous appositional and inverting sutures. Cr, cranial. (*Courtesy of* Dr Clément Paillusseau.)

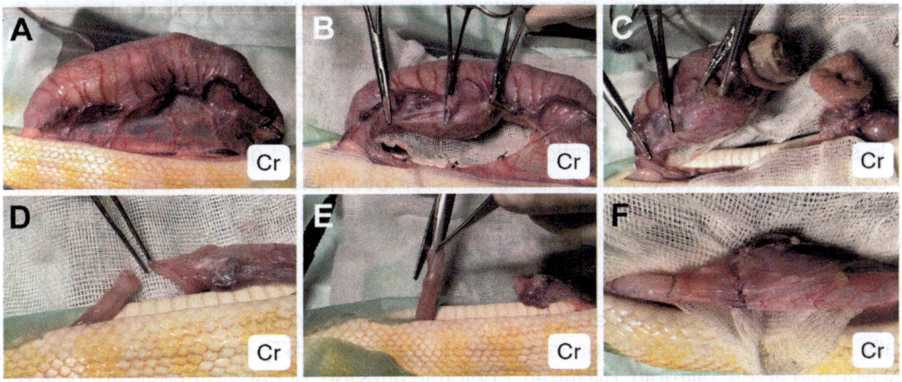

Fig. 14. (*A–F*) Enterectomy in an albino carpet python (*Morelia spilota*). (*A*) Carcinoma. (*B, C*) Segment ligated and transected. (*D, E*) Ends approximated; oblique cut if disparity. (*F*) Anastomosis completed. Cr, cranial. (*Courtesy of* Dr Clément Paillusseau.)

wall.[11] The colon is sutured to the muscular wall, incorporating 3 successive ribs as anchors, except in chelonians where ribs are fused with the carapace. During suturing, the colon is drawn cranially to reduce recurrence risk.

Hepatobiliary System Surgery

Cholecystectomy

This procedure is indicated for gallstones, neoplasia, or chronic bacterial cholecystitis.[40,42–44] After celiotomy, the gallbladder is identified (**Fig. 15**): in chelonians and lizards, it lies within the right hepatic lobe; in snakes, caudal to the liver. The common bile duct is carefully dissected and ligated distally, avoiding pancreatic injury.[42,43] The caudal vena cava can be visualized dorsally.

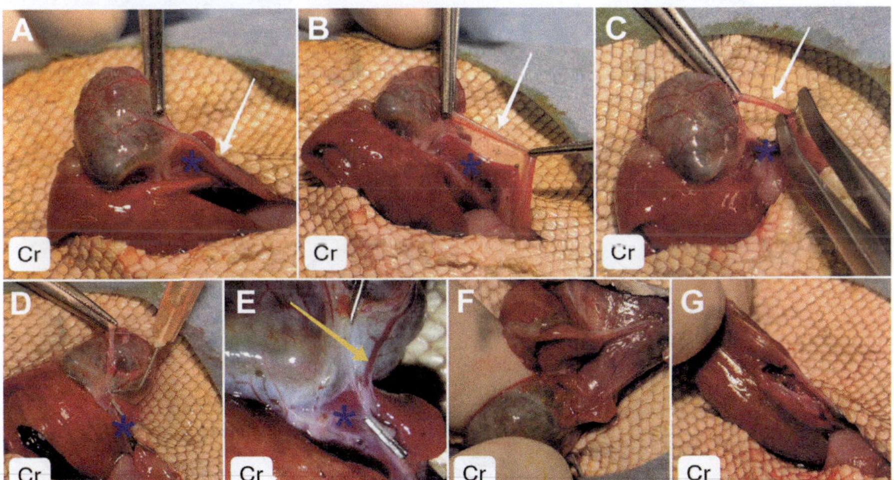

Fig. 15. Cholecystectomy in a bearded dragon (*Pogona vitticeps*). (*A*) Gallbladder identified, closely associated with the vena cava (*blue asterisk*). (*B, C*) Bile duct (*white arrow*) dissected/ligated. (*D*) Gallbladder retracted, serosa dissected using hydrodissection. (*E*) Cystic vein (*yellow arrow*) secured. (*F*) Gallbladder detached. (*G*) Final aspect. Cr, cranial. (*Courtesy of* Clément Paillusseau.)

In lizards and chelonians, the gallbladder is gently pulled ventrally to tension the serosa, which is dissected caudo-cranially using fine scissors or a cotton swab; aspiration of the gallbladder content or hydrodissection (saline instillation in perivenous tissues) may aid separation (personal experience, C.P.). Hemostatic forceps manage vascular supply, and minor parenchymal bleeding is controlled with sponges.[43]

In snakes, the greater separation of liver, vena cava, and gallbladder simplifies the procedure.[44] After ligation, the gallbladder is removed, the coelom rinsed, and closure performed conventionally; in large animals, the biliary duct may be flushed to reduce the risk of retained biliary calculi.

Hepatectomy (biopsies, removal of neoplasia)

Partial hepatectomy is indicated for neoplasia or hepatic abscesses, and diagnostically when liver enzymes (aspartate aminotransferase [AST], sorbitol dehydrogenase [SDH]), bile acids, bilirubin, biliverdin, coelomic effusion, or hepatomegaly suggest pathology. Tissue can be collected for histology, PCR, or microbiology.[40]

All biopsy techniques described in mammals are applicable after conventional celiotomy:

- *Guillotine biopsy*: Performed if the hepatic edge is prominent; if not, 2 notches are made with a clamp, crushing the tissue for hemostasis, and a ligature is placed between them. Only peripheral hepatic parenchyma is sampled.[1]
- *Box suture biopsy*: A suture on a Tapercut (Vicryl® polyglactin 910 suture mounted on a taper-cut needle [Ethicon Inc., Raritan, NJ) needle passes through the liver edge, creating a notch with a knot perpendicular to the edge. A second notch is made 1 to 1.5 cm away, and 1 strand is passed through the first notch before tying.[1] This technique provides better hemostasis and reduces ligature slippage.

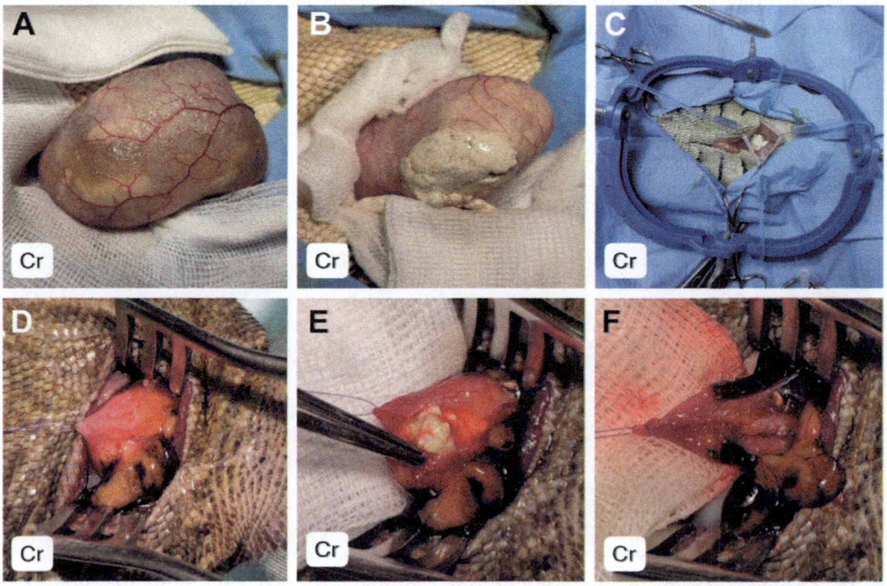

Fig. 16. (*A–F*) Cystotomy in a green iguana (*Iguana iguana*). (*A*) Ventral incision. (*B*) Bladder incision in avascular zone. (*C*) Lonestar® Retractor used. (*D, E*) Same in a Moroccan spiny-tailed lizard (*Uromastyx nigriventris*). (*F*) Two-layer closure. Cr, cranial. (*Courtesy of* Dr Clément Paillusseau.)

- *Punch biopsy*: The punch is inserted at 90° to the liver, rotated clockwise and counterclockwise, then tilted to 45° to detach tissue.[1] Allows sampling of perihilar parenchyma but has higher postoperative bleeding risk.

Alternatively, less-invasive approaches such as endoscopic microbiopsy or ultrasound-guided biopsy can be used depending on case and equipment availability.[45,46]

Urinary Tract Surgery

Cystotomy and partial cystectomy

Cystotomy (**Fig. 16**) is indicated for the removal of calculi, intravesical eggs, bladder trauma, or biopsy in severe cystitis; partial or complete cystectomy may be required for necrosis, neoplasia, or recurrent stones.[27] Only species with a urinary bladder are suitable: chelonians all have 1, snakes and crocodilians do not, and lizards vary (well-developed in green iguanas and skinks, vestigial in agamids).[28] During coelomic surgery, care is needed due to the thin-walled bladder and septic contents. Ventral celiotomy is standard in lizards; chelonians may require prefemoral or transplastron approaches.[27] The bladder is gently exteriorized or the coelom packed with moistened gauze. Incisions are made in less vascular areas, urine is suctioned, and stay

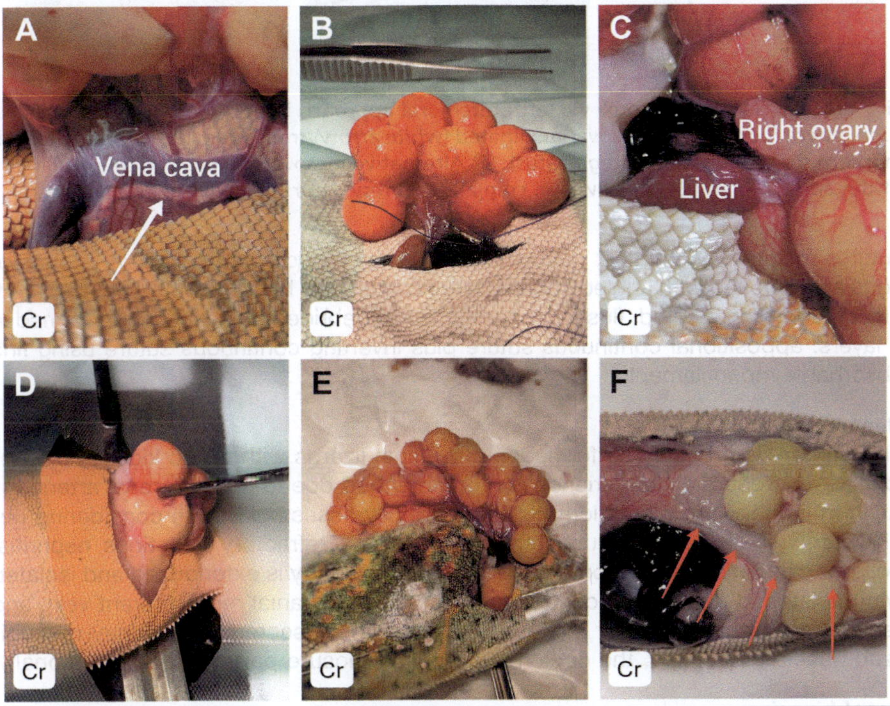

Fig. 17. (*A–F*) Ovariectomy in lizards. (*A*) Ventral approach in a green iguana (*Iguana iguana*). From lateral to medial: right ovary, vena cava, and adrenal gland (*white arrow*) (*B, C*) Same in a bearded dragon (*Pogona vitticeps*). Note the proximity between the right ovary and the right liver lobe in this species. (*D*) Intercostal approach in a panther chameleon (*Furcifer pardalis*). (*E*) Same in a veiled chameleon (*Chamaeleo calyptratus*). (*F*) Pulmonary extensions (*red arrows*) noted. Cr, cranial. (*Courtesy of* Dr Clément Paillusseau.)

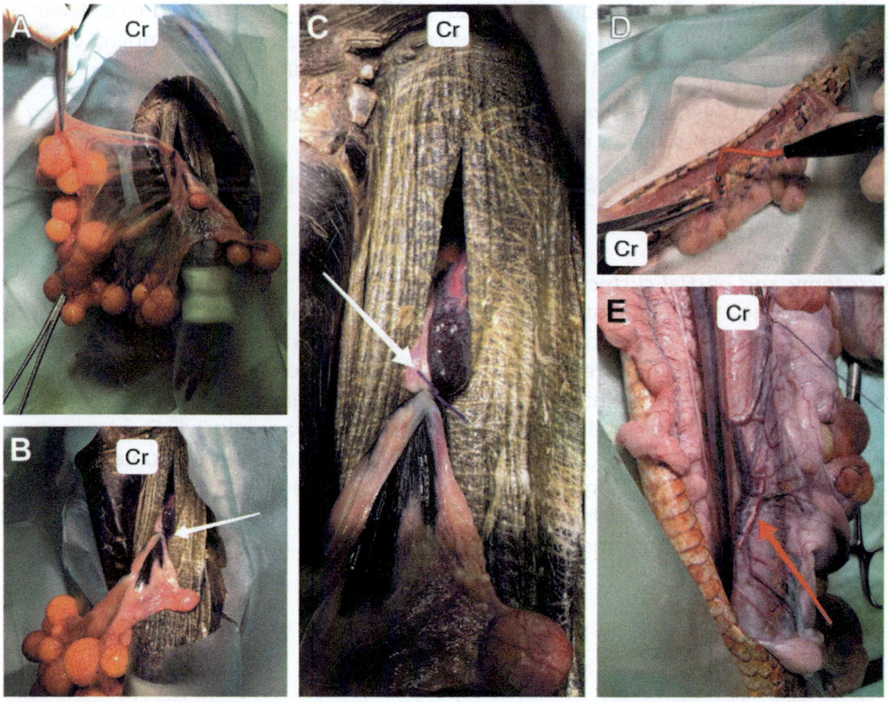

Fig. 18. (*A–E*) (*A*) Ovariectomy via left prefemoral approach in an Asia minor tortoise (*Testudo graeca ibera*). (*B, C*) Mesovarium ligated (*white arrow*)/transected. (*D*) Lateral approach in a corn snake (*Pantherophis guttatus*). (*E*) Alternative mesovarium ligation to avoid injury of the adrenal gland (*red arrow*). Cr, cranial. (*Courtesy of* Dr Clément Paillusseau.)

sutures maintain orientation; marsupialization may reduce contamination. Stones or eggs are removed with angled spoons; large calculi may be fragmented or leveraged. The bladder is inspected, flushed, necrotic tissue debrided, and closure performed in 2 layers: appositional continuous suture plus inverting continuous suture using fine absorbable monofilament.[27]

Nephrectomy

This surgery is primarily performed in snakes; in lizards with pelvic kidneys or chelonians, microsurgical experience is recommended due to multiple renal arteries.[27] As in mammals, renal function must be carefully assessed before considering nephrectomy. Indications include renal neoplasia or refractory infectious nephritis. Following aseptic preparation and celiotomy, the kidney is exteriorized and isolated with moistened gauze. The caudal renal portal vein, cranial renal efferent vein, and renal artery are clamped or ligated; the ureter is transected. The kidney is mobilized, fascia cauterized, the coelom rinsed, and closure performed conventionally.

Renal biopsies

Renal biopsies are indicated when renal disease is suspected from biochemical or ultrasonographic findings.[27] In retrocoelomic kidneys (eg, chelonians), the coelomic membrane is incised to access the parenchyma.[27,28] Guillotine biopsy via celiotomy allows substantial tissue sampling and can facilitate nephrectomy. Less-invasive options include endoscopic microbiopsy or ultrasound-guided biopsy.[28,45]

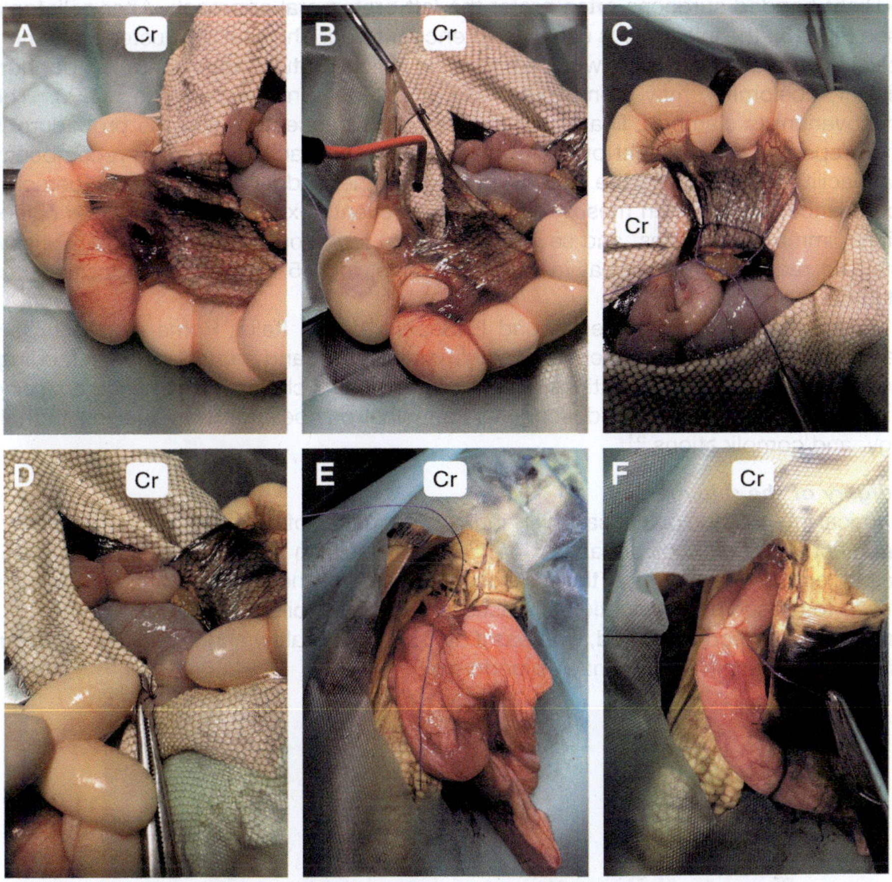

Fig. 19. (*A–F*) Salpingectomy. (*A*) Bearded dragon (*Pogona vitticeps*) with dystocia. Salpinx exteriorized. (*B*) Ligature at fimbrial end and vessels coagulated. (*C*) Alternatively, vascular ligation of the mesosalpinx can be performed. (*D*) Distal duct ligated and excised. (*E, F*) Same procedure in a Russian tortoise (*Testudo horsfieldii*). Cr, cranial. (*Courtesy of* Dr Clément Paillusseau.)

Reproductive Tract Surgery

Ovariectomy

Ovariectomy is indicated for reproductive control or treatment of follicular stasis, oophoritis, torsion, or ovarian neoplasia.[23,34,47–49]

In squamates (**Figs. 17** and **18**), following a celiotomy, ovaries are gently exteriorized with moistened swabs; adhesions are dissected, and the mesovarium clamped and ligated, avoiding the vena cava (right) and adrenal gland (left). In snakes and large lizards, the broad mesovarium requires careful dissection and multiple ligatures. Hemoclips may facilitate hemostasis in large species, while electrocautery can suffice in small species.[34,47,50] The procedure is repeated contralaterally (Video 1).

Special case: endoscope-assisted surgery in chelonians. Endoscopy improves visualization of coelomic organs and ovarian identification, though not essential.[34,48,49,51,52] Bladder aspiration can enhance access. In pond sliders, smaller size aids surgery, and patient positioning (lateral vs dorsal) has little effect.[53]

Right-handed surgeons often prefer the left prefemoral approach. After celiotomy (see **Fig. 18**), the left ovary is usually first encountered. The ovarian cluster is exteriorized via an avascular region, with care to avoid follicle rupture; adhesions from oophoritis or coelomitis may complicate this step (personal experience, C.P.). The mesovarium is clamped, ligated (or clipped), and transected, and the procedure is then repeated for the right ovary from the same approach.[34,52] Dorsal recumbency can facilitate exposure of the right ovary beneath the bladder and intestines (personal experience, C.P.). When mesovarium length prevents exteriorization (aquatic chelonians, immature females, and severe oophoritis), a second right prefemoral incision may be required. An alternative technique involving 45° tilted dorsal position has also been described.[54]

A study on 36 pond sliders found EnSeal®, Alcyon Italia, Roma electrosurgery reduced surgical time, often enabled single-site access, and promoted earlier feeding, with no increase in complications.[55] Another series of 7 chelonians stressed adapting the approach (prefemoral endoscopy vs transplastron coeliotomy) to species, pathology, and complications.[51]

Surgery of the salpinx

Surgical intervention on the salpinx is indicated in cases of dystocia, salpingitis, cesarean section, torsion, or prolapse.[34,47–50,52] The decision between salpingotomy and salpingectomy depends on the macroscopic state of the oviducts and the owner's desire to preserve reproduction. In cases of salpingitis, bilateral resection of oviducts and ovaries is recommended, whereas if oviducts are healthy and fertility preservation is desired, a salpingotomy may be performed.

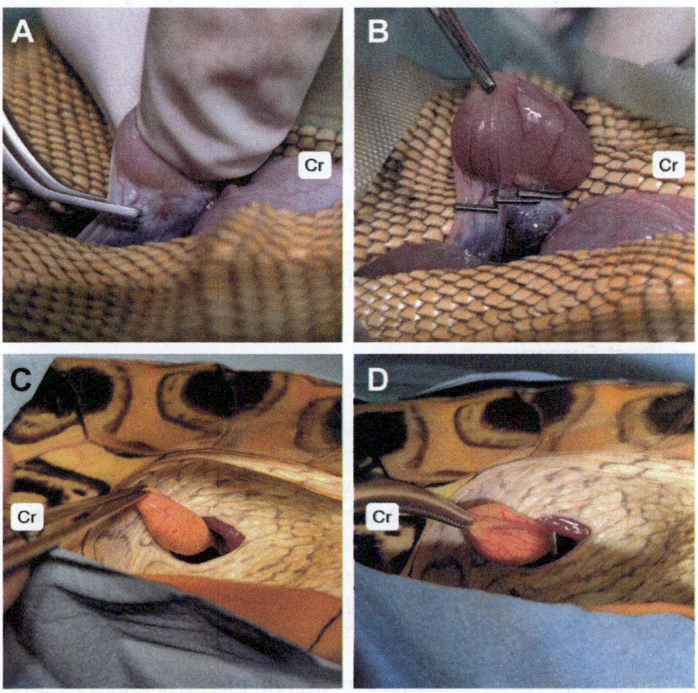

Fig. 20. (*A–D*) Castration in a green iguana (*Iguana iguana*). (*A*) Testis exteriorized. (*B*) Vascular hemoclips applied on mesorchium vessels. (*C, D*) Same procedure in a slider terrapin (*Trachemys scripta*). Cr, cranial. (*Courtesy of* Dr Clément Paillusseau.)

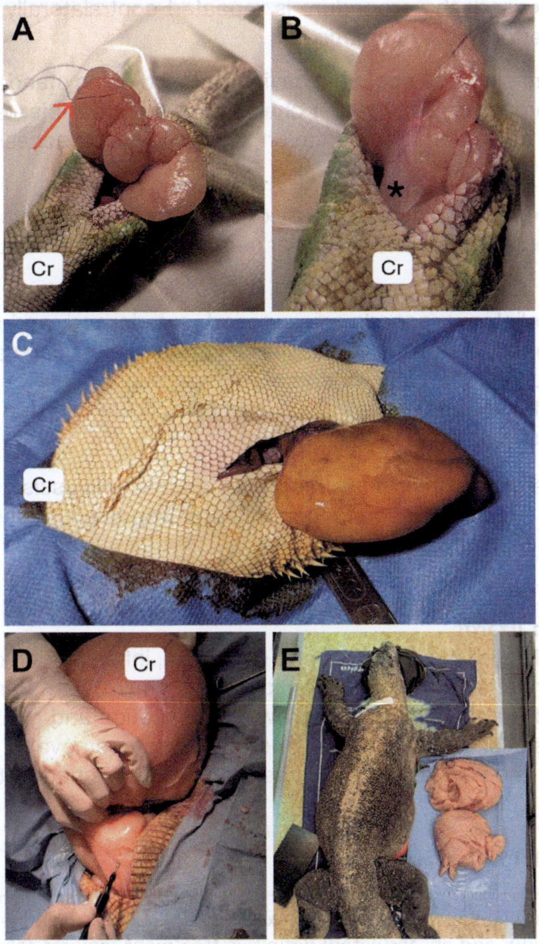

Fig. 21. (*A–E*) (*A*) Removal of the fat pads in a chameleon forest dragon (*Gonocephalus chamaeleontinus*). A stay suture (*red arrow*) is used for convenience. (*B*) In agamids, the ventral aspect of the bladder (*black asterisk*) is attached to the fat pads. (*C*) Same procedure in a bearded dragon (*Pogona vitticeps*). (*D, E*) Same procedure in a Komodo dragon (*Varanus komodoensis*). Cr, cranial. (*Courtesy of* Dr Clément Paillusseau.)

- *Salpingotomy:* In snakes, the coelomic approach is minimized according to egg location. The oviduct is manipulated gently to limit postoperative inflammation, and a longitudinal incision is made along the avascular border opposite the mesosalpinx.[34] Multiple eggs should be extracted through the fewest possible incisions, although several incisions may sometimes be necessary. Closure is performed with monofilament sutures or occasionally left open in small species.
- *Salpingectomy* (**Fig. 19**): The entire oviduct, from the infundibulum to the cervix, is exteriorized. A ligature or hemoclip is placed at the fimbrial end, or electrocoagulation is performed.[34] Mesosalpinx vessels are progressively ligated or coagulated down to the cervix. The distal oviduct is clamped, 2 ligatures (1 simple and 1 transfixing) are placed between clamp and urodeum, and the

oviduct is excised; the procedure is repeated contralaterally. Ipsilateral ovariectomy is performed systematically.

After thorough rinsing, the coelomic cavity is closed using standard techniques.

Prefemoral approach is preferred in chelonians when feasible; large or numerous eggs may require aspiration, fragmentation, or transplastron access.

Orchiectomy

Indications include reproductive or behavioral control (such as intraspecific or interspecific aggression), orchitis, and testicular neoplasia, mainly in lizards and chelonians (**Fig. 20**).[34]

In lizards. After celiotomy, gonads are exposed, exteriorized, and mesorchium vessels ligated or clipped; testes are transected and removed, taking care near the adrenal gland and caudal vena cava. In some species, such as the bearded dragon (*P. vitticeps*), pigmentation of the mesorchium can complicate this step (personal experience, C.P.). Endoscopic castration is possible.[52]

In chelonians. Prefemoral incision with optional endoscopic assistance; contralateral mesorchium may require a second contralateral approach. Transplastron access does not improve testicular exposure.[52,56]

Miscellaneous

Fat pad surgery in lizards

This surgery is indicated in case of fat pad neoplasia, inflammation or morbid obesity with compression effect in the coelomic cavity (**Fig. 21**).[57] Ventral paramedian approach with self-retaining retractor allows identification and gentle exteriorization of the fat pad. Vascular supply is ligated, permitting safe removal.[57] In some species, such as agamids, the ventral aspect of the bladder is attached to the fat pads (personal experience, C.P.).

CLINICS CARE POINTS

- Reptile abscesses require complete capsule excision; simple drainage is ineffective: abscesses are typically caseous and encapsulated; definitive treatment requires complete excision rather than simple drainage.
- Everting skin sutures are preferred because reptile skin inverts easily: reptile skin tends to invert under tension; everting suture patterns are therefore preferred to ensure proper wound apposition.
- Healing is prolonged in reptiles; sutures commonly remain for 6–8 weeks: due to ectothermy and low metabolic rate, wound healing is slow and sutures often need to remain in place for 6–8 weeks.
- Careful identification of the ventral abdominal vein is essential during lizard coeliotomy: the ventral abdominal vein runs along the midline in many lizards and must be identified and preserved to avoid significant hemorrhage.
- Basic surgical principles used in mammals can be applied: fundamental principles of mammalian surgery apply but must be adapted to reptile anatomy and physiology.

DISCLOSURE

The authors have nothing to disclose.

SUPPLEMENTARY DATA

Supplementary data to this article can be found online at https://doi.org/10.1016/j.cvex.2026.04.002.

REFERENCES

1. Johnston SA, Tobias KM. Veterinary surgery: small animal expert consult - E-BOOK: veterinary surgery: small animal expert consult - E-BOOK. Saunders; 2017. Available at: https://books.google.fr/books?id=iGkuDwAAQBAJ.
2. Divers SJ. Surgical equipment, instrumentation, and general principles. In: Divers SJ, Stahl SJ, editors. Mader's reptile and Amphibian medicine and surgery. 3rd edition. W.B. Saunders; 2019. p. 1014–23.e1.
3. Sladky KK, Mans C. Clinical anesthesia in reptiles. J Exot Pet Med 2012;21(1): 17–31.
4. Sladky KK, Mans C. Analgesia. In: Divers SJ, Stahl SJ, editors. Mader's reptile and Amphibian medicine and surgery. 3rd edition. W.B. Saunders; 2019. p. 465–74.e3.
5. Sladky KK. Treatment of pain in reptiles. Veterinary Clinics of North America: Exotic Animal Practice 2023;26(1):43–64.
6. Scheelings TF, Hellebuyck T. Integument. In: Divers SJ, Stahl SJ, editors. Mader's reptile and Amphibian medicine and surgery. 3rd edition. W.B. Saunders; 2019. p. 1042–3.e1.
7. Funk RS, Schnellbacher RW. Snake coeliotomy. In: Divers SJ, Stahl SJ, editors. Mader's reptile and Amphibian medicine and surgery. 3rd edition. Third Edition. W.B. Saunders; 2019. p. 1044–6.
8. Nevarez JG. Crocodilian coeliotomy. In: Divers SJ, Stahl SJ, editors. Mader's reptile and Amphibian medicine and surgery. 3rd edition. W.B. Saunders; 2019. p. 1062–4.e1.
9. Stahl SJ. Lizard coeliotomy. In: Divers SJ, Stahl SJ, editors. Mader's reptile and Amphibian medicine and surgery. 3rd edition. Elsevier; 2019. p. 1047–53.
10. Wüst E, Divers SJ. Chelonian prefemoral coeliotomy. In: Divers SJ, Stahl SJ, editors. Mader's reptile and Amphibian medicine and surgery. 3rd edition. W.B. Saunders; 2019. p. 1054–6.e1.
11. Di Girolamo N, Mans C. Reptile soft tissue surgery. Veterinary Clinics of North America: Exotic Animal Practice 2016;19(1):97–131.
12. McFadden MS, Bennett RA, Kinsel MJ, et al. Evaluation of the histologic reactions to commonly used suture materials in the skin and musculature of ball pythons (Python regius). Am J Vet Res 2011;72(10):1397–406.
13. Pérez-Delgado S, Mozos E, Guerra R, et al. Tissue tolerance to cyanoacrylate adhesives for closure of surgical wounds in *Trachemys scripta* skin. Veterinary Record 2021;188(5):e59.
14. Negrini J, Ginel PJ, Novales M, et al. Clinical and histological findings of cutaneous wound healing in the red-eared slider turtle (*Trachemys scripta elegans*) housed in unheated outdoor enclosures. Vet Dermatol 2016;27(5):413.e106.
15. Kischinovsky M, Divers SJ. Ear. In: Divers SJ, Stahl SJ, editors. Mader's reptile and Amphibian medicine and surgery. 3rd edition. W.B. Saunders; 2019. p. 1028–30.e1.
16. Fleming GJ. New techniques in Chelonian shell repair. In: Current therapy in reptile medicine and surgery. Elsevier Inc.; 2013. p. 205–12. https://doi.org/10.1016/B978-1-4557-0893-2.00016-8.

17. Schmidt V. Abscesses/fibriscesses. In: Divers SJ, Stahl SJ, editors. Mader's reptile and Amphibian medicine and surgery. 3rd edition. W.B. Saunders; 2019. p. 1288–9.e1.
18. Funk RS. Venomoid surgery. In: Divers SJ, Stahl SJ, editors. Mader's reptile and Amphibian medicine and surgery. 3rd edition. W.B. Saunders; 2019. p. 1040–1.e1.
19. Funk RS, Bogan JE. Snake taxonomy, anatomy, and physiology. In: Divers SJ, Stahl SJ, editors. Mader's reptile and Amphibian medicine and surgery. 3rd edition. W.B. Saunders; 2019. p. 50–62.e2.
20. Coimbra FCP, Dobson J, Zdenek CN, et al. Does size matter? Venom proteomic and functional comparison between night adder species (Viperidae: Causus) with short and long venom glands. Comparative Biochemistry and Physiology Part C: Toxicology & Pharmacology 2018;211:7–14.
21. Fry BG, Wroe S, Teeuwisse W, et al. A central role for venom in predation by *Varanus komodoensis* (Komodo Dragon) and the extinct giant Varanus (Megalania) priscus. Proceedings of the National Academy of Sciences 2009;106(22): 8969–74.
22. Fry BG, Winter K, Norman JA, et al. Functional and structural diversification of the anguimorpha lizard venom system. Molecular & Cellular Proteomics 2010;9(11): 2369–90.
23. Stahl S, DeNardo D. Theriogenology. In: Divers SJ, Stahl SJ, editors. Mader's reptile and Amphibian medicine and surgery. 3rd edition. Elsevier; 2019. p. 849–93.
24. Sánchez-Martínez P, Ramirez Pinilla MP, Miranda-Esquivel D. Comparative histology of the vaginal–cloacal region in Squamata and its phylogenetic implications. Acta Zoologica 2007;88:289–307.
25. Stahl S. Clocal scent gland adenitis. In: Divers S, Stahl S, editors. Reptile and Amphibian medicine and surgery. 3rd edition. Elsevier; 2019. p. 1299–300.
26. Couture ÉL, Lung NP, Lair S, et al. Ophidian cloacal scent gland impaction and surgical excision: a case series in six different snake species. J Herpetol Med Surg 2019;28(3–4):81–8.
27. Divers SJ. Urinary tract. In: Divers SJ, Stahl SJ, editors. Mader's reptile and Amphibian medicine and surgery. 3rd edition. W.B. Saunders; 2019. p. 1071–6.e1.
28. Divers SJ, Innis CJ. Urology. In: Divers SJ, Stahl SJ, editors. Mader's reptile and Amphibian medicine and surgery. 3rd edition. W.B. Saunders; 2019. p. 624–48.e2.
29. Kehoe SP, Sanchez-Migallon Guzman D, Avian D, et al. Partial glossectomy in a blue-tongued skink (Tiliqua scincoides) with lingual squamous cell carcinoma. Vol 26. 2016. Available at: https://jhms.kglmeridian.com.
30. Kischinovsky M, Divers SJ. Oral cavity, mandible, maxilla, and beak. In: Divers SJ, Stahl SJ, editors. Mader's reptile and Amphibian medicine and surgery. 3rd edition. W.B. Saunders; 2019. p. 1033–9.e1.
31. Abramjan A, Bauerová A, Somerová B, et al. Why is the tongue of blue-tongued skinks blue? Reflectance of lingual surface and its consequences for visual perception by conspecifics and predators. The Science of Nature 2015;102(7):42.
32. De Meester G, Van Linden L, Torfs J, et al. Learning with lacertids: studying the link between ecology and cognition within a comparative framework. Evolution (N Y) 2022;76(11):2531–52.
33. Cutler D, Divers SJ. Esophagostomy tube placement. In: Divers SJ, Stahl SJ, editors. Mader's reptile and Amphibian medicine and surgery. 3rd edition. W.B. Saunders; 2019. p. 429–31.e1.
34. Stahl SJ. Reproductive tract. In: Divers SJ, Stahl SJ, editors. Mader's reptile and Amphibian medicine and surgery. 3rd edition. W.B. Saunders; 2019. p. 1077–89.e1.

35. McArthur S, Machin RA. Cloacal prolapse. In: Divers SJ, Stahl SJ, editors. Mader's reptile and Amphibian medicine and surgery. 3rd edition. W.B. Saunders; 2019. p. 1090–5.e1.
36. Ortega J, Wyneken J, Garner MM. Aneurysm associated with vascular wall degeneration in bearded dragons (*Pogona vitticeps*). Vet Pathol 2024;61(3): 468–75.
37. Kaiser NC, Greenwood SJ, Gouchie GM, et al. Encephalitozoon pogonae–associated systemic vasculitis in a central bearded dragon (Pogona vitticeps). J Herpetol Med Surg 2021;31(3):168–72.
38. Woodhall H. Successful surgical repair of a spontaneous arterial aneurysm in an inland bearded dragon (Pogona vitticeps). J Herpetol Med Surg 2024;34(2):96–7.
39. Di Girolamo N, Santistevan L, Percival A, et al. Ultrasound-guided transcutaneous glue embolization resolved bilateral temporo-orbital aneurysms in a bearded dragon (Pogona vitticeps) after anatomical characterization via computed tomographic angiography. J Am Vet Med Assoc 2025;263(6). https://doi.org/10.2460/javma.25.02.0065.
40. De Voe R. Gastrointestinal tract. In: Divers SJ, Stahl SJ, editors. Mader's reptile and Amphibian medicine and surgery. 3rd edition. W.B. Saunders; 2019. p. 1068–70.e1.
41. Ballestín A, Akelina Y. Basic and advanced microvascular anastomotic techniques. In: Nikkhah D, Rawlins J, Pafitanis G, editors. Core techniques in flap reconstructive microsurgery: a stepwise guide. Springer International Publishing; 2023. p. 11–8. https://doi.org/10.1007/978-3-031-07678-7_2.
42. Siddle MR, Hanak E, Parker DL, et al. Cholecystectomy for the treatment of enterococcal cholecystitis and cholelithiasis in an inland bearded dragon (*Pogona vitticeps*): a case report. J Exot Pet Med 2020;35:64–8.
43. Pouillevet H, Aymen J, Larouche CB, et al. Diagnosis and surgical management of cholecystolithiasis in two adult inland bearded dragons (Pogona vitticeps). J Herpetol Med Surg 2021;31(1):18–24.
44. Kinney ME, Chinnadurai SK, Wack RF. Cholecystectomy for the treatment of mycobacterial cholecystitis in a pacific gopher snake (Pituophis catenifer). Vol 23. 2013. Available at: https://jhms.kglmeridian.com.
45. Divers SJ. Diagnostic endoscopy. In: Divers SJ, Stahl SJ, editors. Mader's reptile and Amphibian medicine and surgery. 3rd edition. W.B. Saunders; 2019. p. 604–14.e1.
46. Divers SJ. Hepatology. In: Divers SJ, Stahl SJ, editors. Mader's reptile and Amphibian medicine and surgery. 3rd edition. W.B. Saunders; 2019. p. 649–68.e2.
47. Knotek Z, Cermakova E, Oliveri M. Reproductive medicine in lizards. Veterinary Clinics of North America - Exotic Animal Practice 2017;20(2):411–38.
48. Lubian E, Palotti G, Di Ianni F, et al. Disorders of the female reproductive tract in Chelonians: a review. *Animals*. Multidisciplinary Digital Publishing Institute (MDPI) 2025;15(9). https://doi.org/10.3390/ani15091275.
49. Perry SM, Mitchell MA. Reproductive medicine in freshwater turtles and land tortoises. Veterinary Clinics: Exotic Animal Practice 2017;20(2):371–89.
50. Di Girolamo N, Selleri P. Reproductive disorders in snakes. Veterinary Clinics: Exotic Animal Practice 2017;20(2):391–409.
51. Hellebuyck T, Vilanova FS. The use of prefemoral endoscope-assisted surgery and transplastron coeliotomy in Chelonian reproductive disorders. Animals 2022;12(23). https://doi.org/10.3390/ani12233439.
52. Divers SJ. Endoscope-assisted and endoscopic surgery. In: Divers SJ, Stahl SJ, editors. Mader's reptile and Amphibian medicine and surgery. 3rd edition. W.B. Saunders; 2019. p. 615–23.e1.

53. Bardi E, Antolini G, Lubian E, et al. Comparison of lateral and dorsal recumbency during endoscope-assisted oophorectomy in mature pond sliders (*Trachemys scripta*). Animals 2020;10(9):1–8.
54. Di Girolamo N, Studer K, Maranville R, et al. Feasibility, gross postmortem results and participant perception of oblique prefemoral ovariectomy in red eared sliders (*Trachemys scripta elegans*) during a teaching workshop. J Herpetol Med Surg 2022;32(2):130–5.
55. Vetere A, Ablondi M, Gavezzoli M, et al. Comparison of conventional vs. electrosurgical ovariosalpingectomy with the EnSeal® tissue sealer in pond sliders (*Trachemys scripta*): impacts on procedure time, surgical access, and recovery time according to follicular stage. Veterinary Quarterly 2025;45(1):1–9.
56. Chai N. Castration of snakes and lizards by endosurgery 2010;41.
57. Crews J, Gendron K, Sladakovic I, et al. Liposarcoma of the fat body in a bearded dragon (*Pogona vitticeps*). J Herpetol Med Surg 2021;30(4):232–6.

Surgical Conditions of Psittacine and Passerine Birds

Ciro Cococcetta, DMV, Dip ECZM (Avian)[a],
Graham Zoller, DMV, IPSAV (Zoological Medicine), Dip ECZM (Avian)[b,*]

KEYWORDS

- Psittaciformes • Passeriformes • Surgery • Egg binding • Prolapse
- Air sac cannulation • Tracheal surgery • Uropygial gland

KEY POINTS

- Feather cysts can be curetted in patients with high perioperative risk, although total excision including the dermal papilla is the preferred treatment for definitive resolution.
- Cloacal prolapse is common in psittaciformes, secondary to a variety of causes, and may require tissue replacement, cloacopexy and/or cloacoplasty depending on etiology.
- The uropygial gland is mainly affected by adenocarcinoma, the most common epithelial neoplasm. Complete excision including the pygostyle and caudal vertebrae may occasionally be required.
- Tracheotomy and tracheal resection with anastomosis are principal tracheal surgeries. Tracheotomy is indicated for foreign bodies or granulomas, while stenosis or neoplasia may require resection.

INTRODUCTION

Although psittacine and passerine birds are phylogenetically distinct, they are often grouped as *cagebirds* because they share a common lifestyle characterized by close human contact, limited climatic variation, reduced physical activity, exposure to household hazards, and contact with birds from diverse geographic origins. Nutrition and reproduction depend entirely on human management, increasing the risk of husbandry-related disorders. Some of these disorders are surgical conditions, defined here as a disorder for which a surgical procedure can significantly improve the clinical outcome. While surgery may resolve the presenting problem, the underlying cause must be addressed to prevent recurrence.

[a] Centre Hospitalier Vétérinaire (CHV) Saint-Martin, 321 Impasse des Champs, 74350 Allonzier-la-Caille, France; [b] Department of Exotic Pet, OnlyVet Veterinary Hospital Center, 7 rue Jean Zay, 69800 Saint-Priest, France
* Corresponding author.
E-mail address: graham.zoller@gmail.com

Vet Clin Exot Anim 29 (2026) 517–544
https://doi.org/10.1016/j.cvex.2026.04.003 vetexotic.theclinics.com
1094-9194/26/

Abbreviations	
ASC	air sac cannula
FNA	fine-needle aspirate
SCC	squamous cell carcinoma

Both groups share a small body size, which increases perioperative risk due to difficulties of intravenous catheterization, high metabolic rate, sensitivity to minimal blood loss, and the need for refined microsurgical techniques. Adequate preoperative stabilization, appropriate procedure selection, and meticulous tissue handling using microsurgical instruments are therefore critical. This article focuses integrating surgery into a comprehensive clinical framework, addressing indications, stabilization, and adjunct medical and husbandry management.

Surgical Conditions of the Feathers

Fracture of blood feather

Epidemiology and pathophysiology. Developing feathers (*blood feathers*) contain a vascular pulp enclosed within a keratin sheath. Most feathers are supplied by cutaneous arterial branches, whereas primary flight feathers receive blood directly from the radial and ulnar arteries.[1] Damage to the sheath exposes the pulp and may result in rapid blood loss, particularly in birds with coagulopathies or when a primary feather is affected. In a retrospective study of 1454 psittacines, blood feather injuries were reported in 233 birds with 17.6% showing active hemorrhage.[2]

Diagnosis and medical stabilization. Birds typically present with visible hemorrhage. Rapid identification of the affected feather and immediate hemostasis are priorities. Confinement in a quiet, darkened environment may reduce blood pressure. Trimming the distal fragment can decrease movement and discomfort. Coagulation-promoting powders (eg, flour, cornstarch) may be applied locally, or ligation of the proximal fragment can be performed. Caustic agents (eg, silver nitrate) or electrocautery are discouraged due to the risk of follicular damage, impaired feather regrowth, and follicular cysts formation.

Surgical treatment. Definitive treatment generally requires removal of the damaged feather under anesthesia (**Box 1**, **Fig. 1**). Some authors report that extraction can cause follicular trauma and abnormal regrowth, and have suggested to control bleeding with manual pressure.[3]

Prognosis and prevention. Prognosis is favorable. Feather removal controlled bleeding in 23 of 41 cases in 1 study.[2] Experimental data in chickens showed that

Box 1
Technique for the extraction of a fractured blood feather

- Anesthetize the bird if possible.
- Part surrounding feathers for visualization and clear any residual clots to improve grip.
- Use hemostats to firmly grasp the calamus close to the skin.
- Apply slow, constant traction while stabilizing the base of the feather with digital counterpressure.
- Control dermal bleeding with firm pressure or packing the follicle with hemostatic gauze or gel.

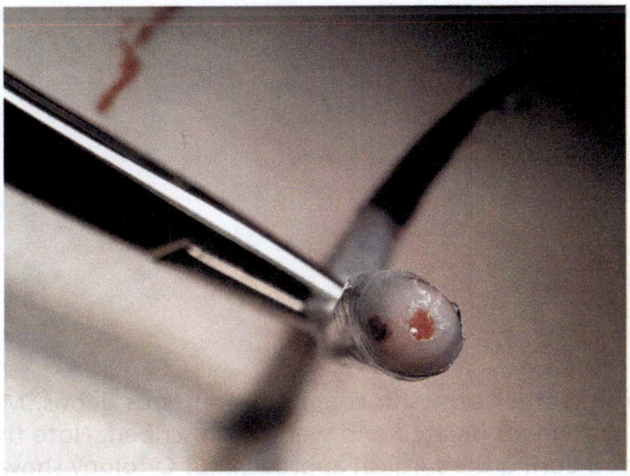

Fig. 1. Extraction of a fractured primary flight feather in a macaw. The calamus was grasped with a needle holder and gently removed with steady traction. The calamus tip and the epidermal collar remain intact. The entry of axial artery is visible. (Image Courtesy of Dr Graham Zoller.)

manual pressure achieved hemostasis within a similar timeframe (3 minutes) but was better tolerated than extraction without anesthesia.[3] Recurrent fracture blood feathers warrants reassessment of diet, environment, and wing-trim design. Imping may be indicated in selected cases.

Feather follicle cyst

Epidemiology and pathophysiology. Feather cysts are common in Fringillidae, particularly canaries, and less frequent in Estrildidae and Sturnidae. In psittacines, they occur commonly in budgerigars,[4,5] but have been reported in cockatoos[6,7] and amazon parrots. In canaries, a hereditary predisposition is suspected, especially in soft-feather breeds, resulting from failure of the feather to emerge through the skin. Benign neoplasms such as feather folliculomas have also been described.[8,9] In other species, follicular dysfunction may be acquired due to infection, malnutrition, or trauma, including feather-destructive behavior.[10,11]

Cysts consist of dysplastic follicles filled with keratinous debris and feather remnants, lined by an epithelial wall.[8] Early lesions contain blood or gelatinous material that becomes compact keratinous material over time. Rupture can lead to secondary infection or hemorrhage.[10]

Diagnosis and medical stabilization. Clinically, cysts present as oval or elongated subcutaneous masses containing yellow-white, caseous, or firm material.[9] (**Fig. 2**A) They may be solitary or multiple and are commonly located on the wings, back, shoulders or chest, potentially impairing flight or causing discomfort. Diagnosis is usually clinical. Fine-needle aspiration may reveal keratinaceous debris, cholesterol crystals, squamous epithelial cells, mixed-cell inflammation or hemorrhage (**Fig. 2**B). Bacterial culture is indicated if infection is suspected. Histopathology may identify underlying neoplasia or chronic follicular dysplasia.[2]

Surgical treatment. Surgery is recommended when cysts cause pain, recurrent infection or functional impairment.[10] Early lesions may be vascular and prone to significant hemorrhage.[12] Delaying surgery until drying of keratin and reduction of inflammation is advisable. Surgical technique depends on lesion number and location (**Box 2**, **Fig. 2**C).

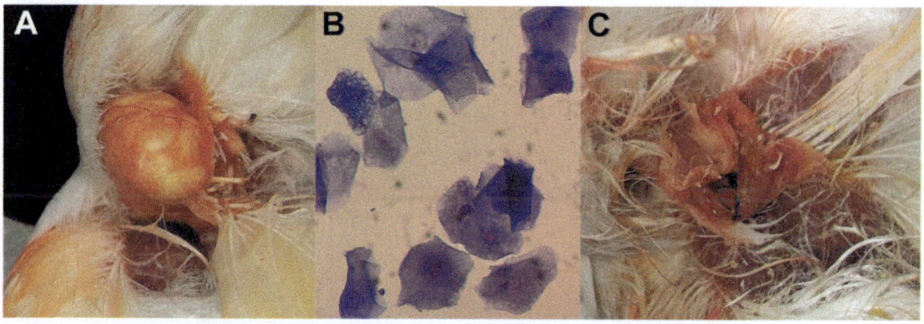

Fig. 2. (*A–C*) (*A*) Large feather cyst with compact keratinous debris. Marsupialization was chosen because the lesion was isolated and well-circumscribed. Note the superficial vessel, which must be avoided during the surgical approach. (*B*) Cytology shows squamous epithelial cells, and keratinous debris without inflammation or infection. (*C*) Postoperative appearance showing a permanent epithelialized stoma for continuous drainage and prevention of recurrence. (Image Courtesy of Dr Graham Zoller.)

Prognosis and prevention. Recurrence is common if the underlying cause persists. In canaries with suspected heritable predisposition, recurrence is expected and affected birds should not be bred.[10] Evaluation of diet, husbandry, and behavioral contributors is essential. Haloperidol has been used to reduce recurrence in birds with feather-destructive behavior.

Surgical Conditions of the Cloaca

Cloacal disease accounted for 3.8% of psittacine cases presented to an exotic referral service.[13] Cloacal prolapse (60.7%), oviductal prolapse (25.6%), cloacal masses

Box 2
Techniques for the surgical management of feather cysts

- *Lancing/curettage:* Indicated for small individual cysts and in cases where decreased invasiveness and short surgical intervention is required. Incise the cyst in an avascular area and remove the keratinous material with curettage. Manage by second intention healing with topical antiseptic (eg, 5% tincture iodine). Associated with a high recurrence rate. Fulguration of the dermal papilla with a radiosurgical unit is effective to prevent new feather growth. However, potential damages to adjacent follicles can lead to the development of feather cysts.[12]
- *Total blade excision:* Removal of the feather follicle is the treatment of choice. Perform a fusiform excision of a piece of skin including the cystic feather follicle taking care to remove the dermal papilla. Perform a radical excision of the whole feather-tract if multiple cysts are present, taking care that the main vascular supply to the tract is located centrally at the cranial third of the pteryla.[84] Suture the surgical wound or manage by second intention healing depending on the size of the wound.
- *Marsupialization:* Indicated when blade excision is not feasible, for example, for large cysts or those attached to bone (wing, tail). Incise the lining of the cyst at the center, parallel to the direction of feather growth. Remove the keratinous material and rinse the cavity. Excise redundant tissue as necessary. Appose the skin to the cyst lining using a simple continuous pattern of monofilament suture.[85]

Use a tourniquet if possible to aid in hemostasis. In case of hemorrhage, hemostatic gauze can aid for hemorrhage control. Radiosurgery is an effective mean to reduce hemorrhage but should be reserved for emergencies as it can damage adjacent follicles.

(20.9%), gastrointestinal prolapse (4.7%), and cloacoliths (2.3%) were most commonly identified. Cloacitis was always secondary. Female birds and cockatoos, particularly *Cacatua alba*, may be predisposed. Understanding cloacal anatomy and the location of major orifices is essential when planning surgical interventions (**Box 3**).

Cloacal masses

Epidemiology and pathophysiology. Cloacal masses reported in psittacines, and less commonly in passerines, include granulomas and neoplasms such as adenocarcinoma, squamous cell carcinoma (SCC), papilloma, fibrosarcoma and lymphoma. Lesions generally arise from the proctodeum. Cloacal papillomas are the most frequent neoplastic condition, particularly in south american psittacines. They are strongly associated with herpesvirus infection, although papillomavirus-associated,[14] or idiopathic cases have been reported.[15] Birds with herpesvirus-associated papillomas may develop multifocal gastrointestinal lesions and are predisposed to pancreatic, biliary or intestinal carcinoma.

Diagnosis and stabilization. Clinical signs include intermittent or persistent vent bleeding (**Fig. 3**A), soiling of vent feathers, straining, prolapse, lethargy, or weight loss. Obstruction is uncommon but possible. Papillomas often follow a cyclic pattern of regression and recurrence.

Direct visualization of the proctodeum can be performed by gentle eversion of the mucosa with moistened cotton-tipped applicators. An otoscope may assist visualization although the field is limited. Rigid cloacoscopy with fluid infusion provides optimal visualization of mucosal surfaces and openings. Papillomas appear cobblestoned, whereas carcinomas are infiltrative and necrotic. Application of 5% acetic acid whiten papillomas. Endoscopic biopsy may be performed, avoiding full-thickness samples.

Diagnostic workup includes complete blood count (CBC), biochemistry (hepatic or pancreatic involvement with papillomatosis), herpesvirus testing, and imaging (contrast radiography or computed tomography [CT]) to assess local infiltration or metastasis.[16]

Box 3
Surgical anatomy and landmarks of the cloaca

The cloaca is a bell-shaped cavity where the distal ends of the digestive, urinary and reproductive tracts connect. It is internally divided by folds into 3 compartments: coprodeum (cranial), urodeum, proctodeum (caudal). The cloacal walls are thin and can easily be traumatized during mass resection and mucosal stripping. The mucosa is richly vascularized and significant bleeding can occur.

- *Coprodeum:* Communicates with the colon cranially and separated from the urodeum by the coprourodeal fold.
- *Urodeum:* It is the smallest compartment where are located the ureteral openings (dorsal, paired at 10 and 2 o'clock), the oviductal opening (left dorsal) in females and ductus deferens openings (dorsolateral, paired) in males, which must be identified and preserved. Ventral approach to the cloaca is recommended. It is separated from the proctodeum by the uroproctodeal fold.
- *Proctodeum:* It houses the phallus (in vasa parrots, *C vasa*) and the opening of the bursa of Fabricius in juveniles. Communicates with the vent caudally, which is the elliptical external opening with a striated sphincter. The vent should be preserved as much as possible during surgical intervention to avoid vent stricture. It is the most common location for papillomas and other cloacal masses.

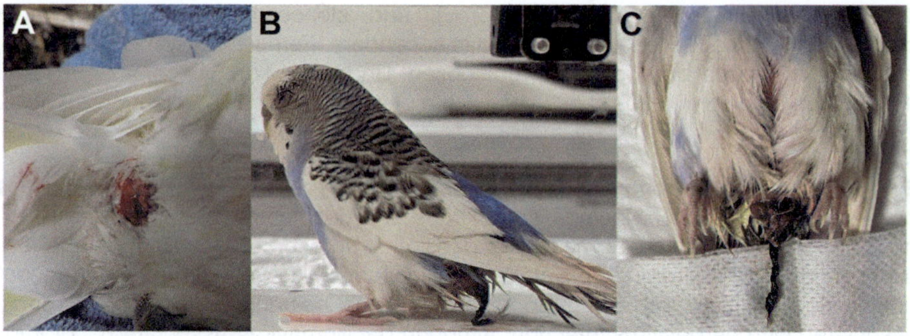

Fig. 3. (*A–C*) (*A*) Cloacal bleeding from a mass in a white cockatoo. (*B*) Prolapsed oviduct in a budgerigar; the bird shows discomfort and surrounding feathers are soiled. (*C*) Close-up of prolapsed tissue showing black discoloration and dehydration, consistent with devitalized tissue. (Image Courtesy of Dr Graham Zoller.)

Surgical treatment. Lesions may be accessed endoscopically or via cloacotomy (**Box 4**). Medical treatments described for papillomas include silver nitrate application, capsicum supplementation,[17] intralesional chemotherapy, topical immunomodulators (eg, imiquimod),[18] and autogenous vaccination.[19] Surgical options include sharp excision,[20] cryosurgery, radiosurgery, laser ablation,[21] and mucosal stripping.[20] (**Box 5**) Hemorrhage is a significant concern due to the rich vascular supply of the cloacal mucosa.

Postoperative care includes topical antimicrobials. Malignant or infiltrative lesions may require adjunct chemotherapy or radiation therapy. Postoperative complications include vent stricture, dehiscence, intestinal entrapment, scarring, dropping retention,

Box 4
Technique for cloacotomy

- Cloacotomy is indicated to obtain a thorough access to the internal structure of the cloaca when lesions cannot be diagnosed or managed endoscopically or medically. It may be necessary for removal of eggs or cloaco/ureteroliths,[22,30] for the resection of deep or extensive inflammatory or neoplastic cloacal lesions,[20,21] and for open reduction of cloacal prolapse.
- Place the bird in dorsal recumbency and insert a moistened cotton bud into the cloaca to outline the lumen.[86] Routine skin preparation (feather plucking and antisepsis) is then performed.
- Perform a ventral midline incision through the skin, vent sphincter muscle, and cloacal mucosa from the vent to the cranial end of the cotton bud with scissors or with the monopolar electrosurgical wire tip.
- Identify proctodeum, urodeum and coprodeum. Locate ureteral openings and take care to preserve them during the intervention (mass excision, cloacopexy, etc.).[22]
- Close the cloacal mucosa with 4-0 monofilament absorbable suture on a taper needle in a simple continuous pattern beginning at the cranial end of the incision.
- Appose the vent sphincter with a single horizontal mattress suture.
- Close the skin over the cloaca and sphincter with a simple continuous pattern using similar material. Closure requires meticulous apposition of mucosa, vent sphincter and skin to minimize postoperative stricture.

Box 5
Technique for mucosal stripping

- Mucosal stripping is indicated for removal of extensive or recurrent cloacal papilloma limited to the mucosa because this technique removes only the diseased mucosa, preserving deeper structures.
- A cloacotomy is performed to approach the cloacal inner structure.
- Dissect carefully the cloacal mucosa from the uroproctodeal fold to the mucocutaneous junction, taking care to preserve the ureteral and reproductive tract openings during dissection.
- Once the mucosa has been removed, appose the caudal edge of the uroproctodeal fold to the skin using a simple continuous pattern using a monofilament rapidly absorbable material.[22]

and inadvertent trauma to cloacal openings. Gentle tissue handling and use of magnification are essential.[22]

Prognosis and prevention. Evidence comparing therapeutic success is limited. Recurrence is common, particularly with herpesvirus-associated papillomas. Weekly application of 50% silver nitrate solution allowed regression of tumors after 2 to 5 weeks of treatment. Local recurrence was observed in 1 of 6 cases.[23] Aggressive surgical treatment remains controversial due to viral etiology and frequent multifocal disease. Prognosis is fair to poor depending on lesion type, extent and response to therapy.

Cloacal obstruction

Epidemiology and pathophysiology. Cloacal obstruction occurs when eggs or cloacoliths block fecal or urinary flow.[24,25] It can be associated with compression of pelvic structures causing paresis, circulatory and metabolic disturbance, and shock.[26] Cloacoliths are firm urate concretions occurring in birds with impaired voiding.[13] They are uncommon and primarily reported in amazon and African gray parrots.[13,25] Egg binding and dystocia are common in small psittacines and passerines.[19] Predisposing factors include environmental stressors, first egg laying, and conditions responsible of muscle dysfunction, compression of the reproductive tract, and abnormal egg formation.[19,24]

Diagnosis and stabilization. Cloacal obstruction is an emergency, particularly in birds under 100 g.[19] Common signs include celomic distension, straining, respiratory compromise, paresis, abnormal droppings, weakness, and cyanotic pelvic limbs.[19] Diagnosis relies on identification of a celomic mass via celomic or digital cloacal palpation. Radiographs can confirm the presence of mineralized intraluminal material, ultrasound may identify soft-shelled eggs,[19] and cloacoscopy can reveal underlying mural lesions. CBC and biochemistry may assist in identifying underlying causes and metabolic consequences.

Stabilization includes fluids, nutritional support, analgesia (eg, butorphanol), and warmth (80°F–90°F). In egg binding, calcium supplementation, oxygen, high humidity (>50%), calm and dark environment, and vent lubrication are recommended. Broad-spectrum antibiotics are indicated if cloacal compromise is suspected.

Surgical treatment. Cloacoliths are removed under anesthesia via the vent when possible or via cloacotomy if required (**Box 6**).

Box 6
Technique for transvent cloacolithiasis removal

- Lubricate the cloaca generously to reduce mucosal trauma and laceration.
- Gently dilate vent and expose the cloacolithiasis.
- Fragment the cloacoliths with mosquito forceps.
- Extract pieces sequentially irrigating as needed. Avoid forceful traction to prevent mucosal laceration.

Management of egg binding depends on timeline, stability and cause. Stable birds with normal egg and no sign of obstruction, adherence or laceration may respond to medical induction of egg-laying (**Box 7**). If medical therapy fails or decompensation occurs, manual extraction is indicated if the egg is well mineralized and percloacal ovocentesis is indicated if the egg is poorly mineralized and visible. Transabdominal

Box 7
Medical and surgical techniques to manage egg-related cloacal obstruction

1. *Medical induction of egg laying*: Provide parenteral calcium supplementation (eg, 50–100 mg/kg intramuscular [IM]). Apply PGE2 (0.02–0.2 mg/kg) topically on the uterovaginal sphincter to relax uterovaginal sphincter and oviductal contraction. [a] Parenteral oxytocin (1–5 UI/kg IM) and prostaglandin E2 (PGF2)α (0.02 mg/kg IM) can be used only if sphincter is opened and there is no mechanical obstruction.[55,60] However, oxytocin often appear deceiving (potentially because birds physiologically have mesotocin) and prostaglandin PGF2α can cause systemic reactions.[87] The egg is usually expelled within 15 minutes when hormonal therapy is effective. If not, administration can be repeated for 24 to 48 hours as long as the bird is not decompensating.
2. *Manual delivery*: Lubricate generously the cloaca with hydric gel and gently dilate the cloacal aperture using lubricated cotton tip applicators with the bird under light anesthesia. An atraumatic eye speculum can be used to maintain the lips of the vent opened. Perform cervical massage to open the uterovaginal sphincter. If necessary, insert a blunt probe gently in a twirling motion to dilate the cervix.[88] Apply gentle digital pressure to the cranial portion of the egg in a caudal direction, taking care not to push dorsally against the kidneys. Potential complications may include egg rupture, displacement of the egg or fragments into an ectopic position, and uterine trauma.[89,90]
3. *Percloacal ovocentesis*: Perform per-cloacal ovocentesis with the bird anesthetized and intubated. Manipulate the egg so that it is visible through the cloaca. Introduce a 16–22G needle through the shell and aspirate the content with a 10 to 20 mL syringe. Soft-shelled eggs will usually collapse with negative pressure while hard-shelled eggs may require manual compression. Remove the shell in one piece or shell fragments piece by piece with small forceps taking care to avoid laceration of the oviduct and cloaca. If eggshell cannot be removed, they can be left in place and should be naturally expelled within 2 to 3 days. Rinse the cloaca, vagina, and oviduct with saline and disinfectant to reduce the incidence of secondary infections. Complications include failure to remove the egg shell, cloacal edema, egg fragmentation, hemorrhage, and laceration with secondary celomitis.[24]
4. *Transabdominal ovocentesis*: Position the egg against the abdominal wall so that other abdominal organs are pushed away. Insert a needle on the ventral abdomen into the egg through the celomic wall and aspirate the content. Hemorrhage, iatrogenic lesion to shell gland or other celomic organs, secondary infections and celomitis can occur.

[a]Special attention should be provided to flushing any excess PGE_2 gel from the cloaca and avoiding contact with droppings, as exposure to PGE_2 gel may cause menstrual irregularities and induce spontaneous abortion in women.

ovocentesis should be avoided as it carries higher risk. If these procedures fail (egg remnants >36 hours), lead to complications (oviduct rupture), or are contraindicated (ectopic eggs, necrosis, torsion), salpingotomy, cloacotomy or salpingohysterectomy are indicated. Bacterial culture and sensitivity and histopathology should be performed on the oviductal tissue.

Prognosis and prevention. Prognosis for cloacolithiasis is fair to excellent if underlying causes are corrected.

In egg-binding, overall success rates is 72.7% with best outcomes associated with higher body weight, preserved mentation, combined medical/mechanical assistance and absence of sedation.[27] After resolution of egg binding, hormonal therapy (leuprolide or deslorelin acetate) and environmental measures (reduce photoperiod, remove real or perceived mate and nest boxes, optimize diet with a special attention to calcium/vitamin D3) should be considered to prevent further laying and allow time for tissues to heal and to address underlying causes. Salpingohysterectomy may be considered for long term control.[28]

Cloacal prolapse

Epidemiology and pathophysiology. Cloacal prolapse is the protrusion of cloacal, oviductal, or colonic tissue through the vent. Causes include sphincter atony,[29] or increased intracelomic pressure from space-occupying lesions or straining secondary to cloacal, urinary,[30] reproductive, gastrointestinal, or behavioral disorders (eg, masturbation or separation anxiety).[31]

Diagnosis and stabilization. Prolapse may be acute or chronic, and associated with hematochezia, tenesmus, respiratory distress, or shock (**Fig. 3**B). Chronic cases often begin as intermittent *winking* of tissue at the vent. Physical examination should assess tissue origin (**Box 8**), viability, and cloacal tone (**Fig. 3**C). Celomic distension may be present depending on the underlying cause.

Evaluation should include saline infusion cloacoscopy (with biopsy if indicated), imaging (radiography, ultrasound, and CT) with contrast, and bloodwork as previously described. Gastrointestinal causes may require fecal wet-mount, Gram stain, and bacteriologic testing of fresh urofeces or cloacal swab. Fluoroscopy can aid assessment of rectal or coprodeal motility and morphology. Idiopathic cases may show no anomalies.

Cloacal prolapse exposes mucosa to trauma and bacterial contamination. Stabilization includes fluids, parenteral antibiotics, warmth, and oxygen as needed. Analgesia is essential and may rely on butorphanol and meloxicam, provided the bird is normohydrated and free of ureteral obstruction. Local anesthesia (eg, lidocaine spray and xylocaine gel), and topical anti-inflammatories (eg, flurbiprofen and dimethylsulfoxide [DMSO]) may reduce discomfort and straining. Prolapsed tissue should be protected

Box 8
Identification of prolapsed tissues

Identification of the origin of the prolapsed tissue is important and relies on a careful assessment of the size and appearance of the structures.[91] Magnification, good lighting and lubricated cotton tip applicator may be required for proper evaluation.

- The uterus can be identified by its longitudinal striations and folds, corrugated aspects, and its origin from the left side of the vent. Presence of egg material should be noted and will provide confirmation.
- Rectal prolapse are midline, smooth and devoid of linear folds or striation. Presence of fecal matter in the lumen will help to identify the gastrointestinal origin of the prolapse.[90]

with water-based lubricants, and topical hypertonic solution may reduce edema. Elizabethan collars may prevent self-trauma.

Therapeutic approach. Emergency reduction is performed once stabilized to prevent infection, trauma, and devitalization (**Box 9**). This may be sufficient in mild cases with viable tissue when the underlying cause is addressed. Severely compromised tissue requires debridement including salpingohysterectomy or intestinal resection-anastomosis.

Cloacopexy is indicated for recurrent or chronic prolapse, when underlying cause persist (eg, cloacal hyperplasia, celomic mass, hypersexuality, sphincter atony) or in idiopathic cases (**Box 10**). Excessive tension must be avoided to prevent colonic entrapment.[32,33] Ventplasty may be combined with cloacopexy to reduce vent diameter and is recommended for vent atony or chronic prolapse (**Box 11**). Cloacoplasty can affect defecation, urination, and egg-laying, requiring close short- and long-term monitoring. Cloacal reduction is reserved for cases with redundant tissue and may be performed alone or in combination with other techniques (**Box 12**).

Prognosis and prevention. Prognosis depends on the organ involved. Survival rate to discharge was 64% for oviductal prolapse and 0% for gastrointestinal prolapse, without significant differences between taxonomic group, sex, or primary cloacal pathology.[13] Recurrence occurred in 29% of oviductal prolapses and is more likely if the underlying cause persists, as continued straining may lead to pexy dehiscence, inadequate adhesion formation and cloacal hypertrophy. Chronic reproductive behaviors may respond to leuprolide acetate or environmental modification. Psychotropic drugs may be indicated in selected cases.[34]

Surgical condition of the uropygial gland

The uropygial gland is one of the few sebaceous glands present in birds, along with the *glandulae auriculares*, and the *glandulae venti*.[35] Anatomically localized at the base of the tail, dorsal to the last caudal vertebrae and the levator caudae muscles. The macroscopic morphology of the glandula uropygialis varies among avian species and in general, the gland is bilobed, but its overall shape shows marked interspecific variation (**Fig. 4**).[36–38] It is a holocrine tubuloalveolar gland with an oily secretion that

Box 9
Reduction of prolapse

- Under general anesthesia, rinse and disinfect prolapsed tissues using chlorhexidine solution or other nontoxic cleansers.
- Repair any laceration and remove any content in the cloaca (egg, cloacolithiasis)
- Replace tissue using a cotton tip applicator generously lubricated with water-based lubricant.
- Apply 2 temporary transcloacal stay sutures using interrupted or mattress suture with 3-0 or 4-0 monofilament, placed perpendicular to the vent approximately one-third and two-third across to avoid immediate recurrence. A purse-string suture is contraindicated because it will impede the normal movements of the cloacal lips during defecation and the bird is more likely to become obstipated. Maintain Q-tips centrally to allow defecation.
- Manage postoperative pain with non-steroidal anti-inflammatory drugs (NSAIDs) or tramadol.
- Remove cloacal sutures within 4 to 5 days (up to 2 weeks if needed) to limit the risk of nerve damage and postsurgical cloacal sphincter atony.

Box 10
Techniques for cloacopexy

Different techniques of cloacopexies have been described and treatment of choice depends on individual circumstances:

- *Percutaneous cloacopexy*: Use this technique for temporary or permanent treatment. Delineate the margins of the cloaca with a lubricated cotton tip applicator and lift it to the celomic wall. Apply 2 to 3 simple interrupted sutures through skin, body wall, and urodeum. This procedure is not recommended due to the risk to trap or perforate ureters, rectum, duodenum or pancreas.
- *Open circumcostal (rib) and sternal cloacopexy*[22,47,91]: Delineate the margins of the cloaca with a lubricated cotton tip applicator. Perform a ventral midline incision over the most anterior portion of the cloaca to access the caudal celom, taking care not to incise the wall of the cloaca. If required, extend incisions parasternally bilaterally to provide access to the last rib. Identify the serosal surface of the cloaca and remove the intracelomic fat on its ventral surface. Preplace sutures with nonabsorbable monofilament material (eg, nylon, dexon, or wire) around the eighth rib (at the junction of the sternal and vertebral portions) bilaterally then through the full thickness of the ventral surface of the urodeum craniolaterally. Tighten the suture to appose the cloacal wall to the rib. The vent should be slightly inverted. If suture create excessive inversion of the vent, use the cartilaginous caudal border of the sternum to anchor the cloaca. Incise or scarify the ventral aspect of the cloaca. Place 2 sutures through the cloacal wall and incorporate them in the abdominal wall closure.
- *Subserosal cloacopexy*[47]: This technique can be used alone if the tension using rib or sternal cloacopexy is too important or in association with the previous techniques to create further attachments. Perform a ventral midline celiotomy as previously described. Make a 2- to 5-mm incision in the ventral cloacal serosa to the level of the submucosa of the coprodeum, parallel to its length, approximately 5 to 10 mm from the midline. Realize a corresponding incision of similar length on the opposite side in the peritoneal surface of the body wall. Preplace 3 to 4 interrupted or simple continuous sutures with 4-0 to 7-0 nonabsorbable monofilament to appose seromuscular incision with the corresponding incision in the abdominal wall. Tie the suture once they are all preplaced and the position of the cloacal is appropriate. Repeat the procedure on the contralateral side.

has several functions, and the composition vary between different species and even between free-living and captivity songbirds.[9,39] It is present in most birds and is relatively large in some aquatic species, but is absent in other species including the ostrich, emu, cassowaries, bustards, frogmouths and many pigeons, woodpeckers, and parrots.[1]

Inflammatory or traumatic insults can obstruct the excretory ducts of the uropygial gland, leading to glandular impaction or abscess formation. Management may be medical or surgical, depending on severity. Typically involves debridement, restoration of duct patency, and the use of antibiotics when indicated.[40,41] In some birds, an underlying neoplastic process may predispose the gland to secondary infection.

Epidemiology and pathophysiology

Distinguishing impaction of the uropygial gland from a suspected neoplasm is often possible on careful inspection; however, when inflammation is present, this differentiation becomes less evident, making cytologic or histologic evaluation essential whenever uncertainty remains.[42] The chronicity of the lesion and the bird's nutritional status should also be considered, as glandular impaction is frequently associated with hypovitaminosis A, leading to squamous metaplasia and hyperkeratosis.[9] Neoplasms of the uropygial gland may be adenomas or carcinomas and are often difficult to distinguish grossly; both appear as enlarging masses at the gland site, sometimes

Box 11
Techniques for cloacoplasty/ventplasty

Before making the incisions, estimate how much tissue needs to be resected to make a normal vent diameter, only large enough to allow 1 to 2 cotton tip applicators to be inserted. Two techniques have been described as below:

- *Symmetric cloacoplasty*:
  - If the reduction in size is mild to moderate, perform a triangular incision over the cranioventral side of the vent with the base of the triangle on the leading edge of the vent, and the point away from it. Spare the sphincter and transverse cloacal muscles if possible. Use bipolar electrosurgery or laser to control hemorrhage. The submucosa is closed with the dermis using simple interrupted absorbable suture placed medial to lateral. If required, the sphincter muscle is closed using a mattress suture in the muscle from cranial to caudal. The dermis and the epidermis are closed in the same fashion.[92]
  - If a larger reduction is required, excise the mucocutaneous border on the lateral third of the dorsal and ventral vent lips, and maintain the middle third untouched. The lateral third of the vent is closed on both sides with one to 2 vertical mattress sutures using fine monofilament absorbable suture transversely. The middle third remains open to allow elimination of feces and urine.[86]
- *Asymmetric cloacoplasty*: Realize a semicircular excision at the mucocutaneous junction from the right side. Perform 2-layer closure using a 6-0 monofilament absorbable material with (1) a full-thickness horizontal mattress to reduce cloacal opening by 50% to 75% and (2) a row of simple interrupted sutures, tension-relieving suture applied. Place a tension-relieving suture to aid in healing of the incision.[92]

ulcerated. In psittacine birds, adenocarcinoma of the uropygial gland is the most commonly diagnosed epithelial tumor, reported predominantly in budgerigars and occasionally in sulfur-crested cockatoos; affected birds typically present with a progressively enlarging, inflamed mass, and the median age at diagnosis is 8 years (range 1–61).[43] Importantly, extirpation of the uropygial gland does not appear to compromise survival in pigeons, hens, or passerine species.[44]

Diagnosis and medical stabilization

Owing to the structural fragility of the gland and the risk of damaging the excretory ducts, some authors advocate complete excision with subsequent histopathologic assessment to confirm the diagnosis and evaluate surgical margins. Specifically, regarding SCC, diagnosis can be obtained by cytology or histopathology.[45] Those type of tumor concerns about their ability to be locally invasive and have a low metastatic rate. They are best treated surgically, with the goal of a complete surgical excision.[46] Appropriate antibiotic coverage and species-specific analgesia should be initiated. The use of protective devices such as Elizabethan collars or suitable body

Box 12
Technique for cloacal reduction

- Perform a ventral midline incision as described previously to expose the cloaca.
- Realize an incision in the ventral aspect of the cloaca cranial to the sphincter, preserving the sphincter and avoiding entry into the ureters and colon.
- Excise excess tissue on from the ventral aspect of the cloaca.
- Close the cloaca with a simple continuous monofilament suture. Closure of the skin is routine.

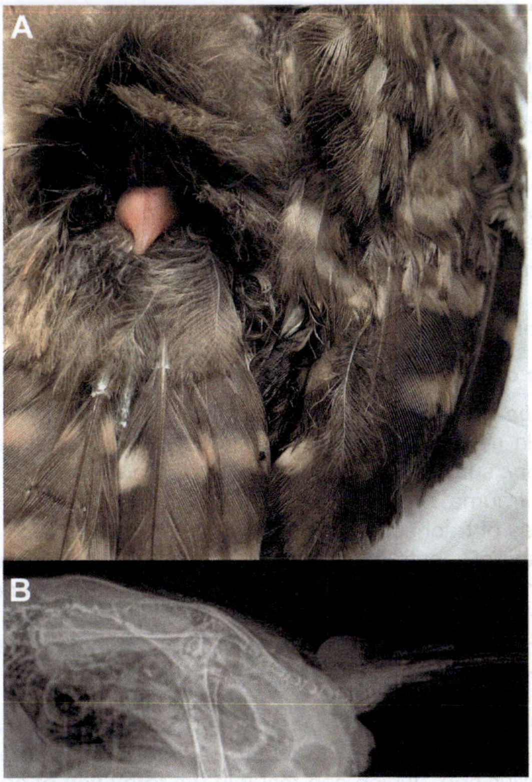

Fig. 4. (*A, B*) (*A*) Normal appearance of the uropygial gland in a little owl (*Athena noctua*). (*B*) Visualization on radiograph. (Image Courtesy of AvianDoc, Collarile and Cococcetta.)

vests is essential to prevent further contamination, local infection, and to avoid self-mutilation of the tail.

Surgical treatment

Definitive treatment usually requires removal of the entire gland under general anesthesia (**Box 13** for technical details).[47] A single case has been reported in the literature in which tail amputation, including the terminal caudal vertebrae and the pygostyle, was required. For detailed information and illustrations of this case, refer to the original publication.[48]

Box 13
Technique for uropygial gland excision

- The gland is surgically excised by creating an incision encircling its base.
- The uropygial gland has a rich blood supply, careful hemostasis is required.
- To remove the whole gland, begin the dissection caudally to cranially.
- Routine closure in cases of small defect (primary apposition).
- If the defect is too large, healing may be allowed by secondary intention using a hydroactive dressing, or alternatively, a skin flap can be applied to cover the defect.

Prognosis and prevention
Limited information is available in the literature regarding outcomes following surgical removal of uropygial gland SCC. However, local radiation therapy using a single strontium probe treatment has been successfully used as the sole therapy in 2 budgerigars (*Melopsittacus undulatus*) with uropygial gland carcinoma and in a cockatiel (*Nymphicus hollandicus*) with a uropygial gland adenoma, with complete resolution and disease-free follow-up at 8, 9, and 2 months, respectively.[46] In another reported case involving a blue-and-yellow macaw (*Ara ararauna*) with uropygial gland adenocarcinoma, surgical tail amputation resulted in an uneventful recovery, with no complications or recurrence observed up to 3.5 months postoperatively.[48] In literature, other treatment such as photodynamic therapy or cryotherapy has been used to reduce or treat SCCs in several avian species.[46]

Surgical Condition of the Lower Respiratory Tract

Air sac cannula/tube
An air sac cannula (ASC) can be used to induce and maintain anesthesia during selected respiratory surgeries (tracheal and syringeal), oral and neck procedures (eg, beak surgery, trauma, or masses at the thoracic inlet), or as an alternative airway in emergency cases of tracheal obstruction.

Common causes of obstruction include postintubation tracheal stenosis,[49,50] foreign bodies, tracheal or syringeal aspergillomas, trauma, and masses at the thoracic inlet.[22,47,49]

When tracheal obstruction is suspected, the air sac tube should be placed in the caudal thoracic or in the abdominal air sacs.[51]

Epidemiology and pathophysiology. One of the principal etiologic agents implicated in tracheal obstruction or stenosis in avian species is fungal infection, particularly caused by *Aspergillus* spp., which can result in the formation of obstructive granulomatous or plaque-like lesions within the trachea or syrinx.[9] Similar lesions could be induced by bacterial infections. Aspirated material, such as seeds, plant fragments, or even a winged insect (*Gelechioidea*) represents additional rarer cause of acute obstruction.[52,53] Tumors of the trachea are rare in birds. Tracheal osteochondroma was recognized in a psittacine bird and resulted in tracheal stenosis.[9] Diffuse ossification with osteopetrosis of tracheal rings in a yellow-crowned parrot (*Amazona ochrocephala*) with a history of chronic respiratory distress and death after development of marked dyspnea.[54]

Tracheal stenosis is also a well-recognized complication of endotracheal intubation, typically developing within 2 to 3 weeks. In a review of 23 postintubation cases, proposed causes included mechanical trauma from the tube, chemical irritation, mucosal desiccation (as reported in rabbits)[55] and, irritating anesthetic gases.[56] Bird species with long necks seem over-represented.[9]

Clinical signs of tracheal obstruction vary with the duration and severity of the blockage.

Acute obstructions cause rapid collapse, weakness, extended neck and wings, marked mouth-breathing with sternal lift, and loud inspiratory sounds. Chronic or slowly developing obstructions produce subtler signs: mild but progressive dyspnea, reduced activity to compensate, decreased or altered vocalization, and worsening respiratory effort as the obstruction advances.[57] These signs, however, are not specific, as lower respiratory tract disease (lungs or air sacs) may appear similar.

Diagnosis and medical stabilization. Endoscopy is the fastest and most accurate diagnostic tool (**Fig. 5**). Radiography and CT scan could be helpful and is some cases

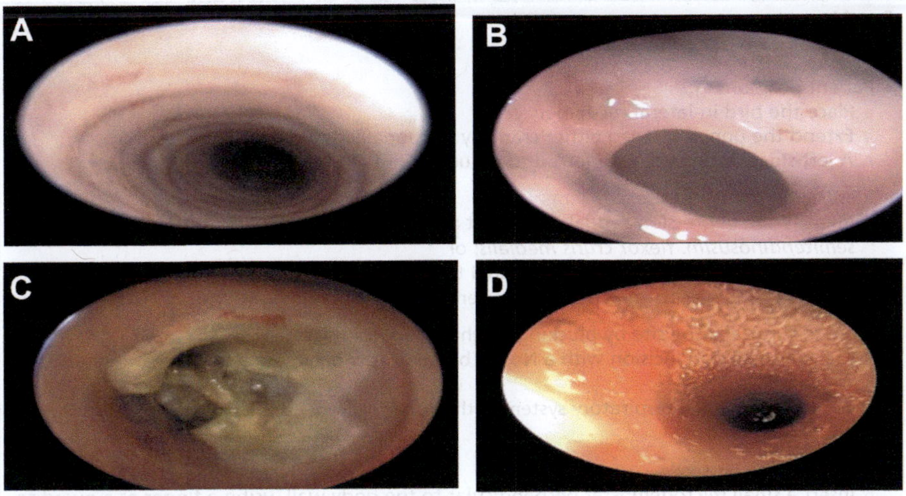

Fig. 5. (*A–D*) (*A*) Normal appearance of the trachea on endoscopy, (*B*) Postintubation stenosis, (*C*) Fungal granuloma, (*D*) Edema and bacterial tracheitis. (Image Courtesy of AvianDoc, Collarile and Cococcetta.)

fundamental to completely investigate the whole respiratory tract (**Fig. 6**). Maintain a calm environment with minimal noise and dim lighting and provide supplemental oxygen. Sedation may be indicated to reduce stress and metabolic demand. All necessary equipment should be prepared in advance to minimize procedure time before air sac cannulation.

Surgical treatment. Preoxygenation may help facilitate the procedure and premedicate the bird or induce with anesthetic gas by mask. Follow the procedure in **Box 14**.

Prognosis and prevention. Antibiotic, antifungal, and analgesic therapies are typically administered, according to the species, either before or immediately after the ASC

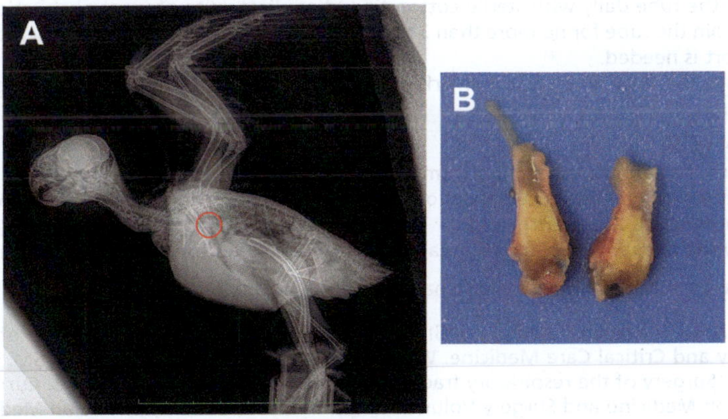

Fig. 6. (*A, B*) Lateral radiographic projection of a cockatiel (*Nymphicus hollandicus*). Area of increased radiopacity few millimeters cranially to the syrinx (*red circle*). (*B*) Macroscopic image of the lesion: granuloma caused by *Pasteurella* spp. (Image Courtesy of AvianDoc, Collarile and Cococcetta.)

Box 14
Technique for air sac tube placement[51,61]

- Patient positioning:
  - Place the bird in lateral recumbency.
  - Extend the uppermost leg either cranially or caudally depending on access.
  - A left-sided approach is preferred to reduce risk of injury to the right liver lobe.
- Identify the insertion site:
  - Identify the depression caudal to the last rib (eighth in parrots), ventral to the *semitendinosus/m. flexor cruris medialis*; or
  - Identify the triangular depression caudal to the pectoral muscle, cranial to the thigh, and ventral to the synsacrum (usually between the seventh and eighth ribs in Psittaciformes).
- Prepare surgically the site by plucking feathers and disinfect:
  - Make a small skin incision with a No. 11 blade of few millimeters to expose the muscular wall.
  - Gently distend the respiratory system with oxygen to reduce the risk of puncturing abdominal organs.
- Penetrate the air sac:
  - Insert a small microhemostat perpendicular to the body wall, using a finger as a guard to avoid penetrate too ventrally.
  - Bluntly penetrate the muscle and air sac (typically felt as 2 *pops* or a sudden loss of tissue tension).
  - Open the hemostats slightly to create a passage.
- Insert the cannula/tube (inner diameter of the tube $\geq$ inner diameter of the trachea):
  - Insert a sterile, fenestrated endotracheal tube segment or air sac cannula through the opening created by the hemostats after they are withdrawn or while kept them open.
  - Confirm airflow using an anesthesiology monitor (capnography); alternatively, when such equipment is not available, a down feather may be used to assess airflow by observing feather movement.
  - If available and possible perform a brief endoscopy or a radiograph.
- Secure the tube:
  - Fix the cannula with sutures (cruciate suture).
  - Add a filter (mask material or filter paper) to prevent aspiration of dust/feathers. Careful in small bird or small diameter tube.
- Monitoring and maintenance:
  - Be aware that $ETCO_2$ readings may drop or disappear due to CO_2 wash-out (open circuit).
  - Clean the tube daily with sterile cotton-tipped applicators to prevent obstruction.
  - Maintain the tube for no more than 3 to 5 days; replace in the contralateral air sac if longer support is needed.
  - Remove the tube when tracheal airflow is restored; confirm by briefly occluding the cannula.
- After removal
  - Culture the cannula tip and perform a brief endoscopic exam of the site.
  - Watch for inflammatory complications (focal fungal granulomas may occur; apply topical amphotericin B if present).
  - Allow the stoma to heal by secondary intention, applying topical ointment as needed.
- Monitor for subcutaneous emphysema, which is usually self-limiting.

From Beaufrère H. Oxygen therapy. In: Graham JE, Doss GA, Beaufrère H, editors. Exotic Animal Emergency and Critical Care Medicine. Wiley; 2021. p. 450–456; and Guzman DSM, Speer BL, Echols MS. Surgery of the respiratory tract. In Speer B, van Zeeland YRA, editors. Current Therapy in Avian Medicine and Surgery Volume II E-Book: Current Therapy in Avian Medicine and Surgery Volume II E-Book. Elsevier; 2025. p. 407–421.[51,61]

placement.[58] In a study considering 84 birds undergoing ASC placement, 4.8% died perianesthetically due to underlying disease. Among survivors, 32.5% experienced ASC-related complications, most commonly loss of patency (23.8%), followed by dislodgement, obstruction, or insufficient cannula diameter. Other complications included subcutaneous emphysema, site infection, minor hemorrhage, and celomic inflammation (<4% each). Only 3 deaths were directly attributable to ASC complications. Median survival after placement was 4 days, with 58.9% of birds surviving to ASC removal and 61% alive at 30 days. Risk factors for complications included exercise intolerance and abnormal respiratory sounds, while intercostal placement and periprocedural antibiotics improved survival. Voice changes at presentation were associated with reduced survival.[58]

Tracheal surgery

The main tracheal surgeries include tracheotomy, tracheostomy, tracheal resection and anastomosis, tracheal stenting,[59] tracheal prosthesis for tracheal collapse,[60] and syringotomy.[61]

Epidemiology and pathophysiology. Tracheal surgery in birds is primarily indicated for the removal of obstructive material such as seeds, granulomas (fungal, bacterial, and parasitic), posttraumatic scarring, or epithelial and mucous neoplasia, all of which may lead to respiratory distress, dyspnea, or changes in vocalization. Foreign material may sometimes be detected by transillumination after wetting the overlying feathers with alcohol, although obstructions located at the syrinx or main bronchi often remain invisible on routine examination.

Diagnosis and medical stabilization. Clinical signs are those already reported in the chapter of air-sac cannulation.

Tracheoscopy, radiography, and CT imaging are useful diagnostic tools for confirming tracheal obstruction. In particular, the CT provides a complete visualization of the whole respiratory system and provides a full-body evaluation. When foreign bodies or masses cannot be resolved through less invasive approaches such as endoscopy or suction,[53] tracheotomy becomes necessary.[62,63] Because surgical access temporarily compromises the airway, air-sac intubation is required to maintain anesthesia during the procedure. Preoxygenation, appropriate sedative drugs, antibiotics, and species-specific analgesia should be considered and implemented as soon as possible.

Surgical treatment. Positioning is common to all the procedures; the bird should be placed in a dorsal recumbency or slightly elevate the cranial portion of the body (~45°); feathers must be plucked to have a sterile skin. Surgically prepare the skin in a standard way. In this article, only tracheotomy, tracheostomy, and tracheal resection with anastomosis are discussed (**Boxes 15–17**).

Prognosis and prevention. Postoperative management typically includes antibiotics, antifungals, opioids, and anti-inflammatories as needed. Cage rest helps prevent trauma to the surgical site.

Removal of the ASC should occur only after temporary occlusion of the cannula; careful monitoring for respiratory distress should be provided following its removal. Endoscopic evaluation is recommended to assess healing and to confirm the absence of granulomas or strictures.[62,64]

Common complications include intraluminal granuloma formation at the suture site, reported as frequent.[22] Additional complications include early postoperative

Box 15
Technique for tracheotomy

- *Skin incision*
  - Incise the skin along the ventral midline of the neck (or slightly lateral to the crop).
  - If doubts in avoiding the crop mucosa, use a probe to inflate a small volume of air into the crop.
  - Dissect subcutaneous tissues to expose the paired muscles (*sternohyoideus, tracheolateralis, sternotrachealis, and cleidotrachealis*); note species variability.
  - Locate the recurrent nerves on the ventrolateral/lateral tracheal surface.
  - Avoid trauma through gentle, precise dissection.
- *Localize the lesion*
  - Use a probe or rigid endoscope to detect or visualize the stenosis/lesion.
  - Use transillumination, radiographic measurements, or CT imaging for preoperative localization.
- *Tracheal incision*
  - Make a transverse incision over the identified site using a No. 11 scalpel or beaver miniblade.
  - Incise approximately 50% of the tracheal circumference on the ventral side.
- Place stay sutures around tracheal rings adjacent to the incision.
- Remove the obstruction (grasping, debridement, suction, or pushing it).
  - If needed may place a transverse hypodermic needle caudal to the lesion to prevent caudal displacement.
  - If needed, by a rigid endoscope confirms the successful removal and assess area.
- *Closure of the trachea*
  - Preplace simple interrupted sutures incorporating 1 to 2 tracheal rings on each side of the incision.
  - Use monofilament absorbable sutures (4–0 to 8–0, eg, PDS).
- *Close the subcutaneous tissue* and skin routinely.

hemorrhage, late tracheal stenosis, surgical site infection, aspiration, and pneumonia. Damage to the recurrent nerves may occur; although this does not cause laryngeal paralysis in birds, it may result in voice change due to their role in innervating esophageal, crop, tracheal, and syringeal muscles.[47,62] Diameter mismatch (especially in macaws and cockatoos) may occur when large cranial tracheal segments are resected, increasing stenosis risk.[62]

For uncomplicated procedures, the prognosis is generally good. When diseased tissue is incompletely removed or further tracheal damage occurs, stenosis may develop and require tracheal resection and anastomosis (**Fig. 7**). Following anastomosis, recurrent or delayed complications are possible; endoscopic and radiographic reassessment at 1, 2, and 6 months postsurgery has been suggested.[62]

Tracheostomy Reported complications of tracheostomy include surgical site dehiscence, subcutaneous emphysema, secondary infections, granuloma formation around the stoma causing reduction in diameter, and mucus accumulation in the lower airway.[62,65] Data from literature suggest a poor prognosis with a survival times ranging from 5 weeks in a hooded vulture (*Necrosyrtes monachus*) and 3 to 5 months in 2 psittacine birds (amazon parrot and blue-and-yellow macaw).[65] Mortality is primarily due to loss of effective airflow through the stoma and recurrence of obstructive airway clinical signs, often leading to euthanasia or spontaneous death.[62]

Box 16
Tracheal resection and anastomosis (reporting only different point from tracheotomy)

- Cranial and caudal to the lesion, bisect a tracheal ring circumferentially using a No. 11 or beaver blade.

Alternative: cut the intratracheal ring tissue one ring cranial and caudal to the affected segment.

- Remove the diseased tracheal segment (from 1 to 15 tracheal rings removed in different species reported in literature).[61]
- Anastomosis preparation
  - Preplace simple interrupted sutures (4–0 to 8–0 monofilament absorbable, eg, polydioxanone) on a tapered needle.
  - Use a minimum of 4 sutures to approximate the tracheal ends.
  - Tighten each suture individually, placing extraluminal knots to achieve proper opposition of tracheal ends.
  - If a large segment has been removed and the distal trachea is smaller, insert the smaller distal end into the proximal end to allow proper alignment.
- Perform routine subcutaneous and skin closure.

Surgical Condition of the Skin

Soft tissue masses are predominantly of neoplastic origin. Bacterial granulomas can also occur, but they are less commonly reported as requiring surgical excision.

Epidemiology and pathophysiology

Cutaneous papillomas are uncommon and may be virally induced in gray parrots, and cockatiels, typically present as papillary facial growths. Although histologic features are similar across species, a viral etiology in cockatiels remains unproven. These

Box 17
Tracheostomy

- Prepare and position the patient as for a tracheotomy.
- Identify the surgical site 1 to 2 cm ventral to the mandible to prevent stoma obstruction during neck flexion.
- Make a transverse incision between the tracheal rings, cutting roughly one-third of the tracheal circumference using a No. 11 or beaver blade.
- Create a second parallel transverse incision to achieve a final stoma length about three times its width.
- Connect the 2 transverse incisions by cutting through the tracheal rings, forming a rectangular stoma.
- A custom stainless-steel stent may be placed to prevent premature closure (reported in concept but not yet formally described).
- Suture the skin to the stoma using 5-0 to 7-0 monofilament absorbable suture on a cutting or reverse-cutting needle.
- Use a simple continuous pattern to secure the stoma edges.

From Guzman DSM, Speer BL, Echols MS. Surgery of the respiratory tract. In Speer B, van Zeeland YRA, editors. Current Therapy in Avian Medicine and Surgery Volume II E-Book: Current Therapy in Avian Medicine and Surgery Volume II E-Book. Elsevier; 2025. p. 407–421; and Lennox A, Nemetz L. Tracheostomy in the Avian Patient. Semin avian exotic pet med. 2005;14:131–134.[61,65]

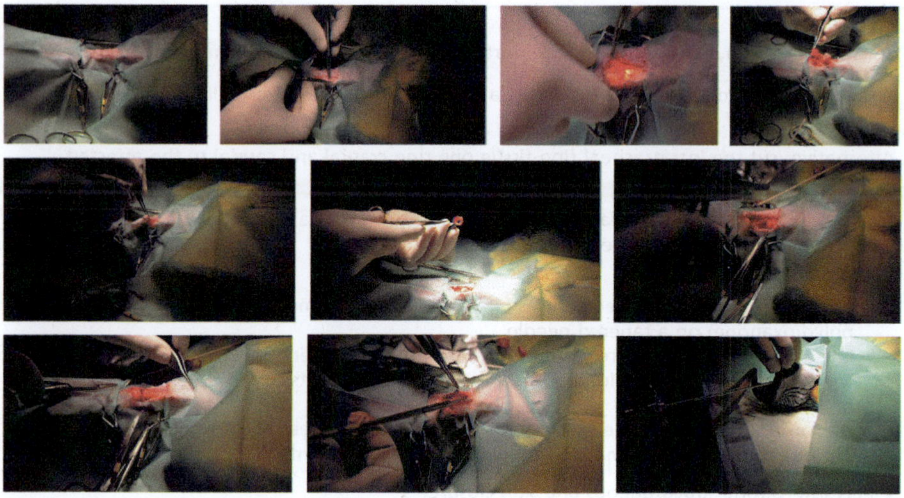

Fig. 7. Step-by-step images of the tracheal resection with anastomosis procedure in a macaw (*Ara ararauna*). (Image Courtesy of AvianDoc, Collarile and Cococcetta.)

lesions consist of frond-like projections covered by proliferative, hyperkeratotic epidermis supported by a delicate vascular stroma.[9]

SCCs are malignant epithelial tumors occurring throughout the body, commonly on feathered skin.[66,67] The beak, the uropygial gland, the phalanges, and the upper gastrointestinal tract (especially the crop) were also reported as possible site.[46] Parrot species such as cockatiels, amazon parrots, and conures are frequently reported, whereas passeriformes appear under-represented in several studies.[5,46,68] However, in the authors' opinion, this may reflect a bias related to the low number of passeriformes submissions for histopathology, particularly among privately owned birds.

Mesenchymal tumors encompass neoplasms of vascular, fibrous, adipose connective tissue, and lymphoma. Gross differentiation between benign and malignant forms is often difficult. Lipomas are benign adipose tumors and liposarcomas are more invasive and metastatic.[69] They are commonly reported neoplasms in avian skin, usually well circumscribed but occasionally infiltrative.[46] They occur most often in obese budgerigars, quaker parrots, amazon parrots, and macaws. They are typically subcutaneous, frequently near the pericloacal region.[70] Concerning the genus *Amazona*, hypotheses of a genetic predisposition and obesity linked to high-energy diets have been proposed to explain the higher prevalence of lipomas observed in these species.[9,46,70,71] Anatomically, lipomas are more frequently reported in the sternum, abdomen, and inner face of the thigh[72]; and pericloacal area.[70]

Fibrosarcomas are malignant common tumors of the skin of pet birds. Fibromas are infrequently diagnosed. Both tumors present as firm nodules or masses, but more they have indistinct margins and more they are aggressive.[9]

Myxosarcomas, rare soft tissue sarcomas, described once in a severe macaw (*Ara severus*).[46]

Xanthomas are non-neoplastic dermal masses composed of lipid-laden macrophages and cholesterol clefts.[73] They occur mainly in gallinaceous birds and most commonly in cockatiels and budgerigars.[74] They easily get confused with neoplastic due to the friable, yellowish-orange, and well vascularized aspect.[9] Clinically those lesions are often extensive and lead to ulceration of the skin or self-mutilation episodes.

In a recent study, the prevalence of adipocytic tumors and xanthomas on necropsy was 1.3%.[73] Adipocytic tumors were observed in 27 genera, with significantly higher odds in *Amazona* followed by *Myiopsitta*, *Melopsittacus* and *Agapornis*, while *Ara* showed lower odds.[73] Age was a significant risk factor for many adipocytic tumors. No association was found between adipocytic tumors and atherosclerosis or hepatic lipidosis. Xanthomas were associated with atherosclerosis but not with hepatic lipidosis.[73]

Diagnosis and medical stabilization

In terms of diagnosis, 2 key considerations must be emphasized: first, many cutaneous and soft tissue masses share a similar gross clinical appearance; second, the degree of malignancy cannot be determined clinically (**Fig. 8**). This necessitates the use of cytology and histopathology for definitive diagnosis. In one study evaluating 59 cases, fine-needle aspirates (FNAs) and impression smears were assessed cytologically and compared with histopathology as the gold standard. Cytology and histopathology fully agreed in 72.8% (43 of 59) of cases. Cytology correctly identified 87.5% (35 of 40) of malignant lesions and 55.6% (5 of 9) of benign processes. No significant difference was found between cytology and histopathology for detecting malignant neoplasia in birds (P=.185). The diagnostic performance of FNAs and impression smears for avian tumors was also comparable.[5]

SCCs behave as locally invasive tumors with low metastatic potential, and complete surgical excision remains the treatment of choice.[68] Because SCCs are relatively resistant to radiation, larger or deeper lesions respond poorly, and intralesional chemotherapy or cryotherapy provide variable results.[46]

Surgical treatment

Surgical excision remains the treatment of choice for squamous cell carcinoma (SCC) and other sarcomas (eg, adipocytic neoplasms). The use of electrosurgery is recommended to ensure effective hemostasis and to minimize blood loss, particularly in small patients.[47]

Key considerations include the following[22,47,70,75]:

- Wide surgical margins are required for effective tumor control.
- Attention to highly vascularized structures is necessary to minimize hemorrhage.
- Some neoplasms may be associated with lipid excess, influencing coagulation.
- For certain tumors, preoperative staging to exclude potential metastases is recommended.

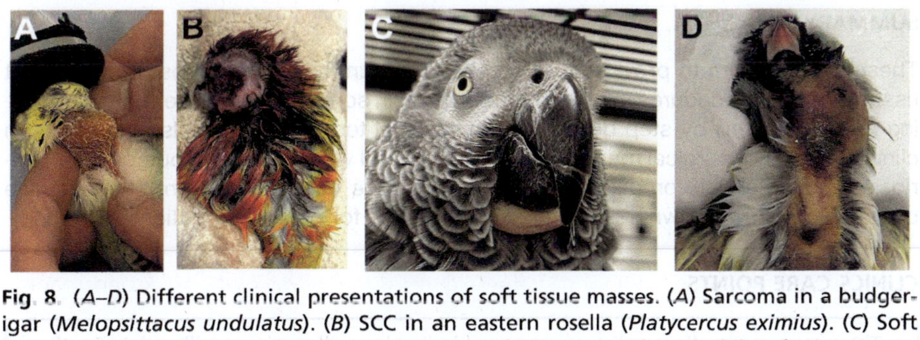

Fig. 8. (*A–D*) Different clinical presentations of soft tissue masses. (*A*) Sarcoma in a budgerigar (*Melopsittacus undulatus*). (*B*) SCC in an eastern rosella (*Platycercus eximius*). (*C*) Soft tissue mass of unknown origin in a gray parrot (*Psittacus erithacus*). (*D*) Soft tissue mass of unknown origin in Gouldian finch (*Erythrura gouldiae*). (Image Courtesy of AvianDoc, Collarile and Cococcetta.)

- Given the association with patient age, a thorough preoperative assessment is advised.
- Owners should be informed of the potential risk of recurrence.
- Consideration of chemotherapy protocols is warranted for partially excised tumors.
- Adequate analgesia and perioperative antibiotic therapy should be provided.
- Protective measures such as collars or vests may be necessary depending on tumor location.
- In cases requiring amputation, patient welfare should be prioritized, and the environment adapted to accommodate functional limitations (eg, perches, feeding stations).

Prognosis and prevention

Regarding sarcomas, the human medical literature provides conflicting data on the prognostic impact of partial versus complete excision.[50,76–78] Some studies suggest that achieving clean margins is not necessarily associated with overall survival in primary extremity soft tissue sarcomas, likely due to the frequent occurrence of internal organ metastases.[79]

From a histopathological perspective, a study on human oral fibrous–epithelial lesions demonstrated that thermal damage at surgical margins varies depending on the instrument used (electrosurgery > laser > cold blade). However, none of the instruments evaluated compromised diagnostic interpretation.[76]

For some tumors like lipomas, management primarily involves dietary modification and increased exercise, as those neoplasms may regress with weight reduction. L-carnitine supplementation has shown preliminary promise in reducing lipoma size in budgerigars.[80] Xanthomas may develop secondary to obesity, hyperlipidemia, and trauma.[81] Vitamin A supplementation may be beneficial, but intervention is only necessary if the mass becomes traumatic or functionally limiting.

Surgical excision is indicated for rapidly growing or symptomatic masses, with histopathology required to distinguish lipomas from liposarcomas, which are more invasive and metastatic.[46]

Conservative surgery is associated with high recurrence due to invasive margins, making wide excision necessary. Postoperative radiation and/or intralesional chemotherapy may be considered when complete excision is not feasible.[82,83] In some cases the localization and the nature of the tumors did not allowed to complete resection and several long-term recurrence occurred over 8 years.[70]

SUMMARY

These sections aim to provide a comprehensive summary of the most frequent soft tissue surgical procedures in psittaciformes and, in some cases, passeriformes, offering not only a step-by-step description of surgical techniques, but also guidance on clinical signs, nonsurgical management options, and when available, outcomes, prognosis, and potential complications. These data are essential not only for effective communication with owners, but most importantly, for optimizing patient welfare.

CLINICS CARE POINTS

- The most common cloacal diseases are egg binding in small species, papillomas in South American birds, and idiopathic prolapse in cockatoos. Management may be medical, surgical, or combined, depending on the underlying cause.

- Cloacal prolapse has multiple causes, including straining from cloacal extracloacal disorder, space-occupying celomic lesions, or sphincter atony from neurologic or system disease.
- Acute dyspnea, stridor and noisy breathing with increased respiratory effort are clinical signs consistent with tracheal obstruction. In cases such as granulomas, the growth may be chronic until a sudden acute deterioration occurs. In all situations, tracheal obstruction is a medical emergency requiring air sac cannulation. Traumatic, infectious or neoplastic causes may require tracheotomy or tracheal resection with anastomosis. When no perioperative or postoperative complications occur, the prognosis is generally favorable.
- Soft tissue masses and neoplasms of the uropygial gland can involve several anatomic structures with variable invasiveness. Cytology and biopsy allow a definitive diagnosis and better surgical planning. Radiographs and CT scans may be recommended to rule out metastasis and to perform preoperative assessment and tumor staging. Squamous cell carcinomas typically show irregular, poorly encapsulated margins, with strong local invasiveness but low metastatic potential. Chemotherapy, photodynamic therapy or cryotherapy may be considered as alternatives or adjuncts to surgical excision, particularly when the surgical site presents healing challenges or when amputation should be avoided.

DECLARATION OF AI AND AI-ASSISTED TECHNOLOGIES IN THE WRITING PROCESS

During the preparation of this work, the authors used ChatGPT to condense, summarize, or help to rephrase text to meet the permitted word count. After using this tool, the authors reviewed and edited the content as needed and take full responsibility for the content of the publication.

DISCLOSURE

The authors have no commercial or financial conflicts of interest to declare. This study was not supported by a grant.

REFERENCES

1. King AS, McLelland J. Birds: their structure and function. Elsevier Science Health Science Division; 1984.
2. White SD, Beaufrère H, Guzman DSM, et al. Cutaneous disorders in captive psittacines, a retrospective study of 1454 cases at a university veterinary teaching hospital (1988–2021). Vet. Dermatol 2025;36(2):205–17.
3. Whitehead MC, Welle KR, Allender MC, et al. Evaluation of treatment for severed blood feathers in chickens (Gallus gallus). Proceedings of the 36th Annual Conference and Expo of the Association of Avian Aeterinarians. 2015. San Antonio, TX. p. 27.
4. Martin LF. Retrospective study on the species distribution and common diseases in exotic pets presented to the Clinic for Zoo Animals, Exotic Pets and Wildlife, University of Zurich from 2005 to 2014. Dissertation. University of Zurich; 2018.
5. Sutherland M, Luk K, Courtman N, et al. Survey of the clinical, cytological, and histopathological features associated with neoplasms in captive avian species in melbourne, Australia. J Avian Med Surg 2023;37(3):243–65.
6. Turner RC, Graham JE, Hahn S, et al. Infraorbital keratin cyst in an umbrella cockatoo (*Cacatua alba*). J Avian Med Surg 2019;33(2):150–4.
7. Harrison GJ. Microsurgical procedure for feather cyst removal in a citron-crested cockatoo (*Cacatua sulphurea citrinocristata*). J Avian Med Surg 2003;17(2): 86–90.

8. Zwart P, Grimm F. Plumafolliculoma (feather cyst) in canaries (Serinus canaria): a benign tumor. 2003; Proceedings of the 7th European AAV Conference 2003, Tenerife. p. 241–247.
9. Raidal S. Integument. In: Schmidt R, Struthers JD, Phalen D, editors. Pathology of pet and aviary birds. 3th Edition. Hoboken (NJ): John Wiley & Sons, Inc.; 2024. p. 405–37.
10. Langlois I. Medical causes of feather damaging behavior. Vet Clin North Am Exot Anim Pract 2021;24(1):119–52.
11. Farris KEH, Doss GA. Use of haloperidol in companion psittacine birds: 19 cases (2012–2022). J Avian Med Surg 2025;38(4):202–7.
12. Ferrell ST. Avian integumentary surgery. Semin avian exotic pet med 2002;11(3): 125–35.
13. Gill KS, Helmer PJ. Cloacal diseases in companion parrots: a retrospective study of 43 cases (2012–2018). J Avian Med Surg 2020;34(4):364–70.
14. Latimer KS, Niagro FD, Rakich PM, et al. Investigation of parrot papillomavirus in cloacal and oral papillomas of psittacine birds. Vet clin path 1997;26(4):158–63.
15. Gartrell B, Morgan K, Howe L, et al. Cloacal papillomatosis in the absence of herpesvirus and papillomavirus in a sulphur-crested cockatoo (*Cacatua galerita*). N Z Vet J 2009;57(4):241–3.
16. Detweiler A, Carpenter JW, Kraft SL, et al. Radiographic diagnosis: avian cloacal adenocarcinoma. Vet Radiol Ultrasound 2000;41(6):539–41.
17. Wissman MA, Parsons B. Internal papillomatous disease. Managing the papilloma-positive breeder bird. afa Watchbird 2000;XXVII(4):26–7.
18. Lennox A. The use of aldara (imiquimod) for the treatment of cloacal papillomatosis in psittacines. EXOTIC DVM 2002;4(3):34–5.
19. Krautwald-Junghanns ME, Kostka VM, Hofbauer H. Observations on the significance of diagnostic findings in egg-binding of Psittaciformes. Vet rec 1998;143-(18):498–502.
20. Antinoff N, Hoefer HL, Rosenthal KL, et al. Smooth muscle neoplasia of suspected oviductal origin in the cloaca of a blue-fronted Amazon parrot (*Amazona aestiva*). J Avian Med Surg 1997;268–72.
21. Dvorak L, Bennett RA, Cranor K. Cloacotomy for excision of cloacal papillomas in a Catalina macaw. J Avian Med Surg 1998;11–5.
22. Mison MB, Bennett RA. Surgery of the avian gastrointestinal tract. In: Bennett RA, Pye GW, editors. Surgery of exotic animals. Hoboken (NJ): Wiley-Blackwell; 2022. p. 178–89.
23. Lekdumrongsak T, Banlunara W. Treatment of cloacal papilloma with 50% silver nitrate solution in chestnut-fronted macaws (*Ara severus*). Thai J Vet Med 2017;47(4):531–5.
24. Abou-Zahr T, Carrasco DC, Jones SL, et al. Percloacal ovocentesis in the treatment of avian egg binding: review of 20 cases. J Avian Med Surg 2019;33(3): 251–7.
25. Beaufrère H, Nevarez J, Tully TN. Cloacolith in a blue-fronted Amazon parrot (*Amazona aestiva*). J Avian Med Surg 2010;24(2):142–5.
26. Albuquerque Átilla HA, Rabelo Rodrigues I, de Souza Lopes E, et al. Distocia em calopsita (*Nymphicus hollandicus*) com complicações metabólicas por isquemia renal: um relato de caso. Pubvet 2019;13(08).
27. Vavlas A, Galusha H, Mayer J, et al. Resolution of egg binding is possible in most client-owned parrots when multiple treatment strategies are considered. J Am Vet Med Assoc 2025;263(5):628–34.

28. Bowles HL. Reproductive diseases of pet bird species. Vet Clin North Am Exot Anim Pract 2002;5(3):489–506.
29. Graham JE, Tell LA, Lamm MG, et al. Megacloaca in a moluccan cockatoo (*Cacatua moluccensis*). J Avian Med Surg 2004;18(1):41–9.
30. Dennis PM, Bennett RA. Ureterotomy for removal of two ureteroliths in a parrot. J Am Vet Med Assoc 2000;217(6):865–8.
31. Zaffarano B. Clinical brief: an interesting prolapse case. Proceedings of the NAVC Conference, January 17-21, 2015, Orlando, Florida, USA. p. 1285–1286.
32. van Zeeland YR, Schoemaker NJ, van Sluijs FJ. Incisional colopexy for treatment of chronic, recurrent colocloacal prolapse in a sulphur-crested cockatoo (*Cacatua galerita*). Vet Surg 2014;43(7):882–7.
33. Radlinsky MG, Carpenter JW, Mison MB, et al. Colonic entrapment after cloacopexy in two psittacine birds. J Avian Med Surg 2004;18(3):175–82.
34. Nemeth NM, Gonzalez-Astudillo V, Oesterle PT, et al. A 5-year retrospective review of avian diseases diagnosed at the department of pathology, university of Georgia. J Comp Pathol 2016;155(2–3):105–20.
35. Konig HE. Avian anatomy 2nd edition: textbook and colour atlas. 5m Publishing Limited; 2016.
36. Montalti D, Gutiérrez AM, Reboredo G, et al. The chemical composition of the uropygial gland secretion of rock dove Columba livia. Comp Biochem Physiol A Mol Integr Physiol 2005;140(3):275–9.
37. Karaavci Funda A, Dortbudak Muhammet B, Demircioglu M, et al. Investigation of glandula uropygialis in different avian species using morphometric and histological methods. Anat Histol Embryol 2024;53(5):e13107.
38. Stangier N, Sandhöfer S, Mosig A, et al. The uropygial gland of the Great Cormorant (P*halacrocorax carbo*): I. Morphology. J Ornithol 2023;164(3):591–603.
39. Grieves LA, Bottini CLJ, Gloor GB, et al. Uropygial gland microbiota differ between free-living and captive songbirds. Sci Rep 2022;12(1):18283.
40. Abou-Zahr T. Avian dermatology. Vet Clin North Am Exot Anim Pract 2023;26(2):327–46.
41. Harrison GJ, Lightfoot TL, Harrison LR, et al. Clinical avian medicine. Spix Publishing; 1994. Incorporated.
42. Ritchie BW, Harrison GJ, Harrison LR. Avian medicine: principles and application. Wingers Pub; 1994.
43. Sutherland M, Luk K, Courtman N, et al. Survey of the clinical, cytological, and histopathological features associated with neoplasms in captive avian species in Melbourne, Australia. J Avian Med Surg 2023;37(3):243–65.
44. Montalti D, Salibian A. Uropygial gland size and avian habitat. Ornitol Neotrop 2000;11:297–306.
45. Goh G, Chong SM, Xie S. Radical surgical excision of dermal squamous cell carcinoma in a pesquet's parrot (*Psittrichas fulgidus*). J Exot Pet Med 2020;35.
46. Robat CS, Ammersbach M, Mans C. Avian oncology: diseases, diagnostics, and therapeutics. Vet Clin North Am Exot Anim Pract 2017;20(1):57–86.
47. Guzman DS-M. Avian soft tissue surgery. Vet Clin North Am Exot Anim Pract 2016;19(1):133–57.
48. Robertson J, Guzman DS, Sinnott D, et al. Modified tail amputation technique in a blue and gold macaw (*Ara ararauna*) with uropygial gland adenocarcinoma. J Avian Med Surg 2020;34(1):57–64.
49. de Matos R, Morrisey JK, Steffey MA. Postintubation Tracheal Stenosis in a Blue and Gold Macaw (Ara ararauna) Resolved With Tracheal Resection and Anastomosis. 2006.

50. Nemeth NM, McHale B, Schmidt R, et al, editors. Pathology of pet and aviary birds. 3th Edition. Hoboken (NJ): John Wiley & Sons, Inc.; 2024. p. 97–142.
51. Beaufrère H. Oxygen therapy. In: Graham JE, Doss GA, Beaufrère H, editors. Exotic animal emergency and critical care medicine. Wiley; 2021. p. 450–6.
52. Cannon MJ. Unusual tracheal foreign body in an African grey parrot. Vet Clin North Am Exot Anim Pract 2006;9(3):551–6.
53. Clayton LA, Ritzman TK. Endoscopic-assisted removal of a tracheal seed foreign body in a cockatiel (*Nymphicus hollandicus*). J Avian Med Surg 2005;19(1): 14–8, 15.
54. Santana CH, Oliveira AR, Carvalho TP, et al. Tracheal stenosis in a yellow-crowned parrot (A*mazona ochrocephala*) due to diffuse ossification and osteopetrosis of tracheal rings. J Comp Pathol 2023;204:7–10.
55. Marfatia S, Donahoe PK, Hendren WH. Effect of dry and humidified gases on the respiratory epithelium in rabbits. J pediatr surg 1975;10(5):583–92.
56. Sykes JMT, Neiffer D, Terrell S, et al. Review of 23 cases of postintubation tracheal obstructions in birds. J Zoo Wildl Med 2013;44(3):700–13.
57. Doneley B. Tracheal obstruction in parrots: an approach to diagnosis and treatment. Proceeding of the 19th AAVAC Annual Conference. 2011; Canberra. p. 123–128.
58. Byron-Chance D, Gomez L, Hollwarth AJ, et al. Outcomes and complications associated with caudal thoracic and abdominal air sac cannulation in 68 birds. J Avian Med Surg 2023;37(2):144–54.
59. Mejia-Fava J, Holmes SP, Radlinsky M, et al. Use of a nitinol wire stent for management of severe tracheal stenosis in an Eclectus parrot (*Eclectus roratus*). J Avian Med Surg 2015;29(3):238–49.
60. McClure SR, Taylor TS, Johnson JH, et al. Surgical repair of traumatically induced collapsing trachea in an ostrich. J Am Vet Med Assoc 1995;207(4):479–80.
61. Guzman DSM, Speer BL, Echols MS. Surgery of the respiratory tract. In: Speer B, van Zeeland YRA, editors. Current therapy in avian medicine and surgery volume II E-book: current therapy in avian medicine and surgery volume II E-book. Elsevier; 2025. p. p407–21.
62. Beaufrer H. Disease of the respiratory tract. In: Speer B, van Zeeland YRA, editors. Current therapy in avian medicine and surgery volume II E-book: current therapy in avian medicine and surgery volume II E-book. Elsevier; 2025. p. p395–406.
63. Westerhof I. Treatment of tracheal obstruction in psittacine birds using a suction technique: a retrospective study of 19 birds. J Avian Med Surg 1995;9(1):45–9.
64. Yaw TJ, Doss GA, Colopy SA, et al. Emergency tracheotomy and subsequent tracheal resection and anastomosis in a blue crane (*Anthropoides paradiseus*). J Am Vet Med Assoc 2020;256(11):1262–7.
65. Lennox A, Nemetz L. Tracheostomy in the avian patient. Semin avian Exotic Pet Med 2005;14:131–4.
66. Klaphake E, Beazley-Keane SL, Jones M, et al. Multisite integumentary squamous cell carcinoma in an African grey parrot (*Psittacus erithacus erithacus).* Vet rec 2006;158(17):593–6.
67. Suedmeyer WK, Henry C, McCaw D, et al. Attempted photodynamic therapy against patagial squamous cell carcinoma in an African rose-ringed parakeet (*Psittacula krameri*). J Zoo Wildl Med 2007;38(4):597–600.
68. Zehnder A, Swift L, Sundaram A, et al. Multi-institutional survey of squamous cell carcinoma in birds. In: Proceedings of the Annual Conference of the Association of Avian Veterinarian 2014 New Orleans (LA). p. 3.

69. Graham JE, Werner JA, Lowenstine LJ, et al. Periorbital liposarcoma in an African grey parrot (*Psittacus erithacus*). J Avian Med Surg 2003;17(3):147–53.
70. Castro PF, Fantoni DT, Miranda BC, et al. Prevalence of neoplastic diseases in pet birds referred for surgical procedures. Vet Med Int 2016;2016:4096801.
71. Reavill DR. Pet bird oncology. Proceding of the Annu 19th AAVAC Conference2011; Canberra. p. 105–122.
72. Filippich LJ. Tumor control in birds. Semin avian exotic pet med 2004;13(1): 25–43.
73. Megan L, Guzman DS, Keel K, et al. Prevalence, anatomical distribution, and risk factors of adipocytic tumors and xanthomas in psittaciformes: 1096 cases (1998-2018). J Avian Med Surg 2024;38(2):108–15.
74. Souza MJ, Johnstone-McLean NS, Ward D, et al. Conjunctival xanthoma in a blue and gold macaw (*Ara ararauna*). Vet ophthal 2009;12(1):53–5.
75. Adair JE, Riggs GL. Treatment of recurrent multifocal cutaneous squamous cell carcinoma in an African grey parrot (*Psittacus erithacus*) with intralesional carboplatin in poloxamer 407. J Avian Med Surg 2022;36(2):200–5.
76. Endo M, Lin PP. Surgical margins in the management of extremity soft tissue sarcoma. Chin clin oncol 2018;7(4):37.
77. Heslin MJ, Woodruff J, Brennan MF. Prognostic significance of a positive microscopic margin in high-risk extremity soft tissue sarcoma: implications for management. J clin oncol 1996;14(2):473–8.
78. Stojadinovic A, Leung DH, Hoos A, et al. Analysis of the prognostic significance of microscopic margins in 2,084 localized primary adult soft tissue sarcomas. Ann Surg 2002;235(3):424–34.
79. Bonvalot S, Levy A, Terrier P, et al. Primary extremity soft tissue sarcomas: does local control impact survival? Ann surg oncol 2017;24(1):194–201.
80. De Voe RS, Trogdon M, Flammer K. Preliminary assessment of the effect of diet and L-carnitine supplementation on lipoma size and bodyweight in budgerigars (*Melopsittacus undulatus*). J Avian Med Surg 2004;18(1):12–8.
81. Lipar M, Horvatek D, Prukner-Radovčić E, et al. Subcutaneous xanthoma in a cockatiel (*Nymphicus hollandicus*) - a case report. Veterinarski arhiv 2011; 81(4):535–43.
82. Lamberski N, Théon AP. Concurrent irradiation and intratumoral chemotherapy with cisplatin for treatment of a fibrosarcoma in a blue and gold macaw (*Ara ararauna*). J Avian Med Surg 2002;16(3):234–8.
83. Ramsay EC, Bos JH, McFadden C. Use of intratumoral cisplatin and orthovoltage radiotherapy in treatment of a fibrosarcoma in a macaw. J Assoc Avian Med 1993;7(2):87–90.
84. Bauck L. Radical surgery for the treatment of feather cysts in the canary. AAV Today 1987;1(5):200–1.
85. Hnilica KA, Patterson AP. Small animal dermatology-E-book: a color atlas and therapeutic guide. Elsevier Health Sciences; 2016.
86. Doneley B. Surgery. In: Doneley B, editor. Avian medicine and surgery in practice : companion and aviary birds. 2nd edition. London UK: CRC Press; 2016. p. 385–419.
87. Zaffarano B. The prolapsed cloaca (and all it contains). Proceeding of the NAVC Conference 2015. p. 1280–1282.
88. Apurva SRS, Bali AS. Manual Manipulation of egg in Indian parrot (A*lexandrian parakeet*) suffering from egg bound condition. The Science World a monthly e magazine 2022;2(11):1766–9.

89. Greenacre CB, Gerhardt L. Psittacine and passerine birds. In: Ballard B, Cheek R, editors. Exotic animal medicine for the veterinary technician. 2017. p. 43–72.
90. Bowles HL. Avian obstetrics I and II. proceeding of the The North American Veterinary Conference 2003 Windsor, CO. p. 1168–1174.
91. Forbes NA. Soft tissue surgery. In: Chitty J, Lierz M, editors. BSAVA manual of raptors, pigeons and passerine birds. BSAVA Library; 2008. p. 143–56.
92. Zaheer O, Beaufrère H, Jajou S, et al. Asymmetrical cloacoplasty for the treatment of chronic cloacal prolapse in Psittaciformes: a case series. J Avian Med Surg 2020;34(2):172–80.

Soft Tissue Surgery of Raptors and Columbiformes

Panagiotis Azmanis, DVM, PhD, DipECZM (Avian), Dip ZOOMED (RCVS)[a,*],
Daniel Calvo Carrasco, LV, CertAVP(ZM), DipECZM(Avian), MRCVS[b]

KEYWORDS

• Raptors • Columbiformes • Soft tissue surgery • Wound management
• Ingluviotomy • Propatagium • Imping • Pododermatitis

KEY POINTS

- Unique anatomic challenges: Avian soft tissue surgery is dictated by distinct anatomy, such as thin, friable skin with extensive skeletal attachments and a diffuse vasculature.
- Species-specific pathologies: Raptors suffer frequently with trauma from flight collisions and interactions, whereas Columbiformes commonly exhibit tissue deficits from predator attacks and ingluvial pathologies.
- Wound classification: Effective surgical planning relies on accurate classification based on etiology, contamination level (class I–IV), and the extension of the lesion.
- Reconstructive importance: Specific procedures like the cervical advancement flap for cranial defects and precise propatagial ligament repair are vital for restoring physiologic function and flight.
- Specialized techniques: Procedures such as imping, tendon repair, and falconry training are essential for physiotherapy and mental preparation for wild and captive raptors.

INTRODUCTION

Soft tissue surgery in avian patients presents a unique set of challenges dictated by distinct anatomy and species-specific physiology. This article focuses specifically on birds of prey and pigeons and present the most prevalent soft-tissue pathologies and their repair. The fundamental principles of the surgical approaches described herein are not exclusive to these orders and could be applied across the wider avian class.

Raptors are carnivorous species that actively hunt and feed on other vertebrates, primarily mammals, reptiles, and smaller birds. Raptors span a nonuniform taxonomic

[a] Dubai Falcon Hospital/ Wadi Al Safa Wildlife Center, Dubai, United Arab Emirates; [b] Veterinary Healthcare and Scientific Programmes, Bird Paradise, Mandai Wildlife Group, Singapore
* Corresponding author. Dubai Falcon Hospital, 22a Street, PO BOX23919, Zabeel 1, Dubai.
E-mail address: azmanis.vet@gmail.com

Vet Clin Exot Anim 29 (2026) 545–567
https://doi.org/10.1016/j.cvex.2026.06.001 vetexotic.theclinics.com
1094-9194/26/

Abbreviation	
CAF	cervical advancement flap

group, and includes birds from 4 different orders: Accipitriformes, Falconiformes, Strigiformes, and Cathartiformes.[1,2]

Raptors frequently present to veterinary clinics and rehabilitation centers with diverse soft-tissue pathologies requiring immediate surgical intervention: wing and body wounds from collisions or entanglement, embedded foreign bodies (hooks and line), crop impactions and infections, and penetrating coelomic injuries. Compared to domestic and pet birds, raptors are nature's athletes and as such require special attention to anesthetic risk, surgical intervention, and rehabilitation.[3]

The order Columbiformes—comprising more than 300 species of pigeons and doves—presents a diverse clinical caseload spanning from the miniature Diamond dove (*Geopelia cuneata*) to the huge Victoria Crowned Pigeon (*Goura victoria*).

Veterinary surgeons encounter these birds in multiple contexts: as high-performance racing athletes, valued companion animals, residents of zoologic institutions, and frequently as wildlife casualties. In contrast to the raptorial species previously discussed, columbids are ecologically defined as prey rather than predators, and are commonly affected by predatory attacks from raptors[4] or domestic carnivores. In fact, specific raptors such as the Peregrine falcon (*Falco peregrinus*) and the Eurasian sparrowhawk (*Accipiter nisus*) have evolved effective strategies specifically to hunt them[4] (**Fig. 1**). Anatomically, the most significant soft tissue feature of this order is the large, bilobulated crop (ingluvies).[5]

The goals of surgical treatment are stabilization, source control (debridement/removal of foreign material), restoration of integumentary continuity, and the return of normal physiologic function, thereby ensuring the welfare of birds and maximizing the release potential of free-living casualties.

PREOPERATIVE ASSESSMENT AND ANESTHESIA

A comprehensive triage and baseline diagnostics are essential to maximize successful outcomes. Key evaluations include body condition assessments, hydration,

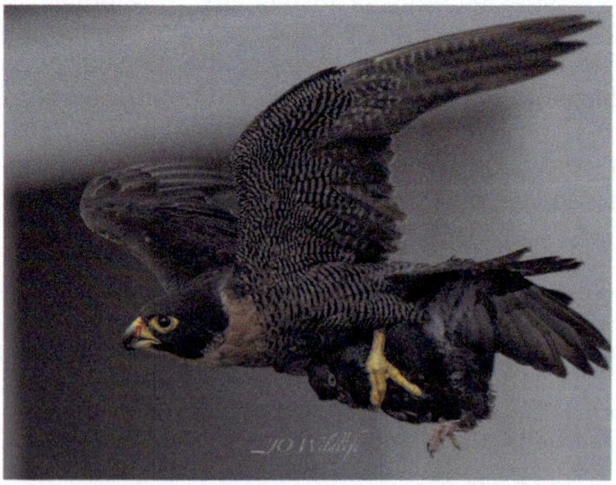

Fig. 1. The "Black Shaheen" or Ernest's Peregrine Falcon (*F peregrinus ernesti*) capturing his specialized aerial prey: a pigeon. (*Courtesy of* Alfred Wong.)

bloodwork (hematology and biochemistry) when feasible, radiographs for radiopaque foreign bodies or fractures, and assessments for concurrent injuries (eg, head trauma and pulmonary compromise). Where available, advanced imaging modalities such as ultrasonography, computed tomography, and fluoroscopy should also be considered to further evaluate soft tissue, internal structures, and complex injuries. It is important that life-threatening conditions,[6] particularly relevant for patients with trauma, are identified, if present, and treated, before addressing more obvious injuries such as wounds, that could be managed while the focus is on stabilization of the patient. Raptors and pigeons are at an increased risk of regurgitation and aspiration; fasting protocols and airway protection should be individualized based on species, body condition, and emergency status.[7] Anesthesia in raptors and pigeons is a major determinant of perioperative outcome and must account for avian respiratory anatomy (rigid lungs, air sacs), high metabolic rates, and species-specific responses to agents. Inhalational anesthesia with isoflurane or sevoflurane delivered in oxygen is commonly used for soft-tissue procedures; careful monitoring (capnography, pulse oximetry, electrocardiogram, and temperature) and preparedness for rapid airway or ventilatory support are required. Sedation protocols for short procedures can reduce risk when combined with local/regional blocks. Pre-emptive analgesia (opioids, nonsteroidal anti-inflammatory drugs where appropriate) should be instituted.[8]

Following patient stabilization, the focus shifts to wound assessment. To effectively perform this evaluation and classify the injury according to established grading scales, it is imperative that the clinician possesses a thorough understanding of both the avian anatomy and the specific physiology of the wound healing process.

AVIAN INTEGUMENT

The avian skin is thinner and more friable than in mammals. It is attached to the muscles in relatively few places, but has extensive attachments to the skeleton, for example, in the limbs. The skin is composed of 2 main anatomic layers, the epidermis and the dermis. The epidermis is entirely avascular with its nutrition derived from the dermis via simple diffusion in areas of thin skin or structural adaptations in thicker more active regions. The dermis comprises fibrous connective tissue with blood vessels, nerves, sensory corpuscles, tendons, smooth muscles linking together feather tracts (apterial muscles), and ectodermal feather follicles with numerous attendant smooth muscles (feather muscles) that subtend the feathers. Avian collagen resembles mammalian collagen; however, fibrils of collagen are neatly arranged in a horizontal orientation with a few vertical fibrils, which creates a much thinner dermis, which contributes to weight reduction and cutaneous pliability during flight.[9]

In birds, the cutaneous vasculature is diffuse, with arteries and veins primarily branching within the deep dermis and forming anastomoses, while arterial-venous connections are limited and aid thermoregulation. Cutaneous arteries supply feather follicles and associated muscles, with major flight feathers having separate radial and ulnar arterial supply, and vessels cross feather tracts randomly. Cutaneous nerves accompany these vessels, supplying sensory and motor fibers to the skin, dermis, and cutaneous muscles, without following feather follicle patterns.[9]

Stages of Wound Healing

Wound healing in mammals is described through 5 stages though in birds (mostly studied in chicken) only 3 distinct have been described and studied: the inflammatory, the proliferative (collagen), and the maturation. The inflammatory stage begins immediately after injury, involving vasoconstriction, vasodilation, and immune cell infiltration to remove debris and bacteria, ending with fibroblast appearance. The proliferative (collagenic) stage starts 3 to 4 days after injury, with fibroblasts producing collagen fibers, new capillaries forming, and epithelial cells migrating over the wound. The maturation stage lasts weeks to months, with collagen remodeling, fiber strengthening, and reduced fibroblast numbers. Healing speed in both birds and mammals depends on factors like contamination, tissue damage, nutrition, vascular supply, and wound care.[10]

Wound Assessment and Classification

Accurate classification of soft tissue injuries is the cornerstone of effective surgical planning. Given the unique properties of the avian integument, specifically its limited elasticity, in specific areas, and rapid metabolic response, wounds must be evaluated not only by their gross appearance but also by their underlying etiology and bacterial burden. The following table (**Table 1**) consolidates the standard veterinary wound classification systems, integrating the degree of contamination with species-specific injury patterns commonly observed in raptors and Columbiformes to guide appropriate therapeutic intervention.

Wound Lavage/Debridement/Closure

Initial steps

Primary management mandates systemic stabilization followed by copious sterile isotonic lavage and meticulous sharp debridement of nonviable tissue under general anesthesia whenever possible. Antiseptic lavage (chlorhexidine 0.05%) has support in the literature[18] for avian wounds is commonly used. Sharp debridement with preservation of viable tissue and maintaining feather follicle integrity, when possible, optimizes healing.[18]

Closure strategy

When contamination is minimal and tissue viability is good, immediate primary closure for contaminated wounds may be attempted. More commonly, delayed primary or secondary closure is elected. Topical therapies (moist wound dressings, advanced wound-healing agents) have been used but water exposure and wild bird housing constraints must be considered for raptors.[18]

Case series/outcomes

Multiple retrospective series document favorable outcomes when early, aggressive debridement and appropriate antimicrobial/analgesic therapy are provided; prognosis depends on extent of tissue loss, contamination, and whether underlying structures (tendons and joints) are involved.[18]

Principles of Avian Soft-tissue Surgery

The principles of soft tissue surgery in birds have been reviewed extensively in recent literature.[19] General principles mirror those in other species, but the clinician should always consider the summarized points in **Table 2**. For further reading on these aspects, please consult the relevant references.[19–22]

Specific Procedures

Trauma-related injuries: wound management and soft tissue repair

Traumatic defects of the integument and deep soft tissues constitute a primary cause of veterinary admission for avian patients. Clinical presentations are variable and may be classified by morphology or etiology, including simple lacerations, extensive crush injuries, thermal burns, and severe necrosis resulting from self-mutilation or

Table 1
Wound classification

Classification System	Category/ Grade	Description and Clinical Management	Key References
I. Etiologic Classification (Based on Mechanism of Injury)	Traumatic lacerations	Acute defects from collisions or predation. Range from epithelial damage to muscle tearing	Redig (2000)[11]
	Puncture wounds	Deep tracts masking underlying damage (eg, cat bites and talons). High infection risk	Cousquer (2003)[12]
	Degloving injuries	Extensive skin separation; common in Columbiformes due to skin fragility ("fright molt" defense)	Bennett (1997)[13]
	Constriction injuries	Ischemic necrosis from entanglement (fibers and hair)	Harcourt-Brown (2002)[14]
II. Surgical Classification (Based on Contamination Level)	Class I: Clean	Aseptic, nontraumatic incisions (eg, lipoma removal)	Fossum (2018)[15]
	Class II: Clean-contaminated	Entry into hollow viscera (eg, Ingluviotomy) with controlled contamination	Fossum (2018)[15]
	Class III: Contaminated	Fresh traumatic wounds (4–6 h) or open fractures	Cousquer (2003)[12]
	Class IV: Dirty/ Infected	Old wounds (6–8 h), devitalized tissue, or predator bites	Fossum (2018)[15]
III. Healing Mechanism	Primary closure	Immediate suturing for clean/ fresh wounds	Bennett (1997)[13]
	Delayed primary/ secondary	Staged debridement or granulation for contaminated/large defects	Redig (2000)[11]
IV. Pododermatitis	Types I–V	Graded from epithelial thinning (I) to osteomyelitis (V)	Remple (1993)[16]
V. Extension of the Lesion	Superficial wounds	Protocol: Clean + topical antimicrobial (silver sulfadiazine/triple Abx) + nonadherent pad + transparent adhesive film (eg, Tegaderm). Follow-up: Reassessment/bandage change in 2–3 d	Martel & Mans (2021)[17]
	Full-thickness wounds	Protocol: Requires extensive bandaging. Tie-over dressings (suture loops + umbilical tape) preferred for waterfowl/ parrots. Topicals: Deep wounds filled with hydrogel/ hydrocolloid. Ionic silver hydrogels (gel/sheets) frequently used to allow	Martel & Mans (2021)[17]

(continued on next page)

Table 1
(*continued*)

Classification System	Category/ Grade	Description and Clinical Management	Key References
		prolonged intervals between changes (reducing stress). Contraindications: Drains rarely used (minimal exudate). Wet-to-dry bandages rarely used (too bulky/frequent changes). Honey/sugar use limited by mess/location	

infection.[25] In both birds of prey and pigeons, a significant number of soft tissue pathologies requiring surgical intervention are directly attributable to traumatic injuries.[26] This prevalence is inextricably linked to the distinct behavioral and ecological niches these groups occupy. For raptors, the physical demands of predation and high-velocity flight predispose them to collision and capture-related trauma, whereas pigeons frequently present with extensive soft tissue deficits sustained during evasion or attacks by predators.

In the author's experience (PA), wounds in raptors can be further related to falconry-managed raptors and free-living raptors. Falconry raptors often suffer wound injuries in their hack pens, in their tethering areas, from their jesses (if inappropriate size) as well as injuries during the hunting, for example, degloving injuries of the head or

Table 2
Avian soft tissue basic principles

Category	Key Considerations and Requirements
Clinical expertise	The clinician must possess a deep familiarity with avian-specific anatomy and physiology, particularly how the avian healing process differs from mammals to select the most suitable surgical techniques
Equipment and technique	Precision is mandatory. Use of microsurgical instruments, surgical loupes, or operating microscopes is recommended to minimize tissue trauma to improve outcomes and recovery times[19–22]
Hemostasis	Critical priority. While birds have a higher relative tolerance for blood loss than some mammals, their small absolute body size means even minor hemorrhage can be life-threatening, and should therefore be minimized using appropriate hemostatic equipment[19,23,24]
Wound assessment	Focus on contamination levels and tissue viability. In wild birds (especially raptors), wounds often present late, necessitating staged management (debridement, lavage, and delayed closure)
Closure strategy	Primary closure is ideal for clean, viable tissue. However, secondary intention or delayed primary closure is frequently required due to high contamination and significant tissue loss
Materials and patterns	Use monofilament sutures (6–0 to 2–0). Tension-reducing patterns like vertical mattress or cruciate are vital to prevent dehiscence. Staples or adhesives may be used as adjuncts

propatagium, puncture wounds by other birds. Moreover, during training raptors might collide with the falconer stooping toward the lure or get "slashing" injuries (linear lacerations) of the chest, the head, the back and toe amputation from the blades of the drones (**Fig. 2**). During molting, raptors kept in communal enclosures (hacking molting pens) might attack each other, or in case the species are not compatible even kill each other. On the other hand, free-living raptors commonly suffer from collisions—blunt trauma (buildings, wind turbines, barbed wire, road traffic), electrocutions, and illegal shotgun wounds.

Classically, the "'golden 'period" for primary closure was defined as the first 6 to 8 hours after injury.[27] However, current veterinary consensus suggests that the degree of contamination and tissue viability are more accurate predictors of outcome than the time elapsed since injury alone.[15] This distinction is particularly relevant for avian wildlife casualties, which frequently present well beyond this traditional timeframe. As noted by Cousquer,[12] strict adherence to time-based rules is often impractical in these patients; instead, they require management strategies that focus on aggressive debridement and wound bed preparation to facilitate successful delayed primary closure. Bite wounds inflicted by dogs and particularly cats are common in avian species, including pigeons.[26]

Medically, bite wounds are classified as contaminated[28] and high-risk due to the deep inoculation of oral flora,[29] necessitating treatment[30] with a high index of suspicion even in the absence of immediate signs. Furthermore, these animals can carry a broad spectrum of zoonotic bacteria[31,32] making it important to understand the diversity of microbial pathogens that may be transmitted to those in contact with them. Mechanically, talon injuries from birds of prey present a parallel challenge. While the initial bacterial load on a talon may be lower than that of the oral cavity, the mechanism of deep tissue puncture creates a similar environment for potential infection. Crucially, the clinician must be aware that the microbial flora of the feet differs significantly

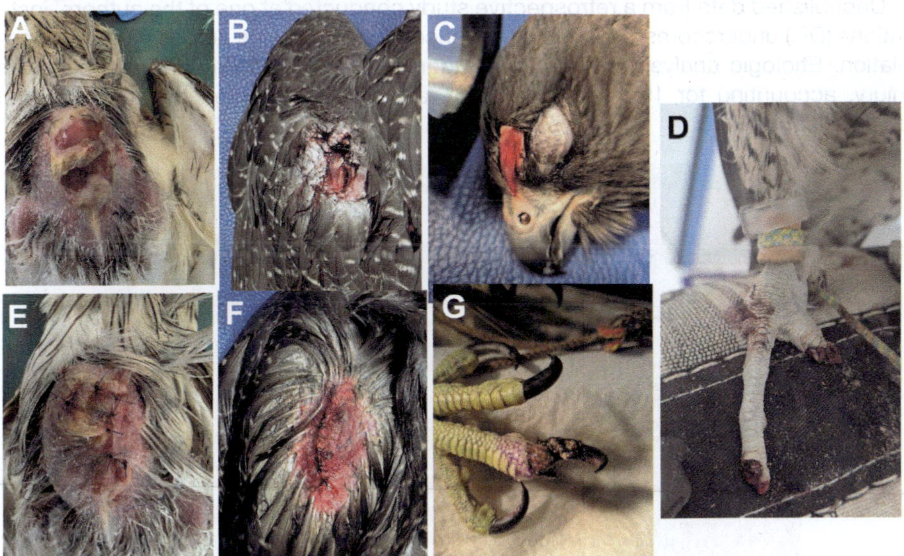

Fig. 2. (*A–G*) Drone propeller injuries. Upper row: Lacerations (*A*) chest, (*B*) dorsal deep biceps, (*C*) eyebrow, and (*D*) toe amputations. Lower row: same injuries after surgical repair (*E–G*).

between captive and free-ranging raptors, with *Staphylococcus aureus* being prevalent in captive environments but rare in healthy wild populations[33,34] complicating the selection of empirical antimicrobial therapy.

The location, extension, complexity, and severity of the injury observed in traumatic injuries will vary widely between individual patients. However, provided the clinician possesses a solid command of the foundational principles previously outlined—specifically the anatomic and physiologic particularities of birds of prey and pigeons, the mechanics of wound healing, and appropriate wound classification—they will be equipped to establish an accurate prognosis and formulate an effective treatment plan for any unique presentation. With this framework in place, the authors have selected a series of commonly encountered injuries, organized by anatomic location and clinical presentation, to illustrate recommended surgical approaches and management strategies.

Head Wounds/Cranial Skin Defects

Injuries to the calvarium can occur in both wild populations and birds under human care, typically resulting from trauma or aggression. The clinical presentation, progression, and management of cranial wounds are intrinsically linked to their etiology, though the decision-making process is rarely binary. Acute impact trauma typically results in degloving injuries where the skin flap remains viable; if addressed early, these defects can often be repaired by simple lavage and reapposition (**Fig. 3**). However, if this same injury presents late, retraction and desiccation of the scalp may render simple apposition impossible. In contrast, wounds resulting from repeated conspecific aggression are characterized by progressive necrosis, often evolving over days, which frequently results in significant tissue loss. Ultimately, the surgical approach cannot be dictated by the mechanism of injury alone but must be determined by a multifactorial assessment that weighs the etiology against the wound's chronicity, the degree of contraction, and the viability of the remaining integument.

Unpublished data from a retrospective study conducted at one of the authors' institutions (DC) underscores the clinical relevance of these injuries across a diverse population. Etiologic analysis revealed that aggression was the predominant cause of injury, accounting for 19 cases, while 15 cases were attributed to other forms of trauma (**Table 3**).

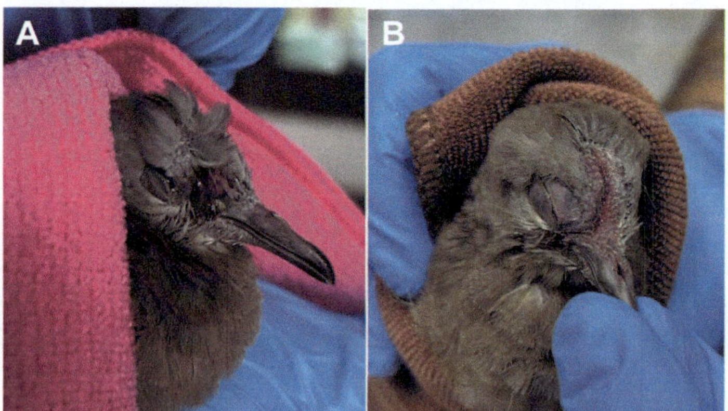

Fig. 3. Fresh head laceration on a wild juvenile eastern spotted dove (*Spilopelia chinensis*). The laceration was located craniodorsally of the right eye (*A*) and was repaired using tissue glue (*B*) with good apposition. (*Courtesy of* Dr D. Calvo Carrasco.)

While simple soft tissue lacerations can be managed by primary closure or might even heal spontaneously, injuries involving cranial exposure frequently progress to chronic, nonhealing wounds.[35,36] This occurs because the exposed, devitalized bone acts as a physical barrier that actively impedes the formation of granulation tissue and epithelial migration.[37,38] Additionally, management is complicated by changes in tissue mechanics: although the calvarial cutis is typically mobile, chronic inflammatory cascades induce marginal fibrosis, resulting in firm adherence to the underlying calvarium.[39,40] This acquired loss of elasticity and mobility renders primary or secondary closure of large defects increasingly difficult. The overall therapeutic choices are summarized in **Table 4**.

Dorsal cervical single pedicle advancement flaps have been well-described for the reconstruction of cranial defects, particularly in larger birds of prey,[25] though the technique was originally detailed across 3 diverse species: the Ring-necked pheasant (*Phasianus colchicus*), Rock dove (*Columba livia*), and Red-tailed hawk (*Buteo jamaicensis*).[41] One author (PA) has used it successfully also to ornamental pheasant species as well as francolins and partridges. The surgical procedure, as described by Gentz,[41] Sanchez-Migallon,[19] and others,[25] involves the elevation of a single pedicle flap via straight or slightly divergent incisions extending caudally from the debrided wound margin (**Fig. 4**).

In the authors' experience (DC), the initial incision length should be at least 1.5 times the length of the defect, consistent with Gentz's recommendations; however, this length may be extended intraoperatively based on tissue tension assessment. Regarding incision geometry, divergent incisions are specifically recommended to broaden the pedicle base, thereby maximizing vascular supply and minimizing the risk of distal flap necrosis. Furthermore, clinicians must carefully evaluate the width of the flap and its proximity to the periocular region. It is the excessive width of the flap or its proximity to the orbits (rather than the incision technique itself) that most frequently results in tension on the upper eyelids, potentially causing distortion or visual impairment. In cases where such tension is inevitable, both authors recommend a staged repair with subsequent tension-relieving procedures.

In the retrospective study conducted by the one of the authors (DC), 63.3% of the presentation cohort required surgical intervention. Among those treated surgically for head wounds, 54.8% underwent a cervical advancement flap (CAF) procedure. Results can be seen in **Table 5**. Consistent with complications described in small animal reconstructive surgery, necrosis of the distal flap tip was the most frequently encountered complication[42] (**Table 6**).

Tendon injuries

Tendon injuries are uncommon in raptors but still require immediate intervention and additional postoperative care. Mostly, the tendons of the hallux or the first/second

Table 3
Prevalence of head injuries in an institute

Order	Percentage (%)
Columbiformes	55
Psittaciformes	17
Galliformes	10

(*Data Courtesy* The data has been taken from Dr D. Calvo Carrasco.)

Table 4
Therapeutic management options according to severity

Severity Grade	Treatment Option	Indication
1	Conservative management	For superficial injuries where soft tissue coverage of the skull remains intact or the defect is minimal
2	Primary closure	For acute wounds where there is no significant loss of integument (use of tissue glue, simple interrupted or horizontal mattress sutures)
3	Advancement flaps	For chronic, nonhealing wounds or lesions where extensive necrosis precludes direct apposition

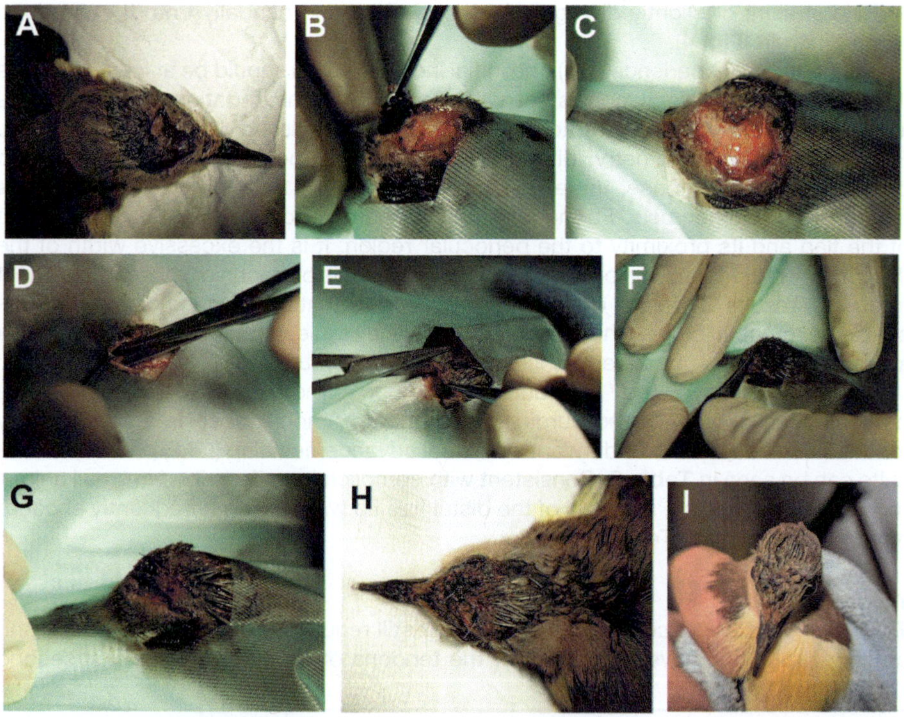

Fig. 4. (*A–I*) Serial images of cervical advancement flap procedure in a Cinnamon ground dove (*Gallicolumba rufigula*) with a traumatic head wound following wound breakdown after a previous surgical repair. (*A*) Appearance of the wound with the skull exposed. (*B*) Removal of debris, scabs, and necrotic tissue followed by debridement of the wound. (*C*) Appearance of the wound following debridement. (*D*) Blunt dissection of the adhesions formed between the skin and underlying soft tissue structures. (*E*) Two lateral incisions extending caudally can be performed with scissors or a blade. (*F*) Testing the apposition to evaluate tension on the surgical site. (*G*) Horizontal mattress sutures are first placed in the rostral edge of the flap. (*H*) Appearance of the flap postsurgically. (*I*) appearance of the wound 10 days after surgery. (*Courtesy of* Dr D. Calvo Carrasco.)

Table 5
Surgical outcome in head injuries after cervical advancement flap

Clinical Outcome Assessment	Percentage (%)	Healing
Favorable	72	Single procedure
Partial favorable	25	Multiple procedures
Unfavorable	3	Death during treatment

(*Data Courtesy* The data has been taken from Dr D. Calvo Carrasco.)

digits are presented in falconry raptors. Tendon injuries might result from prey bite wound, secondary infection or accidental injury. The bird should be admitted directly to the hospital and surgery should be applied immediately after stabilization. Procedural delays frequently result in proximal or distal muscular contraction and tendon retraction within the sheath, significantly complicating surgical localization and tension-free reapposition. Various techniques have been described[49–51] (**Fig. 5**), but there is no controlled study to prove the advantages or disadvantages of each one. Tendon surgery requires excellent microsurgical skills and equipment,[52,53] and common complications are tendon sheath infection, rerupturing, and neural mechanical

Table 6
Other skin flaps and skin grafts

Type of Graft	Species	Clinical Description and Outcome	Reference
Xenograft: Porcine small intestinal submucosa	2 Barn owls, an Umbrella cockatoo, and an American crow	Wounds healed within 6 wk in all 4 birds, with less intensive wound management than that required for healing by second intention. All birds returned to normal function	Hernandez,[43] 2003 JAMS
Xenograft: Fish skin (tilapia) extracellular matrix	1 Marabou stork	Healing was complete after 4 wk	Qabazard et al,[44] JZWM 2024
Nonmesh, full-thickness skin autograft	1 Bald Eagle	After 6 wk, the bird had new feather growth on its dorsal head and was released	Kane JAMS[45] 2019
Full-thickness mesh autograft	1 Ostrich, 2 Great-horned owls	Inguinal fold was used as excision site in both owls. Complete healing was achieved after 2 mo	Hannon et al,[46] 1993 JZWM; Jonhson et al,[47] 1994 JAVMA
Full-thickness allograft	Chickens	Only performed on specific genetic lines in laboratory studies, systematic rejection of the graft	Dietrich et al,[48] 1996

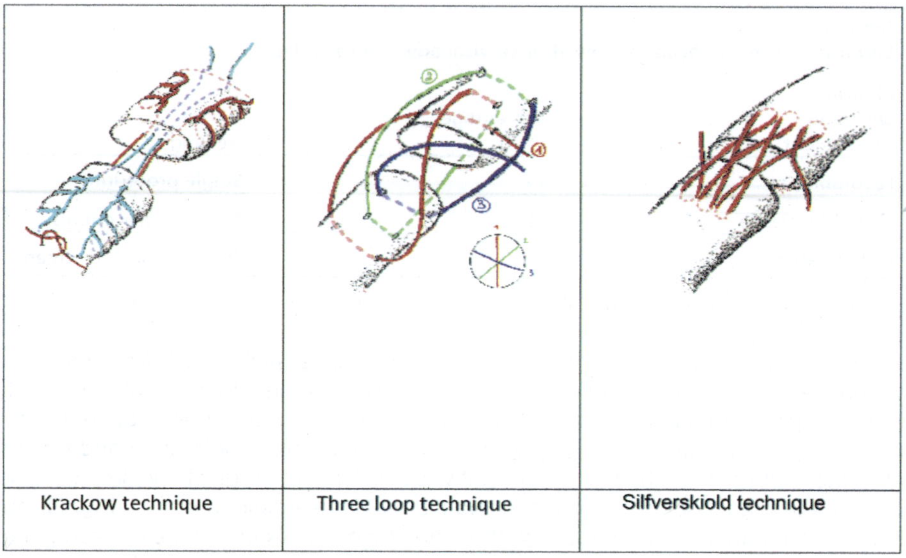

Fig. 5. Different tendon repair suture techniques. (*Courtesy of* Dr P. Azmanis.)

dysfunction after repair. Raptors often feel neuropathic pain and self-mutilate; therefore, a protective hood must be applied for the first week postsurgically.

Propatagium lacerations

This tendon deserves special attention due to its primary clinical importance in flight, which can critically impact its release and survival. The propatagium extends as a triangular fold between the shoulder and the carpus. The propatagium is a dermal bilayer and consists of separate dorsal and ventral layers of fully developed, representative avian integument.[52] Crucially, the leading edge of this structure encloses the propatagial ligament (*ligamentum propatagiale longus*), a collagenous and elastic band responsible for maintaining the tension and airfoil shape necessary for lift generation during flight. Structurally, the *ligamentum propatagiale* is a composite tissue consisting of a central elastic segment-the pars elastica-bordered by proximal and distal collagenous bands, with the specific transition points between these tissue types occurring at variable distances from the shoulder and carpus depending on the species.

Injuries to the propatagium are commonly encountered in free-ranging birds, with general etiologies including collisions with barbed wire fences, predator attacks, and entanglement. A distinct and high-morbidity etiology is the injury caused by abrasive kite strings, known locally as "Manja" encountered mostly in South Asia (India), while sporadic cases occur globally.[54] These strings are often coated with crushed glass, metal, or chemical adhesives to increase their cutting ability. The majority of affected birds are domestic pigeons (*C livia*), followed by Black kites (*Milvus migrans*), but a wide range of species could be affected as endangered vulture species and Magnificent frigatebird (*Fregata magnificens*; **Table 7**, **Fig. 6**).[54–56]

Ingluviotomy, ingluvectomy, and traumatic crop lacerations

Crop disease in raptors (sour crop, chronic impaction, diphtheroid trichomoniasis, and foreign material) can be life-threatening. Medical management (crop lavage, antifungals, antiprotozoals, antibiotics, and supportive care) is first-line when feasible, but

Table 7
General guidelines and recommendations for propatagial tendon repair

Sequence of Actions	Aim	Clinical Description and Outcome	Clinical Note
1	Managing contraction and ligament integrity	Critical surgical objective: Anatomic restoration of the cranial leading edge containing the *ligamentum propatagiale*	Clinical experience suggests that certain species and individuals may tolerate a minor degree of shortening without permanent flightlessness
2	Handling the propatagial ligament	The authors of this review advocate for a less invasive approach than in the past.[57] There is generally no need to isolate or dissect the ligament from the surrounding tissue	The *pars elastica* is readily palpable as a distinct, thickened band within the wound bed and can be effectively sutured "en bloc" with the surrounding adherent tissues. This modification minimizes additional trauma and preserves the vascular supply to the healing ligament
3	Surgical technique and layered closure	*Author (DC) recommends dorsal recumbency and initiation from the ventral aspect*	Leading edge alignment: Re-establish the continuity of the propatagial margin first to anchor the repair
			Deep soft tissue repair: Identify and appose other compromised structures, such as severed muscle bellies or the elbow extension limiting ligament, if affected
			Two-layer skin closure: The integument requires a double-layer closure. The author recommends suturing the ventral skin first to ensure accurate alignment before rotating the wing (if necessary) to address the dorsal surface
4	Postoperative management following reconstruction	A figure-of-8 bandage should be applied for approximately 10 d	
		After bandage removal, patients will require a structured physical therapy (passive and active ROM) under anesthesia	

(*continued on next page*)

Table 7 (*continued*)			
Sequence of Actions	**Aim**	**Clinical Description and Outcome**	**Clinical Note**
		Final rehabilitation: Cage staging or falconry training for several weeks to gain stamina, full range of motion (ROM) and maneuverability	

surgical intervention (ingluviotomy or partial ingluvectomy) is indicated for obstructive impactions, necrotic crop tissue, or penetrative foreign bodies. Surgical technique, if endoscopic removal fails, emphasizes sterile exposure of the crop, limited mucosal incision, removal of debris/foreign body, and careful mucosal and skin closure to

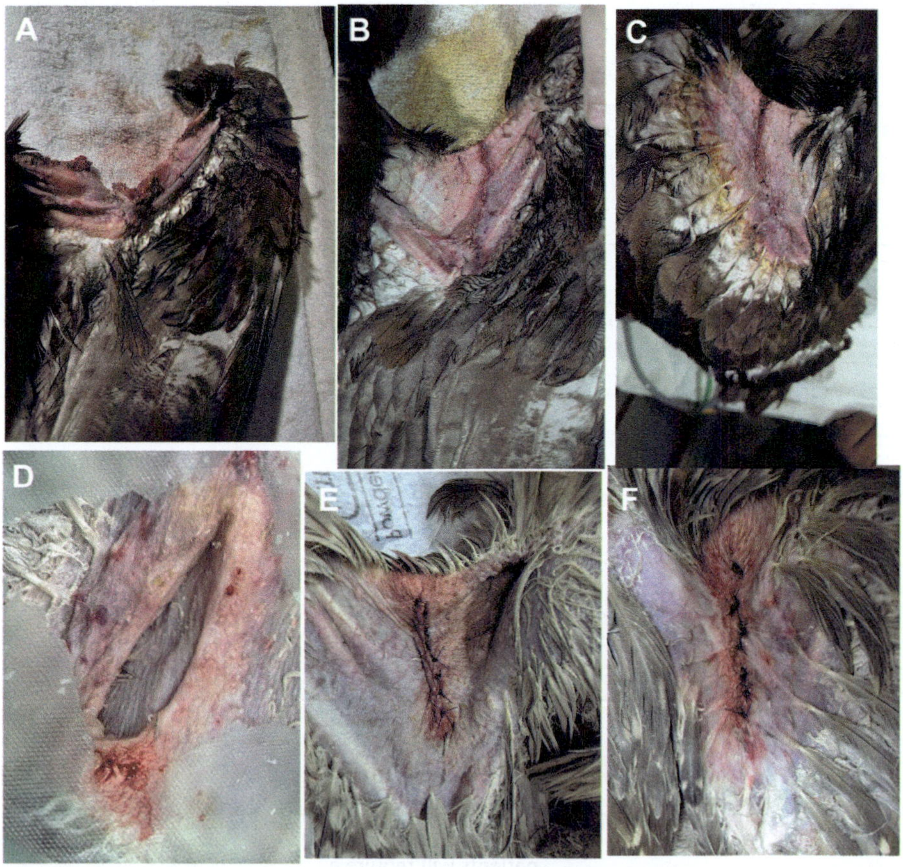

Fig. 6. (*A–F*) Upper row: (*A*) String-related injury on the propatagium of a Black kite (*M migrans*); Ventral (*B*) and dorsal (*C*) aspect of the surgical site following repair. Lower row: chronic drone-related propatagial tear in a Gyrfalcon (*Falco rusticolus*) (*D*); Ventral (*E*) and dorsal (*F*) aspect of the surgical site following repair. (Image (A–C) *Courtesy of* Dr D. Calvo Carasco. Image (E, F) *Courtesy of* Dr P. Azmanis.)

minimize stricture and leakage. Postoperative feeding protocols (small, frequent, easily digestible meals, and monitoring for crop motility) are critical. A postoperative esophageal stenosis in a Harris hawk (*Parabuteo unicinctus*) has been managed successfully with the use of an esophagostomy tube and the gradual application of a high-pressure balloon (Luparello pers com, Azmanis and colleagues in submission). Published case series and reviews describe good outcomes with prompt surgery and attentive postoperative care.[58]

Traumatic crop lacerations are a relatively common lesion observed following impact or window collisions during flight.[59] A study in Brazil identified this injury in 6 animals, with the majority being Columbiformes. This presentation has also been noted in the Kererū, a large native New Zealand species,[59,60] and it has been mentioned by some authors[61] to be very common in pigeons. These authors theorize that "because when [the] crop is filled with food, it expands and touches the skin, even a small concussion can result in its injury." This theory is also suspected by 1 author (PA) in 5 cases of crop injuries after window collision in wild Wood pigeons (*Columba palumbus*) in a city park. Injuries in young birds have also been reported,[61–64] where the trauma is not always witnessed. In these cases, potential causes include foreign bodies[61] and predatory attacks, as well as well-known iatrogenic causes such as tube feeding injuries or thermal necrosis from hot formula administration.

Unpublished data from a preliminary 5 year retrospective study at one of the authors' institutions (DC) identified 26 cases, of which 24 were Columbiformes and 2 were Psittaciformes. Anecdotally, 8 cases were also seen in wildlife casualties, all of which were Columbiformes.

The fundamental principles of crop closure remain consistent whether the defect results from an elective ingluviotomy a chronic fistula, or acute trauma. However, tissue preparation varies by etiology: while clean surgical incisions typically require no modification, traumatic lacerations and fistulas mandate the debridement or 'freshening' of wound edges to expose viable tissue prior to suturing. Anatomically, as a distensible diverticulum of the esophagus, the crop possesses a high tolerance for tissue loss. Nevertheless, clinicians should note that significant resection may reduce the organ's functional volume, thereby limiting the amount of ingesta the patient can consume in a single feeding.

Regarding technique, 1 article[61] evaluated closing in 2 layers versus 1 layer and glue, finding that 2 layers is superior (as previously hypothesized). Some authors recommend closing the crop with a layered closure. Guzman recommends using 5-0 or 6-0 monofilament absorbable suture in a continuous pattern, with a second inverting continuous pattern if required to ensure complete closure.[19] Other authors recommend a single or double-layer continuous pattern but do not consider an inverting closure necessary.[63]

Postoperative complications appear relatively common in Columbiformes, particularly when compared to other species. In the authors' experience, complications are more frequent when closure is delayed; outcomes are superior when the patient is presented shortly after trauma and surgery is performed within the first 24 hours, provided the patient is stable enough to undergo general anesthesia. This contrasts with the delayed surgical repair usually recommended for crop burn fistulas, where the assessment of tissue viability cannot be performed immediately.

Complications such as wound dehiscence, ingluvitis, and septicemia have been reported and appear relatively common. Consequently, the authors recommend early surgical repair for traumatic crop ruptures while concurrently controlling potential secondary bacterial and protozoal infections (commonly *Trichomonas* spp; **Fig. 7**).

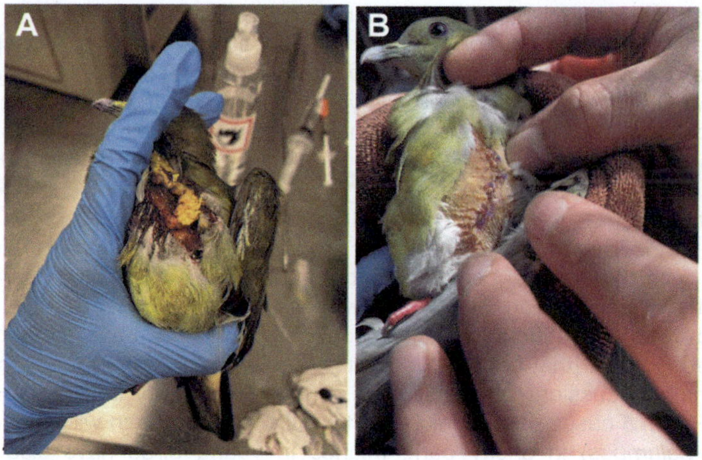

Fig. 7. (*A*, *B*) (*A*, left) Traumatic Crop Rupture in a pink-necked green pigeon (*Treron vernans*); (*B*, right) appearance 10 days postoperative repair performed as an early intervention in 2 layers. (*Courtesy of* Dr D. Calvo Carasco.)

Separately, crop resection has been reported to treat crop ptosis (pendulous crop).[65] However, the authors of this review would caution against this approach. Surgical resection treats the clinical signs but does not address the underlying cause. Delayed crop emptying and secondary pendulous crop are common conditions with various etiologies—particularly in young animals[66] (sometimes called young pigeon disease)—which should be addressed medically rather than surgically.

Keel injuries

Traumatic injuries to the keel are commonly observed in birds with impaired flight capabilities, such as pinioned individuals, or in debilitated, recumbent patients as well as overexcited untrained tethered raptors that hit the ground. These injuries often present as splitting wounds that compromise the skin and underlying soft tissues. While small, superficial defects may be managed conservatively and allowed to heal by secondary intention, larger wounds typically mandate surgical debridement of the necrotic skin, pectoral muscle, and affected bone.

For moderate defects, closure is achieved by suturing the pectoral muscles together over the carina or anchoring them directly to the keel bone, followed by primary skin apposition (**Fig. 8**). However, extensive defects may require reconstruction using a cutaneous axial pattern flap. As described by Ferrell,[9] this technique involves creating 2 lateral thoracic incisions and elevating a flap that preserves the caudal external thoracic artery and vein at its base. The flap is then advanced cranially with minimal tension to cover the defect; the cranial and caudal edges are sutured to the respective corners of the wound, and the remaining margins are closed routinely. Clinicians must be vigilant during the postoperative period, as self-mutilation is a complication frequently observed in birds of prey; these cases can be particularly challenging to manage and often require strict protection of the surgical site.

Imping

Imping[67] refers to the procedure of replacing broken rectrices and remiges (primary and tail feathers). This long-known falconry mastery technique allows the raptor to further hunt or continue its training while it speeds up tremendously the rehabilitation

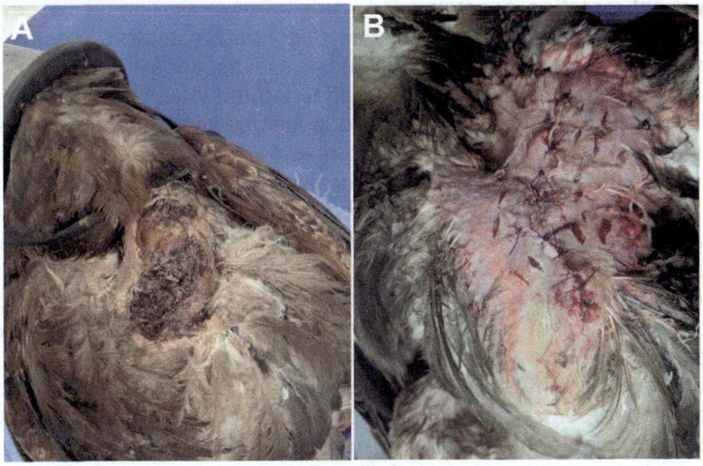

Fig. 8. (*A, B*) Chronic keel injury before (*A*) and after surgical repair and use of relief scarring (*B*) in a Harris hawk. (*Courtesy of* Dr P. Azmanis.)

time of injured wild raptors reducing nosocomial infections or muscle atrophy due to long hospitalization.

The adequate feathers (left or right wing, color, and length) must be obtained by a dead raptor or from a previous molt and adequately preserved until the time to be used. The traumatized feather is cut proximally to its injury, and an internal splint is placed on the cranial feather shaft. The internal splint can be a bamboo stick, a needle, or commercial titanium rods according to the diameter of the shaft. A new feather is measured to the right height and length, and it is fitted on the dorsal aspect of the splint. The overall adaptability, direction, and stability are tested before superglue will be applied on the borders of the attachment. The spot will be dried up with some powder to avoid glue spreading to the adjacent feathers. The stages can be seen in **Fig. 9**.

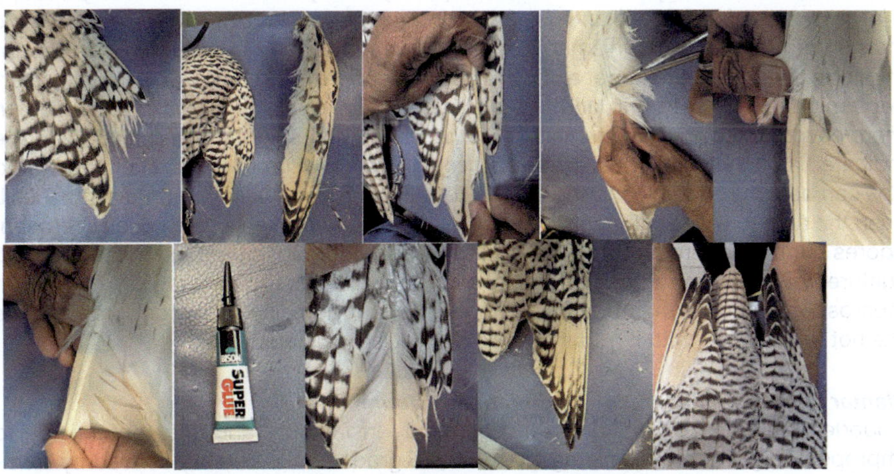

Fig. 9. Imping procedure of the primary feathers of the right wing of a Gyrfalcon. Sequence from upper left to lower right. (*Courtesy of* Dr P. Azmanis.)

Repair intestinal resection–anastomosis

Intestinal resection–anastomosis has been described in raptors mostly to remove foreign bodies (eg, lead fragments and increased ascarids load blockage)[68,69] as well as in rare cases of puncture wounds affecting the intestinal loops with possible risk of peritonitis. The surgical approach and technique itself do not present significant differences than in other species and performed as in the small animals, with care of not flushing the intestinal volume with excessive saline due to the air sac system. Some larger raptors may have increased abdominal fat that might hinder the abdominal approach and the location of the specific loop where the foreign body is located.

Intestinal resection–anastomosis in raptors is primarily indicated for removing foreign bodies, such as lead fragments or obstructive ascarid loads,[68,69] and for treating puncture wounds that carry a risk of peritonitis. Clinical reports have expanded these indications to include complex conditions like ileo-ceco-rectal intussusception, as documented in a Tawny eagle (*Aquila rapax*),[70] and advanced cases of cloacal prolapse where the prolapsed intestinal tissue has become necrotic or devitalized. Although the surgical technique for end-to-end anastomosis, often using 5-0 or 6-0 monofilament absorbable suture, is fundamentally similar to small animal practice, specific avian anatomic constraints must be addressed. A technique was described by Dutton and colleagues,[71] in which sterile, semirigid rubber tubing was placed in the distal colon and removed per-cloaca at the end of the procedure; this facilitated a secure, fluid-tight anastomosis while maintaining sufficient intestinal lumen.

Excessive coelomic fat in larger raptors can significantly hinder the initial abdominal approach and the identification of the affected bowel loop. Most critically, clinicians must avoid flushing the coelom with excessive saline due to the unique interconnected air sac system, which presents a high risk of fluid entry into the respiratory tract. Despite the complexity of these cases, timely surgical intervention can lead to successful clinical outcomes and the eventual release of the bird back into the wild.

Removal of foreign bodies and granulomas from lower respiratory tract (air sac)

Raptors often suffer from bacterial and fungal infections. Aspergillosis is a common fungal disease, which evolves to granuloma formation in the air sacs.[72] Debulking and debridement of granulomas is a common indication for laparoscopic surgery. Granulomas are mostly removed endoscopically if they are small, but if they occupy a larger space of the air sac an open laparotomy is necessary. The normal endoscopic incision at first might be enlarged dorsally and ventrally and a small vaginal dilatator might be used to create larger exit. Crocodile forces, Allis forceps, or flat intestinal forceps might be used to grip and pull-out larger chunks of debris and granulomas. In more severe cases, a fenestration of the rib cage (including the last 2 ribs) might be indicated along with a Lonestar retractor to fully remove granulomas. The fenestrated ribs can be sutured back and the skin as usually apposed. Quite important is to instill/flush the air sac with antifungals in order to avoid possible re-seeding due to remnant spores during the removal. In a case, a 2 port coelioscopic approach and an end loop ligature was used to remove a foreign body from the air sac of a raptor.[73] Although laparoscopic surgery has been described in avian medicine, still most practitioners are not familiarized with it and therefore not yet broadly applied.

Plantar surface management (pododermatitis/bumblefoot)

Pododermatitis is a condition seen commonly in falconry and zoo raptors due to improper weight/exercise management. The 5 grades have been described by Remple.[16] In the early stages, perch hygiene, weight reduction and more training are adequate to resolve the situation. The medium grades (II, III) may require bandages

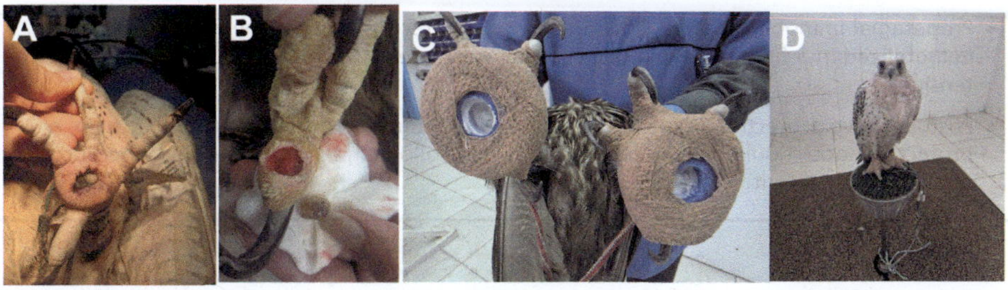

Fig. 10. (*A–D*) Pododermatitis in raptors (*A*) purulent stage IV in a Gyrfalcon (*B*) III in a Steppe eagle (*C*) casting allowing ventilation and ointment application (*D*) simple bandage with propylene foam shoes. (*Courtesy of* P. Azmanis.)

and absorbent padding (from foamy material). In the advanced stages (IV, V) surgery is required (**Fig. 10**). To the author's experience (PA), pododermatitis in falcons has been significantly reduced in the Dubai/UAE compared to the last 2 decades, as result of continuous education and husbandry improvement by the Arab falconers. A less invasive surgical approach (removal of scab, flushing the pus, and mattress suture) has better clinical results than extensive surgical procedures. Although a flap technique has been described,[74] it is rarely needed to be applied in practice but still might prove useful in advanced cases. Wound dressing with manuka honey, hydrocolloid gels, antibiotic creams as well as laser therapy and cold plasma therapy (PA study under submission) and tissue-like regenerative Plasma (TLRP) could promote wound healing, reducing the time of treatment. Although a recent study[75] shows the effectiveness of silicon shoes in chickens, they are not applied in raptors widely anymore as they deem as uncomfortable to stand, perch, and grab food.

SUMMARY

This article details the specific clinical challenges and surgical interventions required for raptors and pigeons, noting that while focused on these groups, the principles are broadly applicable to the wider avian class. The text outlines the necessity of thorough preoperative assessments, individualized anesthesia protocols, and a deep understanding of avian-specific wound healing phases. By categorizing common traumatic injuries and anatomical-specific repairs, such as head wounds, crop lacerations, and propatagial defects, the guide provides a framework for maximizing the survival and release potential of these patients.

CLINICS CARE POINTS

- Hemostasis is critical: Due to small absolute body sizes, even minor hemorrhage can be life-threatening; clinicians should use microsurgical instruments and hemostatic equipment to minimize loss.
- Prioritize triage: Address life-threatening conditions, such as pulmonary compromise or head trauma, before managing obvious but noncritical wounds.
- Surgical precision: Use surgical loupes or operating microscopes to minimize tissue trauma and improve recovery times.
- Air sac safety: Avoid flushing the coelom or intestinal volume with excessive saline during surgery, as fluid can easily enter the interconnected respiratory air sac system.
- Layered crop closure: For ingluviotomy or traumatic ruptures, a layered closure (mucosa and skin) is recommended to prevent leakage, dehiscence, and septicemia.

- Propatagial immobilization: Following propatagial reconstruction, the wing must be immobilized in a figure-of-8 bandage for approximately 10 days to protect the repair from tension.
- Postoperative protection: Raptors are prone to self-mutilation from neuropathic pain; a protective hood should be used for at least 1 week following tendon repairs or other surgical wound management.

DISCLOSURE

The authors of this article has not received any research funding.

REFERENCES

1. Lacasse C. Falconiformes. In: Miller RE, Fowler ME, editors. Fowler's zoo and wild animal medicine, 8. St Louis (MO): Elsevier Saunders; 2015. p. 150–9.
2. Hackett SJ, Kimball RT, Reddy S, et al. A phylogenomic study of birds reveals their evolutionary history. Science 2008;320(5884):1763–8.
3. Samour J. Management of raptors. In: Harrison GJ, Lightfoot T, editors. Clinical avian medicine. Palm Beach (FL): Spix Publishing; 2006. p. 915–55.
4. Donnelly B. Pigeon medicine and surgery. 1st edition. Ames (IA): Blackwell Publishing; 2011.
5. Kettel EF, Yarnell RW, Quinn JL, et al. Raptors, racing pigeons and perceptions of attacks. Eur J Wildl Res 2021;67(73). https://doi.org/10.1007/s10344-021-01513-2.
6. King AS, McLelland J. Digestive system. In: Birds: their structure and function. 2nd edition. London: Baillière Tindall; 1984. p. 86–109.
7. Schoemaker NJ, van Zeeland YRA. Wound care and bandaging techniques. In: Garner MM, Mitchell MA, editors. Exotic animal emergency and critical care medicine. 1st edition. Hoboken (NJ): John Wiley & Sons; 2021. p. 65–88.
8. Longley L. Raptor anesthesia. In: Chitty J, Monks DJ, editors. BSAVA manual of raptors, pigeons and passerine birds. 2nd edition. Gloucester (UK): British Small Animal Veterinary Association; 2016. p. 92–101.
9. Hawkins MG, Griffenhagen GM. Raptor sedation and anesthesia. Vet Clin North Am Exot Anim Pract 2022;25(1):135–61.
10. Ferrell ST. Avian integumentary surgery. Semin Avian Exotic Pet Med 2002;11(3): 125–35.
11. Ritzman TK. Wound healing and management in psittacine birds. Vet Clin North Am Exot Anim Pract 2004;7(1):87–104.
12. Redig PT. Medical management of birds of prey. 3rd edition. St Paul (MN): The Raptor Center; 2000.
13. Cousquer GO. Wound management in the avian wildlife casualty. Vet Nurs J 2003;18(5):13–6.
14. Bennett RA. Soft tissue surgery. In: Altman RB, Clubb SL, Dorrestein GM, et al, editors. Avian medicine and surgery. Philadelphia (PA): WB Saunders; 1997. p. 281–300.
15. Harcourt-Brown N. Radiographic interpretation of the avian wing. Semin Avian Exot Pet Med 2002;11(2):90–100.
16. MacPhail C, Fossum TW. Surgery of the integumentary system. In: Fossum TW, editor. Small animal surgery. 5th edition. Philadelphia (PA: Elsevier; 2018. p. 179–265.

17. Remple JD. Bumblefoot in raptors. In: Redig PT, Cooper JE, Remple JD, et al, editors. Raptor biomedicine. Minneapolis (MN): University of Minnesota Press; 1993. p. 154–60.
18. Martel A, Mans C. Wound care and bandaging techniques. In: Graham JE, Doss GA, Beaufrère H, editors. Exotic animal emergency and critical care medicine. 1st edition. Hoboken (NJ): John Wiley & Sons; 2021. p. 732–7.
19. Burke HF, Swaim SF, Amalsadvala T. Review of wound management in raptors. J Avian Med Surg 2002;16(3):180–91.
20. Sanchez-Migallon Guzman D. Avian soft tissue surgery. Vet Clin North Am Exot Anim Pract 2016;19(1):133–57.
21. Bennett RA. General principles, instruments, and equipment. In: Bennett RA, Pye GW, editors. Surgery of exotic animals. 1st edition. Hoboken (NJ): Wiley-Blackwell; 2022. p. 1–10.
22. McFadden MS. Suture materials. In: Bennett RA, Pye GW, editors. Surgery of exotic animals. 1st edition. Hoboken (NJ): Wiley-Blackwell; 2022. p. 11–22.
23. Phillips H. Magnification surgery. In: Bennett RA, Pye GW, editors. Surgery of exotic animals. 1st edition. Hoboken (NJ): Wiley-Blackwell; 2022. p. 23–34.
24. Kovách AG, Szász E. Survival of pigeon after graded haemorrhage. Acta Physiol Acad Sci Hung 1968;34(4):301–9.
25. Finnegan MV, Daniel GB, Ramsay EC. Evaluation of whole blood transfusions in domestic pigeons (*columba livia*). J Avian Med Surg 1997;11(1):7–14.
26. Rockwell G, Tully TN. Wound management. In: Speer BL, editor. Current therapy in avian medicine and surgery, vol II. 1st edition. St Louis: Elsevier; 2016. p. 777–89.
27. Malik A. Dealing with wild pigeons in practice. Part 1: triage, handling, housing, first aid and euthanasia. Practice 2025;47(8):417–33.
28. Friedrich PL. Die aseptische Versorgung frischer Wunden, unter Mittheilung von Thier-Versuchen über die Auskeimungszeit von Infectionserregern in frischen Wunden. Arch Klin Chir 1898;57:288–310.
29. Young C. Assessing and managing animal and human bites. Wounds U K 2023;19(1):10–6.
30. O'Rourke DP, Lertpiriyapong K. Biology and diseases of reptiles. In: Fox JG, Anderson LC, Otto G, et al, editors. Laboratory animal medicine. 3rd edition. San Diego (CA): Academic Press; 2015. p. 967–1013.
31. Khan MA, Farid M, Sobani ZA, et al. A case of cellulitis of the hands caused by a predatory bird attack. Asian Pac J Trop Biomed 2011;1(2):166–8.
32. Turkmen S, Alinier G, Elmoheen AM, et al. Injuries related to pets, exotic animals, and falconry in Qatar. Qatar Med J 2023;2023(4):27.
33. Magalhães R, Tavares L, Oliveira M. Antimicrobial resistance and virulence potential of bacterial species from captive birds of prey—consequences of falconry for public health. Animals (Basel) 2024;14(6):856.
34. Cooper JE. Veterinary aspects of captive birds of prey. Saul (UK): Standfast Press; 1978.
35. Cooper JE, Needham JR. An investigation into the prevalence of Staphylococcus aureus on avian feet. Vet Rec 1976;98(9):172–4.
36. Harrison GJ. Selected surgical procedures. In: Harrison GJ, Harrison LR, editors. Clinical avian medicine and surgery. Philadelphia (PA): WB Saunders; 1986. p. 580–1.
37. Malley AD, Whitbread TJ. The integument. In: Beynon PH, Forbes NA, Harcourt-Brown NH, editors. Manual of raptors, pigeons and waterfowl. Cheltenham (UK): British Small Animal Veterinary Association; 1996. p. 129–39.

38. Pavletic MM. Basic principles of wound healing. In: Atlas of small animal wound management and reconstructive surgery. 4th edition. Hoboken (NJ): Wiley-Blackwell; 2018. p. 17–46.
39. Hosgood G. Open wounds. In: Johnston SA, Tobias KM, editors. Veterinary surgery: small animal. 2nd edition. St Louis (MO): Elsevier; 2018. p. 1210–20.
40. Cooper JE, Harrison GJ. Dermatology. In: Ritchie BW, Harrison GJ, Harrison LR, editors. Avian medicine: principles and application. Lake Worth (FL): Wingers Publishing; 1994. p. 607–39.
41. Gentz EJ, Linn KA. Use of a dorsal cervical single pedicle advancement flap in 3 birds with cranial skin defects. J Avian Med Surg 2000;14(1):31–6.
42. Logothetou V, L'Eplattenier H, Shimizu N. Complications and influence of cutaneous closure technique on subdermal plexus flaps in 97 dogs (2006–2022). Vet Surg 2024;53(3):546–55.
43. Hernandez-Divers SJ, Hernandez-Divers SM. Xenogeneic grafts using porcine small intestinal submucosa in the repair of skin defects in 4 birds. J Avian Med Surg 2003;17(4):224–34.
44. Qabazard T, Al-Sayegh H. Novel use of Nile Tilapia fish (*Oreochromis niloticus*) skin as xenograft in zoological species. J Zoo Wildl Med 2024;55(3):827–37.
45. Kane LP, Shrader TC, Stice RC. Successful, full-thickness skin graft in a bald eagle (Haliaeetus leucocephalus). J Avian Med Surg 2019;33(2):184–9.
46. Hannon DE, Swaim SF, Milton JL, et al. Full-thickness mesh skin grafts in two great horned owls (*Bubo virginianus*). J Zoo Wildl Med 1993;24(4):539–52.
47. Johnson JH, Schumacher J, McClure SR, et al. Use of a full-thickness autograft on the tarsus of an ostrich. J Am Vet Med Assoc 1994;205(7):1019–20.
48. Dietrich HM, Oliveira-Dos-Santos AJ, Hala K, et al. Skin allograft survival in chicken strains with spontaneous autoimmune diseases. Poult Sci 1996;75(3):285–93.
49. Harcourt-Brown NH. Tendon repair in the pelvic limb of birds of prey. In: Lumeij JT, Remple JD, Redig PT, et al, editors. Raptor biomedicine III. Lake Worth (FL): Zoological Education Network Inc; 2000. p. 217–38.
50. Krackow KA, Thomas SJ, Jones RE. A locking loop suture technique for tendon repair. J Bone Joint Surg Am 1986;68(5):764–5.
51. Silfverskiöld KL, May EJ. Flexor tendon repair in zone II with a new suture technique and an early mobilization program combining passive and active flexion. J Hand Surg Am 1994;19(1):53–60.
52. Calvo Carrasco D. Surgical repair of the flexor digitorum longus of digit 2 on a Harris hawk (Parabuteo unicinctus). In: Proceedings of the European Association of zoo and wildlife veterinarians (EAZWV). 2024. p. 48.
53. Brown RE, Klemm RD. Surgical anatomy of the propatagium. In: Proceedings of the annual conference of the Association of Avian veterinarians. Phoenix (AZ). 1990. p. 176-179.
54. Goldberg DW, Vanstreels RET, Alcala MM, et al. Unforeseen consequences of the COVID-19 pandemic: increased frequency of kite string injuries in magnificent frigatebirds (*Fregata magnificens*) in Rio de Janeiro state, Brazil. Anim Welf 2021;30(2):109–16.
55. Jadhav S, Parasharya BM. Vulture population decline in Gujarat, India with special reference to kite flying. J Threat Taxa 2010;2(3):737–44.
56. Babu S, Subramanya S, Dilawar M. Kite flying: effect of Chinese manja on birds in Bangalore, India. Indian Birds 2015;10(1):13–8.
57. Forbes NA. Soft tissue surgery. In: Samour J, editor. Avian medicine. 3rd edition. St Louis (MO): Elsevier; 2016. p. 294–311.

58. Zheng W, Ruxin D, Yansong G, et al. Diagnosis and treatment of crop inflammation of rough-legged buzzard (*Buteo lagopus*) in Daqing Wildlife Nature Reserve, Heilongjiang Province, China. Thai. J Vet Med 2024;54(4):1–5.
59. Fornazari GA, Saldanha A, Lange RR, et al. Window collisions by birds in Brazil: epidemiologic factors and radiographic and necropsy assessments. J Avian Med Surg 2021;35(3):313–24.
60. Cousins RA. Kereru (*Hemiphaga novaeseelandiae*)—impact injuries, morphometrics, moult and plumage [master's thesis]. Palmerston North (New Zealand: Massey University; 2010.
61. Hussain R, Hussain N, Iqbal N, et al. A study on crop repair by using different ingluviotomy techniques in pigeon. Adv Anim Vet Sci 2020;8(7):753–60.
62. Chaudhary PS, Varshney JP, Deshmukh VV. Surgical correction of crop fistula in baby pigeons. Intas Polivet 2010;11(2):397–9.
63. Basha KMA, Vishal BN, Mahesh V, et al. Traumatic punctured wound of the crop in pigeon (*Columba livia*)—two case reports. Intas Polivet 2010;11(2):402–3.
64. Mison MB, Bennett RA. Surgery of the avian gastrointestinal tract. In: Bennett RA, Pye GW, editors. Surgery of exotic animals. 1st edition. Hoboken (NJ): Wiley-Blackwell; 2022. p. 179–204.
65. Laminou IM. Exérèse du jabot chez le pigeon Mondain: une approche chirurgicale innovante. Rev Afr Sante Prod Anim 2024;2(1):1–6.
66. Schoonheere N, Zoller G. Columbiform pediatrics. Vet Clin North Am Exot Anim Pract 2024;27(2):341–57.
67. Lierz M, Fischer D. Clinical technique: imping in birds. J Exot Pet Med 2011;20(2):131–7.
68. Applegate JR, Van Wettere A, Christiansen EF, et al. Management and case outcome of gastric impaction in four raptors: a case series. J Avian Med Surg 2017;31(1):62–9.
69. Kottferová L, Molnár L, Major P, et al. Removal of foreign bodies from the proventriculus in a young golden eagle (*Aquila chrysaetos*). Acta Vet Hung 2021;69(3):298–302.
70. Sabater M, Huynh M, Forbes N. Ileo coco-rectal intussusception requiring intestinal resection and anastomosis in a tawny eagle (*Aquila rapax*). J Avian Med Surg 2015;29(1):63–8.
71. Dutton TAG, Forbes NA, Calvo Carrasco D. Cloacal prolapse in raptors: review of 16 cases. J Avian Med Surg 2016;30(2):133–40.
72. Azmanis PN, Anzoategui AI, Di Somma A, et al. Retrospective study of aspergillosis in juvenile falcons in United Arab Emirates: prevalence and effect of hybridization. J Zoo Wildl Med 2024;55(4):893–900.
73. Zaheer OA, Beaufrère H. Use of an endoloop ligature and a 2-portal coelioscopic approach for the removal of an arrowhead foreign body in a red-tailed hawk (*Buteo jamaicensis*). J Avian Med Surg 2022;36(1):58–62.
74. Sander S, Whittington JK, Bennett A, et al. Advancement flap as a novel treatment for a pododermatitis lesion in a red-tailed hawk (*Buteo jamaicensis*). J Avian Med Surg 2013;27(4):294–300.
75. Konicek C, Gumpenberger M, Schramel JP. Silicone shoes for the treatment of foot pad dermatitis (bumblefoot) in pet chickens—a retrospective case series. Vet Sci 2020;7(3):113.

Soft Tissue Surgery in Galliformes and Anseriformes

Mikel Sabater González, LV, MRCVS, CertZooMed, DipECZM(Avian)

KEYWORDS

• Galliformes • Anseriformes • Avian • Soft tissue surgery • Surgical principles

KEY POINTS

- Soft tissue surgery in Galliformes and Anseriformes follows established avian surgical principles but requires adaptation to their unique anatomy, physiology and behavior.
- Gentle tissue handling and microsurgical technique are essential to minimize complications such as hemorrhage, dehiscence, and contamination.
- Limited species-specific evidence means surgical success relies heavily on anatomic knowledge and meticulous technique.
- Minimally invasive approaches provide excellent visualization and reduced morbidity.

FUNDAMENTAL PRINCIPLES OF SOFT TISSUE SURGERY

Galliformes and Anseriformes exhibit unique anatomic, physiologic, and behavioral characteristics that influence soft tissue surgical management. Core surgical principles are summarized in **Box 1**.

SOFT TISSUE SURGERIES WITH CLINICAL APPLICATIONS

Digestive Tract Surgery

Surgical management of large oral lacerations or masses ranges from thorough debridement to complete excision and closure. Masses may be removed by sharp surgical excision, cryosurgery, electrosurgery, or chemical cautery.

Sublingual entrapment, reported in a Chinese goose (*Anser cygnoides*), occurs when fibrous material becomes lodged lateral to the frenulum beneath the tongue, forming an intermandibular ventral diverticulum.[8] Chronic cases may require surgery via a ventral intermandibular approach, with removal of impacted material and unilateral or bilateral excision of diverticular tissue, followed by closure to eliminate dead space and prevent recurrence. Marsupialization may be necessary when primary

Exoticsvet, Valencia, Spain
E-mail address: exoticsvet@gmail.com

Vet Clin Exot Anim 29 (2026) 569–586
https://doi.org/10.1016/j.cvex.2026.04.004 vetexotic.theclinics.com
1094-9194/26/

Box 1
Core soft tissue surgical principles in Galliformes and Anseriformes

- Complete anamnesis, physical examination, diagnostics and preoperative stabilization are essential to reduce perioperative morbidity.
- Provide appropriate multimodal analgesia. Follow established avian sedation, anesthesia, and analgesia guidelines, with vigilant perioperative and intraoperative monitoring.[1,2]
- Fasting must be adapted to species and individual needs, and to the planned surgical procedure. In general, fasting chickens and ducks for 3 hours and up to 12 hours for large waterfowl is recommended. Excessive fasting exacerbates catabolic states.
- Position birds to minimize respiratory compromise and reduce risk of aspiration. Provide thermal support to compensate rapid heat loss after feather removal and surgical preparation.
- Maintain strict asepsis and minimize secondary contamination.[3]
- Restrict the use of antimicrobials to evidence-based, medically justified situations.
- Gentle tissue handling and familiarity with microsurgical techniques is necessary. Use microsurgical instruments, sterile cotton-tipped applicators, fine forceps (eg, ring-tip) and sharp fine scissors. Maintain continuous tissue moisture.
- Correct hemostasis is essential. Use direct pressure, monopolar or preferably bipolar electrosurgery to reduce collateral thermal injury, ultrasonic devices, hemostatic agents (solutions, powders, foams, or microfibrillar collagen/thrombin matrices), and microvascular clips. Larger vessels should be ligated with 6-0 to 7-0 absorbable suture.
- Suture selection based on biocompatibility, handling properties, and species-specific behavior. A tenorrhaphy study in chickens demonstrated no significant differences among nylon, polyglyconate, and polybutester in mechanical strength, scar maturation, or tissue reactivity.[4] Research in Columbiformes supports current recommendations for Galliformes and Anseriformes: polydioxanone for visceral and celomic closure; monofilament nylon when suture removal is feasible, or rapidly absorbing monofilaments (eg, poliglecaprone 25) for skin; and selective use of polyglactin 910 where a robust fibrous response is desired, generally avoiding intraluminal applications.[5,6]
- Adequate visualization may require using clear surgical drapes, lightweight retractors (eg, Lone Star retractor), low-flow suction–irrigation systems, surgical loupes with adjustable working distances (24–35 cm) or operating microscopes, and head-mounted light emitting diode (LED) or fiber-optic surgical lights with adjustable intensity.
- Celioscopy provides excellent visualization of internal organs with lower morbidity and faster recovery than open celiotomy. Comprehensive reviews of celioscopy and minimally invasive surgery are published.[7] Limitations include reduced working space due to organomegaly, ascites, or obesity, underscoring the importance of preoperative imaging.

closure is not feasible. Soft, nonfibrous diet must be fed until healing is complete. Prognosis is excellent.

Crop and esophageal surgery are indicated for foreign body removal, repair of lacerations or perforations, and excision of necrotic tissue. Impaction with fibrous material is common in backyard poultry, whereas waterfowl more often ingest linear or metallic foreign bodies.[9] Surgery is performed in dorsal or left lateral recumbency. Diagnostic imaging may aid to localize lesions and minimize incisions. A skin incision parallel to the jugular vein is followed by blunt dissection of subcutaneous tissues. Once the crop or esophagus is exposed, stay sutures are placed and the ingluviotomy/esophagotomy is performed. Impacted material or foreign bodies are removed manually or endoscopically, and the lumen is lavaged (**Fig. 1**). Endoscopy also facilitates intraluminal assessment. Closure is achieved using 5-0 or 6-0 absorbable suture

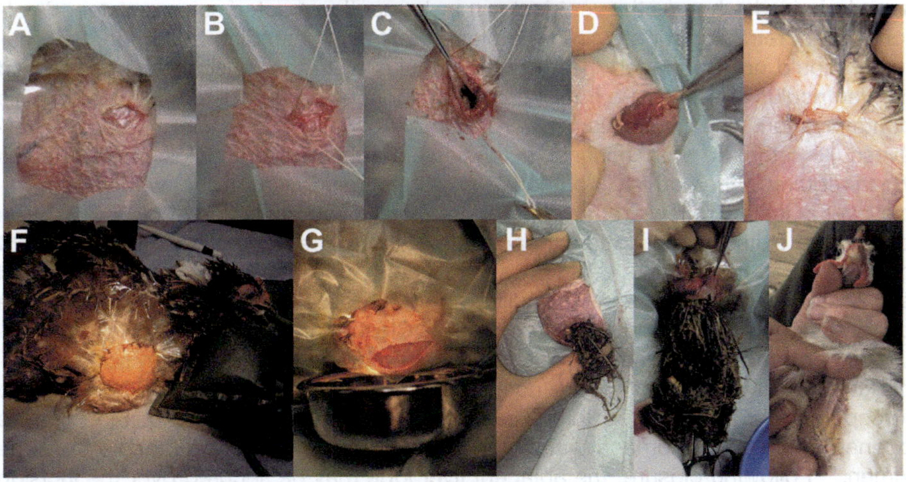

Fig. 1. (*A–J*) Different steps of ingluviotomy and closure in a chicken. (*F–J*) Examples of larger ingluviotomies in a chicken (*F, G*) and in a Guinea fowl (*H–J*).

(eg, polydioxanone) in a simple continuous pattern for mucosal and submucosal apposition, and in an inverting or appositional pattern for the seromuscular layer. Subcutaneous and skin are closed routinely, but a ventral 2 to 3 mm skin opening facilitates drainage. Soft diet feeding must resume after anesthetic recovery. Common complications include leakage, dehiscence, fistula formation, and postoperative crop stasis. Esophagostomy or ingluviostomy tubes may be placed for temporary nutritional support.[10]

Gastric surgery is indicated for foreign body removal, relief of luminal obstructions, full-thickness biopsy, and excision and/or closure of mural lesions. The left paramedian approach provides optimal access to the proventriculus and isthmus (**Fig. 2**). Alternatively, a transverse abdominal or a ventral midline combined with a left paramedial approach may be preferred to access the caudoventral sac of the ventriculus, particularly when the ventriculus is medially displaced.[11] The proventriculus cannot

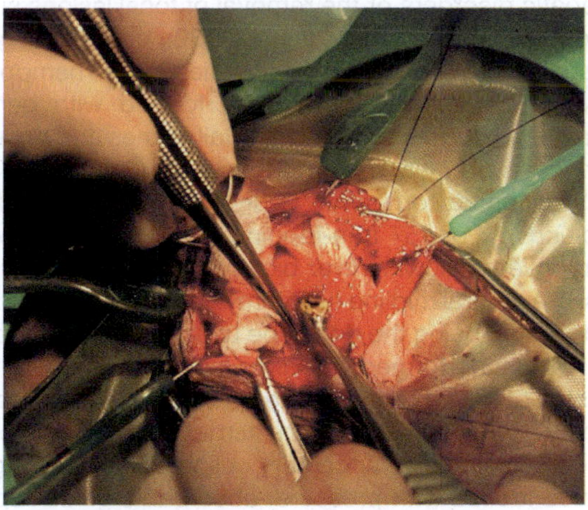

Fig. 2. Gastrotomy in a chicken for foreign body removal.

be exteriorized, whereas the ventriculus may be gently retracted using moistened cotton swabs, retractors or stay sutures placed in its white tendinous portion. Stay sutures should not be placed in the proventriculus or in the muscular component of the ventriculus due to tissue fragility.[11] Moist sponges are useful to minimize celomic contamination. The gastric lumen is preferably accessed by incising the relatively avascular isthmus, with minimal extension into the proventriculus or ventriculus when required. Alternatively, ventriculotomy of the caudoventral sac, where the muscle layer is thinner, allows retrieval of foreign bodies and collection of biopsies.[11] The duodenum exits the caudodorsal sac, which should be generally avoided.[11] Slight clockwise rotation of the ventriculus can improve exposure to the caudoventral sac.[6] Ventriculotomy via ventral midline approach allowed successful removal of a perforating needle in an adult mallard duck.[12] Closure of the isthmus and proventriculus is performed using fine monofilament absorbable suture with closely spaced simple continuous pattern to ensure accurate apposition and prevent leakage. Thumb forceps should not be used to grasp the proventricular wall; instead, they can be opened against the stomach wall while crossing it with the suture needle from the lumen.[11] Following closure, the adjacent liver lobe may be secured over the incision with simple interrupted sutures between the gastric seromuscular layer (separated at least 5 mm from the gastrotomy) and the hepatic capsule.[11] Meticulous ventricular closure with interrupted sutures close together is critical as wall tissues do not invert. Complete ventricular mucosal healing in Japanese quails (*Coturnix japonica*) undergoing caudoventral sac ventriculotomy was confirmed 21 days postsurgery.[13]

Enterotomy with or without enterectomy via ventral midline celiotomy is indicated for foreign body removal, correction of intussusception, and resection of necrotic intestine or masses. After isolating the affected segment with moistened sponges and clamped atraumatically orally and aborally, enterotomy is performed along the antimesenteric border. Then, foreign bodies can be removed and the lumen lavaged before wall closure with 7-0 polydioxanone in a simple continuous appositional pattern. If tissue resection is required, end-to-end anastomosis is achieved with simple interrupted appositional sutures, preferably with slight luminal offset (oblique anastomosis) to reduce stricture risk. Leak testing by fluid injection is not recommended.

Hepatic and Biliary Surgery

Biopsy (surgical, ultrasound-guided or endoscopic-guided) or surgery is indicated for the diagnosis of hepatic disorders or the removal of focal lesions such as abscesses, granulomas, or neoplasia. In common quails (n = 30), ultrasound-guided liver biopsy yielded hepatic tissue in 63.3% of them and one died due to hemopericardium.[14] Surgical liver biopsy and partial hepatectomy performed with gentle handling and adequate hemostasis are well tolerated in both Galliformes and Anseriformes. In Pekin ducks (*Anas platyrhynchos*) (n = 8), repeated biopsies (34) were associated with one perioperative death unrelated to hepatic trauma.[15] In a study with harlequin ducks (*Histrionicus histrionicus*), 7 of 157 free-ranging and 0 of 36 captive individuals died during anesthetic recovery following liver biopsy, but no deaths were attributable to biopsy procedures.[16] A ventral midline celiotomy, just caudal to the sternum, provides optimal access to the liver, being the right lobe usually more accessible. Alternatively, a lateral celiotomy can be performed. The liver location within the hepatic peritoneal cavity requires incision of the surrounding membranes when accessed from the intestinal peritoneal cavity.[17] For resections, the target area is isolated with moistened sponges and transected using bipolar cautery or ligated with fine (eg, 5–0) absorbable suture. Bleeding is controlled with pressure, absorbable gelatin sponges or microfibrillar collagen.[6] Wedge or marginal resections can be obtained with cup-end forceps, scalpel, or curved hemostat, avoiding traction on the fragile hepatic capsule. In harlequin ducks, 3 × 10 mm samples were collected safely.[16] Routine closure is performed. Postoperative risks include hemorrhage and bile leakage.[6]

Bile ducts lie on the caudal visceral surface of each hepatic lobe and must be carefully avoided during surgery, as ligation can result in fibrosing cholangiohepatitis and progressive cholestasis.[18] The right and left liver lobes drain through their respective hepatic duct, which converge into the gallbladder in ducks, geese, and turkeys, or empty directly into the duodenum via hepatoenteric ducts in species without a gallbladder, such as chickens. Surgery of the biliary ducts is generally avoided due to their small diameter and fragility.

Pancreatic Surgery

The avian pancreas has 3 lobes within the duodenal loop. Biopsy or partial resection may be indicated for pancreatitis, cysts, or neoplasia; and is performed via ventral midline celiotomy with gentle exteriorization of the duodenal loop. Ventral lobe sampling is preferred, using suture-fracture or hemostatic clip methods for hemorrhage control.[11] Additional hemostasis is achieved by compression (sutures are rarely required) before routine celomic closure.[6]

Total pancreatectomy is fatal but partial pancreatectomy or biopsy sampling of 1 or 2 lobes is well tolerated. Chickens undergoing 99% pancreatectomy demonstrated a 400% compensatory hypertrophy of the remaining splenic pancreatic lobe within 16 days, maintaining near-normal metabolic parameters aside from transient hyperglycemia.[19] In Pekin ducks (*A platyrhynchos*), subtotal pancreatectomy leaving the splenic lobe intact resulted in temporary diabetes resolving within 12 days.[20] The pancreatic ducts, 1 to 3 per bird, enter the terminal duodenum near the bile or hepatoenteric ducts. Ligation should be avoided because it causes severe acinar atrophy and fibrosis.[21]

Respiratory Tract Surgery

Respiratory surgery is indicated for the diagnosis and management of upper airway obstructions, chronic respiratory infections or traumatic injuries. Minimally invasive procedures are preferred.

Air sac cannulation provides an alternative airway for anesthesia or ventilation in birds with tracheal or syringeal obstruction and during upper airway or head and neck surgery.[22] Excessive celomic fat, ascites, and intracelomic organomegaly may reduce air sac volume, complicating air sac cannulation. Caudal thoracic and abdominal air sacs are most commonly cannulated. With the bird in lateral recumbency, a 0.5 to 1 cm skin incision is made just caudal to the last rib and cranial to the thigh, or between the 2 most caudal ribs. Blunt dissection through the intercostal muscles allows gentle perforation of the air sac wall. A sterile tube (2–3 mm internal diameter for adult chickens or ducks; up to 4–5 mm for large geese) is inserted no more than one-third of the celomic width to avoid visceral injury, secured to the skin and adjacent ribs with finger-trap sutures, and connected to an anesthetic circuit or oxygen source with an oxygen flow of 0.3 L/kg/minute. The endotracheal tube may be clamped or removed to allow ventilation via the cannula, which should be routinely disinfected. Temporary occlusion of the cannula confirms restoration of upper airway patency before removal and routine closure. Postoperative monitoring includes assessment for air leakage, subcutaneous emphysema, or infection.

Despite anatomic descriptions of infraorbital sinus diverticula exist, published surgical reports are limited to infraorbital sinusostomy. This procedure is indicated for the diagnosis and/or treatment of chronic sinusitis refractory to treatment, abscesses, granulomas, and masses affecting this sinus. After a curved incision along the dorsolateral margin of the infraorbital region, the overlying skin is reflected, purulent material is curetted, and the cavity is flushed with sterile saline. Opening the beak may improve access. The sinus opening may be sutured or left open for drainage and healing by secondary intention. Trephination of the beak or skull is rarely required but may be considered in refractory cases.[6]

The choana can be obstructed by foreign bodies, caseous debris, fungal plaques, or neoplasia (**Fig. 3**). With the oral cavity opened, obstructive material/tissue is gently removed, hemorrhage is controlled with gentle pressure or topical epinephrine (1:10,000), and the mucosa is flushed with saline or 0.05% diluted chlorhexidine.

Tracheotomy, with or without tracheostomy, is indicated for persistent upper airway obstruction, tracheal collapse, or removal of foreign material or masses not amenable to medical treatment or endoscopic management. Successful surgical correction of a 1-cm complete tracheal defect in a mallard duck (*A platyrhynchos*) has been reported.[23] Resection and end-to-end anastomosis are indicated for focal stenosis, granuloma, neoplasia, and traumatic avulsion.[24] The bird is placed in dorsal recumbency, with its cranial half elevated and the neck hyperextended 45 to 60°. A ventral midcervical approach and lateralization of the esophagus/crop to the right allows tracheal exposure by blunt dissection of the sternotracheal muscles. Blood vessels

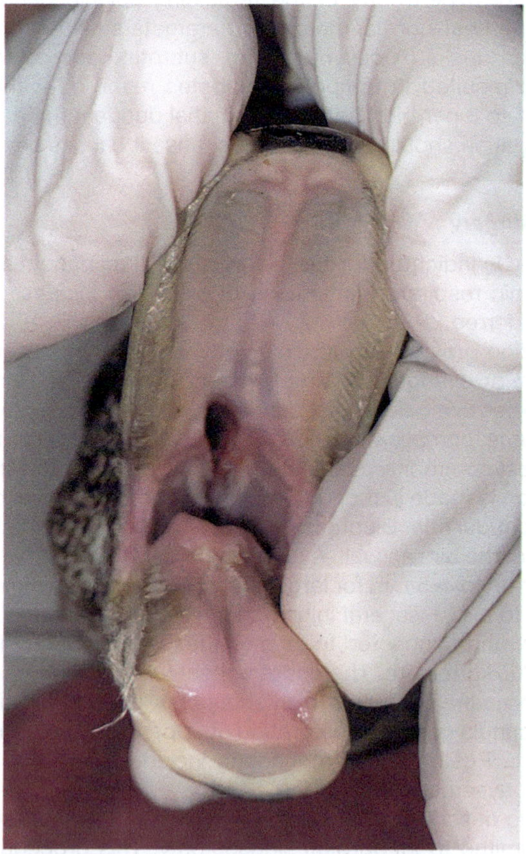

Fig. 3. Healed choanal lesion after foreign body (seed) removal.

between the muscle bellies should be coagulated. Stay sutures facilitate tracheal manipulation. The ventral half of the annular ligament between rings located 4 to 5 rings cranial to the problematic region is transversally incised allowing foreign body or granuloma removal or debridement. Distal tracheal or syringeal procedures may require gentle approximation with a blunt hook passed caudal to the syringeal bifurcation. Tracheal closure is done using 4-0 to 8-0 polydioxanone in a simple interrupted pattern through the annular ligament between one or 2 tracheal rings at both sides of the incision tied externally. Alternating encircling one or 2 rings reduces tension. The sternotracheal muscles or the clavicular air sac do not need suturing. The skin can be closed in a Ford interlocking pattern.[24] A tracheostomy tube or air sac cannulation may be necessary until airway patency is restored. If necessary, multiple tracheal rings (eg, up to 9% of the tracheal length in a mallard duck, and 5 tracheal rings in a goose) can be resected without creating excessive tension following anastomosis.[25,26] Lateral approaches may be advantageous in long-necked species with cranial tracheal lesions.[24]

Pulmonary or air sac wall lesions can be biopsied or excised via a lateral approach to the caudal thoracic or abdominal air sacs. Lesions firmly adhered to the pulmonary parenchyma may require partial debridement under direct visualization when complete excision risks damage to the parabronchial architecture.[24] Alternatively, lung exposure allowing vascular clamping for wedge biopsy can be achieved through a skin incision and blunt muscle dissection at the third intercostal space.[27] Focal pulmonary masses may require partial pneumonectomy, accessed via the caudal thoracic air sac or an intercostal approach transecting part of one or more ribs.[24] Affected lung tissue is gently separated from adjacent structures and vascular clips are applied to control hemorrhage before excising the diseased portion. Additional hemostasis may be achieved applying oxidized regenerated cellulose.[24]

Cardiovascular Surgery

Cardiac surgery is uncommon, and most interventions are diagnostic or palliative. Pericardiocentesis allows drainage and analysis of pericardial effusions.[28] Chronic effusive or constrictive pericarditis refractive to pericardiocentesis may require pericardiectomy. Partial pericardiectomy has been reported in Psittaciformes but not in Galliformes or Anseriformes.[29,30] Experimental bilateral ligation of the common carotid and vertebral arteries in Leghorn hens (n = 37) resulted in a 6% reduction in body weight and four deaths within 2 weeks. No cardiac hypertrophy, neurologic deficits, or behavioral abnormalities were observed in surviving birds.[31]

Female Reproductive Surgery

Although a persistent right oviduct with or without a functional right ovary is present in some birds, most females only have a functional left reproductive system. Reproductive surgery is frequently performed in females presented with egg binding, oviductal impaction, salpingitis, egg yolk celomitis, and cloacal prolapse.[32]

Egg binding (dystocia) refractive to medical management may require direct, percutaneous, or transcloacal ovocentesis. Ovocentesis with a 22 G needle allows egg content aspiration before careful shell collapse and removal with lubricated forceps. Ovocentesis under celioscopic visualization is preferred to prevent mucosal tearing.

Salpingotomy is indicated in egg binding or localized oviductal impactions when reproductive function must be preserved. Via a left lateral or ventral midline approach, the oviduct is incised avoiding major blood vessels, evacuated, lavaged, and closed with fine (4–0 to 6–0) absorbable suture using a simple continuous or interrupted pattern before routine celomic closure. Then, reproductive stimulation must be suppressed for 2 to 4 weeks.[33]

Salpingohysterectomy is indicated for chronic egg laying and oviductal diseases unresponsive to medical management.[34] A left lateral approach provides optimal exposure, while a ventral midline approach allows broader tract evaluation. Following a left lateral celiotomy and incision through the left abdominal air sac, the ovary and oviduct are visualized (**Fig. 4**) The cranial oviduct/infundibulum is gently retracted and suspensory ligament vessels are clipped or cauterized as needed. The cranial, middle, and caudal oviductal arteries may require hemostasis with hemoclips or cautery. Finally, the oviduct is hemoclipped near its junction with the cloaca and excised.[33] Endoscopic salpingohysterectomy has not been described in Galliformes or Anseriformes.

Preovulatory follicles may be removed to reduce the risk ectopic ovulation. The follicular vascular pedicles can be hemoclipped and excised, or twirled free. In chickens, laying pauses proportionally increase with the number of follicles removed.[34] Normal preovulatory follicles appear yellow and contain thick yolk, whereas cystic follicles are pale or translucent and filled with clear fluid. Cystic follicles should be aspirated or excised. If a cyst ruptures, leaked yolk should be removed and analyzed.[33]

Ovariectomy is reserved for severe ovarian disease or hormonal control refractive to medical management. Complete ovariectomy is necessary for permanent reproductive suppression but carries a high risk of hemorrhage due to the ovary close association with the common iliac vein and cranial renal artery.[33] A study of ovariectomy via left lateral celiotomy using a vessel and tissue-sealing device in chickens (10 immatures and 10 adults) concluded the procedure is achievable but carries notable risks of hemorrhage (n = 3) and incomplete ovarian excision (n = 8). Salpingohysterectomy

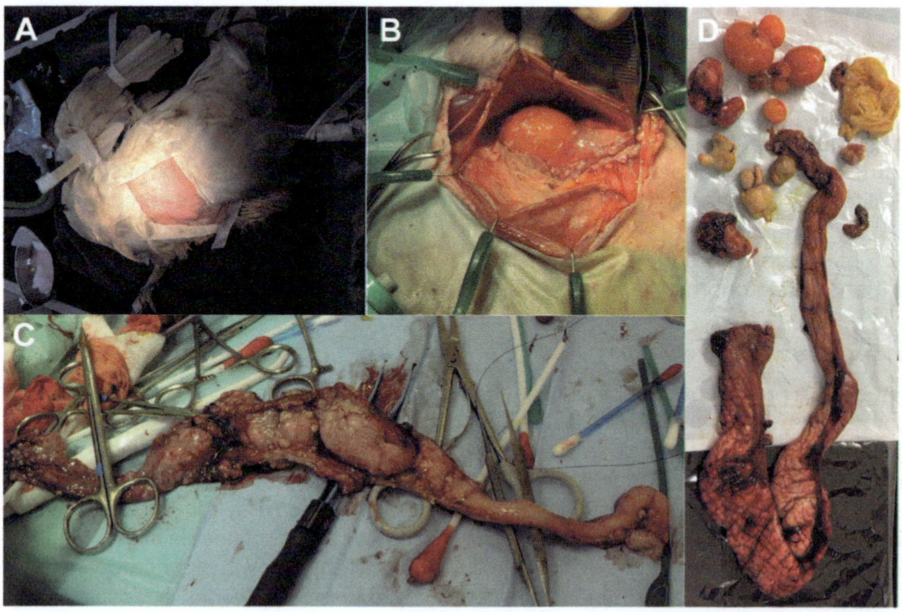

Fig. 4. (*A–D*) Salpingohysterectomy. (*A*) Patient positioning in right lateral recumbency. (*B*) Intraoperative view of the reproductive tract. (*C*) Excised oviduct showing external lesions compatible with of salpingitis and/or neoplasia, and intraluminal impactions. (*D*) Excised oviduct and abnormal preovulatory and postovulatory follicles.

was necessary to facilitate ovarian access in mature birds.[35] A cranial left lateral celiotomy provides optimal exposure of the left ovary, but a ventral midline or combined transverse approaches may be needed for caudal access.[33] The ovary is gently debulked to visualize its attachments to the common iliac vein and associated vessels. Large follicles can be aspirated or detached to minimize bleeding. Vascular control is achieved using vascular clamps, hemostatic clipping, bipolar cautery, radiosurgery or fine (eg, 6–0) absorbable ligatures. Sections of the ovary are sequentially excised or cauterized until the main vasculature, particularly the common iliac vein, is fully identified.[33] In case of advanced or invasive disease, clipping the common iliac vein cranially and caudally to the ovary may be necessary to reduce risk of hemorrhage during complete excision.[33] Alternatively, electrocautery can coagulate follicles, particularly in immature birds, but residual ovarian tissue can regenerate under estrogenic stimulation. Partial resections or laser ablation may be used for debulking in cases of neoplasia where complete excision is unsafe. Potential complications of ovariectomy include severe hemorrhage, and damage to major vessels, adrenals, kidneys, or nerve plexuses.

Male Reproductive Surgery

Surgical castration is rarely performed. Indication includes orchitis, testicular neoplasia or specific testicular hormone-dependent disorders. The effectiveness of orchidectomy alone in reducing undesirable male sexual behaviors remains controversial. In roosters, the procedure has traditionally been performed for caponization.[36] Although caponization has long been believed to create more docile males, evidence from other galliform species (eg, Gambel's quail [*Callipepla gambelii*] and scaled quail [*C. squamata*]) indicates that behavioral outcomes can be inconsistent.[37]

The testicular artery arises from the cranial renal artery and provides most of the arterial blood supply to the testis. An accessory testicular artery may arise directly from the aorta. Venous drainage returns either directly to the caudal vena cava or forms a common stem with the adrenal veins. In Pekin drakes, 2 testicular veins empty directly into caudal vena cava.[38]

Orchidectomy in birds is either performed via a left lateral celiotomy or a ventral midline approach with transverse parasternal/parapubic incisions. To access the testicles via a ventral midline celiotomy, the left abdominal air sac normally overlies the testis and needs to be reflected dorsally or incised.[39] Bipolar electrosurgery is preferred over microsurgical scissors to free the testes from the mesorchium. Approaching the right testis through a left lateral celiotomy requires incision of the interposed mesorchium separating the 2 testes. Each testis is gently retracted ventrally, and one or more hemostatic clips are applied dorsally from caudal to cranial to control hemorrhage from the testicular vessels as close as possible to the vena cava and common iliac vein. Due to restricted space, a right-angled clip applier facilitates placement.[39] The testis is then excised distal to the applied clips. Most common complications of orchidectomy are severe hemorrhage and incomplete removal of testicular tissue.[39] Any residual tissue may be fulgurated using bipolar electrosurgery. Although vessel-sealing devices may improve hemostasis, their use in avian castration has not yet been fully evaluated. Alternatively, if the testicular blood supply is small, a hemostat may be used temporarily instead of a clip; the testis is pulled free, and the hemostat holds the vascular stump for 1 to 2 minutes before release. Direct pressure hemostasis may also be applied. Diode laser excision can be used and may eliminate the need for clip placement.[33] Closure is routine. Minimally invasive orchidectomy has been reported in pigeons but neither in Galliformes nor Anseriformes.[40]

Vasectomy have been described for population control of Canada geese, production of surrogate parents from wild-caught northern Texas bobwhite quail (*Colinus virginianus texanus*) to rear the more endangered masked bobwhite quail (*C virginianus ridgwayi*), and sterilization of immature birds using the Japanese quail (*C japonica*) as a model species.[41–44] In these species, vasectomy has been performed intracelomically through bilateral celiotomy or via endoscopic-assisted techniques. For intracelomic (open) vasectomy, the bird is positioned in lateral recumbency, the left leg is pulled dorsocaudally and the wings secured dorsally. A skin incision is made from the sixth rib to the pubic bone. The superficial medial femoral vessels are cauterized, and the abdominal wall is opened by blunt dissection. The intercostal vessels of the last 2 ribs are cauterized and the ribs transected to expose the coelomic cavity. The abdominal air sac is penetrated to access the *ductus deferens*, which is isolated and gently elevated, before removing 5 to 8 mm. Ligation or clipping of the cut ends is unnecessary. The procedure is repeated on the contralateral side, before routine celomic wall closure. Endoscopic-assisted vasectomy has been reported in Japanese quails.[44] A 5 mm incision at the caudal apex of the triangle formed by the last rib, pubic bone, and *flexor cruris* muscle, or at the midsection of the intercostal space between the last 2 ribs is followed by the introduction of a 2.7 mm endoscope with an operating sheath through the abdominal air sac wall to visualize the *ductus deferens*. The *ductus* is grasped with biopsy forceps, elevated, and a segment of 5 to 8 mm near the epididymis, where the ductus is less closely associated with the ureter, is excised. The procedure is repeated on the opposite side. When performing vasectomies, damaging the common iliac vein or the ureter must be avoided. Vasectomized birds may remain capable of fertilizing eggs until residual sperm stored distal to the vasectomy loses viability. In roosters, experimental occlusion of *ductus deferentes* immediately distal to the *epididymides* resulted in cessation of spermatogenesis within 5 to 7 days.[45] Reported complications of open vasectomy include restoration of luminal continuity of the operated ductus deferens and, consequently, fertility—and inadvertent laceration of the underlying common iliac vein or adjacent ureter.[46]

Anseriformes present an intromittent phallus. In Galliformes, a functional lymphatic intumescence consisting of a median and 2 lateral phallic bodies, on the floor of the lip

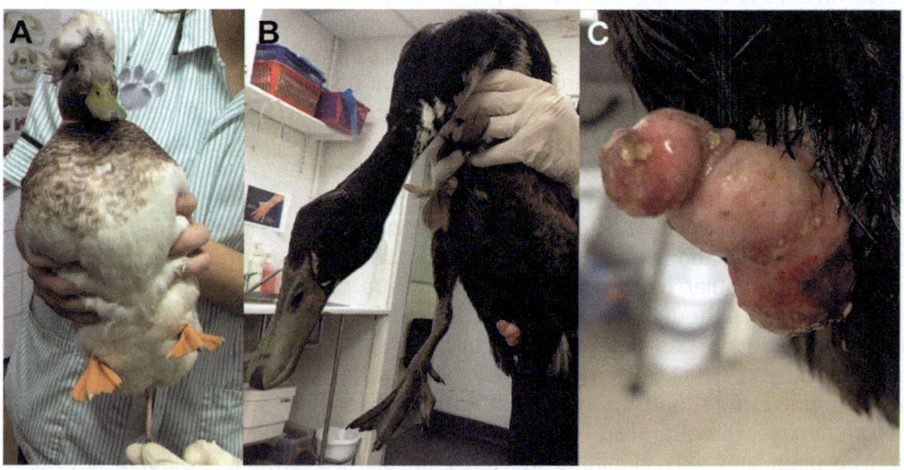

Fig. 5. (*A–C*) (*A*) Phallus prolapse in a crested duck. (*B, C*) Phallus prolapse in an Indian runner duck.

of the vent, called nonintromittent phallus, passes the sperm to the female through the *cloacal kiss*[32] (**Fig. 5**). If recurrent phallus prolapse occurs, it can be tackled with 4-0 monofilament absorbable suture to its resting position within the cloacal mucosa. Severely necrotic phalli may need surgical debridement or partial or total amputation. The portion proximal to the necrotic or severely traumatized region can be ligated using absorbable suture in an encircling pattern before sharp excision.[6]

Urinary Surgery

Urinary tract surgery in Galliformes and Anseriformes is uncommon because its location and close relation with the reproductive and gastrointestinal tracts challenge surgical access, being most urinary procedures diagnostic or palliative.

Renal surgery is generally limited to focal procedures such as biopsy collection and superficial mass removal due to their location within the renal fossae, complex vascular anatomy, and close association with the sacral plexus. Using a left lateral paralumbar fossa approach (commonly endoscopic) or a ventral midline celiotomy, the kidney is identified dorsal to the abdominal air sac. A right lateral approach may be used for unilateral disease.[6] A small incision is made through the abdominal air sac and overlying membranes to expose the serosal surface. 5-F cup biopsies can be taken from the cranial renal division to avoid major vessels. The middle division can also be sampled if the cranial division is obscured by vascular tissue (eg, an active ovary or neoplasia). Hemostasis is achieved with direct pressure or gelatin sponges. Surgical renal biopsy via dorsal pelvic approach was developed in helmeted Guinea fowls (*Numida meleagris*), Japanese quails, Pekin ducks, Indian peafowls, among other avian species, but causes greater tissue damage than other approaches and does not allow full evaluation of the kidneys.[47]

Reports of surgical treatment of ureterolithiasis in birds are limited. Simple ureteral ligation results in ipsilateral renal atrophy.[6] Successful ureterolith removal via right lateral celiotomy has been reported in a hen.[48] With the bird in left lateral recumbency and the right leg pulled forward, an incision was made between the sixth rib and the pubic bone. Fat and viscera were displaced ventrally to expose the dilated right ureter containing a 10-mm calculus and multiple smaller stones. Two ureterotomies were performed and closed with 3 cruciate 4-0 glycomer 631 sutures. Ureterotomy had been previously reported in an Amazon parrot in which one stones was removed via left lateral celiotomy and the second one via ventral midline celiotomy.[49] The ureterotomies were closed with 6-0 polyglyconate suture in a simple continuous suture pattern oversewn with a Cushing's pattern. Extracorporeal shock wave lithotripsy was successful in a Magellanic penguin (*Spheniscus magellanicus*) with renal stones, but its utility may be reduced in species with more developed air sac systems.[50]

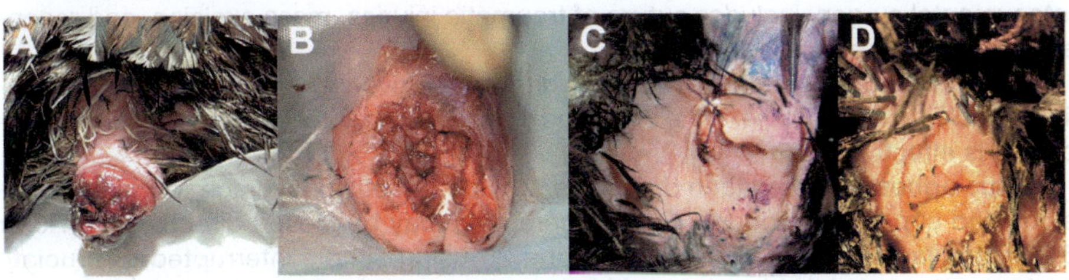

Fig. 6. (*A–D*) (*A*) Cloacal prolapse severely traumatized in a chicken. (*B*) Macroscopic appearance after debridement of necrotic tissue, removal of maggots and disinfection. (*C*) Postoperative appearance immediately after surgical reconstruction. (*D*) Postoperative appearance 2 weeks after surgery.

Cloacal and Vent Surgery

Cloacal surgery is indicated for prolapse management, foreign body removal, cloacolith extraction, trauma repair, and resection of neoplastic or inflammatory lesions (**Fig. 6**). Cloacoscopy is very useful for the evaluation and treatment of cloacal disorders.

Cloacal impaction with uric calculi or inspissated urates is common in dehydrated or obese ducks and turkeys. When conservative treatment fails, surgical removal is necessary. The vent is gently everted to expose the urodeum, and lubricated forceps or microspatulas are used to fragment and extract the calculus. The mucosa is flushed with warm saline, and devitalized tissue is removed.

Cloacopexy may be necessary to correct cloacal prolapses. Open cloacopexy—typically combined with ventplasty—aims to create permanent adhesions between the cloaca and the body wall. A ventral midline celiotomy extended parasternally to access the last ribs, is followed by isolation of the cloacal serosa and removal of fat or connective tissue that might interfere with adhesion formation. Different cloacopexy techniques have been reported in birds. In circumcostal cloacopexy, the cloaca is cranially advanced without tension and sutures secure it to the last rib. In sternal cloacopexy, the sutures pass through the cartilaginous portion of the sternum. Subserosal cloacopexy involves creating paired small incisions in the serosa and submucosa of the coprodeum, placing several sutures to achieve slight vent inversion, and tying these to establish temporary adhesions that will become permanent when sutures degrade. An incorporating cloacopexy may be added by scarifying the ventral cloacal surface and capturing the cloaca within the ventral body wall closure.[51] An incisional colopexy variant—described through a U-shaped celiotomy—allowed colonic stabilization in a cockatoo.[51] Complications of cloacopexy include failure of adhesion leading to reprolapse, dehiscence, excessive cloacal hypertrophy, inadvertent penetration of the cloaca with resulting peritonitis, and entrapment of the colon.[51]

Ventplasty is indicated for resection of traumatic or neoplastic vent lesions, and to prevent prolapse recurrence (generally combined with cloacopexy). Single (cranioventral) or paired (lateral) triangular resections may be required depending on the amount of epidermis and dermis to be excised. The sphincter and transverse cloacal muscles should be avoided. The submucosa is apposed to the dermis with simple interrupted absorbable sutures placed from medial to lateral. Then, mattress sutures are used to attach the sphincter muscle to the dermis, and the epidermis is closed. The resulting vent should allow normal passage of droppings.[51]

Integumental Surgery

Integumental surgery includes suture of traumatic injuries, mass excision, and reconstructive flap procedures.

Gentle aseptic preparation of the skin or preoperative cleaning of wounds with saline, 0.05% diluted chlorhexidine or diluted 1% povidone-iodine, with or without povacrylex, is effective.[3]

Tissue adhesive or collagen dressings provide effective coverage for minor abrasions and superficial wounds. Small lacerations may be closed directly with 4-0 or 5-0 monofilament nylon or poliglecaprone 25 using simple interrupted or cruciate patterns. Prompt debridement and closure of traumatic injuries is essential to prevent secondary infections. Devitalized edges must be sharply excised, and the wound copiously irrigated with sterile saline or Ringer's lactate. Chemical and thermal burn injuries often require conservative management before considering surgical closure. In regions with significant tension, such as the pectoral or thigh area, tension-relieving suture patterns (eg, horizontal mattress, vertical mattress, far-near-near-far pattern, tension-relieving subcutaneous sutures, or stent sutures) and/or tissue flaps can help distribute pressure more evenly. Galliformes have minimal amounts of subcutaneous tissue and sutures must engage both dermis and adjacent fascia for secure closure. Anseriformes have a more developed subcutaneous fat layer, which facilitates undermining for the creation of advancement flaps. To reduce the risk of seroma formation, the subcutaneous layer should be apposed with fine absorbable suture (5–0 polydioxanone suture [PDS]) before skin closure.

Excision of cutaneous and subcutaneous lesions requires margin identification, and when possible, its nature. An elliptical incision is made, incorporating at least 2 to 3 mm margin of normal tissue. Then, the mass is dissected from the surrounding fascia. Hemostasis can be achieved by applying pressure, or using bipolar cautery and/or fine ligatures. This is especially important during the excision of neoplastic or hyperplastic tissue from highly vascular regions (eg, the comb and wattles in chickens, the caruncles in Muscovy ducks or the snood in turkeys). Feather cysts, frequently located in the wing and cervical region of Galliformes, must be excised completely, including the sac, to prevent recurrence before closure by primary, or if small enough, secondary intention. Cystic enlargement, abscessation or neoplasia of the uropygial gland may necessitate partial or complete gland excision. The gland is dorsally approached, dissected, and resected with ligation of its small vascular pedicle, before routine wound closure.

For large excisions, skin advancement, rotation, or transposition flaps are preferred to minimize tension. Local flaps heal well when vascular pedicles are preserved. Rotation flaps up to 90° can effectively cover moderate defects in the thoracic or inguinal regions. When local flaps are inadequate, skin grafts harvested from apterial zones such as the lateral thorax or abdomen can be used. The recipient site must be immobile and free of infection. Success rates are variable but generally good in well-vascularized areas.

Avian integument heals rapidly if kept clean and protected from pecking or self-trauma. Sutures can be removed 7 to 10 days after surgery. In waterfowl, water access should be limited until feathers regrow and skin heals. Technological advances in wound healing in birds have been reviewed.[52]

Pododermatitis is a chronic, often debilitating condition of the plantar surface of the foot caused by repetitive trauma, poor substrate, obesity, or secondary infection bacteria. Advanced stages where abscessation or granulomatous tissue is present (grades III–V), require surgical treatment. After aseptic preparation, the lesion is circumscribed with an elliptical incision, the antigenic capsule is bluntly dissected and excised, and the defect is irrigated with sterile saline before skin closure by primary (simple interrupted or horizontal mattress sutures of 4–0) or secondary intention (requiring repeated disinfection and dressing changes). A padded pressure bandage (nonadhesive dressing with cohesive wrap) aids redistributing weight away from the surgical site. Frequent bandage changes and systemic antibiotherapy are required. Recurrence is common if predisposing factors are not corrected.

Ocular and Periocular Surgery

As ocular and periocular surgery in birds has been reviewed in the Carlo Paoletti and colleagues' article, "Ocular Surgery in Non-Mammalian Species," in this issue, only specific cases are listed in bibliography.[53–61]

Otic Surgery

Myringotomy has been mentioned but not clearly described as part of the treatment for otitis media and interna in birds. Surgical drainage and flushing of the pneumatic cavity of the quadrate bone was reported in a Chinese goose with peripheral vestibular disease.[62]

Neurosurgery

Neurosurgery has rarely been reported. A presumed peripheral cerebral cyst was removed by suction and gentle dissection via craniectomy in a crested Pekin duck.[63]

Reports of peripheral nerve surgery are limited to fracture-associated nerve entrapment and biopsy sampling. When neuromuscular disease is suspected (eg, Marek's disease, nutritional neuropathies, and toxic myopathies), biopsy of peripheral nerve or muscle can aid diagnosis provided their limitations are understood.[64,65] No reported cases of sciatic nerve decompression in Galliformes or Anseriformes were found by the author.

Other Soft Tissue Surgical Procedures

Nonclinical techniques and those considered inhumane or ethically controversial are not discussed in the text but are cited in the bibliography for contextual completeness.[66–72]

CLINICS CARE POINTS

- Fast chickens and ducks for 3 hours, and large waterfowl for up to 12 hours.
- Close the subcutaneous fat layer in Anseriformes with 5-0 polydioxanone suture to prevent postoperative seromas.
- Place ventriculus stay sutures only in the white tendinous portion to avoid tissue tearing.
- Avoid fluid leak testing after enterotomy, and perform oblique anastomoses to prevent strictures.
- When possible, limit tracheal resections to 5 rings in geese and 9% of length in ducks.

DISCLOSURE

The author does not have any commercial or financial conflicts of interest or any funding sources to disclose.

REFERENCES

1. Molter C, Escobar A, Schroeder C. Backyard poultry and waterfowl sedation and anesthesia. Vet Clin North Am Exot Anim Pract 2022;25(1):163–80.
2. Mulcahy DM, Heard DJ. Chapter 21. Ducks, geese, and swans (waterfowl). In: West G, Heard D, Caulkett N, editors. Zoo animal and wildlife immobilization and anesthesia. 3rd edition. Hoboken (NJ): Wiley-Blackwell; 2025.
3. Doden G, Ramachandran A, Kanda I, et al. Saline, chlorhexidine, and povidone-iodine alone or in combination with iodine povacrylex are effective antiseptics in chickens (*Gallus gallus domesticus*). Am J Vet Res 2024;85(7). AJVR.24.01.0005.
4. Jann HW, Stein LE, Good JK, et al. A comparison of nylon, polybutester, and polyglyconate suture materials for long digital flexor tenorrhaphy in chickens. Vet Surg 1992;21(3):234–7.

5. Bennett RA, Yaeger MJ, Trapp A, et al. Histologic evaluation of the tissue reaction to five suture materials in the body wall of rock doves (*Columba livia*). J Avian Med Surg 1997;11:175–82.
6. Echols MC. Chapter 21. Soft tissue surgery. In: Greenacre CB, Morishita TY, editors. Backyard poultry medicine and surgery: a guide for veterinary practitioners. 2nd edition. Hoboken (NJ): Wiley Blackwell; 2021. p. 381–433.
7. Divers SJ. Avian endosurgery. Vet Clin North Am Exot Anim Pract 2010;13(2): 203–16.
8. Grosset C, Sanchez-Migallón Guzmán D, Waymire A, et al. Extraoral surgical correction of lingual entrapment in a Chinese goose (*Anser cygnoides*). J Avian Med Surg 2013;27(4):301–8.
9. Muscatello G. Oesophageal impaction in a Canada goose (*Branta canadensis*). Aust Vet J 1998;76(8):537–40.
10. Huynh M, Sabater M, Brandão J, et al. Use of an esophagostomy tube as a method of nutritional management in raptors: a case series. J Avian Med Surg 2014;28(1):24–30.
11. Mison MB, Bennett RA. Chapter 13. Surgery of the avian gastrointestinal tract. In: Bennett RA, Pye GW, editors. Surgery of exotic animals. Hoboken (NJ): Wiley Blackwell; 2022. p. 175–89.
12. Fereshteh M, Goudarzi M, Khoshnegah J, et al. Successful surgical removal of a perforating ventricular foreign body from a mallard duck (*Anas platyrhynchos*): a case report. J Poultry Sci Avian Dis 2023;1(2):37–41.
13. Ferrell S, Werner J, Kyles A, et al. Evaluation of a collagen patch as a method of enhancing ventriculotomy healing in Japanese quail (*Coturnix coturnix japonica*). Vet Surg 2003;32(2):103–12.
14. Zebisch K, Krautwald-Junghanns ME, Willuhn J. Ultrasound-guided liver biopsy in birds. Vet Radiol Ultrasound 2004;45:241–6.
15. Carp NZ, Saputelli J, Halbherr TC, et al. A technique for liver biopsy performed in Pekin ducks using anesthesia with Telazol. Lab Anim Sci 1991;41:474–5.
16. Mulcahy DM, Esler D. Survival of captive and free-ranging harlequin ducks (*Histrionicus histrionicus*). J Wildl Dis 2010;46:1325–9.
17. Mison MB, Bennett RA. Chapter 11. Approaches to the caudal coelom (abdomen) of birds. In: Bennett RA, Pye GW, editors. Surgery of exotic animals. Hoboken (NJ): Wiley Blackwell; 2022. p. 154–62.
18. Onderka DK, Langevin CC, Hanson JA. Fibrosing cholehepatitis in broiler chickens induced by bile duct ligations or inoculation of *Clostridium perfringens*. Can J Vet Res 1990;54:285–90.
19. Hazelwood RL, Cieslak SR. In vitro release of pancreatic hormones following 99% pancreatectomy in the chicken. Gen Comp Endocrinol 1989;73:308–17.
20. Laurent F, Karmann H, Mialhe P. Insulin, glucagon and somatostatin content in normal and diabetic duck pancreas. Horm Metab Res 1987;19:134–5.
21. Martland MF. Histopathology of the chick pancreas following pancreatic duct ligation. Vet Rec 1986;118:526–30.
22. Pérez Orrico ML, Sabater González M. Anestesia por perfusión de saco aéreo (APA) en aves y su utilidad en oftalmología. Lince (SEOVET) 2022;21:45–52.
23. Adair JE, Riggs GL. Surgical repair of a complete transverse tracheal rupture in a mallard duck (*Anas platyrhynchos*). J Avian Med Surg 2022;35(4):451–6.
24. Pye GW. Chapter 14. Surgery of the avian respiratory system and cranial coelom. In: Bennett RA, Pye GW, editors. Surgery of exotic animals. Hoboken (NJ): Wiley Blackwell; 2022. p. 190–203.

25. Sánchez-Migallón Guzmán D, Mitchell M, Hedlund CS, et al. Tracheal resection and anastomosis in a mallard duck (*Anas platyrhynchos*) with traumatic segmental tracheal collapse. J Avian. Med Surg 2007;21(2):150–7.
26. Clippinger TL, Bennett RA. Successful treatment of a traumatic tracheal stenosis in a goose by surgical resection and anastomosis. J Avian Med Surg 1998;12(4): 243–7.
27. Altman RB. Chapter 41. Soft tissue surgical procedures. In: Altman RB, Clubb SL, Dorrestein GM, et al, editors. Avian medicine and surgery. Philadelphia: WB Saunders; 1997. p. 704–32.
28. Straub J, Pees M, Enders F, et al. Pericardiocentesis and the use of enalapril in a Fischer's lovebird (*Agapornis fischeri*). Vet Rec 2003;152(1):24–6.
29. Fitzgerald BC, Beaufrère H. Cardiology. In: Current veterinary therapy in Avian medicine. Vol I. Philadelphia: WB Saunders; 2016. p. 252–328.
30. Hernandez-Divers SJ, McBride M, Hanley C. Minimally invasive endosurgery of the psittacine cranial coelom. Exot Dvm 2004;6:33–7.
31. McGinnis CH Jr, Ringer RK. Carotid sinus reflex in the chicken. Poult Sci 1966; 45(2):402–4.
32. Calvo Carrasco D, Sabater González M. Reproductive disorders in commonly kept fowl. Vet Clin North Am Exot Anim Pract 2017;20(2):509–38.
33. Echols S, Speer B. Avian reproductive tract diseases and surgical resolutions. Clin Theriogenol 2022;14:32–42.
34. Johnson PA, Brooks C, Wang SY, et al. Plasma concentrations of immunoreactive inhibin and gonadotropins following removal of ovarian follicles in the domestic hen. Biol Reprod 1993;49:1026–31.
35. Sullivan JL, Wakamatsu N, Yin JH, et al. Assessment of a vessel and tissue-sealing device for ovariectomy in chickens to evaluate the potential application of the procedure to other avian species. Am J Vet Res 2021;82(4):310–7.
36. Chen KL, Lee TY, Chen TW, et al. Effect of caponization and different exogenous androgen on hepatic lipid and β-oxidase of male chickens. Poult Sci 2009;88: 1033–9.
37. Hagelin JC. Castration in Gambel's and scaled quail: ornate plumage and dominance persist, but courtship and threat behaviors do not. Horm Behav 2001; 39:1–10.
38. Kremer A, Budras KD. The blood supply of the testis in Pekin drakes (Anas platyrhynchos). Macroscopic, light microscopic, and scanning electron microscopic studies. Anat Anz 1990;171:73–87.
39. Mehler SJ, Bennett RA. Chapter 12. Avian reproductive procedures. In: Bennett RA, Pye GW, editors. Surgery of exotic animals. Hoboken (NJ): Wiley Blackwell; 2022. p. 163–74.
40. Hernandez-Divers SJ, Stahl SJ, Wilson GH, et al. Endoscopic orchidectomy and salpingohysterectomy of pigeons (*Columba livia*): an avian model for minimally invasive endosurgery. J Avian Med Surg 2007;21(1):22–37.
41. Converse KA, Kennelly JJ. Evaluation of Canada goose sterilization for population control. Wildl Soc Bull 1994;22:265–9.
42. Ellis DH, Carpenter JW. A technique for vasectomizing birds. J Field Ornithol 1981;52:69–71.
43. Hundgen K, Raphael B, Sheppard C. Egg fertility among vasectomized and non-vasectomized male resident Canada geese at the Wildlife Conservation Park/ Bronx Zoo. Zoo Biol 2000;19:35–40.
44. Jones RG, Redig PT. Endoscopy-guided vasectomy in the immature Japanese quail (*Coturnix coturnix japonica*). Proc Eur Assoc Avian Vet 2003;117–23.

45. Janssen SJ, Kirby JD, Hess RA, et al. Identification of epididymal stones in diverse rooster populations. Poult Sci 2000;79:569–74.
46. Samour J. Vasectomy in birds: a review. J Avian Med Surg 2010;24(3):169–73.
47. Suedmeyer K, Bermudez A. A new approach to renal biopsy in birds. J Avian Med Surg 1996;10(3):179–86.
48. Modesto F, Guillier D, van Bruggen LW. Successful treatment of ureteral obstructive lithiasis by ureterotomy in a domestic hen. J Avian Med Surg 2022; 36(1):70–7.
49. Dennis PM, Bennett RA. Ureterotomy for removal of two ureteroliths in a parrot. J Am Vet Med Assoc 2000;217(6):865–8.
50. Machado C. Disintegration of kidney stones by extracorporeal shock wave lithotripsy in a penguin. Proc Int Conf Zool Avian Med 1987;343–9.
51. Mison M, Mehler S, Echols MS, et al. Selected coelomic surgical procedures. In: Speer BL, editor. Current therapy in Avian medicine and surgery. St Louis (MO): Saunders; 2016. p. 645–57.
52. Sabater González M, Mayer J. Technological advances in wound treatment of exotic pets. Vet Clin North Am Exot Anim Pract 2019;22(3):451–70.
53. Park SA, Davidson H, Thompson KA, et al. Successful chemical ablation of an intraorbital cyst caused by an eyelid injury and iatrogenic ankyloblepharon formation in a duck. J Am Vet Med Assoc 2018;253(9):1164–8.
54. Houston K, Fontaine C, Dziedzic-Nyrka N, et al. Successful management of a refractory orbital pseudocyst in a Chinese goose using intraorbital gentamicin injection. Vet Ophthalmol 2025;1.
55. Lewin AC, Riedel RM, Queiroz-Williams P, et al. Successful surgical removal of the crystalline lenses in a black-necked swan (*Cygnus melancoryphus*). J Avian Med Surg 2023;37(1):41–5.
56. Busch TJ. Bilateral dermoids in a goose. N Z Vet J 1985;33:189–90.
57. Murphy CJ, Belhorn RW, Buyukmihci NC. Subconjunctival hibernoma in a goose. J Am Vet Med Assoc 1986;189:1109–10.
58. Gilger BC, McLaughlin SA, Smith P. Uveal malignant melanoma in a duck. J Am Vet Med Assoc 1995;206:1580–2.
59. Kennedy FS. An outbreak of conjunctival rhinosporidiosis in swans (*Cygnus* spp.). Proc Assoc Avian Vet 1994;426–7.
60. Kennedy FA, Buggage RR, Ajello L. Rhinosporidiosis in captive swans. J Med Vet Mycol 1995;33:157–65.
61. Sadar MJ, Guzman DS, Burton AG, et al. Mycotic keratitis in a Khaki Campbell duck (*Anas platyrhynchos domesticus*). J Avian Med Surg 2014;28(4):322–9.
62. Delk KW, Mejia-Fava J, Jiménez DA, et al. Diagnostic imaging of peripheral vestibular disease in a Chinese goose (*Anser cygnoides*). J Avian Med Surg 2014;28(1):31–7.
63. Yaw TJ, Jeffery ND, Cain B, et al. Removal of a presumed peripheral cerebral cyst via craniectomy in a crested Pekin duck (*Anas platyrhynchos f. dom*). J Avian Med Surg 2016;30(3):263–8.
64. Cortes AL, Montiel ER, Lemiere S, et al. Comparison of blood and feather pulp samples for the diagnosis of Marek's disease and for monitoring Marek's disease vaccination by real-time PCR. Avian Dis 2011;55:302–10.
65. Sesny Gall L, Kőröci L, Cortes AL, et al. Use of real-time PCR to rule out Marek's disease in the diagnosis of peripheral neuropathy. Avian Pathol 2018;47(4):1–24.
66. Demirkan I, Altin S, Demirkan A, et al. Comparison of the effects of flight restraint in the partridge (*Alectoris chukar*) by tenectomy, capsulectomy or tenectomy plus capsulectomy techniques. Kafkas Univ Vet Fak Derg 2010;16:1017–24.

67. Shaw SN, D'Agostino JJ, Davis MR, et al. Primary feather follicle ablation in common pintails (*Anas acuta acuta*) and a white-faced whistling duck (*Dendrocygna viduata*). J Zoo Wildl Med 2012;43(2):342–6.
68. Peterson RDA, Burmester BR, Fredrickson TN, et al. Effect of bursectomy and thymectomy on the development of visceral lymphomatosis in the chicken. J Natl Cancer Inst 1964;32(6):1343–54.
69. Fagan AB, Kennaway DJ, Oakley AP. Pinealectomy in the chicken: a good model of scoliosis? Eur Spine J 2009;18(8):1154–9.
70. Manangi MK, Clark FD, Coon CN. Improved colostomy technique and excrement (urine) collection for broilers and broiler breeder hens. Poult Sci 2007;86: 698–704.
71. Jirjis FF, Waibel PE, Duke GE, et al. An improved colostomy technique in turkeys. Br Poult Sci 1997;38:603–6.
72. Poppema TF, Duke GE. The effectiveness of ligating or detaching ceca as an alternative to cecectomy. Poult Sci 1992;71(8):1384–90.

Ocular Surgery in Non-mammalian Species

Carlo Paoletti, DVM, Dipl ECZM (Small Mammals); Postgraduate University Diploma in Microsurgical Techniques (Faculty of Medicine, Sorbonne University, Paris)[a,*], José Rosas-Navarro, DVM, Dipl ECZM (Small Mammals); Postgraduate University Diploma in Microsurgical Techniques (Faculty of Medicine, Sorbonne University, Paris)[a], María Luisa Pérez Orrico, LV, MRCVS, C.E.S. Ophtalmologie Vétérinaire ENVT, ECVO Residency Trained Clinician[b], Aure-Eline Grillot, DVM, Dipl ECVO[c]

KEYWORDS

• Veterinary ophthalmic surgery • Exotic animal ophthalmology • Striated iris
• Mydriasis • Spectacle disorders • Nictitating membrane • Scleral ossicles
• Phacoemulsification

KEY POINTS

- Ophthalmic surgery in fish, amphibians, reptiles, and birds requires species-specific planning due to their major anatomic and physiologic particularities.
- Corneal disease, spectacle disorders, cataracts, and painful end-stage ocular disease are among the most common surgical indications across nonmammalian taxa.
- Surgical decision-making must incorporate husbandry, environmental parameters, and anesthesia protocols tailored to each species.
- Techniques such as keratectomy, lensectomy, phacoemulsification, spectaculotomy, enucleation, and exenteration are feasible but require magnification, delicate instrumentation, and strict postoperative care.
- Early recognition and appropriate intervention are essential to prevent systemic complications, optimize comfort, and preserve function whenever possible.

Video content accompanies this article at http://www.vetexotic.theclinics.com.

INTRODUCTION

Ophthalmic surgery in nonmammalian species presents distinctive challenges driven by marked anatomic and physiologic differences from mammals. Fish, amphibians,

[a] Exotic Animal Department, Centre Hospitalier Vétérinaire AniCura-ADVETIA, 9 Avenue Louis Breguet, 78140 Vélizy-Villacoublay, France; [b] Hospital Veterinario, Universidad Católica de Valencia (UCV), Exoticsvet, Valencia, Spain; [c] Department of Ophthalmogy, Centre Hospitalier Vétérinaire AniCura-ADVETIA, 9 Avenue Louis Breguet, 78140 Vélizy-Villacoublay, France
* Corresponding author. Exotic Animal Department, Centre Hospitalier Vétérinaire AniCura-ADVETIA, 9 Avenue Louis Breguet, 78140 Vélizy-Villacoublay, France
E-mail address: carlovet@gmail.com

Vet Clin Exot Anim 29 (2026) 587–605
https://doi.org/10.1016/j.cvex.2026.04.008 **vetexotic.theclinics.com**

Abbreviation	
SIS	small-intestinal submucosa

reptiles, and birds exhibit unique ocular structures including rigid or highly spherical lenses, fragile or ultrathin corneas, spectacles, scleral ossicles, and striated irides that influence diagnostics, anesthesia, and surgical planning. These species also differ widely in environmental needs and healing strategies, requiring clinicians to tailor perioperative management to optimize outcomes and minimize stress and morbidity. Understanding species-specific adaptations is fundamental for selecting appropriate surgical techniques, ensuring patient comfort, and achieving functional recovery.

Ocular Surgery in Fish

Fish ophthalmology reflects unique adaptations: the cornea contributes little to refraction, while a spherical, high–index lens provides almost all optical power, and light adaptation depends on retinomotor rather than pupillary mechanisms.[1]

Clinically, agnathans seldom require intervention; cartilaginous fish occasionally undergo surgery for trauma or parasitism, and teleosts remain the primary focus.[2–4]

Perioperative considerations

Fish anesthesia is most commonly achieved by adding the anesthetic directly to the water, allowing rapid absorption through the gills (Video 1).

For large species, topical application on the gills can further speed induction. Alternative routes include intramuscular, intravenous, or intraperitoneal injections, as well as oral administration via stomach tube or medicated food, though onset may be variable.

If the fish must remain out of the water, anesthesia can be maintained by gently pumping a diluted anesthetic solution over the gills. During anesthesia, monitoring should include assessment of reflexes, response to stimuli, and heart rate.

Recovery should take place in clean, anesthetic-free water. Many different anesthetic agents can be used in fish; further information can be found in the article, "Soft Tissue Surgery in Fish" in this issue, and for detailed information on their selection and dosage, reference should be made to specialized veterinary texts.

Anatomic considerations

Teleost eyes are structurally supported by scleral cartilage and ossicles, which provide rigidity and stability to the globe.[2]

The cornea retains the same basic organization seen in other vertebrates—epithelium, stroma, Descemet's membrane, and endothelium, but in many species the epithelium accounts for nearly half of the total thickness, a feature believed to limit osmotic flux and compensate for the absence of eyelids.[2]

Spectacles have been described in several fish groups and show remarkable diversity, ranging from a simple lid skin covering the cornea, to a subspectacular space separating dermal and scleral cornea, and finally to a fused eyelid structure that creates a tertiary spectacle.[1]

The iris of most teleosts also departs significantly from the mammalian model, lacking muscular fibers and therefore true pupillary light reflexes.[2]

In species where pupillary movements are present (elasmobranchs), they are slow, sometimes consensual[2] and largely controlled through cholinergic innervation.[2]

Corneal disease

Corneal disease is one of the most frequent surgical indications in teleosts: ulcers typically require debridement under anesthesia with cyanoacrylate patching to prevent perforation, and outcomes depend on strict water-quality control, medicated immersion, and antimicrobial support.[2] Corneal lipidosis may necessitate superficial keratectomy, but durable resolution hinges on correcting husbandry.[5]

The use of liquid nitrogen cryosurgery for the treatment of corneal masses has been reported.[2]

Lens surgery

Cataract is a major cause of visual impairment in fish, arising from environmental and nutritional factors, osmotic imbalance, parasitism, genetic predisposition, elevated temperature, and environmental pollution.[2]

From a surgical perspective, cataract removal is technically challenging. Phacoemulsification has been attempted in sturgeons and isolated teleosts,[2] but the extreme density of fish lenses limits its feasibility, and some authors discourage its use.[2] Intracapsular or extracapsular lensectomy remains the preferred option, with intracapsular extraction favored to reduce postoperative inflammation and the risk of panophthalmitis.[2]

Lens luxation, either traumatic or secondary to systemic disease, has also been described and may necessitate lensectomy or enucleation to prevent secondary glaucoma.[2]

Enucleation

Enucleation is considered a last-resort ophthalmic procedure in fish, primarily indicated in cases of ocular pain or advanced ocular disease. A common predisposing condition is exophthalmia, which most frequently results from infections.[2] Other reported causes include ectopic thyroid tissue,[2] trauma, nutritional deficiencies, and neoplasia.[2]

Intraocular tumors are rare in fish, with retinoblastoma being the only consistently reported malignancy.[2] Nevertheless, isolated case reports have described other neoplasms successfully managed by enucleation, such as a uveal iridophoroma in a betta fish (*Betta splendens*)[6] and a primary ocular chondrosarcoma in a discus (*Symphysodon aequifasciatus*).[7]

Clinically, exophthalmia predisposes the globe to trauma and may lead to blindness through stretching of the optic nerve. When the condition becomes severe, progressive, or unresponsive to treatment, enucleation is indicated.[2]

Other situations in which enucleation is warranted include intraocular neoplasia[6,7] and cases of end-stage ocular pain.

When pathology extends beyond the globe or orbital contamination is suspected, exenteration is preferred, as it allows en bloc removal of all orbital contents, albeit with a higher risk of hemorrhage.[8] In such cases, a thorough assessment of disease extent, including appropriate imaging, is essential before planning surgery (**Fig. 1**).

Standard enucleation in teleosts is performed under general anesthesia, most commonly via a transconjunctival approach. The procedure begins with a periocular incision at the orbital rim, followed by dissection of scleral cartilage and periocular connective tissues. Extraocular muscles are transected close to their origins to mobilize the globe, and the optic nerve together with associated vessels is severed. Hemorrhage is generally minimal but may require ligation or cautery in larger species or chronic inflammatory states. The orbit can be packed with absorbable gelatin sponges and left to reepithelialize, while postoperative care involves systemic antimicrobials and anti-inflammatory therapy.[2,9]

When exenteration is indicated, all orbital contents—including extraocular muscles, fat, and connective tissue—are removed en bloc (**Fig. 2**). Due to the higher hemorrhagic risk, hemostasis is achieved through direct pressure, cautery, or topical

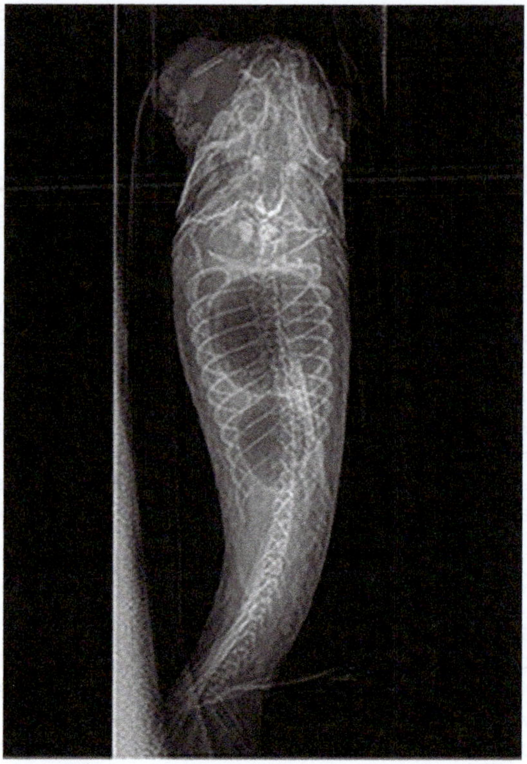

Fig. 1. Presurgical radiograph of a goldfish (*Carassius auratus*) presented with a left ocular mass. (Image Courtesy of Dr Carlo Paoletti.)

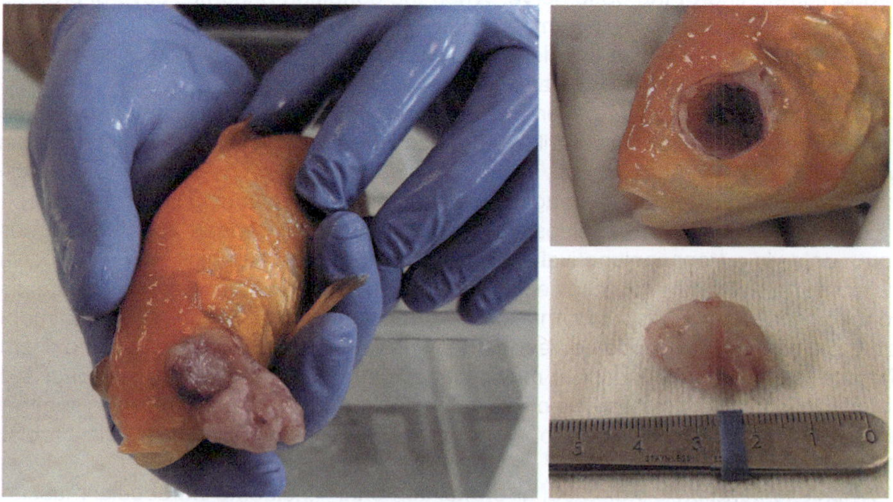

Fig. 2. Enucleation performed for an ocular neuroblastoma in a goldfish (*Carassius auratus*). (Image Courtesy of Dr Carlo Paoletti.)

hemostatic agents such as collagen powder or phenylephrine. Depending on species and defect size, the orbit may be left open, packed with a protective paste (eg, Orabase®), or covered with an advancing skin flap.[8]

Ocular Surgery in Amphibians

Vision plays a critical role in terrestrial anurans in which blindness may result in anorexia and welfare concerns. In contrast, urodeles and aquatic anurans rely more heavily on olfaction in addition to vision, whereas caecilians depend primarily on olfaction and rostral tentacles with only minimal visual input.[10]

Amphibian ocular surgery must be tailored to species-specific physiology and husbandry: permeable skin, distinctive ocular anatomy, and environmental requirements drive case planning, anesthesia, and recovery.[11]

Accordingly, surgical planning in anurans must consider the thin barrier between the globes and the oral cavity, as well as the role of globe retraction and protrusion in swallowing. Disruption of this membrane can impair feeding and may lead to anorexia.[10]

Anesthesia and monitoring

General anesthesia is most often induced with immersion in buffered tricaine methanesulfonate. Sensitivity varies widely among species and developmental stages, so continuous monitoring is essential. Alternative protocols (other immersion baths, topical, inhalant, or injectable methods) are selected case by case.[12]

Preoperative preparation

Amphibian skin is thin and highly absorptive, so surgical field preparation must be minimal and nonirritating: sterile saline or very dilute chlorhexidine are preferred. Povidone–iodine should be avoided in larvae and neotenic taxa, where iodine exposure may induce metamorphosis[10]; this same permeability also means drug administration requires precise dilution, as even topical preparations can achieve systemic exposure through the skin.[10,13,14]

Intraoperative principles

Because amphibian skin is fragile and easily torn, the use of fine instruments, magnification, and careful closure techniques is essential. Interrupted sutures with slowly absorbable monofilament reduce tension and bacterial wicking, while controlled postoperative environments are necessary due to the prolonged healing process.[10]

Corneal surgery

Because the amphibian cornea is extremely thin and prone to perforation, corneal ulcers are generally not managed with debridement or keratoplasty as first-line treatments.[15] Since aquatic environments rapidly dilute topical medications, alternative approaches are often required. Temporary tarsorrhaphy, third-eyelid flaps, and application of butyl cyanoacrylate have been described in the literature as supportive measures to safeguard the globe and maintain corneal surface integrity during the epithelial healing process.[16]

Lipid keratopathy is a corneal disease documented in captive populations of amphibians, typically associated with underlying husbandry imbalances (**Fig. 3**).[15,17,18] While metabolic keratopathies such as corneal lipidosis in other species may occasionally require superficial keratectomy, in amphibians this condition tends to remain chronic, and long-term control depends primarily on correcting environmental and dietary factors.[15] Phototherapeutic keratectomy using laser ablation has been reported in other contexts,[19] and in the authors' opinion may represent a potential option for future investigation.

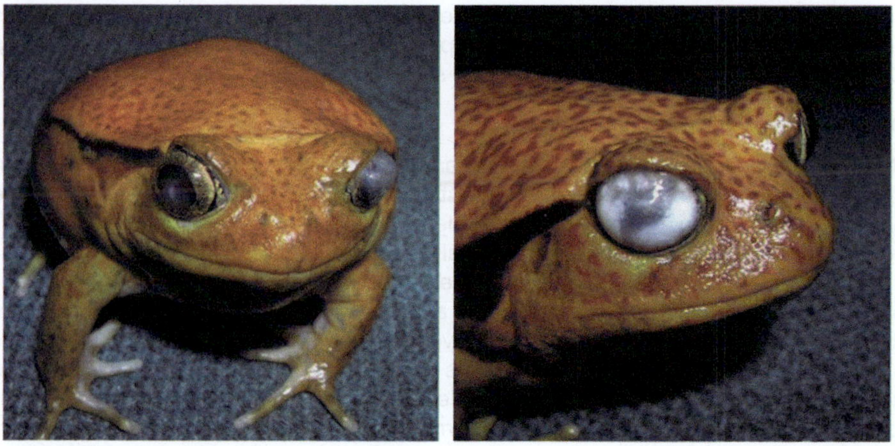

Fig. 3. Corneal lipidosis in a tomato frog (*Dyscophus guineti*). (Image Courtesy of Dr Carlo Paoletti.)

Cataract surgery

Cataracts are most frequently reported in anurans, and surgical planning must account for a shallow anterior chamber and eyelids close to the limbus. Corneal entry slightly posterior to the limbus is recommended to avoid proximity to the eyelids, which can complicate suturing. Mydriasis is achieved once the patient is anesthetized.[15]

Due to the typically dense nature of amphibian cataracts, aspiration tends to be of limited effectiveness. A small (<22-gauge) phacoemulsification needle with a divide-and-conquer technique is preferred, with closure using very fine (9–0 to 11–0) absorbable sutures. Postoperative non-steroidal anti-inflammatory drugs use remains controversial.[15] Lens material removal without intraocular lens implantation is considered sufficient because many amphibians regenerate functional lenses.[15] Two case reports describe lens removal in a milk frog (*Trachycephalus resinifictrix*) via a 180° limbal incision, Snellen loop extraction, and 9-0 nylon closure,[20] as well as successful phacoemulsification in an American toad (*Anaxyrus americanus*).[21]

Enucleation

Enucleation is considered a salvage procedure for amphibians with irreversible blindness or painful intraocular disease, including retrobulbar neoplasms or abscesses.[15] The surgery is anatomically challenging: anurans lack a hard palate and rely on ventral globe compression for swallowing, so enucleation may impair feeding. Bilateral procedures are strongly discouraged, as bilateral retractor bulbi denervation increased swallowing effort significantly in frogs.[15] During surgery, placement of gauze in the oral cavity can help stabilize the globe in species that retract the eyes to assist swallowing. After local anesthetic infusion, the conjunctiva is incised and extraocular muscles dissected, with care to avoid the oral cavity and facial vein.[16] The optic nerve and vessels are transected, hemorrhage is controlled with pressure or hemostatic sponges, and closure is achieved with temporary tarsorrhaphy or, in some cases, second-intention healing.[16,21]

True ocular neoplasms are rare in amphibians but have been reported, including a corneal/retrobulbar epithelioma in the European common frog (*Rana temporaria*),[22] an ophthalmic adenocarcinoma in an African clawed frog (*Xenopus laevis*),[23] and a corneal dermoid in a red-eyed tree frog (*Agalychnis callidryas*),[24] all successfully managed with enucleation.

A final indication for enucleation is painful glaucoma, as the use of carbonic anhydrase inhibitors in amphibians may result in transdermal absorption, potentially disrupting systemic acid–base balance and causing harmful effects.[25]

Ocular Surgery in Reptiles

Before considering ophthalmic surgery in reptiles, correct husbandry and stabilize the patient because a large proportion of ocular surface disease and delayed healing is husbandry-driven and may improve without operative intervention.[26–32]

Surgical planning must then be anatomy-led: striated irides make topical mydriatics unreliable; intact spectacles block topical penetration; many squamate corneas are ultrathin; and a Harderian-based tear film occupies a subspectacular space with species-specific outflow, absent in chelonians. These determinants dictate drug-delivery route, watertight low-tension closure, and strict postoperative environmental control.[29]

Diagnostic localization and imaging

Localization of ocular lesions relies on adequate magnification and precise plane identification: a slit lamp or operating microscope is essential to differentiate anterior chamber disease from subspectacular pathology in spectacled species, where nasolacrimal duct patency is best evaluated by fine-gauge fluorescein injection into the subspectacular space with confirmation of intraoral dye egress (**Fig. 4**), and ultrasonography further delineates intraocular and retrobulbar structures with minimal physical restraint.[26–29]

Anesthesia and mydriasis

Because topical mydriatics are ineffective in striated irides, reliable dilation is achieved under general anesthesia using intracameral neuromuscular blockade (eg, curare or D-tubocurarine), often supplemented with viscoelastic-assisted mechanical dilation.[28–30,33]

However, in turtles, the topical use of rocuronium bromide alone or combined with phenylephrine has been reported as a safe and effective alternative.[34,35]

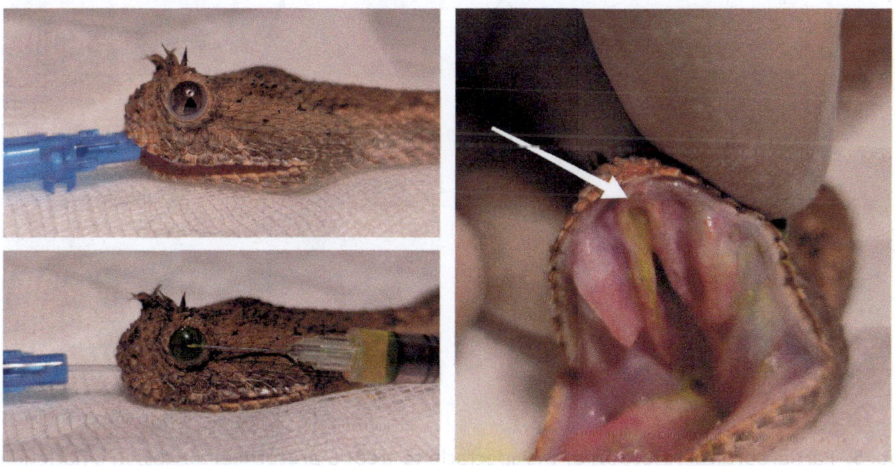

Fig. 4. Jones test performed by subspectacular fluorescein injection in a many-horned adder (*Bitis cornuta*) to assess nasolacrimal duct patency. White arrow: distal opening of the nasolacrymal duct. (Image Courtesy of Dr Clément Paillusseau.)

When the spectacle is present, topical therapy will not reach intraocular targets, so perioperative protocols should favor systemic medications or precisely delivered local therapy (eg, intracameral or subspectacular routes) over additional topical dosing.[31]

In large chelonians with mobile lids but poor tolerance for frequent handling, subpalpebral lavage systems can provide reliable topical delivery.[36]

Eyelid surgery

Eyelid repair in reptiles, usually trauma-related, aims to restore anatomy and limit scarring. Small defects close well with 6-0 or 7-0 braided coated sutures, while larger ones may require blepharoplasty or sliding grafts.[29] Successful eyelid reconstruction has been reported in a leopard gecko (*Eublepharis macularius*). with congenital ankyloblepharon.[37]

Spectacle disorders and surgery

Spectacle debridement or partial spectaculectomy is indicated for abrasions, substrate entrapment, or subspectacular abscesses. A lateral spectaculotomy involving up to 25% to 30% of the spectacle allows flushing and antibiotic therapy, with the wound left open for drainage (**Fig. 5**). Healing occurs within weeks, and complete spectacle regeneration is typically achieved in about 3 months.[29]

Spectacle avulsion rapidly causes corneal desiccation and therefore requires immediate tectonic coverage, typically achieved with mucosal, collagen, or amniotic membrane grafts sutured to the remaining edges, to protect the corneal epithelium until a new spectacle regenerates.[29,30]

For clean avulsions where a mechanical shield that synchronizes with shedding is desirable, a porcine small-intestinal submucosa (SIS) graft secured over the cornea can bridge the defect; in a Brazilian rainbow boa (*Epicrates cenchria cenchria*), the graft shed at the first ecdysis (~30 days) and the spectacle fully regenerated by the next ecdysis (~39 days).[38]

In cases of extensive avulsion complicated by infectious keratomalacia, a 2-layer amniotic membrane construct—consisting of a deep disk tucked under the spectacle remnant and fibrin-glued to the cornea, plus a superficial disk spanning the defect

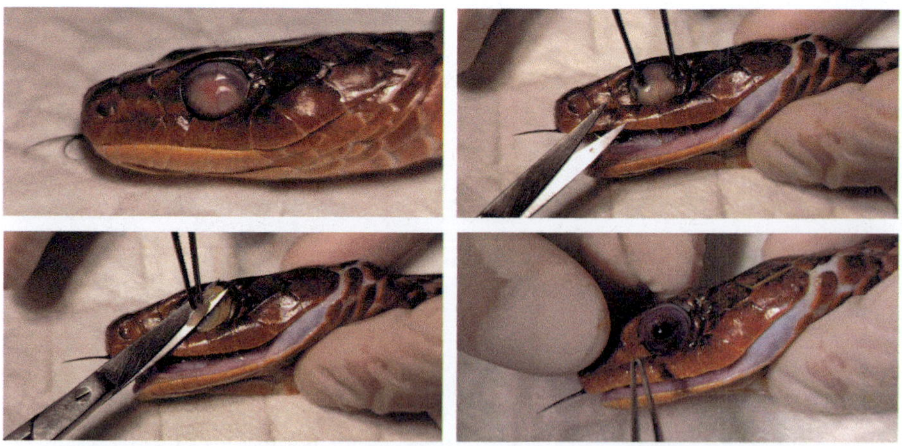

Fig. 5. Partial surgical resection of the spectacle to treat a precorneal abscess in a harlequin snake (*Chironius scurrula*). Although the approach shown was effective, the gold-standard technique involves resection of a small triangular wedge from the ventral third of the spectacle. (Image Courtesy of Dr Cléménr Paillusseau.)

secured with sparse 9-0 sutures and fibrin glue—restored a sealed surface and achieved spectacle continuity and corneal clarity within 4 months.[39]

In practice, SIS provides durable mechanical shielding for uncomplicated avulsions, whereas amniotic membrane is preferred for infected, melting corneas requiring anti-inflammatory and antiprotease support.

In spectacled species, pseudobuphthalmos results from obstruction of the nasolacrimal duct, leading to fluid accumulation in the subspectacular space and an apparent ocular enlargement. Management requires either relief of the obstruction or surgical creation of an alternative drainage pathway (conjunctivoralostomy/buccostomy), typically maintained with a Silastic tube™ for up to 6 weeks.[40]

Corneal surgery

Deep corneal ulcers or lacerations can be managed with 8/0 to 10/0 sutures, cyanoacrylate adhesives, or conjunctival grafts. In chelonians and lizards, a third eyelid flap may be used for severe lesions, though this approach limits visualization and exerts pressure on the globe during healing.[39]

In reptiles, firm infectious corneal plaques can be gently lifted off the cornea when loosely attached; where the plaque is very adherent, a superficial keratectomy is required, followed by culture-guided topical antibiotic therapy and correction of systemic or nutritional factors.[31,39]

In rapidly progressive melting keratitis with perforation and severe anterior uveitis, prompt enucleation may be indicated to reduce septic risk given the grave globe prognosis.[41]

Cataract surgery

Cataract surgery in reptiles is rarely reported,[30] and when performed it is most often performed using irrigation–aspiration techniques because of the typically soft lens consistency.[29]

In spectacled reptiles, an additional step is necessary: the spectacle must be incised and reflected before accessing the cornea and anterior chamber.[29,33]

Outcomes reported in snakes confirm feasibility but highlight anticipated issues: postoperative uveitis can occur yet typically responds to medical therapy, whereas small globes and prior spectacle scarring may necessitate larger spectaculectomies that prolong healing.[42]

In large lizards, phacoemulsification has produced stable visual recovery with uncomplicated healing (**Fig. 6**).[43,44]

In turtles, phacoemulsification is reported to have successful outcome but can be challenging to perform.[45]

Enucleation

Enucleation is indicated when vision and comfort cannot be preserved.[29]

In reptiles with mobile eyelids, the surgical approach parallels that used in mammals: a lateral canthotomy facilitates exposure, followed by transconjunctival enucleation or, alternatively, a modified evisceration similar to that performed in birds, which preserves the rigid scleral shell to minimize postoperative enophthalmos.[46]

Because periocular soft tissue is sparse, closure is performed in a single layer (4–0 to 7–0) with slightly everted skin edges to reduce inversion and dysecdysis (**Fig. 7**).[29,47]

In species with a fused spectacle, the globe and spectacle are removed en bloc, the optic vasculature clamped, and the wound left to granulate by secondary intention over 4 to 6 weeks under topical antibiotic coverage (**Fig. 8**).[29,47]

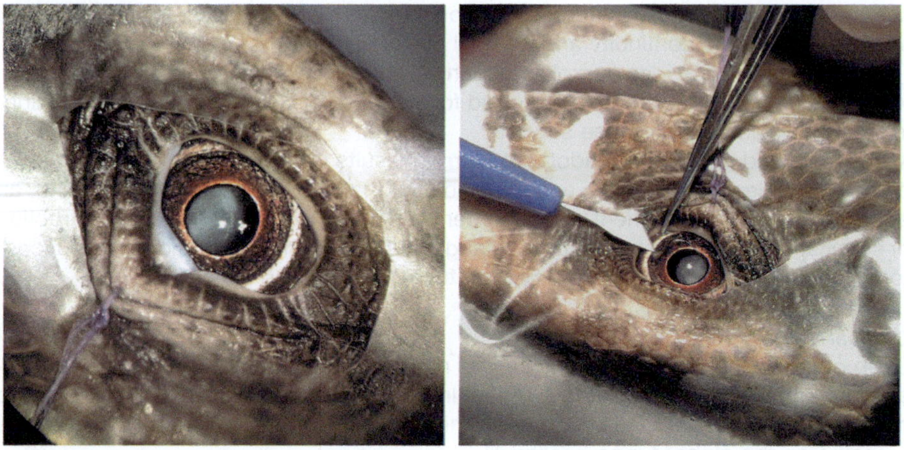

Fig. 6. Patient positioning and surgical field preparation before extracapsular cataract removal in a savannah monitor (*Varanus exanthematicus*). (Image Courtesy of Dr Clémént Paillusseau.)

Favorable outcomes are reported, including a panther chameleon (*Furcifer pardalis*) resuming normal hunting within 48 hours and remaining well at 1 year.[48]

When the surgical wound cannot be closed, the fixation of SIS to periocular skin is reported to facilitate healing of the wound by secondary intention.[49]

Exenteration has been described in a case of periorbital adenocarcinoma in a central bearded dragon (*Pogona vitticeps*), but the tumor recurred soon after surgery.[50]

Other

Successful surgical removal of a dacryops dorsal to the globe has been described in a red-eared slider (*Trachemys scripta elegans*). The skin of the upper eyelid was excised and careful dissection of the cyst was performed, being able to spare the globe. After

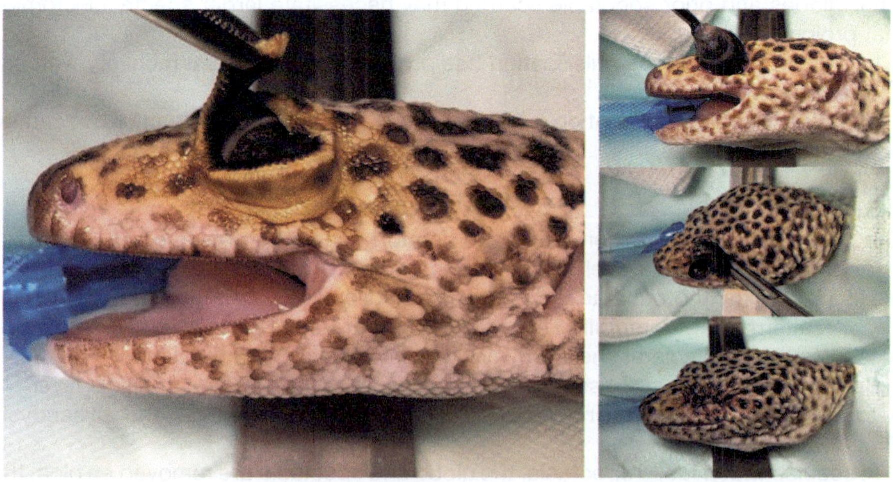

Fig. 7. Enucleation performed to manage eyelid laceration and corneal perforation in a leopard gecko (*Eublepharis macularius*). (Image Courtesy of Dr Clémént Paillusseau.)

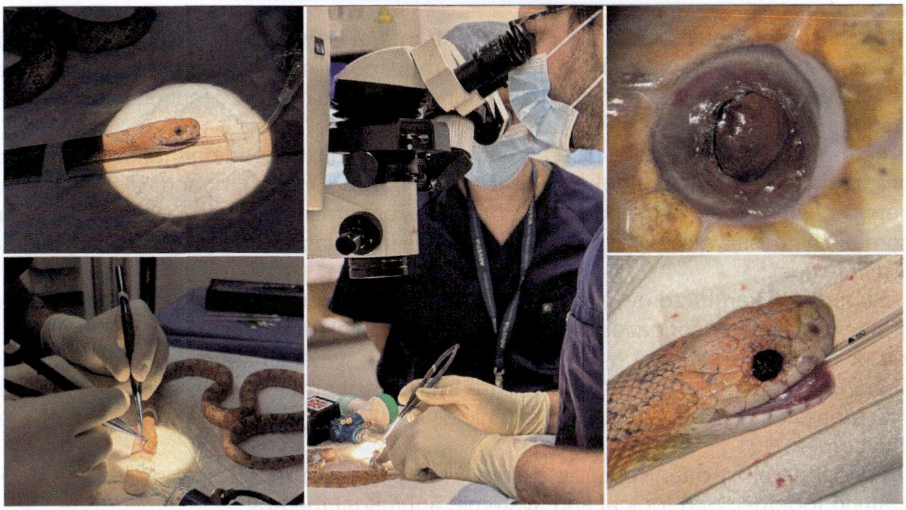

Fig. 8. Enucleation performed for a spectacle lesion with concurrent corneal desiccation in a corn snake (*Pantherophis guttatus*). The use of an operating microscope is essential for ophthalmic surgery. (Image Courtesy of Dr Carlo Paoletti.)

healing, the upper eyelid movements were restricted, but eyelid closure was complete, ocular motility was normal, and the eye was visual.[51]

Avian Ocular Surgery

Avian ocular surgery is dictated by anatomy and physiology that differ markedly from mammals: large, relatively rigid globes with a limbal ring of scleral ossicles, a striated and voluntarily controlled iris, a powerful nictitating membrane, and tear dynamics dominated by the Harderian and lacrimal glands with drainage into the oronasal cavity.[52,53]

These traits influence examination, anesthesia, exposure, tissue handling, and the choice among globe-sparing, shell-sparing, or globe-removal procedures, and they also explain why early, decisive surgical intervention is often required when caseous inflammation, structural failure, or mass effect limit medical therapy.

Eyelid surgery

Eyelid disorders are recognized in birds, though their prevalence varies by etiology.[54]

Surgical repair of eyelid defects has been described, although the thin structure of the avian eyelid generally precludes the use of double-layered closure.[54]

Successful outcomes depend on meticulous technique, with tension-free single-layer closure and, when necessary, sharp excision or curettage of proliferative or caseous lesions to restore a smooth margin. A successful case of bilateral acquired ankyloblepharon secondary to thermal injury has also been reported in a young cockatiel.[54]

Improvement of symblepharon causing third eyelid protrusion with consequences on vision has been reported.[55]

Surgical management of adnexal disorders requires careful consideration of avian blink mechanics. Unlike mammals, in most birds the lower eyelid is the dominant mobile structure, while the nictitating membrane provides a powerful sweeping motion across the cornea. For this reason, temporary partial tarsorrhaphy is generally preferred over third-eyelid flaps when protecting nonhealing erosions, recent grafts, or over operated corneas.[53]

Corneal surgery

Corneal surgery must account for the thin stroma, a Bowman-like layer, and the rigid limbus with overlapping ossicles. Incisions require millimetric precision, and sutures should be placed very superficially with buried knots to minimize friction with the nictitating membrane.[53,54,56]

For nonhealing superficial ulcers, meticulous epithelial debridement has proven its efficacy in a laughing kookaburra (*Dacelo novaeguineae*.),[57] and diamond-burr debridement and a thin cyanoacrylate bandage, or ultrashallow grid keratotomy (given corneal thinness) was useful in a refractory case in a hyacinth macaw (*Anodorhynchus hyacinthinus*).[58]

Superficial keratectomy and/or corneal grafting (conjunctival pedicle or bridge grafts) are reserved for cases unresponsive to medical therapy, such as delayed healing or malacic or stromal ulcers of variable depth, where tectonic support may be needed. Keratectomy allows definitive removal of abnormal or infected corneal tissue and promotes healing, but can be technically challenging in some species due to the thin cornea.[53,56]

Fungal keratitis often requires a combined approach of surgical debridement or grafting together with topical and systemic antifungal therapy.[53,54,56]

Keratoplasties have been successfully performed, including penetrating keratoplasties with conjunctival grafts in 2 great horned owls (*Bubo virginianus*)[59] and fresh homologous corneal grafting in a Californian brown pelican (*Pelecanus occidentalis californicus*).[60]

Graft failure was reported in a great horned owl (*Bubo virginianus*) following escape, ultimately necessitating exenteration.[61]

Enucleation

Globe removal is indicated for blind and painful eyes caused by perforation, panophthalmitis, intraocular tumors, or end-stage glaucoma.

The large globe, short optic nerve, and thin interorbital septum make enucleation technically demanding and increase traction and hemorrhage risks; careful exposure, meticulous hemostasis, and dead-space control are essential.[53,54]

Due to the large size of the avian eye and the presence of prominent scleral ossicles, enucleation may result in significant disfigurement and, in some cases, alter the balance of the head because of the change in weight.[53]

Nevertheless, it remains a primary surgical option in raptors. The procedure can be performed via either a lateral or transaural approach, as reported in owls, and in certain cases incision and collapse of the globe may facilitate the surgery.[54]

Traction on the optic nerve must be minimized, since the contralateral nerve is highly vulnerable to avulsion, and a lethal oculocardiac reflex has been reported.[54]

Once the globe, nictitating membrane, conjunctiva, lacrimal and harderian glands, and eyelid margins are removed, closure is generally achieved with a single cutaneous layer of absorbable or nonabsorbable suture.[54]

Modified evisceration

Modified evisceration is a valid alternative to enucleation. By preserving the scleral shell, it enables eyelid closure, shortens anesthesia, reduces hemorrhage and optic chiasm traction risk, and maintains head symmetry. In psittacines, reports show smooth healing and lasting results, supporting its use as an effective option in selected cases.[46,53,54]

The procedure follows the initial steps of an enucleation but, after removal of the eyelid margins, third eyelid, and associated glands, a 360° limbal keratectomy is performed to excise the entire cornea. The scleral shell is preserved, the uvea, lens, vitreous, retina, and pecten are removed, and finally the eyelids are closed. This technique generally causes less intraoperative bleeding than enucleation.[53]

Conjunctival removal is controversial, and in raptors conjunctiva may be preserved if nasolacrimal drainage is intact, though some recommend excision.[53,54]

Post-evisceration in birds can be complicated by several conditions. Rarely, fluid accumulation in the scleral shell may occur due to residual secretory tissue and may require excision or the use of sclerosing agents such as polidocanol.[53]

Recurrent orbital cysts have also been reported; in a duck and a goose, such cysts following evisceration were successfully managed with intraorbital gentamicin injection.[62,63] In addition, orbital emphysema has been described in an ostrich, in which a nasolacrimal–oropharyngeal one-way valve mechanism was suspected; in similar cases, punctal ligation and orbital decompression may be required.[64]

Evisceration with prosthesis

Evisceration with intrascleral prosthesis has been described in raptors and parrots but carries significant risks, including corneal ulceration, implant extrusion, and intraocular infection, frequently leading to secondary enucleation. Prosthetic implantation is generally discouraged as it provides no functional benefit and adds surgical risks.[53,54]

Neoplasia

In avian ophthalmology, the management of ocular and periocular neoplasia prioritizes the preservation of vision whenever possible and the maintenance of comfort when vision cannot be restored. Regardless of the approach, appropriate management is essential to prevent local recurrence and potential systemic dissemination of the neoplastic process. Enucleation remains the treatment of choice for intraocular lesions confined to the globe, such as uveal malignant melanoma[65] and iridociliary adenoma.[66]

In contrast, exenteration is reserved for malignant or invasive orbital disease, where the lesion extends beyond the globe into adjacent orbital tissues. This radical and definitive procedure involves removal of all orbital contents—including the globe, extraocular muscles, and surrounding soft tissues—to achieve complete excision with tumor-free margins (**Fig. 9**).

When the eyelids are not affected, they may be preserved to facilitate closure and improve postoperative outcome. Retrobulbar tumors, such as the adenocarcinoma

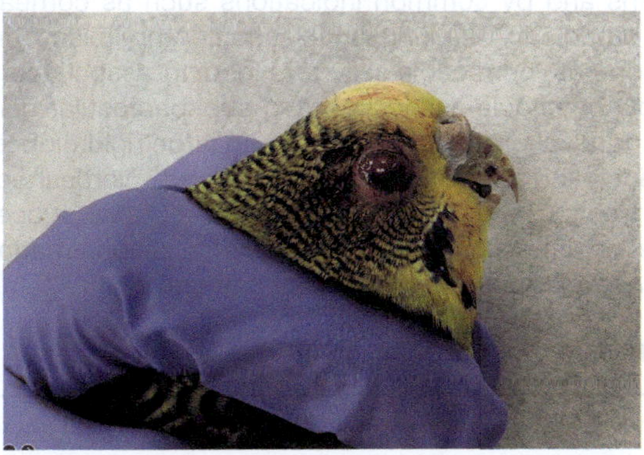

Fig. 9. Conjunctival carcinoma necessitating exenteration in a budgerigar (*Melopsittacus undulatus*). (Image Courtesy of Dr Carlo Paoletti.)

reported in a common buzzard (*Buteo buteo*),[67] exemplify conditions in which exenteration would be considered appropriate.

Mydriasis, cataract and lens surgery

Cataract and lens luxation are recognized in birds and, in suitable cases, both can be managed surgically.

In order to perform lens or vitreous surgery, mydriasis should be obtained. Predictable intraoperative dilation is achieved with general anesthesia to suppress voluntary iris tone; intracameral neuromuscular blockade and viscoelastic may be added, since topical parasympatholytics are unreliable with a striated iris.[53,54]

Topical rocuronium bromide reliably produces mydriasis in various bird species and is generally safe; transient local ocular effects are rare, but care is needed to avoid systemic effects.[68–72] The surgeon should consult species-specific literature regarding drug use, as safety and efficacy may vary between species and may not be established in all cases, particularly for bilateral application.

Cataract and lens surgery rely on the soft avian lens and its ciliary–capsular fusion (annular pad). Because of the small size of the avian eye, conventional extracapsular extraction techniques are generally challenging, and surgical planning must take these anatomic constraints into account. After chamber stabilization and controlled capsulotomy, most cataracts in small to midsized birds are removed by irrigation–aspiration; phacoemulsification is reserved for dense lenses. The implantation of intraocular lenses has been reported in several bird species.[54,73–77]

In aquatic species, postoperative infection has been reported, warranting close monitoring.[78]

Postoperative care

Postoperative management focuses on comfort, surface protection, infection control, and early rehabilitation. Topical and/or systemic antibiotics are administered as indicated to prevent secondary infection. Intraocular inflammation is usually mild, and visual recovery is rapid when structural integrity is preserved.[56]

SUMMARY

Non-mammalian ophthalmic surgery requires detailed knowledge of taxon-specific ocular anatomy and physiology. A key cross-taxonomic feature is the striated, voluntarily controlled iris, which limits the effectiveness of topical mydriatics and often necessitates anesthesia-based or intracameral dilation. Fish surgery is influenced by a rigid high-index lens and by common indications such as corneal disease or end-stage intraocular pathology requiring enucleation. Amphibians present challenges related to fragile corneas, permeable skin, and feeding-associated globe mechanics. Some reptiles show spectacle-associated and subspectacular disorders that affect corneal, lens, and adnexal procedures. Birds, with large rigid globes, scleral ossicles, and a powerful nictitating membrane, require refined microsurgical technique and careful control of traction and hemostasis. Across all taxa, successful surgery depends on precise anesthesia, environmental optimization, magnification, delicate instrumentation, and strict postoperative management.

CLINICS CARE POINTS

- Non-mammalian eye surgery requires species-specific anatomic and physiologic planning.
- Striated iris musculature limits topical mydriasis; anesthesia, intracameral, or neuromuscular blockade may be required.

- Fish, amphibians, reptiles, and birds present unique corneal, lens, and adnexal challenges.
- Spectacle disorders, subspectacular disease, and thin corneas shape reptile and amphibian care.
- Successful outcomes depend on precise anesthesia, magnification, and tailored perioperative management.

DECLARATION OF AI AND AI-ASSISTED TECHNOLOGIES IN THE WRITING PROCESS

During the preparation of this work the authors used Generative AI. After using this tool, the authors reviewed and edited the content as needed and take full responsibility for the content of the publication.

DISCLOSURE

The authors have nothing to disclose.

SUPPLEMENTARY DATA

Supplementary data to this article can be found online at https://doi.org/10.1016/j.cvex.2026.04.008.

REFERENCES

1. Williams DL. Ocular surface biology and disease in fish. Vet Clin Exot Anim Pract 2019;22(1):81–95. Medical and surgical management of ocular surface disease in exotic animals.
2. Parker-Graham CA, Stevens BN, Ang JHM, et al. Ophthalmology of osteichthyes: bony fish. In: Montiani-Ferreira F, Moore BA, Ben-Shlomo G, editors. Wild and exotic animal ophthalmology: volume 1: invertebrates, fishes, amphibians, reptiles, and birds. Cham: Springer International Publishing; 2022. p. 61–104.
3. Williams D. Ophthalmology of cartilaginous fish: skates, rays, and sharks. In: Montiani-Ferreira F, Moore BA, Ben-Shlomo G, editors. Wild and exotic animal ophthalmology: volume 1: invertebrates, fishes, amphibians, reptiles, and birds. Cham: Springer International Publishing; 2022. p. 47–59 [Internet].
4. Williams DL. Ophthalmology of agnatha: lampreys and hagfish. In: Montiani-Ferreira F, Moore BA, Ben-Shlomo G, editors. Wild and exotic animal ophthalmology: volume 1: invertebrates, fishes, amphibians, reptiles, and birds. Cham: Springer International Publishing; 2022. p. 41–5.
5. Hadfield CA. Ocular signs. In: Hadfield CA, Clayton LA, editors. Clinical guide to fish medicine. Hoboken (NJ): Wiley-Blackwell; 2021. p. 350–3.
6. Crevoiserat L, Katzenstein N, LaDouceur EEB. Uveal iridophoroma in a betta fish (*Betta splendens*). J Comp Pathol 2024;215:71–5.
7. Magi GE, Renzoni G, Piccionello AP, et al. Primary ocular chondrosarcoma in a discus (*symphisodon aequifasciatus*). J Zoo Wildl Med 2013;44(1):225–31.
8. Wildgoose WH. Exenteration in fish. Exot Dvm 2007;9:25–9.
9. Sladakovic I, Divers SJ. Surgery and endoscopy. In: Clinical guide to fish medicine [Internet]. 2021. p. 213–32.
10. Gjeltema JL. Introduction to ophthalmology of amphibia. In: Montiani-Ferreira F, Moore BA, Ben-Shlomo G, editors. Wild and exotic animal ophthalmology: volume 1: invertebrates, fishes, amphibians, reptiles, and birds. Cham: Springer International Publishing; 2022. p. 107–20.

11. Wright KM. Chapter 75 - overview of amphibian medicine. In: Mader DR, editor. Reptile medicine and surgery. 2nd edition. St Louis (MO): W.B. Saunders; 2006. p. 941–71. https://doi.org/10.1016/B0-72-169327-X/50079-1. Available at: https://www.sciencedirect.com/science/article/pii/B072169327X500791.
12. Sladakovic I, Divers SJ. 52 - amphibian anesthesia. In: Divers SJ, Stahl SJ, editors. Mader's reptile and amphibian medicine and surgery. 3rd edition. St Louis (MO): W.B. Saunders; 2019. p. 480–5.e1. https://doi.org/10.1016/B978-0-323-48253-0.00052-0. Available at: https://www.sciencedirect.com/science/article/pii/B9780323482530000520.
13. Llewelyn VK, Berger L, Glass BD. Percutaneous absorption of chemicals: developing an understanding for the treatment of disease in frogs. J Vet Pharmacol Therapeut 2016;39(2):109–21.
14. Scott G, Louis MM, Balko JA, et al. Pharmacokinetics of transdermal flunixin meglumine following a single dose in marine toads (*Rhinella marina*). Vet Med Int 2020;2020(1):8863537.
15. Boss C, Plummer CE. Ophthalmology of amphibia: caecilians, salamanders, frogs, toads, and relatives. In: Montiani-Ferreira F, Moore BA, Ben-Shlomo G, editors. Wild and exotic animal ophthalmology: volume 1: invertebrates, fishes, amphibians, reptiles, and birds. Cham: Springer International Publishing; 2022. p. 121–41.
16. Vergneau-Grosset C, Weber IIIES. Amphibian surgery. In: Surgery of exotic animals. 2021. p. 63–73.
17. Nodolf S, Moore BA, Bliss TN, et al. Lipid keratopathy in a group of zoo-housed California tiger salamanders (*Ambystoma californiense*). J Herpetol Med Surg 2025;35(4):211–8.
18. Moore BA, Gjeltema J. Once in a blue moon: lipid keratopathy and intrastromal hemorrhage in a mission golden-eyed tree frog (*Trachycephalus resinifictrix*). Vet Ophthalmol 2019;22(6):933–6.
19. Prando FAS, Pereira JS, Medeiros RS, et al. Use of automated central lamellar superficial keratectomy in the treatment of chronic pigmentary superficial keratitis in dogs. Arq Bras Med Vet Zootec 2022;74.
20. Chai N. Surgery in amphibians. Vet Clin Exot Anim Pract 2016;19(1):77–95.
21. Kilburn JJ, Bronson E, Shaw GC, et al. Phacoemulsification in an american toad (*Anaxyrus americanus*). J Herpetol Med Surg 2019;29(1–2):17–20.
22. Reichenbach-Klinke H, Elkan E. Tumors, benign and malignant. In: The principal diseases of lower vertebrates. Academic Press; 2013.
23. Williams DL, Whitaker BR. The amphibian eye: a clinical review. J Zoo Wildl Med 1994;25(1):18–28. Located at: JSTOR.
24. Abarca JG, Estrella-Morales J, Alvarado-Fernández JC, et al. Diagnosis and surgical removal of a corneal dermoid in a red-eyed tree frog, *Agalychnis callidryas* (Anura, Hylidae), from the Tenorio volcano, Costa Rica. J Herpetol Med Surg 2024;34(4):211–5.
25. Scheid P, Siffert W. Effects of inhibiting carbonic anhydrase on isometric contraction of frog skeletal muscle. J Physiol 1985;361(1):91–101.
26. Berkowski WM, Plummer CE. Ophthalmology of Testudines: turtles and tortoises. In: Montiani-Ferreira F, Moore BA, Ben-Shlomo G, editors. Wild and exotic animal ophthalmology: volume 1: invertebrates, fishes, amphibians, reptiles, and birds. Cham: Springer International Publishing; 2022. p. 271–97.
27. Fleming KS. Ophthalmology of anguimorpha and iguania: chameleons, monitors, dragons, iguanas, and relatives. In: Montiani-Ferreira F, Moore BA, Ben-Shlomo G, editors. Wild and exotic animal ophthalmology: volume 1: invertebrates, fishes,

amphibians, reptiles, and birds. Cham: Springer International Publishing; 2022. p. 205–29.
28. Fleming KS. Ophthalmology of scinciformata and laterata: skinks, lizards, and relatives. In: Montiani-Ferreira F, Moore BA, Ben-Shlomo G, editors. Wild and exotic animal ophthalmology: volume 1: invertebrates, fishes, amphibians, reptiles, and birds. Cham: Springer International Publishing; 2022. p. 183–203.
29. Lawton MPC. 91 - eye. In: Divers SJ, Stahl SJ, editors. Mader's reptile and amphibian medicine and surgery. 3rd edition. St Louis (MO): W.B. Saunders; 2019. p. 1024–7.e1. https://doi.org/10.1016/B978-0-323-48253-0.00091-X. Available at: https://www.sciencedirect.com/science/article/pii/B978032348253000091X.
30. Millichamp NJ. Ophthalmology of serpentes: snakes. In: Montiani-Ferreira F, Moore BA, Ben-Shlomo G, editors. Wild and exotic animal ophthalmology: volume 1: invertebrates, fishes, amphibians, reptiles, and birds. Cham: Springer International Publishing; 2022. p. 231–69 [Internet].
31. Smith Fleming KM. Ocular surface disease in reptiles. Vet Clin Exot Anim Pract 2019;22(1):109–21.
32. Wiggans KT, Moore BA. Ophthalmology of gekkota: geckos. In: Montiani-Ferreira F, Moore BA, Ben-Shlomo G, editors. Wild and exotic animal ophthalmology: volume 1: invertebrates, fishes, amphibians, reptiles, and birds. Cham: Springer International Publishing; 2022. p. 167–81.
33. Ledbetter EC, de Matos R, Riedel RM, et al. Phacoemulsification of bilateral mature cataracts in a Texas rat snake (*Elaphe obsoleta lindheimeri*). J Am Vet Med Assoc 2017;251(11):1318–23.
34. Petritz OA, Westermeyer HD, Whitehead MC, et al. Effective mydriasis in juvenile loggerhead turtles (*Caretta caretta*) following topical administration of rocuronium bromide and 10% phenylephrine. Vet Ophthalmol 2020;23(1):37–43.
35. Tucker-Retter EK, Petritz OA, Westermeyer HD. Mydriasis in eastern box turtles (*Terrapene carolina carolina*) following topical administration of proparacaine, 10% phenylephrine, and rocuronium bromide. Vet Ophthalmol 2025;28(1):48–57.
36. Cummings CO, Nevarez JG, Carter RT. Successful use of a subpalpebral lavage system for management of bilateral uveitis and conjunctivitis in a sulcata tortoise (*Centrochelys sulcata*). J Herpetol Med Surg 2021;31(2):101–6.
37. Rival F. Congenital ankyloblepharon in a leopard gecko (*Eublepharis macularius*). Vet Ophthalmol 2015;18(s1):71–3.
38. Wojick KB, McBride MP. Successful treatment of spectacle avulsion in a brazilian rainbow boa (*Epicrates cenchria cenchria*) by using a porcine small intestinal submucosal graft. J Herpetol Med Surg 2018;28(1–2):23–8.
39. Ledbetter EC, Marion JS, Morrisey JK. Amniotic membrane grafting for traumatic complete spectaculectomy and keratomalacia in a Boelen's python (*Simalia boeleni*). Vet Ophthalmol 2021;24(3):295–300.
40. Sabater M, Pérez M. Congenital ocular and adnexal disorders in reptiles. Vet Ophthalmol 2013;16(1):47–55.
41. Vieu S, Jondeau C, Bott M, et al. Corneal perforation associated with *Providencia rettgeri* in an African helmeted turtle (*Pelomedusa subrufa*). J Herpetol Med Surg 2023;33(3):134–8.
42. Eisenbarth JM, Nelms S, Sim RR, et al. Phacoemulsification for cataract management in two snakes. J Herpetol Med Surg 2021;31(3):189–96.
43. Colitz CMH, Lewbart G, Davidson MG. Phacoemulsification in an adult Savannah monitor lizard. Vet Ophthalmol 2002;5(3):207–9.

44. Myers G, Webb T, Corbett CR, et al. Phacoemulsification for removal of bilateral cataracts in a black water monitor (*Varanus salvator macromaculatus*). J Herpetol Med Surg 2011;21(4):96–100.
45. Westermeyer HD, Cook AG, Harms C, et al. Phacoemulsification cataract surgery in the loggerhead turtle (*Caretta caretta*): surgical technique and outcomes in 10 cases. Vet Ophthalmol 2019;22(5):644–50.
46. Berry A, Graham K, Sladakovic I. Evisceration as an alternative to enucleation in four pet psittacine birds. J Avian Med Surg 2025;39(1):31–8.
47. Diehl KA, McKinnon JA. Eye removal surgeries in exotic pets. Vet Clin Exot Anim Pract 2016;19(1):245–67.
48. Linda Nógrádi A, Szentgáli Z, Cope I. Unilateral enucleation in a panther chameleon (*Furcifer pardalis*). J Herpetol Med Surg 2018;28(3–4):72–5.
49. Cleymaet AM, Ehrhart E, Sadar MJ, et al. Unfolding the diagnosis of subspectacular fluid opacity in a corn snake (*Pantherophis guttatus*). Vet Ophthalmol 2020; 23(4):754–9.
50. Darrow BG, Johnstone McLean NS, Russman SE, et al. Periorbital adenocarcinoma in a bearded dragon (*Pogona vitticeps*). Vet Ophthalmol 2013;16(s1): 177–82.
51. Allgoewer I, Göbel T, Stockhaus C, et al. Dacryops in a red-eared slider (*Chrysemys scripta elegans*): case report. Vet Ophthalmol 2002;5(3):231–4.
52. Koening HE, Liebich HG, Klupiec C. The eye (organum visus). In: Avian anatomy: textbook and color atlas. 2nd edition. 5m Publishing; 2016.
53. Moore BA, Fernandez-Juricic E, Hawkins MG, et al. Introduction to ophthalmology of Aves. In: Montiani-Ferreira F, Moore BA, Ben-Shlomo G, editors. Wild and exotic animal ophthalmology: volume 1: invertebrates, fishes, amphibians, reptiles, and birds. Cham: Springer International Publishing; 2022. p. 321–48. https://doi.org/10.1007/978-3-030-71302-7_16.
54. Vallone LV, Kern TJ. Avian ophthalmology. In: Veterinary ophthalmology. 6th edition. Pondicherry India: Wiley-Blackwell; 2021. p. 2055–84.
55. Williams DL, Flach E. Symblepharon with aberrant protrusion of the nictitating membrane in the snowy owl (*Nyctea scandiaca*). Vet Ophthalmol 2003;6(1):11–3.
56. Griggs A. Ocular surface disease in birds. Vet Clin Exot Anim Pract 2019;22(1): 53–68.
57. Sabater M, Pérez M. Management of a unilateral non-healing corneal ulcer and uveitis in a laughing kookaburra (*Dacelo novaeguineae*). Vet Rec Case Rep 2014;2(1):e000127.
58. Waugh L, Pucket J, Cole GA, et al. Management of a nonhealing, superficial corneal ulcer in a hyacinth macaw (*Anodorhynchus hyacinthinus*). J Avian Med Surg 2017;31(3):239–43.
59. Gionfriddo JR, Powell CC. Primary closure of the corneas of two great horned owls after resection of nonhealing ulcers. Vet Ophthalmol 2006;9(4):251–4.
60. Lynch GL, Scagliotti RH, Hoffman A, et al. Penetrating keratoplasty in a California brown pelican. Vet Ophthalmol 2007;10(4):254–61.
61. Andrew SE, Clippinger TL, Brooks DE, et al. Penetrating keratoplasty for treatment of corneal protrusion in a great horned owl (*Bubo virginianus*). Vet Ophthalmol 2002;5(3):201–5.
62. Houston K, Fontaine C, Dziedzic-Nyrka N, et al. Successful management of a refractory orbital pseudocyst in a Chinese goose using intraorbital gentamicin injection. Vet Ophthalmol 2025. https://doi.org/10.1111/vop.70101.

63. Park SA, Davidson H, Thompson KA, et al. Successful chemical ablation of an intraorbital cyst caused by an eyelid injury and iatrogenic ankyloblepharon formation in a duck. J Am Vet Med Assoc 2018;253(9):1164–8.
64. Rogers CM, Blue-McLendon A, Scott EM, et al. Self-limiting orbital emphysema following ocular evisceration and demonstration of nasolacrimal-oropharyngeal communication in a South African ostrich (*Struthio camelus australis*). J Avian Med Surg 2020;34(4):396–401.
65. Darden JE, Hoppes SM, Aceino AM, et al. Uveal malignant melanoma in a hybrid macaw parrot (*Ara chloropterus* × *Ara militaris*). J Avian Med Surg 2021;35(3): 367–73.
66. Thielen LE, Sledge DG, Hess L. Ocular iridociliary adenoma in a Congo African grey parrot (*Psittacus erithacus*). J Avian Med Surg 2019;33(3):278–84.
67. Bertram CA, Halter L, Feyer S, et al. Retrobulbar adenocarcinoma with subconjunctival extension in a common buzzard (*Buteo buteo*). J Avian Med Surg 2022;36(1):78–84.
68. Cantero F, Ortillés Á, Peña MT, et al. Safety and efficacy of unilateral topical application of rocuronium bromide in healthy scops owls (*Otus scops*). Vet Ophthalmol 2021;24(2):169–76.
69. Barsotti G, Briganti A, Spratte JR, et al. Safety and efficacy of bilateral topical application of rocuronium bromide for mydriasis in European kestrels (*Falco tinnunculus*). J Avian Med Surg 2012;26(1):1–5.
70. Baine K, Hendrix DVH, Kuhn SE, et al. The efficacy and safety of topical rocuronium bromide to induce bilateral mydriasis in hispaniolan Amazon parrots (*Amazona ventralis*). J Avian Med Surg 2016;30(1):8–13.
71. Rhim H, Jung S, Kim N, et al. Application of topical rocuronium bromide dosing by ocular size in four species of wild birds. J Vet Sci 2023;24(4):e59.
72. Susanti L, Kang S, Lee E, et al. Efficacy of topical rocuronium bromide as a mydriatic agent in domestic pigeons (*Columba livia*). J Vet Med Sci 2021;83(3):501–6.
73. Lewin AC, Riedel RM, Queiroz-Williams P, et al. Successful surgical removal of the crystalline lenses in a black-necked swan (*Cygnus melancoryphus*). J Avian Med Surg 2023;37(1):41–5.
74. Carter RT, Murphy CJ, Stuhr CM, et al. Bilateral phacoemulsification and intraocular lens implantation in a great horned owl. J Am Vet Med Assoc 2007;230(4): 559–61.
75. Church ML, Priehs DR, Denis H, et al. Technique, postoperative complications, and visual outcomes of phacoemulsification cataract surgery in 21 penguins (27 eyes): 2011-2015. Vet Ophthalmol 2018;21(6):612–21.
76. Sigmund AB, Jones MP, Ward DA, et al. Long-term outcome of phacoemulsification in raptors—A retrospective study (1999-2014). Vet Ophthalmol 2019;22(3): 360–7.
77. Sritrakoon N, Sutasha K, Kasorndorkbua C, et al. Bilateral cataracts extraction by lens aspiration and foldable intraocular lens implantation in a Black kite (*Milvus migrans*). Open Vet J 2021;11(3):441–6. PubMed PMID: 34722209; PubMed Central PMCID: PMC8541732.
78. Rodrigo SGT, Bliss CD, Alcántar Hernández BE. Incisional infection postphacoemulsification in a chilean flamingo (*Phoenicopterus chilensis*). J Avian Med Surg 2021;35(2):204–9.

Ocular Surgery in Small Mammals

Carlo Paoletti, DVM, Dipl ECZM (Small Mammals); Postgraduate University Diploma in Microsurgical Techniques (Faculty of Medicine, Sorbonne University, Paris)[a,*], José Rosas-Navarro, DVM, Dipl ECZM (Small Mammals); Postgraduate University Diploma in Microsurgical Techniques (Faculty of Medicine, Sorbonne University, Paris)[a], María Luisa Pérez Orrico, LV, MRCVS, C.E.S. Ophtalmologie Vétérinaire ENVT, ECVO Residency Trained Clinician[c], Aure-Eline Grillot, DVM, Dipl ECVO[b]

KEYWORDS

- Small mammal ocular surgery • Microsurgical techniques • Corneal and lens surgery
- Nasolacrimal surgery • Enucleation and exenteration • Retrobulbar abscess
- Phacoemulsification • Harderian gland surgery

KEY POINTS

- Surgical management in small mammals requires mastery of microsurgical techniques due to their extremely thin corneas, compact orbits, and extensive retrobulbar vasculature.
- Rabbits commonly require surgery for nasolacrimal obstruction, Harderian gland prolapse, corneal ulcers, and cataracts, with phacoemulsification remaining the gold standard technique, when feasible for the latter.
- Hystricomorph rodents frequently need surgical intervention for dental-related retrobulbar abscesses, nonhealing corneal ulcers, and traumatic or infectious orbital disease.
- Ferrets may require surgical treatment of corneal disease, conjunctival masses, cataracts, and orbital conditions.
- Rodents often require enucleation or exenteration for trauma, infection, or neoplasia, with meticulous hemostasis being essential due to their prominent retrobulbar venous plexuses.

Video content accompanies this article at http://www.vetexotic.theclinics.com.

[a] Exotic Animal Department, Centre Hospitalier Vétérinaire AniCura-ADVETIA, 9 Avenue Louis Breguet, 78140 Vélizy-Villacoublay, France; [b] Department of Ophthalmology, Centre Hospitalier Vétérinaire AniCura-ADVETIA, 9 Avenue Louis Breguet, 78140 Vélizy-Villacoublay, France; [c] Hospital Veterinario, Universidad Católica de Valencia (UCV), Exoticsvet, Valencia, Spain
* Corresponding author. Exotic Animal Department, Centre Hospitalier Vétérinaire AniCura-ADVETIA, 9 Avenue Louis Breguet, 78140 Vélizy Villacoublay, France
E-mail address: carlovet@gmail.com

Vet Clin Exot Anim 29 (2026) 607–627
https://doi.org/10.1016/j.cvex.2026.04.011 vetexotic.theclinics.com
1094-9194/26/

INTRODUCTION

Ocular surgery in small mammals requires a detailed understanding of species-specific anatomy, physiology, and disease patterns. Rabbits, hystricomorph rodents, ferrets, and myomorph rodents present unique surgical challenges due to thin corneas, shallow orbits, and extensive retrobulbar venous plexuses, all of which increase the risk of intraoperative hemorrhage and iatrogenic trauma. Many ocular conditions in these species arise from dental disease, nasolacrimal obstruction, exposure keratitis, or infectious processes, requiring a comprehensive diagnostic approach before surgical intervention. Advances in microsurgical techniques, imaging, and perioperative care have expanded the feasibility of procedures such as phacoemulsification, dacryocystorhinography-guided nasolacrimal surgery, and orbitotomy in selected cases. Mastery of fine instrumentation, magnification, and hemostasis is essential to safely perform ophthalmic surgery and optimize both visual and clinical outcomes.

Ocular Surgery in Rabbits

Ocular surgery in rabbits requires meticulous planning due to their anatomic and physiologic particularities. The orbit contains a large retrobulbar venous plexus closely associated with the deep lobe of the Harderian gland, posing a significant risk of intraoperative hemorrhage. The optic foramina, approximately 5 mm in diameter, are confluent or minimally separated by a thin layer of presphenoid bone, allowing for the potential bilateral spread of an initially unilateral infection.[1]

The nasolacrimal system, consisting of a single inferior punctum and a sharply curved duct near the maxillary incisors, is particularly prone to obstruction, often secondary to dental disease, and presents challenges for surgical manipulation.[2,3]

During ophthalmic procedures, specific anesthetic and pharmacologic considerations are required. Around 40% of rabbits possess atropine esterases, which reduces the efficacy of atropine for mydriasis; thus, 1% atropine with 10% phenylephrine or 0.5% to 1% tropicamide/cyclopentolate is preferred instead.[4]

Atracurium may be used to achieve ocular centration but requires close monitoring for hypotension and hypothermia due to histamine release. Reversal with neostigmine and glycopyrrolate is effective, and continuous hemodynamic monitoring is essential.[5]

Eyelid lesions in rabbits may be congenital, acquired, traumatic, infectious or neoplastic in origin. Blepharitis may result from bacterial or viral (eg, Shope's fibroma virus and myxomatosis) infection, leading to erythema, crusting, nodular lesions, and periocular alopecia. Conformational defects such as entropion or ectropion are occasionally observed, particularly in French Lop rabbits, and may cause chronic irritation, conjunctivitis, and/or corneal ulceration. In such cases, blepharoplasty may be useful to restore normal eyelid anatomy and function, preventing further corneal damage. Among neoplasia, the most frequently reported eyelid tumors include squamous cell carcinoma, squamous papilloma, Meibomian gland adenoma, Shope's fibroma, and melanoma. These lesions typically present as nodular or ulcerated masses at the eyelid margins. Surgical excision is the treatment of choice, but it should always be preceded by a thorough staging assessment to evaluate the extent of local invasion and rule out regional metastasis, and must be followed by reconstructive eyelid surgical techniques similar to the ones reported in domestic carnivores.[6]

Prolapse of the deep lobe of the Harderian gland, located ventromedially in the orbit, requires precise microsurgical dissection and hemostasis due to its close proximity to the orbital venous sinus (**Fig. 1**). Repositioning procedures such as the modified Morgan pocket technique or gland anchoring to the orbital rim have been successfully used to restore gland position (Videos 1–6).[7]

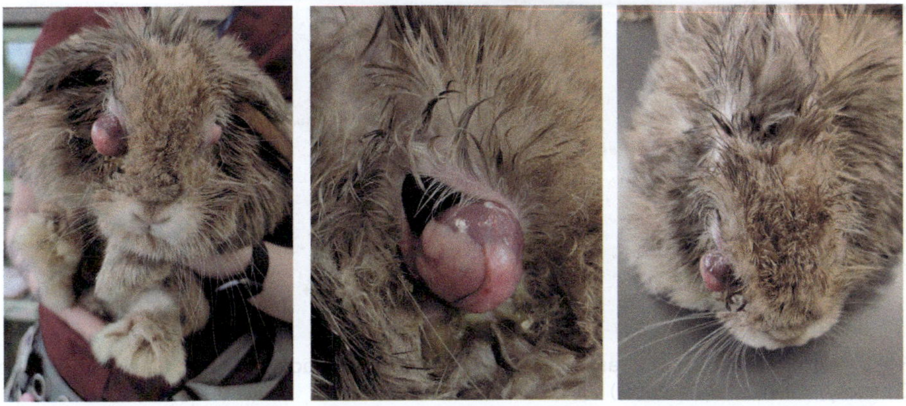

Fig. 1. Prolapse of the third eyelid gland in a rabbit. (Image Courtesy of Dr Carlo Paoletti.)

Dacryocystitis is another frequent indication for surgical intervention and is commonly associated with dental disease or chronic rhinitis. Treatment involves nasolacrimal duct flushing combined with topical and systemic antimicrobials. Computed tomography or radiography with nasolacrimal duct contrast administration (dacryocystorhinography) aids in identifying obstructions. Extraction of the affected incisor may be necessary when reserve crown elongation causes duct compression.[3,8,9] A prevalence of 6.7% of dacryocystitis was reported in a retrospective study based on the medical records of rabbits examined at a single first-opinion/referral exotics clinic in the United Kingdom.[10]

The authors have identified cases of dacryocystitis associated with dacryoliths located within the lacrimal sac (**Fig. 2**). These concretions, typically responsible for chronic or recurrent obstruction, may require surgical removal when conservative management fails. A transcutaneous approach allows removal of the dacryolith by accessing the nasolacrimal duct before its entry into the maxillary bone (**Fig. 3**).

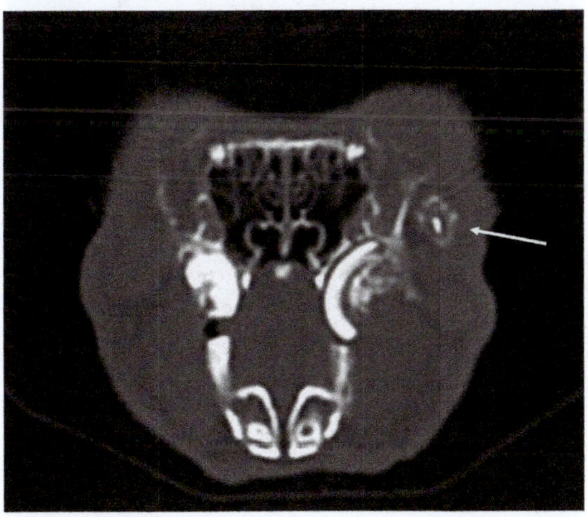

Fig. 2. Large dacryolith, indicated by the arrow, causing complete obstruction of the left nasolacrimal duct in a rabbit. (Image Courtesy of Dr Carlo Paoletti.)

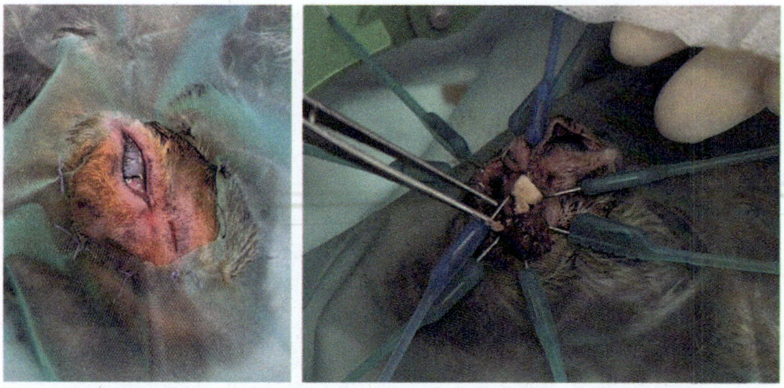

Fig. 3. Surgical removal of a large dacryolith from the nasolacrimal duct of a rabbit. (Image Courtesy of Dr Carlo Paoletti.)

When indicated, microsurgical reconstruction or marsupialization of the duct can be performed to restore tear drainage (Videos 7–9). Less commonly, nasolacrimal obstruction may result from neoplastic infiltration, which may require surgical exploration and excision.[11]

Conjunctival overgrowth (pseudopterygium or conjunctival centripetalization) presents as nonadherent conjunctival tissue extending circumferentially from the limbus (**Fig. 4**). Simple excision is ineffective due to frequent recurrence. Two main surgical approaches are described: the Stades technique, involving radial centrifugal incisions

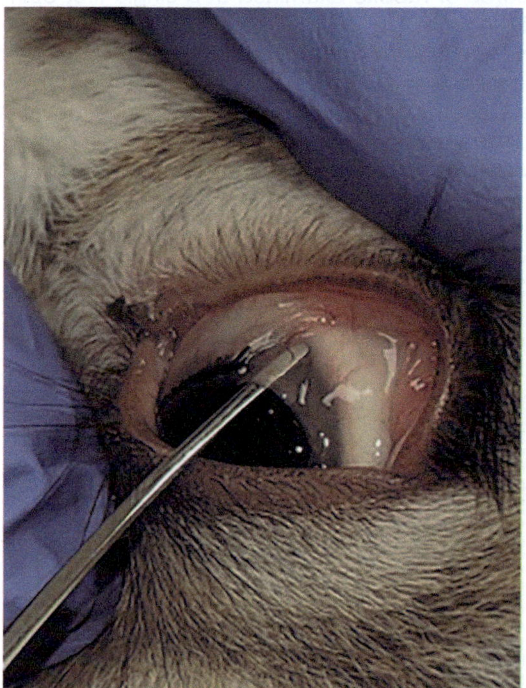

Fig. 4. Pseudopterygium (centripetal conjunctival overgrowth) in a rabbit. (Image Courtesy of Dr Carlo Paoletti.)

of the conjunctival fold with transpalpebral 7-0 polypropylene horizontal mattress sutures and postoperative corticosteroids, providing recurrence-free outcomes for up to 72 months,[12] and a modified method consisting of complete resection to the limbus, inversion of cut edges with Lambert 6-0 polyglactin 910 sutures, and postoperative steroid and cyclosporine therapy, which also achieves long-term resolution.[13,14] Recently, 2 cases of atypical adherent conjunctival overgrowth with corneal adhesion were reported, one successfully treated with adhesiolysis and a modified Stades' technique.[15]

Indolent corneal ulcers characterized by nonadherent epithelial edges are initially managed with mechanical debridement using a sterile swab or diamond burr. If reepithelialization fails, grid or punctate keratotomy can be performed to enhance epithelial adhesion. The use of bandage contact lenses or corneal collagen shields supports healing and improves comfort (**Fig. 5**).[16,17]

A recent case report described the first documented instance of naturally occurring bullous keratopathy in a dwarf rabbit. An infectious origin with secondary rupture of Descemet's membrane was suspected as the underlying cause of the corneal edema. Treatment included temporary tarsorrhaphy, along with topical antibiotics, antifungal agents, and anti-inflammatory medications, which led to resolution of the edema and infection.[18]

Cataracts in rabbits may be congenital, senile, traumatic, or secondary to bacterial or parasitic (*Encephalitozoon cuniculi*) infections, being the latter often associated with phacoclastic uveitis following anterior lens capsule rupture (**Fig. 6**).[19] The preferred treatment is phacoemulsification. Good outcomes are reported with or without intraocular lens implantation (**Fig. 7**).[20–22] When surgery is contraindicated, *E. cuniculi* associated cataracts are managed medically with topical corticosteroids or non-steroidal anti-inflammatory drugs and systemic fenbendazole or albendazole.[23] Enucleation is reserved for painful or refractory cases.

A recent case report documented the first case of bilateral cataracts associated with persistent hyperplastic primary vitreous/persistent hyperplastic tunica vasculosa lentis in a dwarf rabbit. Due to financial constraints, surgical treatment via

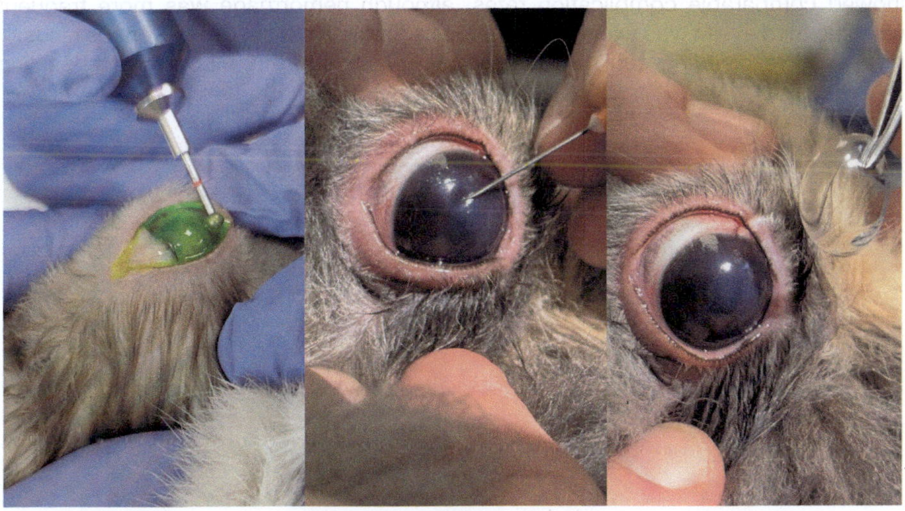

Fig. 5. Diamond-burr debridement, punctate keratotomy, and placement of a bandage contact lens in a rabbit. (Image Courtesy of Dr Carlo Paoletti.)

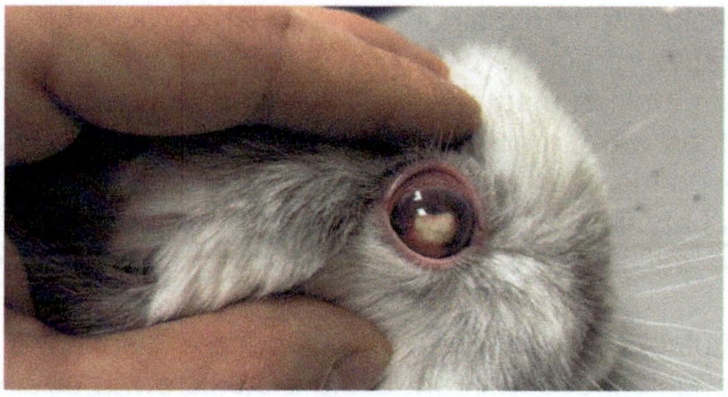

Fig. 6. Phacoclastic uveitis in a rabbit. (Image Courtesy of Dr Carlo Paoletti.)

phacoemulsification was performed on only 1 eye and was successful, with no major complications. Intraocular lens implantation was not attempted because of anatomic limitations. Postoperatively, vision was restored, and no significant complications were observed during follow-up.[24]

In glaucomatous eyes where medical treatment fails, transscleral cyclophotocoagulation can be performed. For unresponsive and painful eyes, definitive treatment options include intravitreal injection of gentamicin combined with dexamethasone, intrascleral prosthesis placement, or enucleation (**Fig. 8**, Video 10).[25,26]

Enucleation is indicated for irreversibly blind or painful eyes resulting from perforated corneal ulcers, globe rupture, panophthalmitis, chronic uveitis, intraocular neoplasia, refractory glaucoma, or exophthalmos secondary to orbital or retrobulbar disease (**Fig. 9**). Classically, the subconjunctival technique is preferred because meticulous dissection close to the sclera minimizes intraoperative hemorrhage and improves visualization. The standard procedure includes a lateral canthotomy, 360° conjunctival peritomy, transection of extraocular muscles, clamping and transection of the optic pedicle, and excision of the eyelid margins, palpebral conjunctiva, and third eyelid, followed by layered closure (**Fig. 10**).[27–29] In a retrospective case series in rabbits, subconjunctival enucleation—with or without third-eyelid removal—showed comparable complication rates, although hemorrhage was more frequent when the third eyelid was excised, reflecting its proximity to the orbital venous sinus.[30] Intraoperative bleeding can be reduced using a LigaSure™ bipolar vessel-sealing

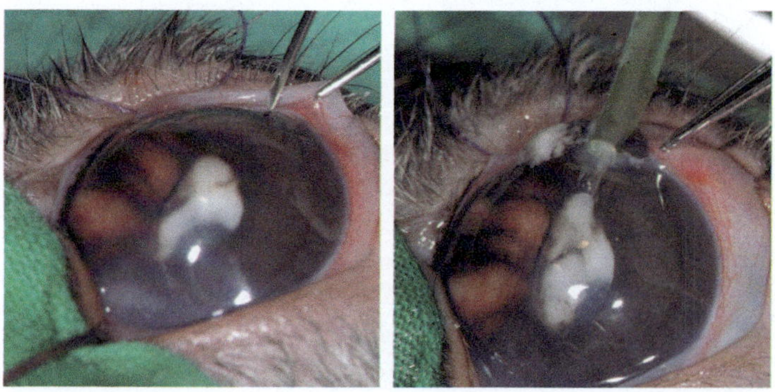

Fig. 7. Phacoemulsification in a rabbit with phacoclastic uveitis. (Image Courtesy of Dr E. Huguet Baudin (Oftalmovet Valencia), Dr M. Sabater González, Dr M. L. Pérez Orrico.)

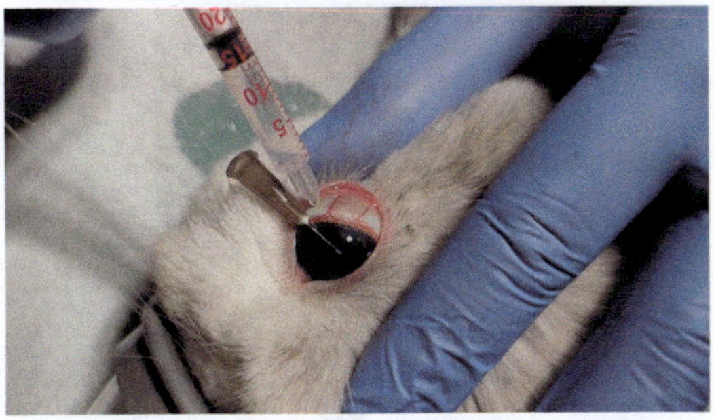

Fig. 8. Intravitreal injection of gentamicin in a rabbit. (Image Courtesy of Dr Carlo Paoletti.)

device, which effectively seals and transects extraocular muscles, the optic pedicle, and the base of the third eyelid.[1] Postoperative serous or mucoid discharge and transient swelling have been reported in approximately 40% of cases, usually resolving within 3 months.[30] However, the authors did not observe these complications in their clinical experience. A transpalpebral approach is preferred in cases involving corneal or conjunctival infection to prevent orbital contamination, whereas exenteration is reserved for extensive periocular disease or abscessation extending beyond the globe.[27] Recently, a modified lateral enucleation technique specifically adapted for small companion animals, including rabbits, has been reported.[31] This modification omits ligation or clamping of the optic nerve, based on the anatomic configuration of the rabbit orbit, in which the external ophthalmic artery provides extensive anastomotic blood supply. This vascular arrangement renders optic nerve clamping unnecessary and potentially harmful. Under general anesthesia, the rabbit is positioned in lateral recumbency. A lateral canthotomy is performed to expose the periocular tissues, followed by blunt dissection of the eyelids and subconjunctival tissues, and sharp incision of the skin close to the eyelid margin. The globe is then rotated medially to visualize the posterior segment, and the optic nerve is transected directly with curved scissors, without prior ligation. Closure involves apposition of the Tenon's capsule and periocular tissues using absorbable sutures, followed by suturing of the palpebral skin margins. No intraoperative or postoperative complications were observed. Intraoperative blood loss was minimal, and all animals healed uneventfully within 2 weeks.

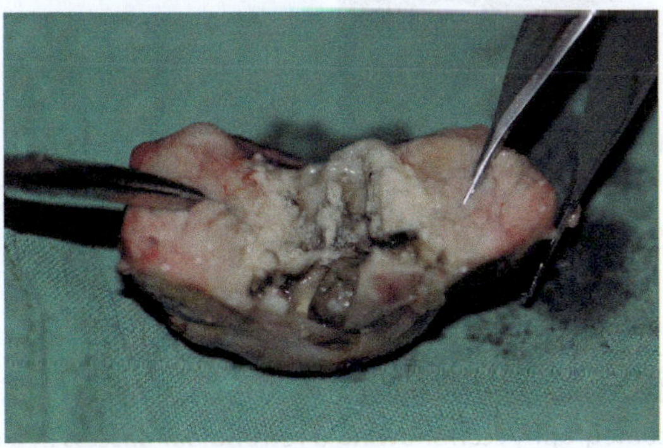

Fig. 9. Purulent panophthalmitis in a rabbit. (Image Courtesy of Dr M. Sabater González and Dr M. L. Pérez Orrico.)

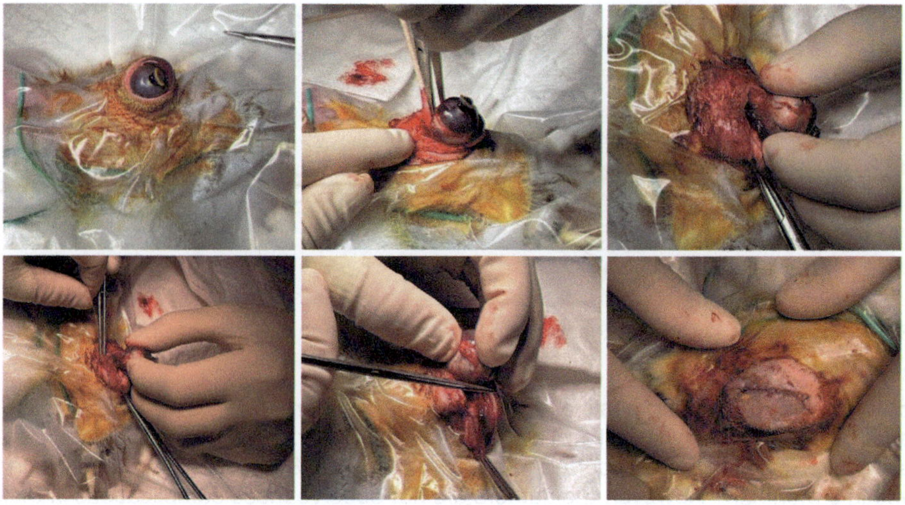

Fig. 10. Enucleation in a rabbit. (Image Courtesy of Dr Carlo Paoletti.)

Retrobulbar abscesses, the most common cause of exophthalmos in rabbits, are odontogenic in 71% of cases. Combined intraoral and extraoral drainage with aggressive debridement and long-term systemic antibiotics achieves resolution in 78% of cases (**Fig. 11**).[32] Marsupialization of abscesses is also reported to be effective.[33] Endoscopic curettage with tooth extraction represents an effective minimally invasive option,[34] while in severe or recurrent cases, exenteration may be required.

Ocular Surgery in Hystricomorph Rodents

Ocular surgery in hystricomorph rodents requires exceptional precision due to their small globe size and delicate ocular structures. The compact orbit, thin cornea, and species-specific anatomic peculiarities significantly constrain surgical access and increase the risk of iatrogenic complications. The Harderian gland, particularly large in these rodents and closely associated with the optic nerve, must be handled with

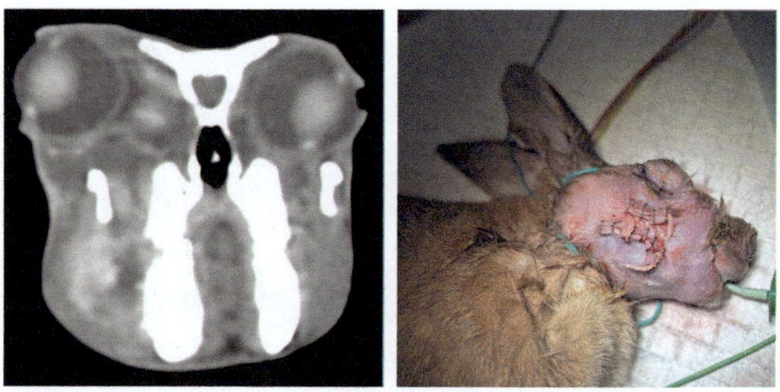

Fig. 11. Computed tomography scan showing a retrobulbar abscess in a rabbit. A suborbital surgical approach allowed successful drainage and preservation of the eye. (Image Courtesy of Dr Carlo Paoletti.)

extreme care to avoid vascular or glandular injury during retrobulbar or orbital procedures.[35]

Adnexal surgical procedures include correction of entropion and posttraumatic eyelid defects,[36] resection of trichiasis,[25] and excision of dermoids involving the cornea or conjunctiva.[37,38]

Prolapse of the nictitating gland should be managed with repositioning techniques to preserve tear function. Dacryocystitis secondary to dental disease has been described in these species. Surgical treatment of the dental lesion and topical medical therapy resulted in partial resolution of the ocular discharge.[39]

Benign periocular enlargements such as *pea-eye* or *fatty-eye*, associated with hypertrophy of the zygomatic or lacrimal glands in Guinea pigs, generally require surgery only when they are symptomatic.[40]

Corneal surgery is indicated for traumatic or chronic nonhealing ulcers, exposure keratitis, and secondary infections. In Guinea pigs and chinchillas, the cornea is extremely thin and occupies most of the palpebral fissure, making microsurgical precision essential to prevent perforation.[41,42]

After infection control, mechanical debridement or grid keratotomy can be performed to promote epithelial adhesion and healing.[43]

In severe cases, particularly when associated with exposure keratitis or exophthalmos, temporary tarsorrhaphy with a single horizontal mattress suture (5–0 or 6–0 nylon)[40] or enucleation may be required to protect the cornea and/or relieve pain.[44]

Cataract is considered the most common intraocular disorder in hystricomorph rodents. It is reported in 14% to 27% of chinchillas, in approximately 17% of Guinea pigs, and accounts for up to 80% of ocular pathology in degus. Reported causes vary among species and include age-related, inherited, and diabetic cataracts (**Fig. 12**).[45]

Phacoemulsification has been successfully performed in a chinchilla, achieving functional visual recovery despite the absence of intraocular lens implantation.[46] However, in other small herbivorous rodents, cataract extraction has not been documented, likely owing to the technical challenges associated with the procedure, remaining enucleation as the preferred treatment of painful or end-stage cases.[25,44]

Enucleation is the most commonly performed ocular surgery in these species and is indicated for painful, blind, or nonresponsive eyes affected by infection, trauma, glaucoma, severe cataract, or intraocular neoplasia (**Figs. 13** and **14**).[25,44]

In Guinea pigs and chinchillas, it is frequently required in association with retrobulbar abscessation secondary to dental disease. Computed tomography is

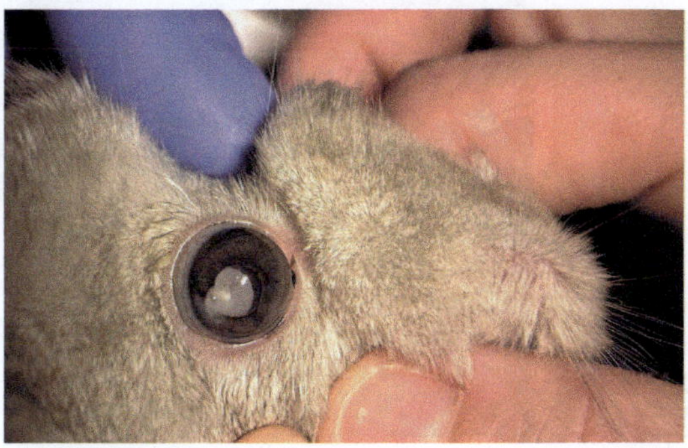

Fig. 12. Suspected traumatic cataract and posterior lens luxation in a chinchilla. (Image Courtesy of Dr Carlo Paoletti.)

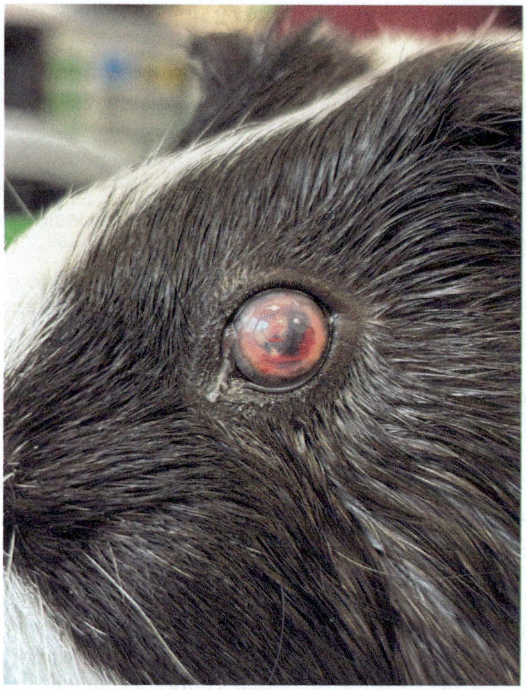

Fig. 13. Suspected intraocular neoplasia in a Guinea pig. (Image Courtesy of Dr Carlo Paoletti.)

recommended to assess the extent of infection and to guide tooth extraction and abscess drainage, performed either before or concurrently with enucleation. During the procedure, the presence of the orbital venous plexus must be carefully considered to minimize intraoperative hemorrhage.

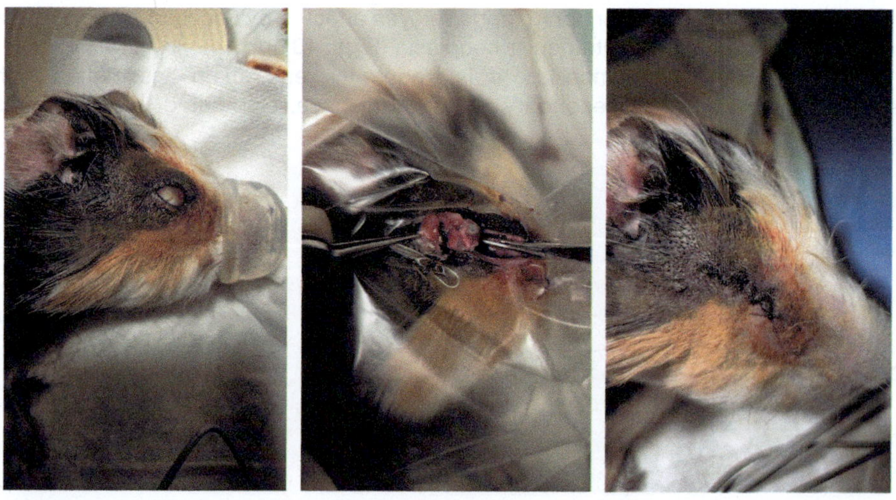

Fig. 14. Enucleation for panophthalmitis in a Guinea pig. (Image Courtesy of Dr Aurélie Latre-Grüss.)

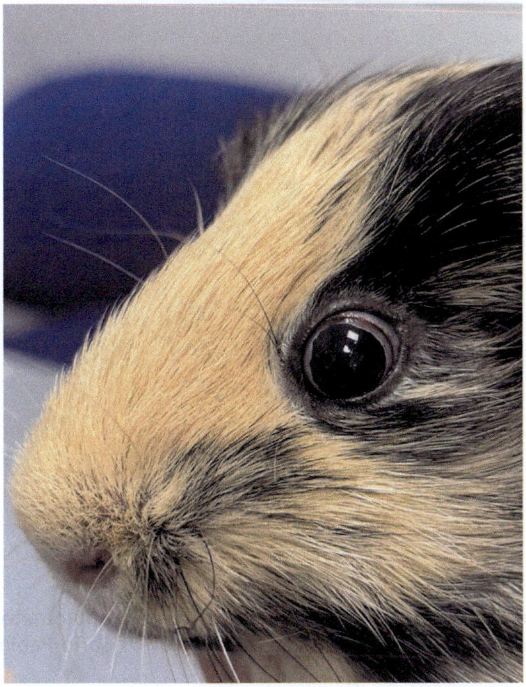

Fig. 15. Choristoma of the ciliary bodies in a Guinea pig. (Image Courtesy of Dr Carlo Paoletti.)

In rare cases, orbital surgery may also be performed for space-occupying lesions. Successful excision of an orbital *Taenia coenurus* cyst has been reported in a chinchilla, resulting in complete recovery.[47]

In Guinea pigs, rare intraocular and periocular neoplasms have been reported, including intraocular osteosarcoma,[48] T-cell lymphoma,[49] palpebral liposarcoma[50] and conjunctival lymphoma,[51] all managed surgically with variable outcomes. Osseous metaplasia/choristoma of the ciliary bodies may form vascularized intraocular masses and induce secondary glaucoma, for which enucleation is indicated when painful or associated with corneal pathology (**Fig. 15**).[52]

Ferrets Ocular Surgery

Ocular surgery in ferrets requires careful consideration of the species' unique anatomy and the diverse range of ocular and orbital conditions encountered. The nictitating membrane is rich in vascular and lymphoid tissue, features that warrants particular caution during surgical excision of the third eyelid or associated masses.[25] This structure may also be involved in lymphomatous infiltration, typically associated with systemic disease in ferrets.

Other adnexal disorders such as distichiasis can cause ocular irritation, epiphora, and conjunctivitis; in these cases, surgical excision of aberrant cilia and their follicles results in complete resolution of clinical signs.[53]

Infectious conjunctivitis, particularly that caused by *Mycobacterium avium* or *Mycobacterium genavense*, may lead to chronic granulomatous inflammation requiring biopsy or surgical debridement for diagnosis and management (**Fig. 16**).[46]

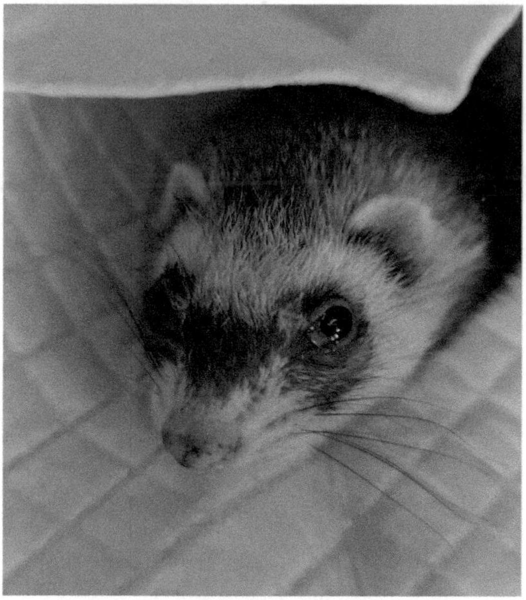

Fig. 16. Ferret presenting with conjunctivitis. In cases of granulomatous inflammation, a conjunctival biopsy is recommended. (Image Courtesy of Dr Carlo Paoletti.)

Corneal disease is another indication for surgical intervention in ferrets. Ulceration, trauma, and corneal dystrophy may occur. A recent case report described a 2-year-old female with bilateral descemetocele secondary to corneal dystrophy, successfully treated in both eyes using small intestinal submucosa grafting combined with a conjunctival pedicle flap, resulting in complete healing and preservation of vision.[54]

In instances of exposure keratitis or exophthalmos, temporary tarsorrhaphy can be applied to protect the cornea and facilitate epithelial healing.[25,55]

Cataracts are very common in this species, with one study reporting 47% of prevalence in 11 to 12-month-old ferrets and some degree of lens opacification in almost all animals by 18 months of age.[56]

Cataracts are surgically manageable in this species, with extracapsular extraction and, more effectively, phacoemulsification being described.[25,57]

Although the small globe and shallow anterior chamber increase technical difficulty and risk of intraoperative trauma, irrigation–aspiration using a reduced-diameter handpiece has been successfully employed. Since appropriately sized intraocular lenses are unavailable, ferrets remain aphakic but typically maintain satisfactory visual function. Reported postoperative complications include anterior uveitis and lens regeneration requiring secondary irrigation and aspiration several months after surgery.[57]

Orbital and globe surgeries are most often required in cases of exophthalmos secondary to retrobulbar or orbital masses, such as zygomatic salivary gland mucocele[58,59] or neoplasia.[60]

Due to the deep orbital anatomy, these lesions frequently remain undetected until they cause marked globe displacement. Depending on the underlying pathology, orbitotomy or enucleation may be indicated, with intraoperative bleeding controlled using direct compression, gelatin sponge packing, or topical thrombin.[60]

Enucleation or exenteration is also performed in cases of nonresponsive glaucoma, severe trauma, or intraocular neoplasia, where meticulous hemostasis is essential due to the presence of the retrobulbar venous plexus.[60]

Ocular Surgery in Myomorph Rodents

Ocular surgery in myomorph rodents presents distinct challenges related to their small orbital anatomy, delicate periocular structures, and extensive venous networks. In rats, mice, and hamsters, a prominent retrobulbar venous plexus poses a risk of hemorrhage during ocular procedures. Moreover, shallow orbits, thin corneas, and large lenses limit intraocular access and demand precise microsurgical techniques.[42,61,62]

The iris in these species is highly vascularized, particularly in hamsters, increasing the risk of intraoperative bleeding. The rudimentary third eyelid offers little to no protection during anesthesia or manipulation, predisposing to exposure keratitis.[63]

In rats and mice, intraocular surgery is technically limited by narrow chambers and lack of a pars plana, making procedures such as iridectomy or phacoemulsification challenging (**Fig. 17**).[61]

Enucleation represents the most common ophthalmic surgical procedure in myomorph rodents and is indicated for painful, irreversibly blind, or end-stage ocular disease such as severe infection, glaucoma, or neoplasia.[25,57]

Tight restraint during examination can induce transient exophthalmos and secondary corneal damage, emphasizing the need for minimal manipulation and gentle tissue handling.[64] Proptosis—frequent in small rodents, especially hamsters should initially

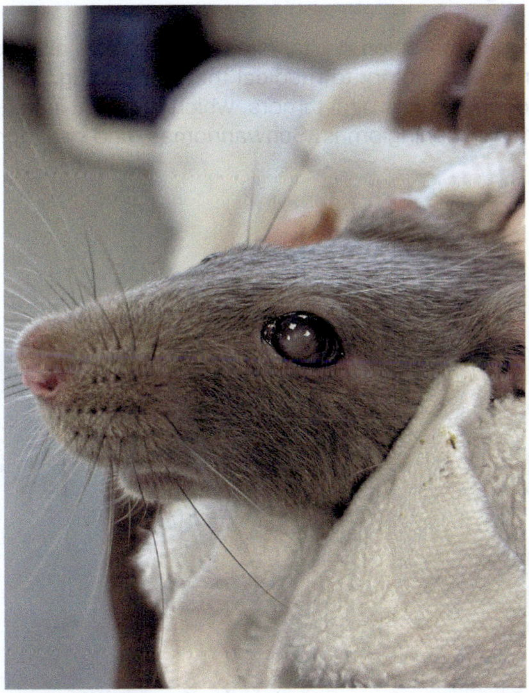

Fig. 17. Cataract surgery in myomorph rodents is particularly challenging because their extremely narrow ocular chambers and the absence of a pars plana severely limit intraocular access. (Image Courtesy of Dr Carlo Paoletti.)

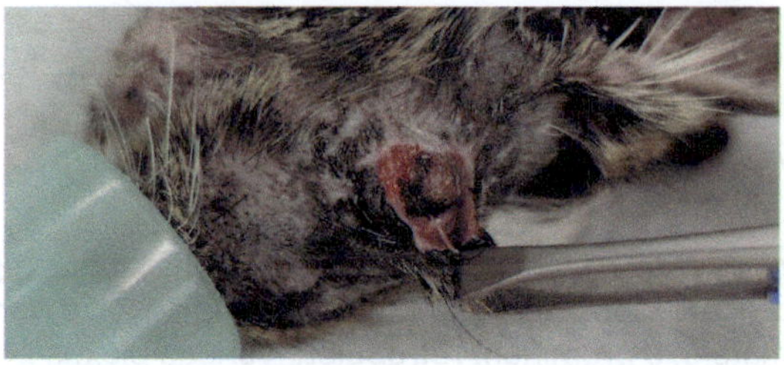

Fig. 18. Ocular desiccation in a degu (*Octodon degus*). (Image Courtesy of Dr Carlo Paoletti.)

be managed with temporary tarsorrhaphy to protect the cornea and maintain ocular position. Enucleation becomes necessary when the eye becomes desiccated or necrotic (**Fig. 18**).

For enucleation, the transconjunctival approach is preferred to minimize hemorrhage. A lateral canthotomy is performed, followed by a circumferential incision 1 to 2 mm from the limbus through the bulbar conjunctiva and Tenon's fascia to the sclera. The extraocular muscles are transected close to their insertions, and the optic nerve is severed. Although clamping or ligation of the entire retrobulbar contents has been described, the dense venous plexus in these species makes this approach technically challenging. Some authors therefore recommend proptosing the globe before removal, followed by hemostasis using cellulose or gelatin sponges and gentle pressure. After removal, the residual conjunctiva is excised, and the eyelid margins, Harderian gland, and third eyelid are removed before suturing the lids closed.[65,66]

Exenteration is indicated when orbital infections such as abscesses or Harderian gland inflammation are refractory to medical therapy[25,67] **Fig. 19**, Videos 11 and 12 and also in cases of ocular or orbital tumors, which primarily include Harderian gland adenomas, optic nerve meningiomas, Schwannomas, and melanomas.[68–71]

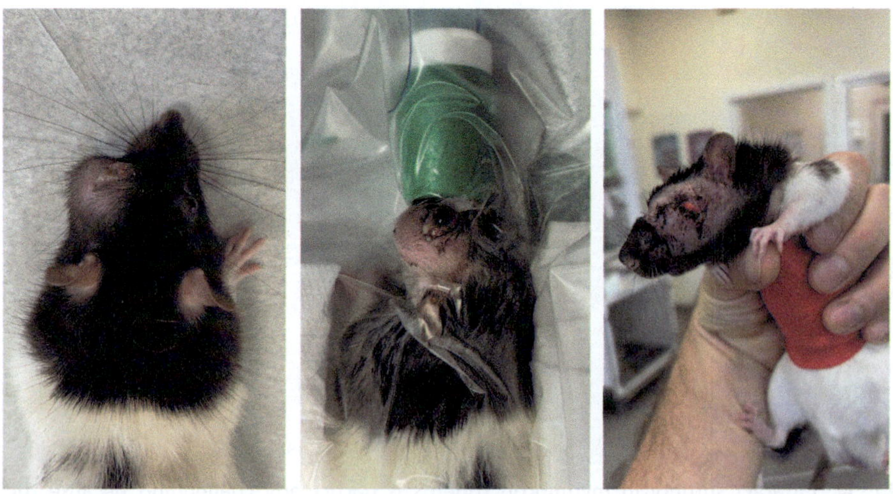

Fig. 19. Enucleation performed in a rat for a suborbital abscess. (Image Courtesy of Dr Carlo Paoletti.)

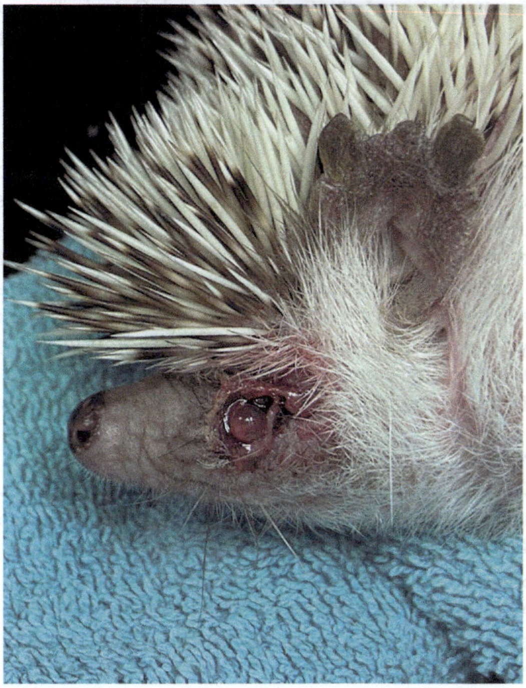

Fig. 20. Corneal perforation with lens prolapse in an African pygmy hedgehog (*Atelerix albiventris*). (*Image Courtesy* of Dr. M. Sabater González, Dr. M.L. Pérez Orrico and Dr. J. MacHale.)

OCULAR SURGERY IN HEDGEHOGS AND SUGAR GLIDERS

Ocular surgery in hedgehogs and sugar gliders is infrequently reported and generally indicated for traumatic, infectious, or space-occupying orbital disease.

In hedgehogs, ocular surgery is most often required for trauma-induced conditions such as proptosis and corneal ulceration. The combination of a shallow orbit, wide palpebral fissure, and prominent eyes predisposes these animals to proptosis even after minor facial trauma or improper handling (**Fig. 20**).[72,73]

Because orbital space is limited, enucleation is frequently necessary, as globe replacement is rarely successful.[72] The presence of a large orbital venous sinus poses a significant risk of hemorrhage during enucleation or other orbital surgeries, requiring meticulous hemostasis.[74,75]

Corneal ulcers, usually secondary to trauma or exposure keratitis, are another common indication for surgery. When medical therapy fails, debridement, grafting, or temporary tarsorrhaphy may be performed to restore corneal integrity.[76,77]

Less commonly, orbital tumors, including acinic cell and lacrimal ductal carcinomas, have been surgically addressed, although prognosis remains poor.[73,78]

Additional ocular conditions such as hyphema, vitreous hemorrhage, panophthalmitis, and meibomian cysts have been described, but these are typically managed medically rather than surgically.[72,75]

In sugar gliders, ocular surgery primarily addresses corneal ulcers, conjunctivitis, and retrobulbar abscesses, often secondary to trauma, inadequate husbandry, or dental disease. Corneal ulcers may require debridement or grafting, followed by careful postoperative hydration and infection control. Retrobulbar abscesses are typically treated with surgical drainage combined with systemic antibiotic therapy to reduce recurrence.[79]

SUMMARY

Small mammal ophthalmic surgery relies on precise microsurgical technique and species-specific perioperative planning. Rabbits commonly require surgery for nasolacrimal obstruction, Harderian gland prolapse, corneal ulcers, and cataracts. Hystricomorph rodents frequently need intervention for dental-related retrobulbar abscesses, nonhealing corneal disease, or orbital pathology. Ferrets often undergo surgical management of corneal lesions, conjunctival masses, cataracts, and orbital disease, whereas rodents typically require enucleation or exenteration due to small globe size and limited intraocular access. Across all taxa, successful outcomes depend on careful anesthesia, magnification, meticulous hemostasis, and tailored postoperative care.

CLINICS CARE POINTS

- In rabbits, nasolacrimal obstruction and corneal or lens disease are common surgical indications; preoperative imaging greatly enhances surgical planning.
- Hystricomorph rodents frequently present with dental-related retrobulbar disease; correcting the underlying dental pathology is essential for successful surgical outcomes.
- Phacoemulsification in ferrets is feasible but technically demanding due to the small globe and shallow anterior chamber.
- In rodents, the small orbital size and relatively large lens make intraocular surgery impractical, and enucleation is the only surgical procedure reported.
- Across species, optimal outcomes require careful anesthesia, adequate magnification, and meticulous hemostasis throughout surgery and recovery.

DECLARATION OF AI AND AI-ASSISTED TECHNOLOGIES IN THE WRITING PROCESS

During the preparation of this work the authors used Generative AI. After using this tool, the authors reviewed and edited the content as needed and takes full responsibility for the content of the publication.

DISCLOSURE

The authors have nothing to disclose.

SUPPLEMENTARY DATA

Supplementary data to this article can be found online at https://doi.org/10.1016/j.cvex.2026.04.011.

REFERENCES

1. Moore BA, Robertson J, Tarbert DK, et al. A novel surgical technique for enucleation in rabbits to reduce the risk of intra- and post-operative orbital hemorrhage. Vet Ophthalmol 2020;23(2):409–13.
2. Fritz J, Gaillot H, Ruel Y. Helical computed tomographic-dacryocystography in adult pet dwarf rabbits: procedure and normal appearance. Vlaams Diergeneeskundig Tijdschrift 2020;89(6). https://doi.org/10.21825/vdt.v89i6.17412.

3. Marini RP, Foltz CJ, Kersten D, et al. Microbiologic, radiographic, and anatomic study of the nasolacrimal duct apparatus in the rabbit (*Oryctolagus cuniculus*). Lab Anim Sci 1996;46(6):656–62.
4. Kovalcuka L, Nikolajenko M. Changes in intraocular pressure, horizontal pupil diameter, and tear production during the use of topical 1% cyclopentolate in cats and rabbits. Open Vet J 2020;10(1):59–67.
5. Adami C, Sanchez RF, Monticelli P. Use of atracurium and its reversal with neostigmine in 14 pet rabbits undergoing ophthalmic surgery: a retrospective study. Vet Rec 2019;184(14):443.
6. Stades FC, van der Woerdt A. Diseases and surgery of the canine eyelid. In: Veterinary ophthalmology. 6th edition; 2021. p. 923–87.
7. Eaton JS. Ophthalmology of lagomorpha: rabbits, hares, and pikas. In: Montiani-Ferreira F, Moore BA, Ben-Shlomo G, editors. Wild and exotic animal ophthalmology, vol. 2. Cham: Springer International Publishing; 2022. p. 367–402. https://doi.org/10.1007/978-3-030-81273-7_17. Mammals [Internet].
8. Florin M, Rusanen E, Haessig M, et al. Clinical presentation, treatment, and outcome of dacryocystitis in rabbits: a retrospective study of 28 cases (2003–2007). Vet Ophthalmol 2009;12(6):350–6.
9. Harcourt-Brown F. Chapter 11 - ophthalmic diseases. In: Harcourt-Brown F, editor. Textbook of rabbit medicine. Burlington: Butterworth-Heinemann; 2002. p. 292–306. https://doi.org/10.1016/B978-075064002-2.50014-X. Available at: https://www.sciencedirect.com/science/article/pii/B978075064002250014X.
10. Hedley J, Ede V, Dawson C. Retrospective study identifying risk factors for dacryocystitis in pet rabbits. Vet Rec 2022;191(5):e1903.
11. Miwa Y, Nakata M, Takimoto H, et al. Spontaneous intranasal tumours in rabbits: 7 cases (2007-2019). J Small Anim Pract 2021;62(5):379–84.
12. Stades FC, Neumann W, Boevé MH. Konjunktivale strikturen beim kaninchen. In: Praktische augenheilkunde für den tierarzt. 1st edition. Schlütersche; 1996. p. 102.
13. Allgoewer I, Malho P, Schulze H, et al. Aberrant conjunctival stricture and overgrowth in the rabbit. Vet Ophthalmol 2008;11(1):18–22.
14. Kim JY, Williams DL, Rho KS, et al. Surgical correction of aberrant conjunctival overgrowth in a rabbit: a case report. Ir Vet J 2013;66(1):18.
15. Khelik I, Johnson JG, McCool E, et al. Aberrant conjunctival overgrowth with corneal adhesions in two pet rabbits (*Oryctolagus cuniculus*). J Exot Pet Med 2023;46:32–7. Located at: CABI Databases.
16. Andrew SE. Corneal diseases of rabbits. Vet Clin Exot Anim Pract 2002;5(2):341–56.
17. Eshar D, Wyre NR, Schoster JV. Use of collagen shields for treatment of chronic bilateral corneal ulcers in a pet rabbit. J Small Anim Pract 2011;52(7):380–3.
18. Irving W, Whittaker C, Caruso K, et al. Bullous keratopathy in a dwarf rabbit (*Oryctolagus cuniculus domesticus*). J Exot Pet Med 2023;47:23–6.
19. Giordano C, Weigt A, Vercelli A, et al. Immunohistochemical identification of *Encephalitozoon cuniculi* in phacoclastic uveitis in four rabbits. Vet Ophthalmol 2005;8(4):271–5.
20. Sanchez RF, Becker R, Dawson C, et al. Calculation of posterior chamber intraocular lens (IOL) size and dioptric power for use in pet rabbits undergoing phacoemulsification. Vet Ophthalmol 2017;20(3):242–9.
21. Sanchez RF, Everson R, Hedley J, et al. Rabbits with naturally occurring cataracts referred for phacoemulsification and intraocular lens implantation: a preliminary study of 12 cases. Vet Ophthalmol 2018;21(4):399–412.

22. Sritrakoon N, Jitsophakul K, Areevijittrakul L, et al. Cataract surgery in pet rabbits: clinical presentation, treatment, and long-term outcomes. Animals 2025;15(19): 2898.
23. Suter C, Müler-Doblies UU, Deplazes P, et al. Prevention and treatment of *Encephalitozoon cuniculi* infection in rabbits with fenbendazole. Vet Rec 2001;148(15): 478–80.
24. Morera C, Costantino I, Caivano D, et al. Bilateral cataract associated with persistent hyperplastic primary vitreous and persistent hyperplastic tunica vasculosa lentis (PHPV/PHTVL) in a dwarf rabbit. J Exot Pet Med 2024;51:43–7.
25. van der Woerdt A. 40 - ophthalmologic diseases of small mammals. In: Quesenberry KE, Orcutt CJ, Mans C, et al, editors. Ferrets, rabbits, and rodents. 4th edition. Philadelphia: W.B. Saunders; 2020. p. 583–94. https://doi.org/10.1016/B978-0-323-48435-0.00040-X. Available at: https://www.sciencedirect.com/science/article/pii/B978032348435000040X.
26. Yuschenkoff D, Graham J, Pumphrey SA. Diagnosis and treatment of glaucoma in client-owned rabbits (*Oryctolagus cuniculus*): 16 eyes from 11 rabbits (2008–2019). J Exot Pet Med 2020;34:67–71.
27. Bennett RA. Rabbit soft tissue surgery. In: Surgery of exotic animals. 2021. p. 240–76. https://doi.org/10.1002/9781119139614.ch17 [cited 2025 Nov 25].
28. Diehl KA, McKinnon JA. Eye removal surgeries in exotic pets. Vet Clin Exot Anim Pract 2016;19(1):245–67.
29. Sanchez-Migallon Guzman D, Szabo Z, Steffey MA. 32 - soft tissue surgery: rabbits. In: Quesenberry KE, Orcutt CJ, Mans C, et al, editors. Ferrets, rabbits, and rodents. 4th edition. Philadelphia: W.B. Saunders; 2020. p. 446–66. https://doi.org/10.1016/B978-0-323-48435-0.00032-0. Available at: https://www.sciencedirect.com/science/article/pii/B9780323484350000320.
30. Hiebert K, Mans C, Eaton S. Subconjunctival enucleation with or without third eyelid removal may present a viable enucleation technique in rabbits: 18 cases (2014–2022). J Am Vet Med Assoc 2023;261(9):1368–73.
31. Allgoewer I, Soukup P. Modified lateral enucleation technique—Surgery without ligation or clamping of the optic nerve: technique description, complication rate and risk factors, and intraoperative blood loss estimation in companion animals. Vet Ophthalmol 2025;28(2):425–37.
32. Levy I, Mans C. Long-term systemic antibiotics and surgical treatment can be an effective treatment option for retrobulbar abscesses in rabbits (*Oryctolagus cuniculus*): 21 cases (2011–2022). J Am Vet Med Assoc 2023;261(10):1488–94.
33. Thomas A, Kazakos G, Pardali D, et al. Surgical management of orbital abscesses in domestic rabbits (*Oryctolagus cuniculus*): a report of seven cases. J Hellenic Vet Med Soc 2020;71(3):2251–60.
34. Martínez-Jiménez D, Hernández-Divers SJ, Dietrich UM, et al. Endosurgical treatment of a retrobulbar abscess in a rabbit. J Am Vet Med Assoc 2007;230(6): 868–72.
35. Gasser K, Fuchs-Baumgartinger A, Tichy A, et al. Investigations on the conjunctival goblet cells and on the characteristics of glands associated with the eye in the Guinea pig. Vet Ophthalmol 2011;14(1):26–40.
36. Monk C. Ocular surface disease in rodents (Guinea pigs, mice, rats, chinchillas). Vet Clin Exot Anim Pract 2019;22(1):15–26.
37. Otto G, Lipman NS, Murphy JC. Corneal dermoid in a hairless Guinea pig. Lab Anim Sci 1991;41(2):171–2.
38. Wappler O, Allgoewer I, Schaeffer EH. Conjunctival dermoid in two Guinea pigs: a case report. Vet Ophthalmol 2002;5(3):245–8.

39. Hisey EA, Rodriguez P, Tarbert DK, et al. Contrast computed tomography dacryocystorhinography identifies nasolacrimal duct obstruction secondary to chronic dental disease in two *Chinchilla langera*. Vet Ophthalmol 2025;28(6):983–9.
40. Williams D, Sullivan A. Ocular disease in the Guinea pig (*Cavia porcellus*): a survey of 1000 animals. Vet Ophthalmol 2010;13(s1):54–62.
41. Cafaro TA, Ortiz SG, Maldonado C, et al. The cornea of Guinea pig: structural and functional studies. Vet Ophthalmol 2009;12(4):234–41.
42. Rodriguez-Ramos Fernandez J, Dubielzig RR. Ocular comparative anatomy of the family Rodentia. Vet Ophthalmol 2013;16(s1):94–9.
43. Mans C, Donnelly TM. 22 - chinchillas. In: Quesenberry KE, Orcutt CJ, Mans C, et al, editors. Ferrets, rabbits, and rodents. 4th edition. Philadelphia: W.B. Saunders; 2021. p. 298–322. https://doi.org/10.1016/B978-0-323-48435-0.00022-8. Available at: https://www.sciencedirect.com/science/article/pii/B9780323484350000228.
44. Müller K, Eule JC. Ophthalmic disorders observed in pet chinchillas (*Chinchilla lanigera*). J Exot Pet Med 2014;23(2):201–5.
45. Holmberg BJ. Ophthalmology of Hystricomorpha: porcupines, Guinea pigs, degus, chinchillas, and relatives. In: Montiani-Ferreira F, Moore BA, Ben-Shlomo G, editors. Wild and exotic animal ophthalmology, vol. 2. Cham: Springer International Publishing; 2022. p. 403–36. Mammals [Internet].
46. Doden G, Patson C, Duensing K, et al. Conjunctivitis associated with *Mycobacterium avium* in a North American ferret (*Mustela putorius furo*). J Exot Pet Med 2023;45:28–9.
47. Holmberg BJ, Hollingsworth SR, Osofsky A, et al. *Taenia coenurus* in the orbit of a chinchilla. Vet Ophthalmol 2007;10(1):53–9.
48. Gomez-Rios JA, Rodríguez-Reyes AA, Ramírez-Lezama J, et al. Primary intraocular osteosarcoma with pulmonary metastasis in a Guinea pig (*Cavia porcellus*). J Exot Pet Med 2019;28:121–7.
49. Steinberg H. Disseminated T-cell lymphoma in a Guinea pig with bilateral ocular involvement. J Vet Diagn Invest 2000;12(5):459–62.
50. Quinton JF, Ollivier F, Dally C. A case of well-differentiated palpebral liposarcoma in a Guinea pig (*Cavia porcellus*). Vet Ophthalmol 2013;16(Suppl 1):155–9.
51. Allgoewer E, Ewringmann C, Pfleghaar S. Pfleghaar. Lymphosarcoma with conjunctival manifestation in a Guinea pig. Vet Ophthalmol 1999;2(2):117–9.
52. Schäffer EH, Pfleghaar S. Secondary open angle glaucoma from osseous choristoma of the ciliary body in Guinea pigs. Tierarztl Prax 1995;23(4):410–4.
53. Verboven CAPM, Djajadiningrat-Laanen SC, Kitslaar WJP, et al. Distichiasis in a ferret (*Mustela putorius furo*). Vet Ophthalmol 2014;17(4):290–3.
54. Cattaneo A, Bersanetti G, Guandalini A. A bilateral corneal descemetocele as a consequence of corneal dystrophy in a ferret (*Mustela putorius furo*). Vet Rec Case Rep 2024;12(2):e837. https://doi.org/10.1002/vrc2.837.
55. Myrna KE, Girolamo ND. Ocular examination and corneal surface disease in the ferret. Vet Clin Exot Anim Pract 2019;22(1):27–33.
56. Good KL. Ocular disorders of pet ferrets. Vet Clin Exot Anim Pract 2002;5(2):325–39.
57. Schlesener BN, Taylor R, Ledbetter EC. Phacoemulsification of a unilateral immature cataract with lens regeneration in a juvenile ferret (*Mustela putorius furo*). J Exot Pet Med 2024;51:5–8.
58. Miller PE, Pickett JP. Zygomatic salivary gland mucocele in a ferret. J Am Vet Med Assoc 1989;194(10):1437–8.

59. Thas I. Acquired salivary mucoceles in two domestic ferrets (*Mustela putorius furo*). Vet Rec Case Rep 2014;2(1):e000051.
60. McBride M, Mosunic CB, Barron GHW, et al. Successful treatment of a retrobulbar adenocarcinoma in a ferret (*Mustela putorius furo*). Vet Rec 2009;165(7): 206–8.
61. Popescu RM, Ober C, Sevastre B, et al. Complications of cataract surgery in Wistar rats undergoing treatment with tamsulosin. Exp Ther Med 2019;17(1):137–46. PubMed PMID: 30651774; PubMed Central PMCID: PMC6307455.
62. Saadi-Brenkia O, Hanniche N, Lounis S. Microscopic anatomy of ocular globe in diurnal desert rodent *Psammomys obesus* (Cretzschmar, 1828). J Basic Appl Zool 2018;79(1):43.
63. Ramos MF, Baker J, Atzpodien EA, et al. Nonproliferative and proliferative lesions of the ratand mouse special sense organs (ocular [eye and glands], olfactory and otic). J Toxicol Pathol 2018;31(3_Suppl):97S–214S.
64. Miwa Y, Mayer J. 26 - hamsters and gerbils. In: Quesenberry KE, Orcutt CJ, Mans C, et al, editors. Ferrets, rabbits, and rodents. 4th edition. Philadelphia: W.B. Saunders; 2021. p. 368–84. https://doi.org/10.1016/B978-0-323-48435-0.00026-5. Available at: https://www.sciencedirect.com/science/article/pii/B9780323484350000265.
65. Szabo Z. 33 - soft tissue surgery: rodents. In: Quesenberry KE, Orcutt CJ, Mans C, et al, editors. Ferrets, rabbits, and rodents. 4th edition. Philadelphia: W.B. Saunders; 2021. p. 467–82. https://doi.org/10.1016/B978-0-323-48435-0.00033-2. Available at: https://www.sciencedirect.com/science/article/pii/B9780323484350000332.
66. Wilding LA, Uchihashi M, Bergin IL, et al. Enucleation for treating rodent ocular disease. J Am Assoc Lab Anim Sci 2015;54(3):328–32. PubMed PMID: 26045460; PubMed Central PMCID: PMC4460947.
67. Zaffarano BA, Allbaugh RA, Whitley EM. Bilateral Harderian gland abscesses in a Syrian dwarf hamster (*Mesocricetus auratus*). J Exot Pet Med 2015;24(2):209–14.
68. Greaves P, Faccini JM. Spontaneous fibrous histiocytic neoplasms in rats. Br J Cancer 1981;43(3):402–11.
69. Krinke G, Fix A, Jacobs M, et al. Eye and Harderian gland. In: Mohr U, editor. International classification of rodent tumors. The mouse [Internet]. Berlin, Heidelberg: Springer Berlin Heidelberg; 2001. p. 347–59.
70. Kurotaki T, Tomonari Y, Kanno T, et al. Malignant amelanotic melanoma behind the left eye in a female Crj:CD(SD)IGS rat: a case report. Vet Pathol 2008;45(5): 681–4.
71. Yoshitomi K, Boorman GA. Spontaneous amelanotic melanomas of the uveal tract in F344 rats. Vet Pathol 1991;28(5):403–9.
72. Wheler CL, Grahn BH, Pocknell AM. Unilateral proptosis and orbital cellulitis in eight African hedgehogs (*Atelerix albiventris*). J Zoo Wildl Med 2001;32(2): 236–41.
73. Kuonen VJ, Wilkie DA, Morreale RJ, et al. Unilateral exophthalmia in a European hedgehog (*Erinaceus europaeus*) caused by a lacrimal ductal carcinoma. Vet Ophthalmol 2002;5(3):161–5.
74. Hamlen H. Retro-orbital blood collection in the African hedgehog (*Atelerix albiventris*). Lab Anim 1997;34–5.
75. Turner PV, Brash ML, Smith DA. Hedgehogs. In: Turner PV, Brash ML, Smith DA, editors. Pathology of small mammal pets. 2017. p. 387–416.
76. Gardhouse S, Eshar D. Retrospective study of disease occurrence in captive African pygmy hedgehogs (*Atelerix albiventris*). Isr J Vet Med 2015;70:32–6.

77. Williams D, Adeyeye N, Visser E. Ophthalmological abnormalities in wild European hedgehogs (*Erinaceus europaeus*): a survey of 300 animals. Open Vet J 2017;7(3):261–7.
78. Fukuzawa R, Fukuzawa K, Abe H, et al. Acinic cell carcinoma in an African pygmy hedgehog (*Atelerix albiventris*). Vet Clin Pathol 2004;33(1):39–42.
79. Johnson-Delaney C. 27 - sugar gliders. In: Quesenberry KE, Orcutt CJ, Mans C, et al, editors. Ferrets, rabbits, and rodents. 4th edition. Philadelphia: W.B. Saunders; 2021. p. 385–400. https://doi.org/10.1016/B978-0-323-48435-0.00027-7. Available at: https://www.sciencedirect.com/science/article/pii/B9780323484350000277.

Skin Surgery in Exotic Companion Mammals

Dario d'Ovidio, DVM, MS, SpecPACS, PhD, DECZM (Small Mammals)[a,b,*],
Lucas Flenghi, DMV, DECZM (Small Mammals)[c],
Paul Raymond, DMV, DECZM (Small Mammals)[d]

KEYWORDS

• Exotic companion mammals • Cutaneous disorders • Surgery • Skin tumors
• Wound management • Trauma • Burns • Cutting-edge treatments

KEY POINTS

- Cutaneous infectious and non-infectious disorders are very common in exotic companion mammals (ECMs).
- Main indications for skin surgery in ECMs include the excision of tumors, the repair of wounds, lacerations and burns, as well as the treatment of integumentary infections.
- New treatments and technologies are available for the management of wounds, trauma and burns, although their clinical efficacy has yet to be demonstrated.
- Considering the anecdotal nature of these therapies, patient's response monitoring is crucial in animals treated with new technologies.

INTRODUCTION

Exotic companion mammals ([ECMs]; eg, ferrets, rabbits, and rodents) are commonly affected by several cutaneous, infectious and noninfectious, conditions including neoplasia, infections and traumatic injuries.[1] Skin (including mammary glands) and subcutaneous neoplasia are reported to be among the most frequently diagnosed conditions in rabbits as well as ferrets (up to 20% in older animals) and rodents.[2–4] Skin surgery is a useful mean required for both diagnostic (eg, biopsy) and therapeutic purposes (eg, mass excision, wound repair, among others). Although commonly performed, some important considerations should be kept in mind when performing skin surgery in ECMs. ECMs' skin is elastic, thin and covered by a dense fur. Therefore, great caution should be paid during aseptic preparation (eg, hair clipping), skin

[a] Private practitioner, Exotic Pet Service, Via C. Colombo 118, 80022 Arzano, Naples, Italy; [b] CDVet, Laboratorio Analisi Veterinarie, Roma, Italy; [c] Private practitioner, Exotic Clinic - Sevetys, Nandy, France; [d] Cordeliers Clinic, Exotic Medicine Service, 29 Av. du Maréchal Joffre, 77100, Meaux, France
* Corresponding author.
E-mail address: dariodovidio@yahoo.it

Vet Clin Exot Anim 29 (2026) 629–648
https://doi.org/10.1016/j.cvex.2026.04.005 vetexotic.theclinics.com

Abbreviations	
ECMs	exotic companion mammals
NIRF-ICG	near-infrared fluorescence angiography with indocyanine green
TBSA	total body surface area

handling, and surgical approach (eg, incision) to prevent skin damage, reduce post-surgical pain and self-inflicted wound trauma.[5] Luckily new technologies and surgical instruments are now available for skin surgery in such patients. The aim of this article is to provide the reader with the most updated information on skin surgery (anatomy, planning, techniques, and complications) and new technologies for the management of a variety of dermatologic surgical conditions in ECMs.

ANATOMY, PHYSIOLOGY, AND MAIN INDICATIONS

ECMs share many integumentary anatomic and physiologic similarities with other pets (eg, dogs and cats) and are frequently used as animal models for human skin disease. The mammalian skin is composed of 3 layers namely the epidermis, the dermis and the hypodermis (subcutis). The epidermis is the outmost layer that provides protection and acts as a physical barrier. It is 4-layered (*stratum basale*, *stratum spinosum*, *stratum granulosum*, and *stratum corneum*) and avascular. The dermis is the middle layer that provides strength, elasticity, and serves as substrate for the epidermis. It is composed of 2 layers (*stratum papillare* and *stratum reticulare*) and it is rich in blood vessels and nerves. The hypodermis or subcutis is the inner layer that provides thermal insulation and connects the outer layers with the underlying muscles, bones and organs. It is made of adipose (variably distributed across species) and connective tissue and is particularly thick in males (eg, ferrets) compared to females to protect animals during mating fights.[6] Despite the skin features common to all mammals, some important species-specific differences should be considered when approaching these patients and/or preparing for surgical treatments of skin conditions.

- Ferrets have a very thick dermis, abundant adipose tissue and numerous sebaceous glands.[4,6]
- Rabbit have abundant adipose tissue, a thin and delicate skin and large ear pinnae.[6]
- Rodents have a fragile skin (predisposed to dehiscence). In rat-like rodents, between the scapulae, in the ventral neck, in the axillary and inguinal regions, the adipose tissue is prominent whereas in cavy-like rodents (eg, guinea pigs and chinchillas) it is scarce.[6]

Main indications for skin surgery in ECMs include the excision of masses, the repair of (traumatic) wounds, lacerations, and burns, as well as the treatment of cutaneous infections (eg, abscesses, pododermatitis, and so on). Less frequent indications include correction of congenital defects and revision of old scars.

Due to their thin epidermis, only few layers of cells, predisposition of some species to disrupt and remove sutures (eg, small rodents), and contraindications in using Elizabethan collars (eg, increased stress, risk of entrapment, limited visual field, and inability to carry out coprophagy), ECMs are challenging patients for skin surgery compared with other small pets.[7] Therefore, gentle manipulation of tissues, minimization of incision length, adequate size and type of suture material and pattern (eg, intradermal suture pattern), good surgical skills, and effective analgesic management are key factors to reduce the risk of postoperative self-trauma.[7] The use of skin staples and tissue glue in ECMs can also be considered where traction is not present.[7]

Diagnostics and Preoperatory Planning

Before planning a surgical treatment, a detailed history (traumatic injury, fight or presence of other animals in the house, and lifestyle of the pet) including specific information about the origin and timing along with the general health pet's condition, should be collected. Following a dermatologic examination, specific diagnostic test will help achieve a final diagnosis. Cytologic evaluation of fine-needle aspirates may provide preliminary information on benign and/or malignant cutaneous masses.[1] However, histopathologic and immunohistochemical evaluation of skin biopsy samples will provide a definitive diagnosis. Imaging methodologies such as radiography, ultrasonography, computed tomography, or magnetic resonance imaging will provide either information about the extension of the lesion (eg, infiltration of a neoplastic mass) and the stage/grade the condition (eg, pododermatitis) or plan the most appropriate therapeutic approach. Finally, blood work including a complete blood count (CBC), serum biochemical analysis, and a hormonal panel will help detect systemic spreading.

Surgery of Skin Tumors

Background

Skin tumors are frequently diagnosed in small mammalian species. Incidence and prevalence of these tumors vary according to specie, sex, age, and other factors like fur color. Frequently treated tumors in small mammalian species include: mast cell tumors, basal cell tumors, soft tissue sarcoma, apocrine scent gland adenoma and adenocarcinoma, squamous cell carcinoma, benign follicular tumors (trichoepitheliomas), melanocytic tumors, epitheliotropic T-cell lymphoma. A study on cutaneous and subcutaneous tumors in small mammals highlighted a high incidence of malignancies. Fibrosarcomas were the most prevalent tumors in rats, degus, African pygmy hedgehogs, and chinchillas. They were also the second most common tumors in rabbits and hamsters.[8] In rabbits, cutaneous tumors are seen mainly in middle-aged to older individuals, and the majority of these tumors are benign, with the most commonly identified being trichoblastoma (trabecular type).[8–10]

Mast cell tumor is the most frequent cutaneous neoplasm diagnosed in ferret.[8,10] In ferret, this tumor has a benign behavior, does not spread locally or metastasize, and presents a good prognosis. Its surgical excision with good margins is curative.

Despite being a rare diagnosis, benign and malignant peripheral nerve sheath tumor are seen in ferrets. These tumors affect skin and subcutis and may be found anywhere on the animal's body, but head is a common affected site.[11] Their growth rate and anatomic location may complicate complete surgical removal. Mammary tumors and lipomatous neoplasms are not true integumentary tumors but their surgical excision and subsequent wound closure, can represent a challenge in rabbits, guinea pigs and rats. Early diagnosis of malignant lesions should be achieved by fine needle aspiration test or biopsy. Tumor removal options include incisional biopsy and excisional biopsy. A surgeon can choose to perform wide margins or no margins excision according to presumptive or definitive diagnosis, and stage of the disease (**Fig. 1**).

Surgical planning

Before surgery, different factors should be assessed: skin tension, elasticity, thickness. These can vary according to species, age, sex, individual factors and body region. Some obese female rabbits for example, may need a plasty after losing weight, because of loose skin in abdominal area impairing the normal flow of urine (**Fig. 2**). Skin elasticity is greater in hamsters and lower in guinea pigs. Wound closure, reepithelialization, and granulation tissue fill are delayed or decreased with aging in many

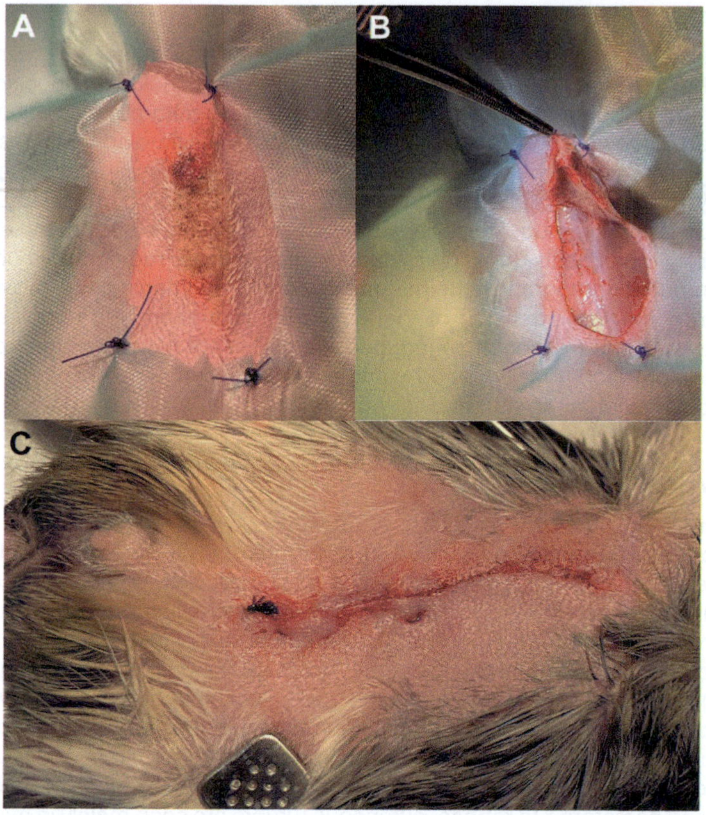

Fig. 1. (*A–C*) Excision of a neoplasia of the ventral marking gland in a gerbil. A wide surgical excision should be performed if an adenocarcinoma is suspected. (*A*) The ventral marking gland is ulcerated and bleeds. (*B*) Subcutaneous tissue is dissected and the gland is excised. (*C*) The wound is closed with intradermal sutures. (Image Courtesy of Dr Paul Raymond.)

strains of mice, rats and New Zealand White rabbits.[12] In most species, especially ferrets, skin is thicker in the dorsal cervical region and thinner on the ventrum.

Skin incision method

The method of skin incision is a very important choice. The surgical site may be extremely vascularized, or situated in a delicate location (eg, eyelid, perianal, or perivulvar area). Skin incisions are frequently made with cold scalpel and some concerns remain regarding electrocautery: excessive scaring, delayed healing and increased infection compared to cold scalpel incisions. Electrocautery is a widely used tool and has the advantage of reducing blood loss during incisions. There have been major technological advances in electrosurgery, modern electrosurgical generators produce a pure sinusoidal cut waveform making this technique safe and precise.[13] Studies have found no significant difference in wound infection rates or scar cosmesis, identified between cold scalpel and electrocautery.[14] Because of the reduced bleeding, electrocautery significantly reduces the incision time. In conclusion, concerns regarding the use of electrosurgery for skin incisions are unfounded and the choice of incision method remains only a matter of surgeon preference.[15]

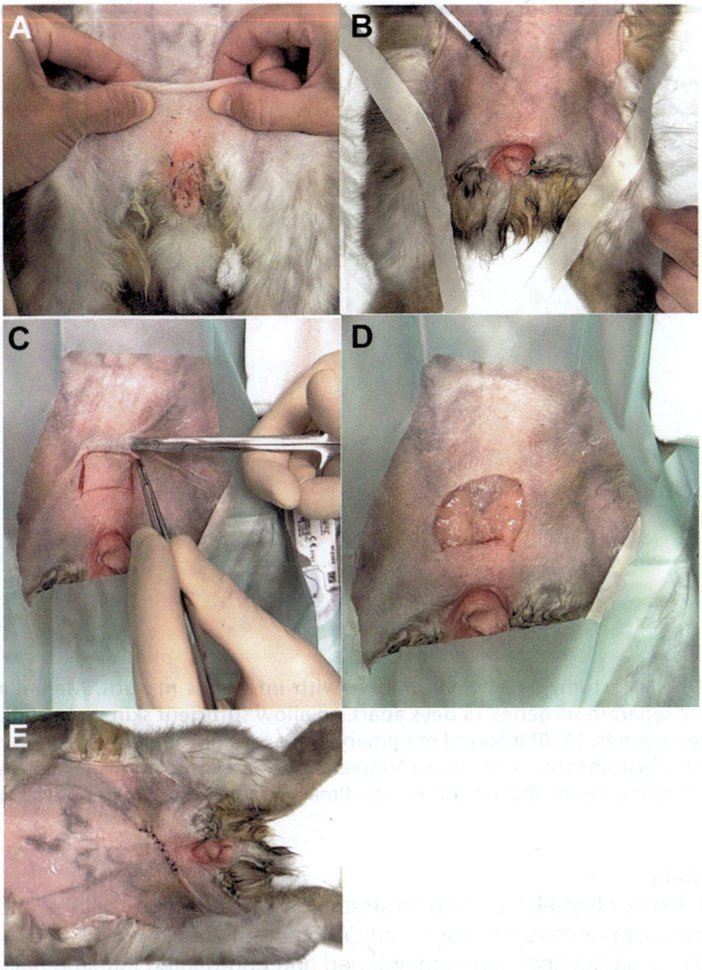

Fig. 2. (*A–E*) Skin surgery on an 8 year old overweight female rabbit with urinary scalding secondary to excess skin buildup following weight loss. (*A*) Evaluation of the size of the skin fold that should be surgically removed. (*B*) Local skin anesthesia on the surgical site. (*C–E*) semicircular skin incision is made and the excessive skin is excised. (*E*) Simple closure of the surgical wound. (Image Courtesy of Dr Paul Raymond.)

Treatment options

Radiation therapy should be used when indicated, to reduce tumor size before surgery, or after excision to minimize risks of recurrence.

Skin tension relief may be obtained through relaxing incisions performed near a defect, subdermal or subcuticular sutures.[16] These sutures bring skin edges into apposition, facilitating wound closure (**Fig. 3**). In the same manner, walking sutures may be used to advance skin margins closer from each other at the center of the defect. Adjustable horizontal mattress suture technique uses continuous intradermal suture anchored at one or both ends, with a button secured on the skin surface. Traction is applied on the suture and progressively tightens the gap.

In case a simple closure is not an option, several reconstructive techniques may be attempted: skin stretching, local flap, axial pattern flap, free skin graft.

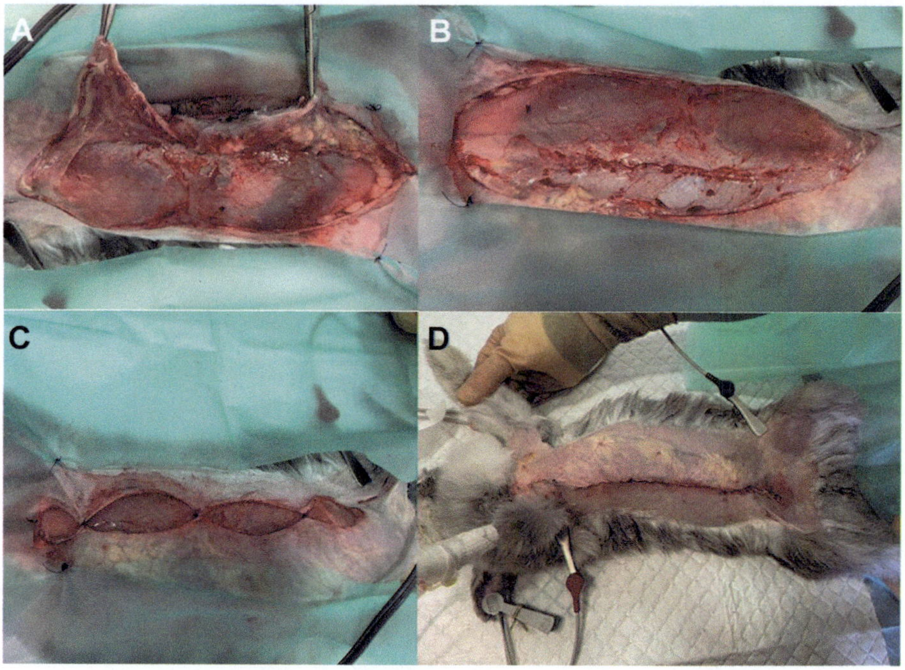

Fig. 3. (*A–D*) Mastectomy in a female rabbit with infectious mastitis. Mammary tissue is removed in 2 separate surgeries 15 days apart, to allow sufficient skin mobilization to close both surgical wounds. (*A, B*) Infected mammary tissue is removed, skin tension is reduced by dissection of subcutaneous tissue. (*C, D*) Simple closure is chosen and cutaneous sutures are performed to bring closer the wound edges. (Image Courtesy of Dr Paul Raymond.)

Skin stretching

Skin stretching involves skin's ability to stretch beyond its natural or inherent elasticity. Chronic stretching force is naturally seen during pregnancy, obesity, and skin growth over tumors. Collagen fibers are straightened and compacted longitudinally in the direction of the stretching force.[16] This method needs time and can only be used in planned surgeries. Continuous tension may be locally maintained for hours to days. Several methods may be used. This list includes but is not limited to: simple suture techniques, skin stretchers involving external self-adherent skin pads with Velcro; or inflatable expanders slowly inflated with saline over time and placed under healthy skin, adjacent to the defect. Expander placed subcutaneously in the rabbit research model, causes considerable skin stretch but interferes with cutaneous blood supply.[17] An external stretching device has been used in a rabbit suffering from a degloving injury covering approximately 30% of its dorsum.[18] The external skin-stretching device was left in place for 72 hours and maintained continuous, adjustable tension on the skin via skin pads and elastic cables through Velcro. External skin stretchers may also be used after surgery when a large wound is closed under excessive tension. The device is usually kept 3 to 5 days after surgery.

Skin flaps

Skin flaps are used when a large wound caused by trauma or oncological resection, cannot be easily closed (**Fig. 4**). A piece of skin that has its own blood supply and

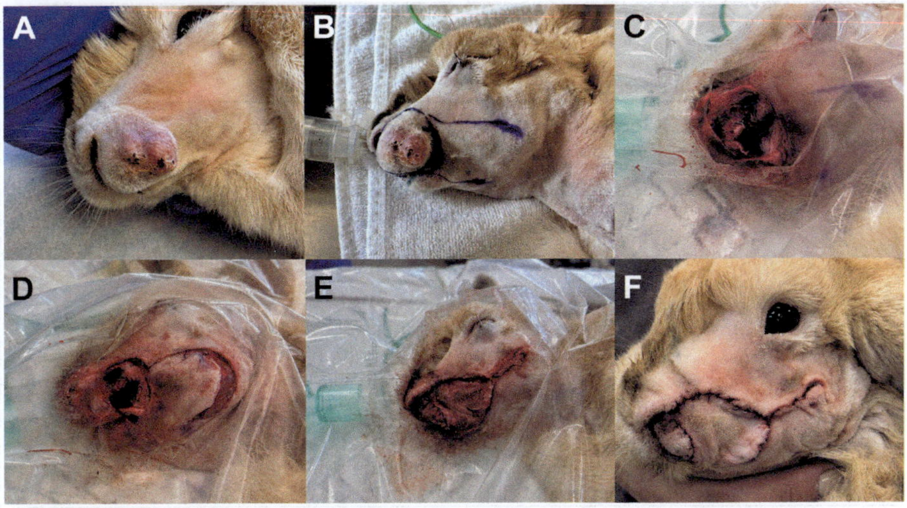

Fig. 4. (*A–F*) Maxillofacial reconstructive surgery in the rabbit: (*A*) Preoperative clinical presentation of an ulcerated nasolabial mass (*B*) Marking of incision lines (*C*) Tumor excision following circular incision and dissection (*D*) Preparation of the cutaneous flap through incision of mobilization lines (*E*) Reconstruction with cutaneous flap and sutures (*F*) Immediate postoperative result with restoration of the maxillofacial profile. (Image Courtesy of Dr Carlo Paoletti.)

originating from an area of relative abundance, is transposed over a large defect, facilitating closure and healing of that wound. Skin flaps may be classified according to the location, the blood supply and their shape (**Table 1**). When performing skin surgery, knowing the anatomic location of tension lines helps minimize tension on wound itself. Description of these lines is scarce in small mammalian species. Anatomic landmarks are often extrapolated from knowledge of dogs and cats.

Single-pedicle advancement flaps have their blood supply entering the flap at the base. Local flaps are very common and are created adjacent to the defect.

Skin flaps containing a direct cutaneous artery are called axial pattern flaps, while majority of skin flaps are subdermal plexus flaps. A flap with a directly embedded cutaneous artery is more likely to survive. Also, the wider a flap, the more likely it is to contain cutaneous branches. Conversely, the viability of a cutaneous flap is limited by its length. The longer a flap, the more likely it is to necrotize and will increase the risk of dehiscence at its tip.

Transposition flaps involve incising non-contiguous donor tissue and rotating it around intact adjacent tissue to close a defect. If the flap covers intact skin between donor and recipient site it is named interpolation flap.

The skin of rats being very loose, this specie has been used as skin flaps technique models in human medicine.[19,20] In Guinea-pigs, a study demonstrated that previously recommended 2:1 flap length:base width ratio was insufficient in most cases.[19] Larger flaps (3.5:1) are preferred. 3:1 was suggested to be the most consistent flap viability ratio in rats 20 3:1 was also a satisfactory ratio in rabbit animal model, using 2 skin flaps of the lower abdominal wall for the study of neo-vaginoplasty in humans.[21]

Skin grafts

Skin graft is a fragment of tissue that is neither vascularized nor innervated. It includes the epidermis and part or all of the dermis. Depending on the relationship between

Table 1
Examples of local skin flaps[6]

Flap	Description
Advancement flap:	A local flap that is moved over the defect to be filled using a sliding motion.
V-Y advancement flap	A V-shaped incision is made to lengthen the local flap. One edge of the incision is then stretched so that the V becomes a Y, and the incision is sutured over the defect. This flap, unlike other advancement flaps, is not detached but mobilized by deep peripheral dissection.
Transposition flap	The tissue is stretched and then repositioned to repair the defect. Transposition is only possible with narrow-pedicled flaps, which are longer than they are wide and therefore have greater mobility but also greater fragility.
Z-plasty	A Z-plasty involves creating a local transposition of 2 or more triangular flaps. This technique combines the aspects of an advancement flap and a rotation flap.
Rotation flap	In the case of a rotation flap, arcuate incisions and counter-incisions are made to increase the width or length of the flap, as well as its mobility. It can then be rotated before being stretched to the defect to be repaired.

From Paterson S. Structure and function of mammal skin. In: Skin Diseases of Exotic Pets. Blackwell Science Ltd; 2006:175–184.[6]

donor and recipient, several types of skin grafts are distinguished: autograft (graft performed on the same individual), homograft or allograft (graft between individuals of the same species), heterograft or xenograft (graft between individuals of different species). Punch skin grafting involves taking small pellets of skin to graft them. Mesh grafting involves cutting parallel rows of staggered slits to create a mesh/mesh-like structure. This increases the surface area covered by the skin sample and creates a route for drainage of blood or serum from under the graft.

- Full thickness autografts was performed for research purpose in rabbits,[22] immune competent rat,[23] mouse,[24] and guinea pig.[25] Correct placement of a protective bandage is a key step toward proper healing. Folded gauze and adhesive bandage can be used to protect and limit movements of the graft.[24] Other reasons for graft failure can be poor preparation of the graft, or incorrect positioning in the graft bed.
- Xenografts are poorly documented in exotic mammalian species. Acellular dermal matrix has shown efficacy in wound reconstruction and healing, in both human and veterinary medicine. Intestinal submucosa, peritoneal membrane, and amniotic tissue are derived from porcine, bovine, or human cadavers.[26] In veterinary medicine, porcine small intestine submucosa meshes has widely been used to replace missing extracellular matrix in mammalian skin. Recently, acellular fish skin grafts obtained from North Atlantic cod have successfully served as skin substitute, facilitating second-intention wound healing following wide surgical tumor excision in dogs.[27] The grafts are interestingly rich in omega-3 fatty acids, among other components. The omega-3 fatty acids have antibacterial and anti-inflammatory properties, serving as a physical antibacterial barrier. Omega-3 polyunsaturated fatty acids given orally as supplements have

shown antineoplastic properties linked to the immunomodulatory and anti-inflammatory effects.[28] It is unknown if acellular fish skin grafts present identical properties. Tilapia skin acellular dermal matrix showed good healing properties in rat skin wound repair model.[29] Tilapia skin is rich in type I collagen, providing good biomedical scaffold structure, mechanical strength, biodegradability and biocompatibility, which is conducive to cell infiltration, adhesion and growth.[27]

Management of Trauma/Burns

Presentation

Burn wound cases are rarely observed in small mammalian species. Main causes of spontaneous burn injuries in these patients involve electric heating pads (**Fig. 5**), hot water bottles, electrosurgical ground pads, hot water scalding, and abuse or malicious intent by humans.[30] Much of burn injury research is performed on animal models. In experimental settings, burn wounds are generated from direct contact with a heated metal, electricity, and heated water.[31]

Patients with severe burns will have significant fluid losses due to loss of the skin barrier. In case of extended burn, surgical treatment should be delayed. First step is estimating the degree and severity of a burn in order to calculate fluid resuscitation requirements. Wallace's Rule of 9s is a simple tool used to assess the total body surface area (TBSA) involved in burn human patients.[32] This method uses a percentage of body surface area as a multiple of 9 to determine the extent of burns. Other techniques involve using the palmar surface as a percentage of body surface (approximates 1%), or a credit card (worldwide standardized surface equal to 45 cm2).[32] Then the %TBSA can be easily calculated by dividing the burned surface area by the total body surface area.

A more precise diagnosis of burn injuries using body mapping chart was obtained with computed tomography (CT) images in dogs.[33] As a general rule, systemic consequences should be expected in patients with greater than 20% TBSA burns.

Pathophysiology

Four degrees are used to qualify the depth of a burn, from superficial lesion to involvement of subcutaneous tissues, including muscles and bone.[30] A burn wound may continue to deepen for several days after the traumatic event because of the compromised vascularization. Aggressive fluid therapy is the most important treatment. Decreased cardiac output and preload lead to significant cardiovascular depression.

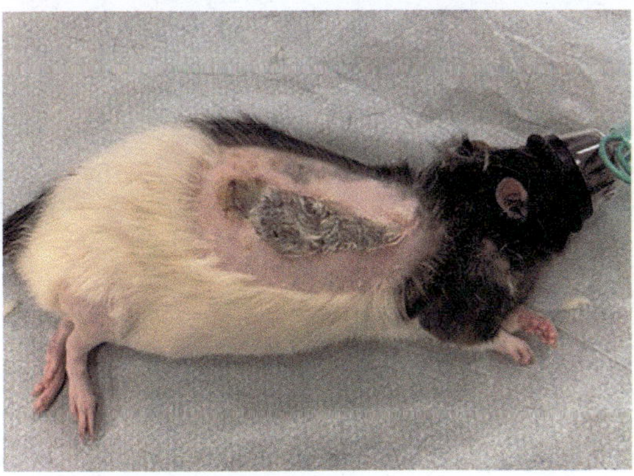

Fig. 5. Skin burn in a rat caused by prolonged contact on an overheating electric pad during surgery. (Image Courtesy of Dr Carlo Paoletti.)

Burn shock may occur in patients with more than 15% to 20% TBSA and lack or delayed appropriate fluid resuscitation.

Initial stabilization and surgical treatments of burn wound patients

Isotonic crystalloids are used for initial fluid resuscitation. The use of natural or synthetic colloids in burn care fluid therapy is controversial. Their use has not proven benefit yet.

In superficial wounds, common treatments include cold water irrigation, pain management, topical antimicrobials and daily monitoring of wound progression until reepithelialization. Dressings are generally not needed.[30]

Surgery is the treatment of choice and should be initiated without delay in deep burn injury. Deep burn injury can either be full-thickness or deep partial-thickness burn.[34]

In deep partial thickness injury, debridement, bacterial culture, topical antimicrobials, and proper dressing should be performed.[30] Surgical treatment may include skin grafts or flaps. Healing of partial thickness injuries involves contraction and epithelialization.

Full thickness burns benefit of early surgical excision and skin grafts or flaps are often needed.

Debridement is a treatment used for common traumatic wounds but also for thermal injuries.

- Enzymatic debridement is mostly used in human medicine.
- Mechanical debridement includes wet-to-wet and wet-to-dry bandaging. This technique allows removal of necrotic tissue and maintains a healthy wound bed. If the wound is compromising the patient, is very large or full thickness, a surgical excision of the lesion may be attempted after initial stabilization (**Fig. 6**).

Two techniques allow excision of burnt tissue: fascial excision and tangential excision.[34] Fascial excision or full thickness excision, means removal of cutaneous and subcutaneous tissue starting at the periphery of the wound. This technique creates a good bed for skin grafting. Tangential excision is a dissection of thin layers of dermis, performed until a viable bed is reached.

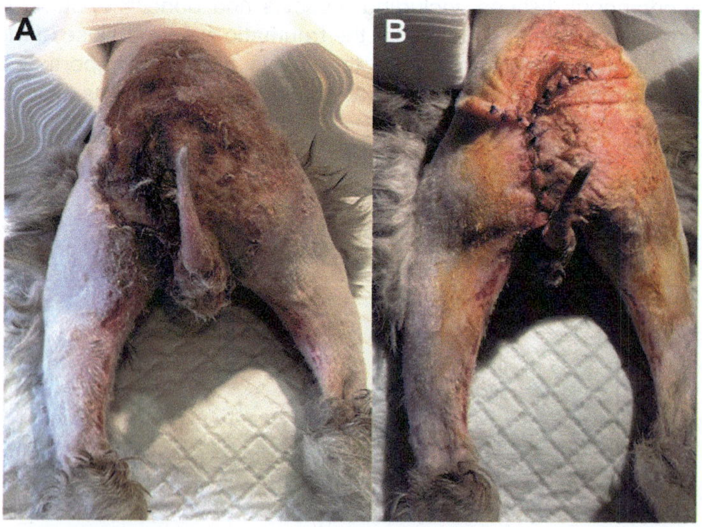

Fig. 6. (*A,B*) Surgical excision of a deep necrotic lesion following mechanical debridement in a rabbit. (Image Courtesy of Dr Paul Raymond.)

Wound healing

Wound healing may vary according to species. Small mammals are generally able to produce vitamin C, which has a key role in collagen synthesis, thus enhancing wound healing.[35] However, the guinea pig is an exception because it lacks L-gulonolactone oxidase, an enzyme required for vitamin C biosynthesis; therefore, dietary vitamin C supplementation is essential in this species. In mice, hair follicles are rich in progenitor cells, which facilitates rapid skin healing and keratinization.[36] Their skin also contains antimicrobial peptides called defensins.[37] In rats, the primary healing mechanism is wound contraction, while in humans it is reepithelialization.[31]

Surgical Complications

Grafts and flaps

Postoperative complications include prolonged inflammation, infection, dehiscence, hematoma, seroma formation, all of which result in failure to heal.[38] The size of the wound influences the risk and severity of complications. Avascular necrosis is a common complication of skin flaps. In case of partial skin flap necrosis, excision of necrotic areas is advised so the remainder of the flap may survive. Total flap necrosis is rare. Local edema is normal and may be observed if a flap is rotated over 90°. This may be observed a few days until venous drainage is restored and should not be misinterpreted for necrosis.

Revascularization of the graft is one of the most important factors in the process of engraftment. Bandage related complications are frequently observed with skin grafts.[27] Skin grafts are covered with bandages to prevent displacement of the graft and auto-mutilation during the process of revascularization. The bandage should be sufficiently but not excessively constrictive. Plastic strips band-aids have been successfully used for this purpose in rat model.[24]

Burn injury

Risks of wound infection and sepsis are reduced by performing early surgical excision, culture and antimicrobial therapy. Blood loss is a common surgical complication, mostly with tangential excision method. Coagulation screening should be performed before surgery and appropriate fluid therapy, whole blood, packed red blood cells, and/or fresh frozen plasma should be administered as indicated. Recurrent anesthesia and prolonged anesthetic time can lead to weight loss, poor body condition, and death, most importantly in ECMs. Wound dehiscence can occur secondary to infection, improper wound closure technique with excessive tension, self-trauma, hypoproteinemia, hypovolemia, or administration of drugs that interfere with healing.[16] Prolonged periods of ischemia, lack of an early angiogenic stimulus in the burn, decreased concentrations of fibroblasts in burn wound fluid, edema, and continued hyperemia are common complications.[30] Other complications include patient status and comorbidities. Obese patients and older patients present higher risks of diabetes, hypertension, cardiac disease, and pulmonary disease; altered pharmacokinetics and pharmacodynamics; but also altered immune responses.[39] These comorbidities may alter proper wound healing and lead to grave complications or even death of the patient.

New Postoperative Support Technologies in Cutaneous Surgery in Small Mammals

Background

Beyond the technical performance of the surgical intervention itself, optimization of the postoperative phase largely determines the final quality of cosmetic and functional outcome. Several contemporary technological modalities have established themselves as effective complementary tools to support the biological processes of wound healing and tissue integration following surgical intervention. The technologies described here represent scientifically validated adjuvants for improving cutaneous surgical outcomes in domestic small mammals.

Matrices and biomaterials: foundations for tissue reconstruction

When a surgical intervention creates significant skin defects or when tissue integrity must be restored quickly, the use of support matrices becomes a relevant strategy. Animal-derived organic matrices (VetBioSISt , Permacol) provide a 3-dimensional structural framework that allows cells to progressively colonize the surgical site.[40] These devices promote granulation tissue formation, limit undesirable scar contracture phenomena, and improve exudate absorption.[41–44] Their use also reduces dependence on conventional dressings, which often demonstrate biologically inferior performance.[42]

Negative pressure therapy: optimization of graft take and management of surgical wounds

Negative pressure technology modifies the local wound environment by creating a controlled microenvironment.[45,46] This system functions by generating controlled negative pressure that fulfills several functions: removal of excess fluid, reduction of interstitial edema, improvement of local vascularization, and direct mechanical stimulation of fibroblastic structures.[45–47]

In the specific context of surgical reconstructions, this technology proves particularly useful for increasing the success rates of grafts and flaps by decreasing complications related to seroma formation.[48–50] Experimental data from various animal models (mice, rat, and rabbit) reveal acceleration of neovascularization processes, more efficient restoration of essential vascular structures, and faster reorganization of extracellular architecture following intervention.[51–54]

The ability to space dressing changes at prolonged intervals also provides important practical advantages for postoperative management.[48]

Certain clinical situations nevertheless constitute contraindications: coagulation disorders, directly exposed tumors, uncontrolled deep infectious foci, as well as certain sensitive anatomic locations.[47,55]

Platelet-rich plasma: biological catalysts of wound healing

The use of platelet-rich plasma relies on the principle that platelets contain bioactive molecules involved in the early phases of the coagulation and tissue repair cascade patient.[56] When isolated and concentrated, these cells release a range of biochemical mediators capable of accelerating several critical stages of postsurgical regeneration: progressive epithelialization of the cutaneous surface, establishment of new capillary networks, and development of functional granulation tissue.[56,57]

Laser therapy: cellular modulation of wound healing

Laser therapy exploits the use of nonionizing light radiation to activate specific cellular metabolic processes. Selected wavelengths effectively penetrate tissue layers, interacting with intracellular elements involved in adenosine triphosphate production (ATP), cell signaling, and the activation of fibroblasts and keratinocytes.[58,59]

At the postoperative level, this approach results in modulation of inflammatory intensity, reinforcement of angiogenic processes, improved quality of scar tissue formation, and better organization of collagen fibrils.[40,58–60] Application protocols vary considerably in terms of power and frequency, with research suggesting the existence of a therapeutic window beyond which beneficial effects diminish or reverse.[61,62]

As a complement to surgical debridement or flap reconstruction, laser therapy amplifies tissue regeneration mechanisms, creating optimal therapeutic synergy. Its clinical efficacy, well-established in the treatment of pododermatitis and myiasis in rabbits (**Figs. 7** and **8**), results in accelerated wound healing and significant pain reduction.[40,63]

Essential precautions include protecting ocular structures and managing local thermal heating, which is particularly important in animals with heavily pigmented skin.[64]

Hyperbaric oxygenation therapy: metabolic and vascular optimization

The increase in partial pressure of dissolved oxygen in blood plasma constitutes the fundamental mechanism of this therapeutic modality.[65] Repeated exposure to a hyperoxic environment generates a cascade of biological adaptations, notably improved cellular energy availability, stimulation of vasoactive molecule synthesis, potentiation of antimicrobial activity of phagocytes, and acceleration of endothelial proliferation.[40,66]

In the postoperative context, these combined mechanisms produce objective acceleration of skin closure and improved perfusion of the scar tissue territory. Therapeutic protocols generally involve multiple weekly sessions of hyperbaric exposure, with each session exceeding 1 hour of exposure.[40,67–70]

Despite its demonstrated efficacy in several experimental models and clinical applications, widespread adoption of this technology remains limited by major economic considerations, particularly the acquisition and maintenance costs of necessary equipment.[40,67–70]

Electrical stimulation: electric fields to direct cellularity

The application of low-intensity microcurrents allows creation of an exogenous electrical gradient at the surgical site. This potential difference influences directional migration of various cell populations: anodes attract certain immune cell lineages

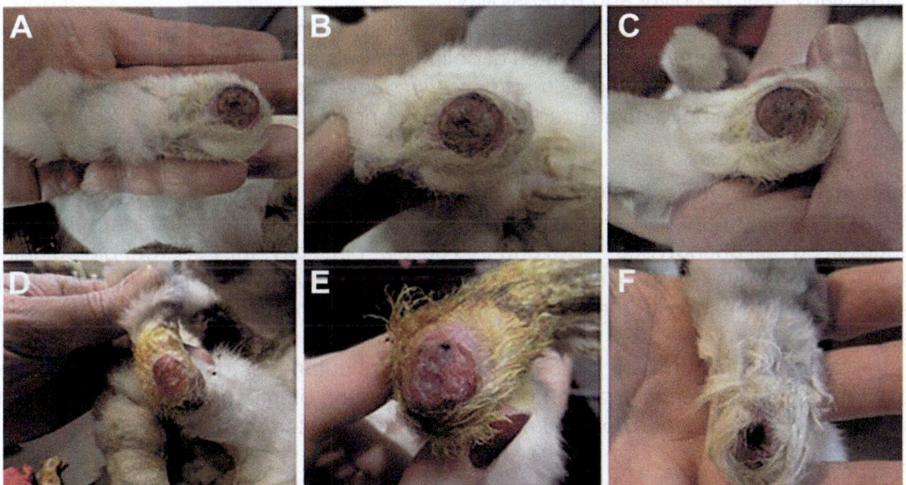

Fig. 7. (*A–F*) A 2-year-old female rabbit with a history of a nonsurgically managed and healed calcaneal fracture developed grade 3 pododermatitis on her foot. Laser therapy was initiated at 3 sessions per week, with settings of 50% intensity, 12,888 J, and 2.05 J/cm^2. (*A, B*) Clinical images of the foot at the initial consultation before starting laser therapy. (*C*) Day 2. (*D*) Day 6. (*E*) Day 19. (*F*) Two months after initiation. (Image Courtesy of Dr Lucas Flenghi.)

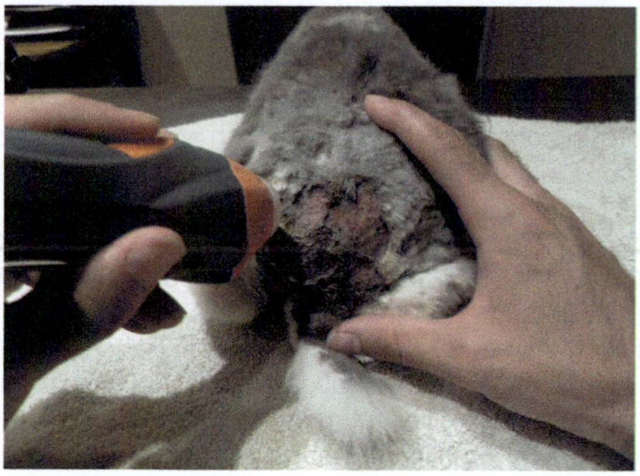

Fig. 8. Laser therapy for a myiasis wound in a rabbit. (Image Courtesy of Dr Lucas Flenghi.)

(phagocytes and polymorphonuclear leukocytes) while cathodes promote migration of extracellular matrix-producing cells (fibroblasts).[71]

When appropriately applied during the postoperative period, this technology potentiates structural protein deposition in scar tissue, improves the quality of vascular reconstructions, and increases the viability of skin grafts. Modalities can be continuous or administered in pulsed fashion according to the targeted therapeutic objectives.[72]

Therapeutic ultrasound: controlled mechanical and thermal effects

The localized application of low-power ultrasound simultaneously generates physical and biological phenomena: transmission of mechanical energy creating tissue micromovement and localized heat production slightly increasing tissue temperature. These 2 mechanisms work together to improve the mechanical properties of skin scars, particularly their flexibility and extensibility.[71,73,74]

At the histologic and functional level, this modality promotes improved vascularization of scar tissue, better organization of collagen fibrils, and acceleration of the matrix remodeling process following skin surgery.[75,76] Nevertheless, the risks of excessive heating or application to devitalized tissue require rigorous patient selection and treatment monitoring.[64,77]

Mesenchymal stroma cells: tissue regeneration through intrinsic cellularity

Mesenchymal stroma cells possess the intrinsic capacity to differentiate into multiple specialized cell phenotypes.[46] Beyond this cellular plasticity, they secrete biologically active molecules capable of modulating the inflammatory environment at the surgical site, regulating inappropriate immune responses, and reducing postoperative pain sensation.[78]

Implantation of such cells directly within surgical cutaneous defects produces acceleration of the reepithelialization process, diminution of inflammatory infiltrate, and increased collagen deposition, ultimately resulting in faster wound healing.[78]

Practical Considerations and Limitations

Applying these techniques requires careful adaptation to the specific needs of small mammals: equipment selection, dosage adjustment, frequency/duration, and greater vigilance for complications. Contraindications and pain management must be considered at each stage. While these innovations are generating great enthusiasm, it remains imperative to keep a critical mindset, temper expectations, and prioritize proven techniques according to the clinical context.

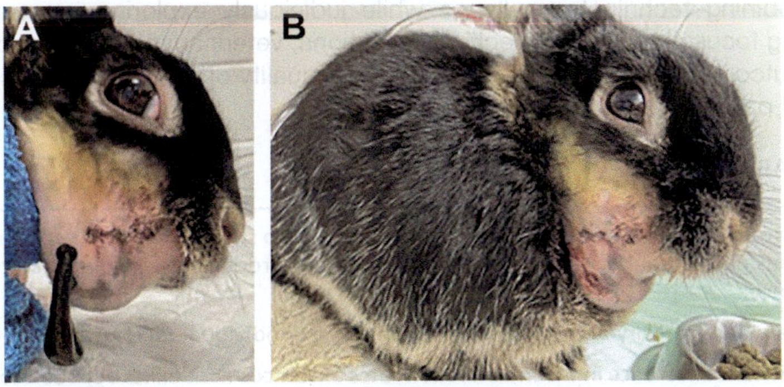

Fig. 9. (*A, B*) Hirudotherapy in a rabbit following postsurgical subcutaneous mandibular hematoma. (*A*) The medicinal leech (*Hirudo medicinalis*) is attached on the skin surface. (*B*) The submandibular hematoma is reduced after hirudotherapy. Edema and loose skin persist even after treatment. (Image Courtesy of Dr Paul Raymond.)

Several new technologies already successfully tested in dogs and cats have yet to see published clinical use in exotic companion mammals.

- Near-infrared fluorescence angiography with indocyanine green (NIRF-ICG): used to map flap vascularization and guide reconstructions in dogs and cats. To date, this technology has not been reported in exotic companion mammals for surgery or wound management.[79,80]
- Powered electroceutical dressings: these produce local microcurrents and have proven effective for chronic infected wounds in dogs and cats. Clinical use in exotic companion mammals isn't documented yet, though, as discussed conventional electrical stimulation has been studied in some laboratory species.[81]
- Maggot debridement therapy: well-established in dogs and cats, but no published equivalent yet in exotic companion mammals.[82]
- Hirudotherapy is employed in human and veterinary medicine to manage early postoperative venous congestion after skin flap surgery, reducing edema and improving microsurgical flap survival. In veterinary practice, it has been used in domestic carnivores, but its use has not been reported in ECMs[83] (**Fig. 9**).
- Complex composite auricular flaps: innovative techniques used for facial reconstruction in dogs, absent from the exotic companion animal literature.[84]

These techniques show strong potential to expand the therapeutic arsenal in exotic companion mammals, but clinical validation in these species is still pending, despite growing enthusiasm for reconstructive surgery and advanced wound management in this field.

SUMMARY

Skin surgery in exotic companion mammals requires a nuanced understanding of species–specific characteristics. The fragile epidermis and predisposition to some skin tumors, incidental injuries, or self-trauma, necessitate meticulous surgical approaches and rigorous postoperative monitoring.

Advances in reconstructive techniques have substantially expanded therapeutic possibilities. The emerging technologies presented offer promising potential for optimizing wound healing, although their clinical use remains largely anecdotal and requires robust validation.

By combining technical excellence while judiciously exploring innovations and maintaining focus on species-specific adaptations, veterinarians can provide optimal surgical outcomes and significantly enhance the quality of life for our exotic companion animal patients.

CLINICS CARE POINTS

- Skin anatomy presents important variations according to species: ferrets have numerous sebaceous glands; rabbit have abundant adipose tissue; rodents are predisposed to dehiscence.
- Skin characteristics vary according to species, age, sex, individual factors, and body region.
- No significant difference in wound infection rates or scar cosmesis exists between cold scalpel and electrocautery.
- Skin surgery is often indicated when a cutaneous mass, a trauma, a burn injury is diagnosed.
- Skin stretching, local flap, axial pattern flap, and free skin graft are reconstructive options to be used for wound management when a simple closure is not possible.
- Assisted-healing technologies and ultrahigh-performance next-generation biomaterials are the most recent treatment options for postsurgical wound managements in ECMs.

DISCLOSURE

The authors have nothing to disclose.

REFERENCES

1. d'Ovidio D, White S, Santoro D. Problem-oriented approach in exotic companion mammals. Vet Clin Exot Anim Pract 2023;26(2):309–26.
2. Sarvi J, Eshar D. Rodent dermatology. Vet Clin Exot Anim Pract 2023;26(2):383–408.
3. Van Zeeland Y. Rabbit oncology. Vet Clin Exot Anim Pract 2017;20(1):135–82.
4. Halck ML, Schoemaker NJ, Van Zeeland YRA. Ferret dermatology. Vet Clin Exot Anim Pract 2023;26(2):359–82.
5. Szabo Z, Bradley K, Cahalane AK. Rabbit soft tissue surgery. Vet Clin Exot Anim Pract 2016;19(1):159–88.
6. Paterson S. Structure and function of mammal skin. In: Skin diseases of exotic pets. Blackwell Science Ltd; 2006. p. 175–84.
7. Capello V. Common surgical procedures in pet rodents. J Exot Pet Med 2011;20(4):294–307.
8. Otrocka-Domagała I, Paździor-Czapula K, Fiedorowicz J, et al. Cutaneous and subcutaneous tumours of small pet mammals—retrospective study of 256 cases (2014–2021). Animals 2022;12(8):965.
9. Bertram CA, Bertram B, Bartel A, et al. Neoplasia and tumor-like lesions in pet rabbits (*oryctolagus Cuniculus*): a retrospective analysis of cases between 1995 and 2019. Vet Pathol 2021;58(5):901–11.
10. Von Bomhard W, Goldschmidt MH, Shofer FS, et al. Cutaneous neoplasms in pet rabbits: a retrospective study. Vet Pathol 2007;44(5):579–88.
11. Williams BH, Wyre NR. Neoplasia in ferrets. In: Ferrets, rabbits, and rodents. Elsevier; 2020. p. 92–108. https://doi.org/10.1016/B978-0-323-48435-0.00008-3.
12. Kim DJ, Mustoe T, Clark RA. Cutaneous wound healing in aging small mammals: a systematic review. Wound Repair Regen 2015;23(3):318–39.

13. Wu AY, Baldwin TJ, Patel BC, et al. Healing comparison of porcine cutaneous incisions made with cold steel scalpel, standard electrosurgical blade, and a novel tissue dissector. Med Res Innov 2017;1(5). https://doi.org/10.15761/MRI.1000124.
14. Aird LNF, Brown CJ. Systematic review and meta-analysis of electrocautery versus scalpel for surgical skin incisions. Am J Surg 2012;204(2):216–21.
15. Franchi M, Ghezzi F, Benedetti-Panici PL, et al. A multicentre collaborative study on the use of cold scalpel and electrocautery for midline abdominal incision. Am J Surg 2001;181(2):128–32.
16. Hedlund CS. Large trunk wounds. Vet Clin North Am Small Anim Pract 2006;36(4):847–72. https://doi.org/10.1016/j.cvsm.2006.02.003.
17. Timmenga EJF, Schoorl R, Bos JD, et al. An improved model for tissue expansion and flap research in the rabbit. Br J Plast Surg 1989;42(3):301–5.
18. Bostrom B, Wilson H, Radlinsky M. The use of an external skin-stretching device for wound management in a rabbit (oryctolagus cuniculus). J Exot Pet Med 2006;15(2):145–9.
19. Nógrádi AL, Csatári D, Cope I, et al. Use of skin flaps for reconstructive surgery in Guinea pigs (*Cavia porcellus*). Vet Rec 2022;191(11):e2183. https://doi.org/10.1002/vetr.2183.
20. Serin M, Bayramicli M. Experimental rat flap models. In: Amr S, editor. Issues in flap surgery. InTech; 2018. https://doi.org/10.5772/intechopen.69923.
21. De Souza JP, Rosito TE, Delcelo R, et al. Vaginal reconstruction with two lower abdominal skin flaps in rabbits: histological and macroscopic evaluation. Eur J Obstet Gynecol Reprod Biol 2012;160(2):179–84.
22. Donoff RB, Grillo HC. The effects of skin grafting on healing open wounds in rabbits. J Surg Res 1975;19(3):163–7.
23. Zhai Q, Zhou F, Ibrahim MM, et al. An immune-competent rat split thickness skin graft model: useful tools to develop new therapies to improve skin graft survival. Am J Transl Res 2018;10(6):1600–10.
24. Cheng CH, Lee CF, Fryer M, et al. Murine full-thickness skin transplantation. JoVE J 2017;(119):55105. https://doi.org/10.3791/55105.
25. Lewin ML, Peck SM. Pigment studies in skin grafts on experimental animals. J Invest Dermatol 1941;4:483–504.
26. Petrie K, Cox CT, Becker BC, et al. Clinical applications of acellular dermal matrices: a review. Scars, Burns & Healing 2022;8:20595131211038313. https://doi.org/10.1177/20595131211038313.
27. Naghi R, Maxwell EA, Carrillo AJ, et al. Acellular fish skin May be used to facilitate wound healing following wide surgical tumor excision in dogs: a prospective case series. JAVMA (J Am Vet Med Assoc) 2023;261(10):1547–54.
28. Amaro GM, Da Silva ADT, Tamarindo GH, et al. Differential effects of omega-3 PUFAS on tumor progression at early and advanced stages in TRAMP mice. Prostate 2022;82(16):1491–504.
29. Lv K, Wang L, He X, et al. Application of tilapia skin acellular dermal matrix to induce acute skin wound repair in rats. Front Bioeng Biotechnol 2022;9:792344. https://doi.org/10.3389/fbioe.2021.792344.
30. Garzotto C, Clarke D. Burn injury. In: Aronson LR, editor. Small animal surgical emergencies. 1st edition. Wiley; 2022. p. 586–99. https://doi.org/10.1002/9781119658634.ch53.
31. Abdullahi A, Amini-Nik S, Jeschke MG. Animal models in burn research. Cell Mol Life Sci 2014;71(17):3241–55.

32. Malic CC, Karoo ROS, Austin O, et al. Resuscitation burn card—A useful tool for burn injury assessment. Burns 2007;33(2):195–9.
33. Henriksson A, Kuo K, Gerken K, et al. Body mapping chart for estimation of percentage of body surface area in mesocephalic dogs. J Vet Emerg Crit Care 2022; 32(3):350–5.
34. Ismail Aly ME, Dannoun M, Jimenez CJ, et al. Operative wound management. In: Total burn care. Elsevier; 2018. p. 114–30.e2. https://doi.org/10.1016/B978-0-323-47661-4.00012-5.
35. Gad AAM, Sirko A. L-gulono-γ-lactone oxidase, the key enzyme for L-Ascorbic acid biosynthesis. CIMB 2024;46(10):11057–74.
36. Joost S, Annusver K, Jacob T, et al. The molecular anatomy of mouse skin during hair growth and rest. Cell Stem Cell 2020;26(3):441–57.e7.
37. Ganz T. Defensins: antimicrobial peptides of vertebrates. C R Biol 2004;327(6): 539–49.
38. Charlesworth T. The use of skin flaps in small animal reconstructive surgery. Companion Animal 2015;20(12):686–93.
39. Rowan MP, Cancio LC, Elster EA, et al. Burn wound healing and treatment: review and advancements. Crit Care 2015;19(1):243.
40. Sabater González M, Mayer J. Technological advances in wound treatment of exotic pets. Vet Clin Exot Anim Pract 2019;22(3):451–70.
41. MacLeod TM, Sarathchandra P, Williams G, et al. Evaluation of a porcine origin acellular dermal matrix and small intestinal submucosa as dermal replacements in preventing secondary skin graft contraction. Burns 2004;30(5):431–7.
42. Schallberger SP, Stanley BJ, Hauptman JG, et al. Effect of porcine small intestinal submucosa on acute full-thickness wounds in dogs. Vet Surg 2008;37(6):515–24.
43. Prevel CD, Eppley BL, Summerlin DJ, et al. Small intestinal submucosa: utilization as a wound dressing in full-thickness rodent wounds. Ann Plast Surg 1995;35(4): 381–8.
44. Kalin M, Kuru S, Kismet K, et al. The effectiveness of porcine dermal collagen (Permacol®) on wound healing in the rat model. Indian J Surg 2015;77(S2): 407–11.
45. Knapp-Hoch H, De Matos R. Clinical technique: negative pressure wound therapy-general principles and use in Avian species. J Exot Pet Med 2014; 23(1):56–66.
46. Buote NJ. Updates in wound management and dressings. Vet Clin Small Anim Pract 2022;52(2):289–315.
47. Howe LM. Current concepts in negative pressure wound therapy. Vet Clin Small Anim Pract 2015;45(3):565–84.
48. Stanley BJ. Negative pressure wound therapy. Vet Clin Small Anim Pract 2017; 47(6):1203–20.
49. Argenta LC, Morykwas MJ. Vacuum-assisted closure: a new method for wound control and treatment: clinical experience. Ann Plast Surg 1997;38(6):563–76 [discussion: 577].
50. Stanley BJ, Pitt KA, Weder CD, et al. Effects of negative pressure wound therapy on healing of free full-thickness skin grafts in dogs. Vet Surg 2013;42(5):511–22.
51. Wu M, Liu Q, Yu Z, et al. Negative-pressure wound therapy induces lymphangiogenesis in murine diabetic wound healing. Plast Reconstr Surg 2023;151(4): 779–90.
52. Chen SZ, Li J, Li XY, et al. Effects of vacuum-assisted closure on wound microcirculation: an experimental study. Asian J Surg 2005;28(3):211–7.

53. Rigotti G, Chirumbolo S, Cicala F, et al. Negative pressure from an internal spiral tissue expander generates new subcutaneous adipose tissue in an in vivo animal model. Aesthetic Surg J 2020;40(4):448–59.
54. Jacobs S, Simhaee DA, Marsano A, et al. Efficacy and mechanisms of vacuum-assisted closure (VAC) therapy in promoting wound healing: a rodent model. J Plast Reconstr Aesthetic Surg 2009;62(10):1331–8.
55. Bayer LR. Negative-pressure wound therapy. In: Orgill DP, editor. Interventional treatment of wounds. Springer International Publishing; 2018. p. 193–213. https://doi.org/10.1007/978-3-319-66990-8_12.
56. Abdullah BJ, Atasoy N, Omer AK. Evaluate the effects of platelet rich plasma (PRP) and zinc oxide ointment on skin wound healing. Ann Med Surg 2019; 37:30–7.
57. Sultana M, Akter M, Yesmin N, et al. Wound healing effects and antibacterial properties of heterologous platelet-rich plasma on Staphylococcus aureus induced septic wounds in rabbits. J Adv Vet Anim Res 2022;9(3):481.
58. Poyton RO, Ball KA. Therapeutic photobiomodulation: nitric oxide and a novel function of mitochondrial cytochrome c oxidase. Discov Med 2011;11(57):154–9.
59. Pryor B, Millis DL. Therapeutic laser in veterinary medicine. Vet Clin Small Anim Pract 2015;45(1):45–56.
60. Melo VAD, Anjos DCSD, Albuquerque Júnior R, et al. Effect of low level laser on sutured wound healing in rats. Acta Cir Bras 2011;26(2):129–34.
61. Al-Watban FAH, Zhang XY, Andres BL. Low-level laser therapy enhances wound healing in diabetic rats: a comparison of different lasers. Photomed Laser Surg 2007;25(2):72–7.
62. Mendez TMTV, Pinheiro ALB, Pacheco MTT, et al. Dose and wavelength of laser light have influence on the repair of cutaneous wounds. J Clin Laser Med Surg 2004;22(1):19–25.
63. Mayer J, Ness RD. Laser therapy for exotic small mammals. In: Riegel RJ, Godbold JC, editors. Laser therapy in veterinary medicine. 1st edition. Wiley; 2017. p. 285–97. https://doi.org/10.1002/9781119220190.ch26.
64. Thompson E. Debridement techniques and non–negative pressure wound therapy wound management. Vet Clin Small Anim Pract 2017;47(6):1181–202.
65. Bhutani S, Vishwanath G. Hyperbaric oxygen and wound healing. Indian J Plast Surg 2012;45(02):316–24.
66. Edwards ML. Hyperbaric oxygen therapy. Part 1: history and principles. J Vet Emerg Crit Care 2010;20(3):284–8.
67. Korn HN, Wheeler ES, Miller TA. Effect of hyperbaric oxygen on second-degree burn wound healing. Arch Surg 1977;112(6):732.
68. Bilic I, Petri NM, Bezic J, et al. Effects of hyperbaric oxygen therapy on experimental burn wound healing in rats: a randomized controlled study. Undersea Hyperb Med 2005;32(1):1–9.
69. Hatibie MJ, Islam AA, Hatta M, et al. Hyperbaric oxygen therapy for second-degree burn healing: an experimental study in rabbits. Adv Skin Wound Care 2019;32(3):1–4.
70. Sheikh AY, Rollins MD, Hopf HW, et al. Hyperoxia improves microvascular perfusion in a murine wound model. Wound Repair Regen 2005;13(3):303–8.
71. Bélanger A. Therapeutic electrophysical agents: evidence behind practice. 2nd edition. Wolters Kluwer Health/Lippincott Williams & Wilkins; 2010.
72. Kloth LC. Electrical stimulation for wound healing: a review of evidence from in vitro studies, animal experiments, and clinical trials. Int J Low Extrem Wounds 2005;4(1):23–44.

73. Paliwal S, Mitragotri S. Therapeutic opportunities in biological responses of ultrasound. Ultrasonics 2008;48(4):271–8.
74. Pavletic MM. Topical wound care products and their use. In: Atlas of small animal wound management and reconstructive surgery. 1st ed. Wiley; 2018. p. 53–94. https://doi.org/10.1002/9781119267539.
75. Meirer R, Brunner A, Deibl M, et al. Shock wave therapy reduces necrotic flap zones and induces VEGF expression in animal epigastric skin flap model. J Reconstr Microsurg 2007;23(4):231–6.
76. Da Costa Gonçalves A, Barbieri CH, Mazzer N, et al. Can therapeutic ultrasound influence the integration of skin grafts? Ultrasound Med Biol 2007;33(9):1406–12.
77. Davidson JR. Current concepts in wound management and wound healing products. Vet Clin Small Anim Pract 2015;45(3):537–64.
78. Pelizzo G, Avanzini MA, Icaro Cornaglia A, et al. Mesenchymal stromal cells for cutaneous wound healing in a rabbit model: pre-clinical study applicable in the pediatric surgical setting. J Transl Med 2015;13(1):219.
79. Eiger SN, Bertran J, Reynolds PS, et al. Use of near-infrared fluorescence angiography with indocyanine green to evaluate direct cutaneous arteries used for canine axial pattern flaps. Vet Surg 2024;53(6):1073–82.
80. Quinlan ASF, Wainberg SH, Phillips E, et al. The use of near infrared fluorescence imaging with indocyanine green for vascular visualization in caudal auricular flaps in two cats. Vet Surg 2021;50(3):677–86.
81. Heald R, Salyer S, Ham K, et al. Electroceutical treatment of infected chronic wounds in a dog and a cat. Vet Surg 2022;51(3):520–7.
82. Dawson KA, Mickelson MA, Blong AE, et al. Management of severe burn injuries with novel treatment techniques including maggot debridement and applications of acellular fish skin grafts and autologous skin cell suspension in a dog. JAVMA (J Am Vet Med Assoc) 2022;260(4):428–35.
83. Kermanian CS, Buote NJ, Bergman PJ. Medicinal leech therapy in veterinary medicine: a retrospective study. J Am Anim Hosp Assoc 2022;58(6):303–8.
84. Price JB, Wood CJ, Liptak JM. The pinna composite flap for wound reconstruction in a dog. Vet Surg 2021;50(8):1704–8.

Surgical Management of Ear Diseases in Rabbits

Emma Monge, DVM, DECZM (Small Mammals)[a,*],
Charly Pignon, DVM, DECZM (Small Mammals)[b]

KEYWORDS

• Rabbit • Otitis • Ear canal ablation • Bulla osteotomy

KEY POINTS

- Otitis externa and media are common in rabbits, especially lop-eared breeds, due to conformational canal stenosis and poor ventilation.
- Surgery is indicated when clinical signs of otitis externa are recurrent or refractory to medical therapy.
- In case of otitis media, by extension otitis interna if not yet present could occur rapidly, and therefore surgical approach to the tympanic bulla is mandatory.
- The most common postoperative complications are minor, typically consisting of wound dehiscence and delayed healing.
- Neurologic complications such as facial nerve paresis/paralysis, and less commonly vestibular dysfunction, can occur postoperatively but are usually transient.

INTRODUCTION

Ear disease is frequently encountered in pet rabbits, with otitis externa and otitis media representing the most clinically relevant entities. Because these disorders are often chronic at presentation, medical therapy alone seldom provides durable resolution. Surgical approaches tailored to lagomorph anatomy offer long-term control when the middle ear is involved or when signs recur despite appropriate medical management. Species-specific anatomic features must guide case selection and perioperative planning.

[a] Department of Zoological Medicine, Ecole Nationale Vétérinaire de Toulouse-INRAE, UMR IHAP VIRAL, France; [b] Exotics Medicine Service, Ecole Nationale Vétérinaire d'Alfort, Maisons-Alfort, France
* Corresponding author. Department of Zoological Medicine, Ecole Nationale Vétérinaire de Toulouse-INRAE, UMR IHAP VIRAL, 23 chemin des Capelles, 31300 Toulouse, France.
E-mail address: emma.monge@envt.fr

Vet Clin Exot Anim 29 (2026) 649–667
https://doi.org/10.1016/j.cvex.2026.04.012 **vetexotic.theclinics.com**

Abbreviations	
CT	computed tomography
LECAR	lateral ear canal resection
LECARBOM	lateral ear canal resection and bulla osteotomy with marsupialization
PECALBO	partial ear canal ablation and lateral bulla osteotomy
PECAWBO	partial ear canal ablation without bulla osteotomy
PMMA	polymethylmethacrylate
TECALBO	total ear canal ablation and lateral bulla osteotomy
VBO	ventral bulla osteotomy

EAR ANATOMY

The external ear of the rabbit includes large, thin, highly vascular pinnae that contributes to thermoregulation and sound reception.[1] Another proposed role is absorbing shock that might interfere with vision during high-speed locomotion.[2] The external canal is supported by annular, auricular, and scutiform cartilages (**Fig. 1**) and follows a J-shaped course toward the tympanic membrane; unlike dogs and cats, rabbits do not have distinct vertical and horizontal canal segments.[3] In lop-eared rabbits, a conformational gap and kink between the tragus and the annular cartilage narrow

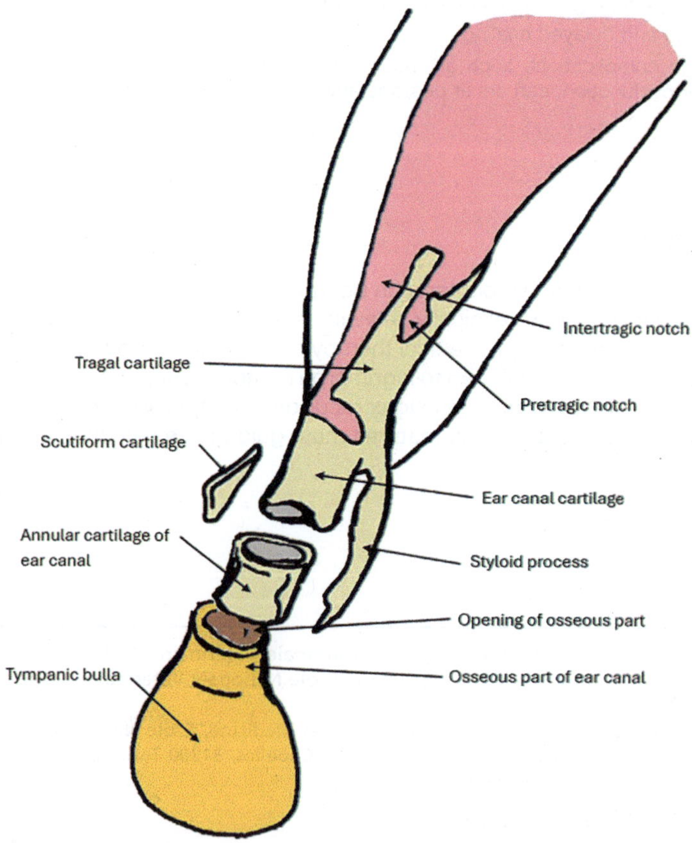

Fig. 1. Rabbit ear anatomy—cartilages of the ear. (Image Courtesy of Dr Emma Monge.)

the canal and impair ventilation and drainage, which promotes cerumen retention and recurrent otitis; erect-eared breeds are less predisposed because their canals do not have this stenosis and ventilate more effectively.[4,5] The tympanic bulla is relatively large, and the *pars tensa* lies immediately deep to the annular cartilage, which often requires sedation or general anesthesia for adequate visualization. The facial nerve courses close and lateroventrally to the bulla (**Figs. 2** and **3**), which explains why transient facial spastic paresis can complicate both disease and surgery.[1,3] The vestibular apparatus resides within the petrous temporal bone, so progression to the inner ear may produce a vestibular syndrome and nystagmus.

DIAGNOSTICS

Definitive diagnosis of rabbit ear disease cannot rely on clinical signs alone. A complete work-up begins with bilateral otoscopy, ideally using videoendoscopy (**Fig. 4**) to allow simultaneous inspection and therapeutic flushing of the canal, documentation, and guided myringotomy when indicated. Because the tympanic membrane

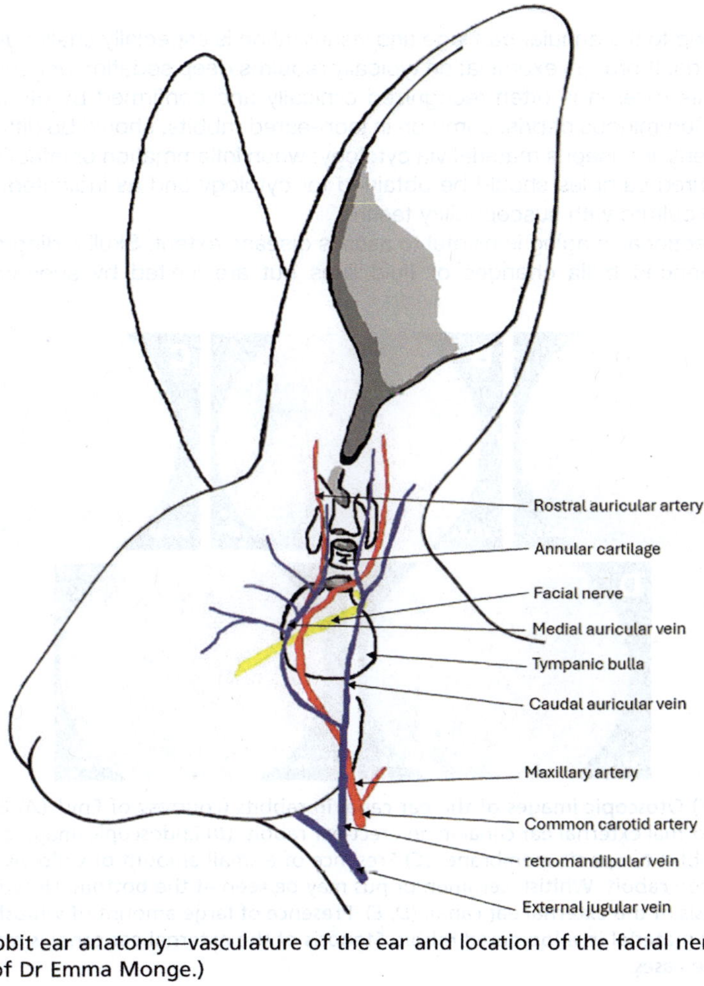

Fig. 2. Rabbit ear anatomy—vasculature of the ear and location of the facial nerve. (Image Courtesy of Dr Emma Monge.)

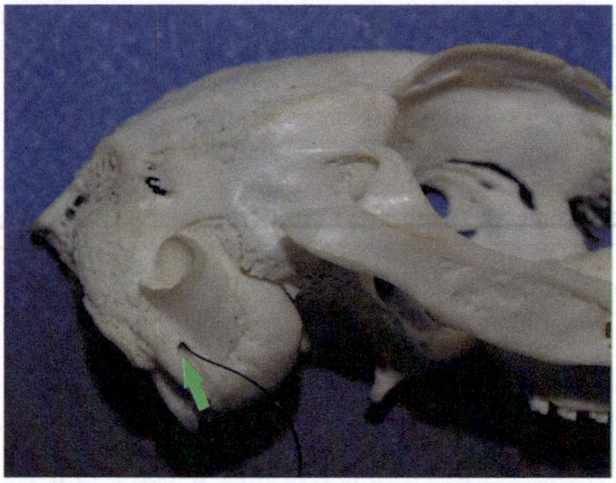

Fig. 3. Photograph of a rabbit skull showing the stylomastoid foramen (*green arrow*) and the course of the facial nerve indicated by a black thread. (Image Courtesy of Dr José Rosas-Navarro.)

lies just deep to the annular cartilage and visualization is especially challenging in lop-eared breeds, thorough examination typically requires deep sedation or general anesthesia. Otitis externa is often recognized clinically and confirmed by otoscopy and cytology. Ceruminous debris, common in loop-eared rabbits, should be differentiated from purulent or caseous material via cytology; when inflammation or infection is suspected, paired samples should be obtained for cytology and as indicated, bacterial and fungal culture with susceptibility testing.

Cross-sectional imaging is pivotal to assess disease extent. Skull radiographs may reveal advanced bulla changes or fluid lines but are limited by superimposition.

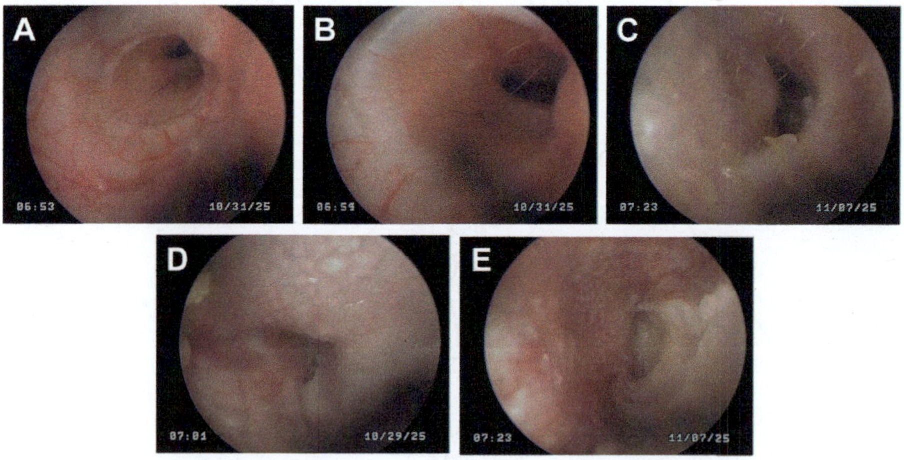

Fig. 4. (*A–E*) Otoscopic images of the ear canal in rabbits (courtesy of EnvT (*A*) Endoscopic view of a normal external ear canal in an erect-ear rabbit. (*B*) Endoscopic image of a normal erect-ear rabbit tympanic membrane. (*C*) Presence of a small amount of yellowish cerumen in a lop-eared rabbit. Whitish cerumen or pus may be seen at the bottom. Noted the moderate stenosis of the external ear canal. (*D, E*). Presence of large amount of whitish cerumen or purulent material in a lop-eared rabbit. Stenosis of the external ear canal is more important is these cases.

Computed tomography (CT) is the modality of choice for evaluating the tympanic bullae (**Fig. 5**) and detecting middle/inner ear involvement, and in many rabbits can be performed conscious or under light sedation with diagnostic image quality.[6] CT assists in surgical planning, prognostication, and triage by identifying external canal occlusion, tympanic membrane deviation/rupture, bulla filling, wall thickening, osteitis/lysis, and periauricular changes; intravenous contrast can further delineate mucosal enhancement, soft-tissue swellings, and abscessation. A CT-based grading system provides reproducible, 4 tier (I–IV) classifications for both otitis media and external canal material load, facilitating standardized nomenclature, communication, and outcome studies; severe (grade IV) otitis media commonly correlates with heavy external canal material.[7] CT is also useful to screen for underlying dental or upper respiratory disease. Otitis media is frequently subclinical.[6]

Middle-ear sampling via myringotomy or bulla osteotomy guides targeted antimicrobial therapy, which is important because antibiotic penetration into the bulla is poor.

Otitis interna is usually diagnosed in rabbits with peripheral vestibular signs after exclusion of relevant differentials such as *Encephalitozoon cuniculi* or *Toxoplasma gondii*.[8]

SURGERY OF THE PINNA

Otectomy

Indications

Rabbits' ears can be seriously injured during a fight between mates, followed by bites and other trauma. Lacerations of the ear are possible following an ear stuck in the cage of the animal. If the cartilage is severely affected or if the loss of skin is too great, an otectomy has to be considered. Some cases of serious frostbite have also been reported in animals living outside. In this case, the purpose of the otectomy is to prevent any spread of necrosis. The other indications of otectomy are neoplasia (melanoma for example), necrosis of the pinna (after IV catheterization or complication of surgical procedure with vascular injuries).

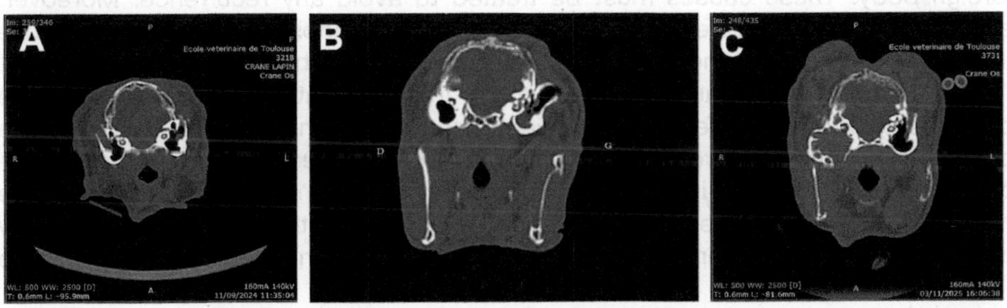

Fig. 5. (*A–C*) CT image of otitis externa and otitis media in rabbits (*A*). Transverse CT images at the level of the tympanic bulla in a lop-eared rabbit with bilateral otitis externa. Both external ear canals are expanded with a soft tissue–attenuating material and ectasia of the base of the right external ear canal are noted. (*B*) Transverse CT images at the level of the tympanic bulla in an erect-ear rabbit presented for chronic rhinitis. The left tympanic bulla is filled with soft tissue–attenuating material, but the normal structure of the bulla is maintained. (*C*) Transverse CT images at the level of the tympanic bulla in a lop-eared rabbit with bilateral otitis externa and right otitis media. The right external ear canal is replaced by a large soft tissue–attenuating mass that expands from the left middle ear, causing local disruption and lysis of the right tympanic bulla. (Image Courtesy of EnvT.)

Surgical technique

To perform an otectomy, also called pinnectomy (**Fig. 6**), the animal is anesthetized, then the ear is totally shaved.[9] The cutaneous incision is previously marked with a marker to ensure a harmonious contour of the ear. The ear is surgically prepared. The vascularization of the ear can be visualized using a transilluminator. It is possible to mark the ear vessels with a marker to minimize the risk of accidental injury; however, some of these vessels will inevitably need to be transected during the procedure. To prevent bleeding, ligations of the most important vessels are performed using a monofilament absorbable suture material. The skin is incised on each side following the predefined line. The cutaneous bleeding is stopped by pressure gauze soaked with a few drops of epinephrine. The skin is dissected 5 mm to the base of the ear to separate it from the cartilage. The cartilage is cut 5 mm back from the skin using scissors. The skin is then sutured using an interrupted pattern with a monofilament absorbable suture material.

Postoperative care

A bandage is made to protect the sutures. Gauze sponges are rolled on themselves and placed inside the ear. The ear is "wrapped" around the gauzes. The entire ear is then wrapped in gauze bandage material and fixed with tape. The animal is discharged with an analgesic (meloxicam). A wound check and a bandage change are performed on days 7 and 14. The stitches are removed on day 14.

Complications

The wound can dehisce if the cartilage has not been shortened enough from the skin. In this case, the cartilage puts too much pressure on the surgical wound which prevents good healing.

Ear Hematoma

Etiology

The othematoma or ear hematoma seems infrequent in the rabbit.[10] The cause is most often due to self-injury when the animal scratches or shakes his ears. The underlying causes may be an inflammatory process, a parasitic infection, or the presence of a foreign body. These causes must be treated to avoid any recurrence. Moreover, ear's anatomy in lop-eared rabbit (longer and more mobile ears) may predispose them to ear hematoma. The hematoma usually appears on the inner surface of the ear.

The branches of the caudal auricular artery that penetrate inside the cartilage are often the source of the bleeding. Bleeding continues as long as there is no pressure balance between blood pressure and pressure within the hematoma. This painful process causes an increase in pruritus and discomfort, causing the rabbit to shake the head and traumatize the ear further, thereby exacerbating the hematoma. Eventually the pressure within the hematoma may increase and stop the bleeding. In this mature

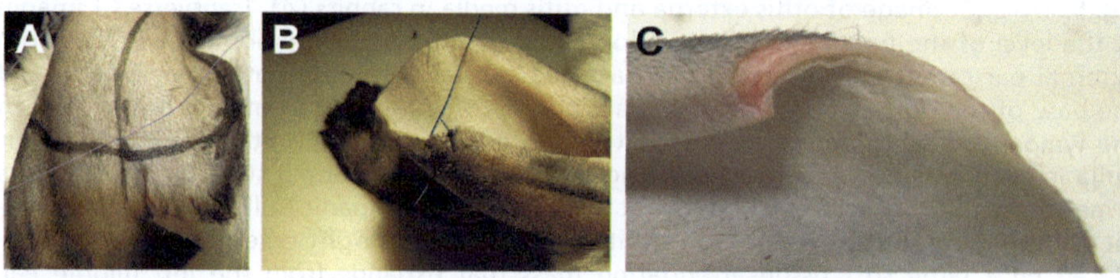

Fig. 6. (*A–C*) Partial pinnectomy in a rabbit. (Image Courtesy of EnvA.)

hematoma, fibrin is lysed leading forming a serohemorrhagic fluid. If the othematoma is not treated, it can lead to thickening and significant deformation of the ear.

Surgical technique

On an anesthetized animal, the ears are shaved and then surgically prepared. The skin on the side of the hematoma is incised along its entire length. Serohemorrhagic fluid and fibrin are removed. The inside of the wound is rinsed with warm saline fluid. If needed, a flap of skin is excised along the incision so that the edges can properly face each other when they are affixed to the cartilage. Single points crossing the ear through the cartilage are made using a 2-0 diameter nonresorbable monofilament sutures (**Fig. 7**). The stitches are made parallel to the major axis of the ear over the entire area that has been separated from the cartilage. The incised skin is left open in order to drain any new collections.

Postoperative care

A bandage similar to that used during the otectomy is made. The bandage is changed daily until there is no more serohemorrhagic fluid production and then the bandage is changed every 3 days. The bandage and the stitches are removed 14 days after the surgery.

Complications

Injury to the auricular vessels may occur during suture placement. If the underlying cause of the othematoma has not been treated or if the number of stitches is not enough to be able to flatten the skin on the cartilage, then, the othematoma may recur.

SURGERY OF THE EXTERNAL EAR CANAL

Lateral Ear Canal Resection or Lateral Ear Canal Ablation

Indications

Lateral ear canal resection (LECAR)/lateral ear canal ablation is indicated for otitis externa refractory to medical therapy, especially when the canal is filled with soft tissue/cerumen or purulent material that is difficult to clear. It is particularly relevant in lop-eared rabbits with conformational stenosis and poor ventilation/drainage, and in cases of ectasia of the base of the external ear canal (in lop-eared rabbits), para auricular empyema, obstructive external canal masses (eg, benign or malignant neoplasia) confined to the external ear. Case selection should integrate otoscopy/videoendoscopy, cytology $\pm$ culture, and CT to confirm that disease is limited to the external

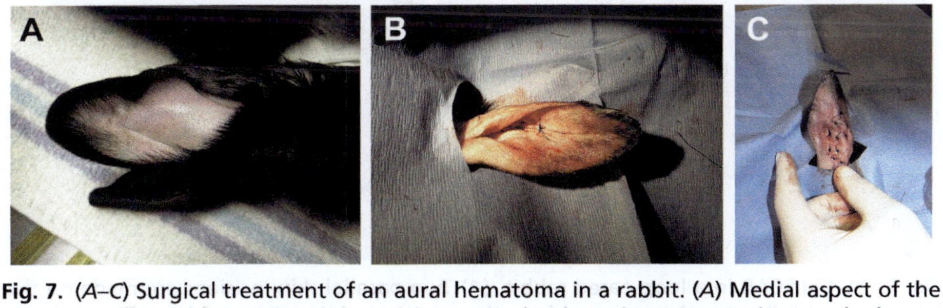

Fig. 7. (*A–C*) Surgical treatment of an aural hematoma in a rabbit. (*A*) Medial aspect of the pinna revealing the aural hematoma. (*B*) A vertical S-shaped incision made over the hematoma to allow drainage and removal of blood clots and fibrinous material and full-thickness mattress sutures are placed parallel to the incision. The incision is left open to allow continued drainage. (*C*) Appearance of the lateral aspect of the pinna after placement of the mattress sutures. (Image Courtesy of EnvA.)

canal and to exclude or document middle-ear involvement that would alter the surgical plan.

Surgical technique

Under general anesthesia, and after the rabbits is positioned in lateral recumbency, the side of the face and both sides of the pinna are clipped and prepared with povidone-iodine (temporary blepharorrhaphy to protect the cornea). Two parallel skin incisions are made on the lateral aspect following the ear canal from the proximal of the pinna to the ear base. Care is taken not to damage the blood vessels that supply the pinna. Bipolar electrosurgery could be used to control bleeding. A cotton tip swab is inserted into the ear canal down to the junction of the ear canal cartilage and annular cartilage. The swab is tilted laterally to create a slight protuberance in the skin, which serves as a reference point to localize the annular cartilage. A mark is made over the protuberance, and an incision is made 1.0 to 1.5 cm ventral to the mark to join the lateral parallel skin incisions. The subcutaneous tissues are dissected from the auricular cartilage, and the skin flap is excised. The tragal and ear canal cartilages are exposed using Stevens scissors for dissection. Straight blunt Mayo scissors are used to create 2 parallel cuts in the lateral wall of the tragal and ear canal cartilages. The cartilage flap is transected ventrally at the opening of the annular cartilage and excised. Care is taken to separate the ear canal epithelial lining from the tragal and ear canal cartilages along the cut edge of the ear canal so that it can be reattached to the skin without tension on the wound. The skin and the subcutaneous tissue are sutured with a monofilament absorbable suture material at the edge of the annular cartilage marking the opening of the equivalent of the horizontal canal.[11–13]

The remaining ear canal is then cleaned and rinsed with warm saline to eliminate purulent debris. The free edge of the vertical portion of the ear remaining canal is sutured to the skin using single interrupted pattern with the same suture as previously (**Fig. 8**). During this step, it is important to check that the remaining part of the scutiform cartilage does not exert too much tension on the sutures. If necessary, it is dissected, and a thin flap is removed. At the end of the surgery, the base of the ear canal (the curved part of the J) is in direct communication with the external environment, reducing the accumulation of debris and thus allowing easier cleaning.

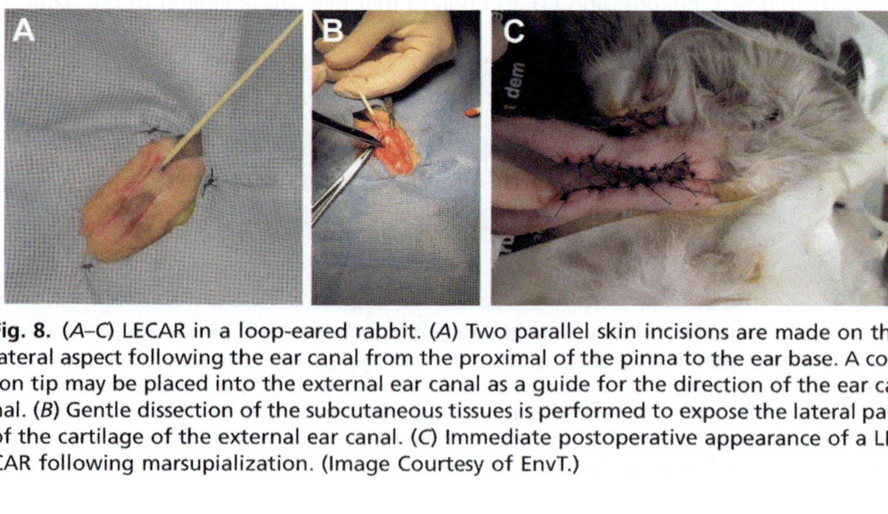

Fig. 8. (*A–C*) LECAR in a loop-eared rabbit. (*A*) Two parallel skin incisions are made on the lateral aspect following the ear canal from the proximal of the pinna to the ear base. A cotton tip may be placed into the external ear canal as a guide for the direction of the ear canal. (*B*) Gentle dissection of the subcutaneous tissues is performed to expose the lateral part of the cartilage of the external ear canal. (*C*) Immediate postoperative appearance of a LECAR following marsupialization. (Image Courtesy of EnvT.)

Postoperative care

Postoperative care consists of analgesia, systemic, and local antibiotic therapy. The remaining part of the ear canal is rinsed with saline using a fine syringe to remove the crusts and the remaining pus.

The animal needs to be seen in consultation 1 week after surgery to check the healing of the surgical wound and to remove, after moistening with warm saline, the accumulation of crusts around the sutures. The sutures can be removed 2 weeks after the surgery (**Fig. 9**).

Complications

The wound facing the cartilage can dehisce if it has not been cut short enough and exerts too much pressure on the sutures (**Fig. 10**). There is a risk of bleeding if the rostral or caudal auricular veins are punctured. If pressure hemostasis is not possible, ligation of these vessels may result in necrosis of the ear pinna. Therefore pressure or the use of hemostatic sponges is preferred. In a recent multicase series of 25 rabbits treated with lateral ear canal resection, 7 of 25 developed postoperative complications.[13] Reported issues included wound swelling/erythema, profuse mucopurulent discharge with whitish fibrinous deposits, and severe crust formation with localized wound infection confirmed cytologically in one case; suture dehiscence occurred in 3 of 25. One rabbit had prolonged nonhealing at day 131 due to multidrug-resistant *Staphylococcus aureus* surgical-site infection requiring extended non-steroidal anti-inflammatory drugs (NSAIDs)/antiseptics/antibiotics. Eighteen of 25 showed no recurrent otic signs during follow-up and owners reported improved activity/quality of life; 2 of 25 developed late recurrence (at 543 and 762 days) managed medically.[13]

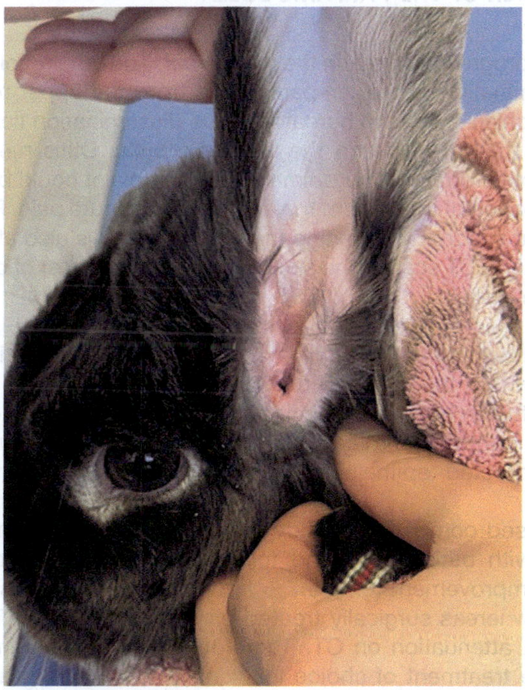

Fig. 9. Aspect of LECAR surgery in a lop-eared rabbit after complete healing. (Image Courtesy of EnvT.)

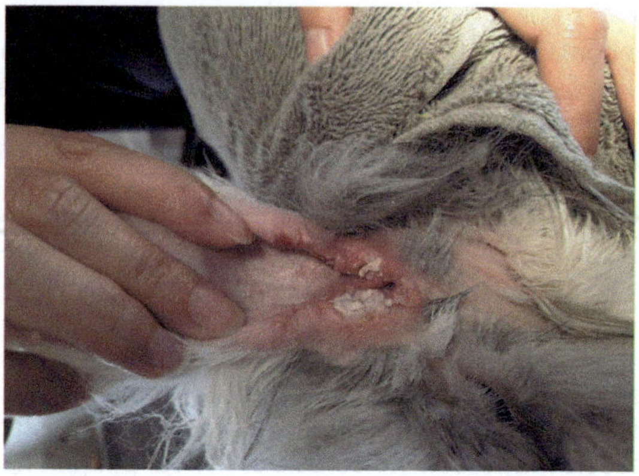

Fig. 10. Postoperative complication of wound dehiscence after a LECAR procedure in a lop-eared rabbit. (Image Courtesy of EnvT.)

Most LECAR complications are localized, wound related, and medically manageable, but clinicians should counsel owners about the possibility of delayed healing, dehiscence, resistant-organism infection, and late recurrence, and schedule close early rechecks to debride crusts, maintain canal patency, and adjust antimicrobials based on culture.

SURGICAL APPROACH OF THE TYMPANIC BULLA

Indications

Otitis externa can progress and reach the middle ear. The other etiology for middle ear infection is contamination of the tympanic bulla from the upper respiratory system through the Eustachian tube, and hematogenous dissemination (less probable). This infection includes the eardrum and the tympanic bulla. Otitis media is considered very painful for rabbits like for other animals. The complaint could be only depression and anorexia. Palpation of the base of the ear may elicit acute pain. Rabbits could present with vestibular syndrome (meaning that the inner ear is also affected) but that is not always the case. A CT scan of the skull is the diagnostic test of choice to allow the visualization of the bulla.[6]

While medical therapy (including systemic antibiotics and anti-inflammatory drugs) may offer transient clinical improvement, it is rarely curative once infection has established within the middle ear. The caseous nature of exudate and the poor vascular perfusion of the bulla limit antibiotic penetration and clearance of infectious debris. In contrast, surgical management enables direct removal of inspissated pus and infected epithelium, thereby restoring aeration and preventing recurrence.

A recent CT-based comparative study quantified these differences objectively.[14] Among 46 ears with otitis media and follow-up imaging, medically treated ears showed minimal improvement (only 5.7% improved, 17.1% worsened, and 77.1% remained static), whereas surgically treated ears improved in 54.5% of cases, with resolution of bulla attenuation on CT. Therefore, early surgical intervention should be considered the treatment of choice for confirmed otitis media in rabbits, especially when CT reveals bulla involvement or chronic changes refractory to medical therapy.

Lateral Ear Canal Resection and Bulla Osteotomy with Marsupialization

Surgical technique

The first steps of this surgery are the same as the ones described previously for the LECAR.[12] After the tragal and ear canal cartilages flap are transected and excised, a plastic Lone Star Retractor is placed to expose the annular cartilage. The annular cartilage is bluntly freed from the surrounding tissue and excised using Stevens scissors, exposing the osseous part of the ear canal. Micro-Friedman rongeurs are used to remove the lateral aspect of the acoustic meatus and enlarge the tympanic bulla opening. Care must be taken during this step to avoid damaging the facial nerve which is medioventrally positioned to the bulla. If there is bone lysis or tympanic wall thickening (grades III and IV) based on 3D images of the CT scan, the affected fragments are resected using micro-Friedman rongeurs. The tympanic cavity is curetted (Volkmann curette, single-ended oval 3 mm scoop, 18 cm) to remove debris, pus, and epithelial lining, which are submitted for bacterial culture and antibiotic susceptibility. Care is taken to avoid aggressive curettage dorsomedially where the vestibular or oval window of the inner ear is located. The tympanic cavity is then gently flushed with warm sterile saline. The bulla can be inspected with a 1.9 or 2.7 mm diameter rigid endoscope to ensure remaining debris and pus are removed. The epithelial layer of the exposed ear canal is sutured to the skin overlying the pinna. Subcutaneous tissue around the bulla osteotomy opening is marsupialized to the surrounding skin using monofilament absorbable suture material n a simple interrupted pattern (**Fig. 11**). The skin wound around the tympanic bulla opening heals by 2 to 3 weeks (**Fig. 12**). Fibrous tissue from the surrounding scar begins lining the tympanic bulla and eventually covers the opening (**Fig. 13**).

Postoperative care

Pain treatment must be continued and reevaluated daily until the animal eats by himself. The continuous infusion of fentanyl, lidocaine, and ketamine is gradually decreased over 1 to 2 days, and if the animal is comfortable, can be replaced with buprenorphine. Meloxicam is added to the regimen. While awaiting culture and sensitivity results, empirical antibiotic therapy could be initiated with oral azithromycin. Second-line options, such as marbofloxacin or enrofloxacin, could be considered based on the antibiogram.

The surgical wound is gently flushed with saline one to twice daily. Hospitalization time after surgery ranged from 2 to 15 days, with a median time of 3 days.[12]

The rabbit is discharged, with pain medications, antibiotics, and surgical wound flush, only when he is able to eat by himself and he is comfortable. Weekly rechecks are made to monitor the surgical wound healing.

Complications

Multiple complications are described after this type of surgery. It is important to take the time to discuss them with the owner.

The risks related to this surgery are a lesion of the facial nerve, leading to a facial hemiparalysis or hemiparesis, a lesion of the vestibular apparatus during the curettage of the tympanic bulla leading to a vestibular syndrome and hemorrhage by damaging and ligation of the rostral veins or auricular arteries leading to small necrosis of the ear with a partial dehiscence of the wound. Partial dehiscence typically occurred within 7 days with a 2 to 4 mm margin of necrosis noted along the incision extending less than 1 cm on the pinna. In these cases, necrotic tissue should be debrided and healing by secondary intention is usually completed by 21 days. If a

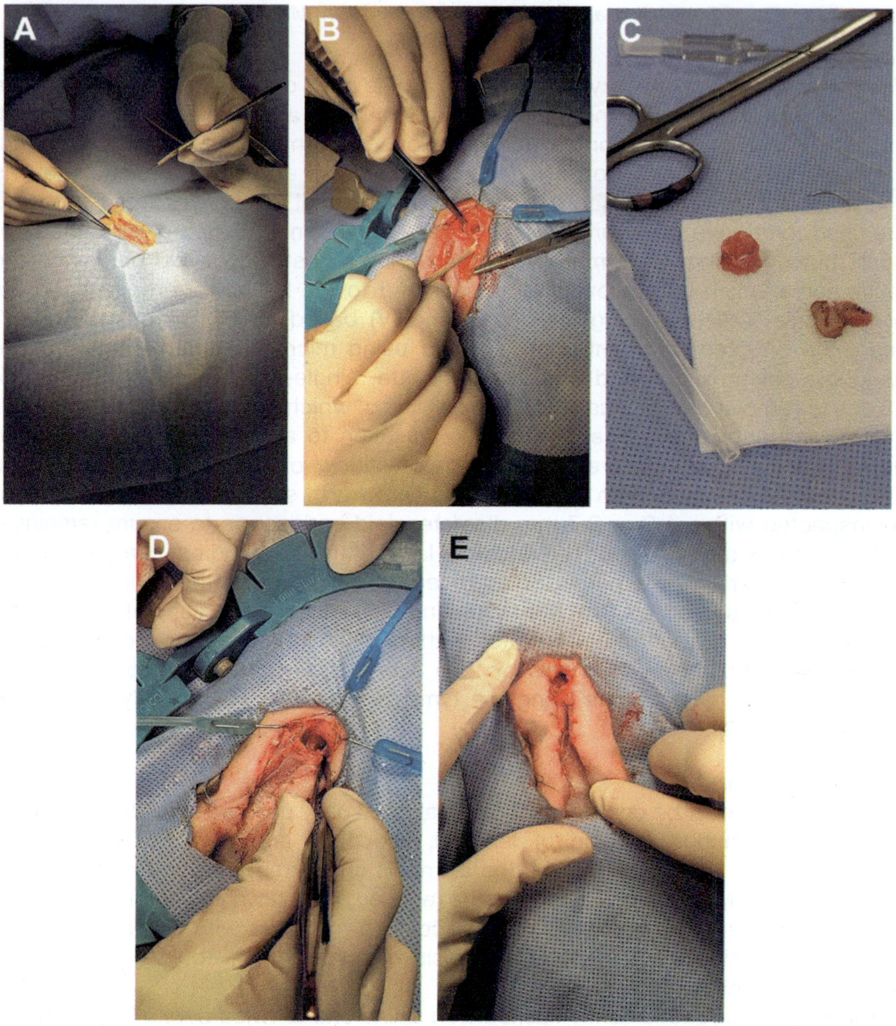

Fig. 11. (*A–E*) LECARBOM in a rabbit. (*A*) Two parallel skin incisions are made on the lateral aspect following the ear canal from the proximal of the pinna to the ear base. A cotton tip may be placed into the external ear canal as a guide for the direction of the ear canal. (*B*) After resection of the lateral part of the auricular cartilage (as in LECAR procedure) and placement of a Lone Star Retractor, the annular cartilage is gently dissected to be completely exposed. (*C*) Complete removal of the annular cartilage. (*D*) Visualization of the opening of the osseous part of ear canal. (*E*) Immediate postoperative appearance of a LECARBOM following marsupialization. (Image Courtesy of EnvT.)

head tilt is already present, there is also a risk that the head tilt does not fully improve or does not improve at all. In a retrospective study, on 44 ears, complications were found in 12 ears (7 wound dehiscence/necrosis, 1 head tilt, 2 transient facial nerve paralysis, 2 para-auricular abscesses).[12] Overall, the rate of complication is lower than in dogs undergoing a total ear canal ablation and lateral bulla osteotomy (TECALBO).[15]

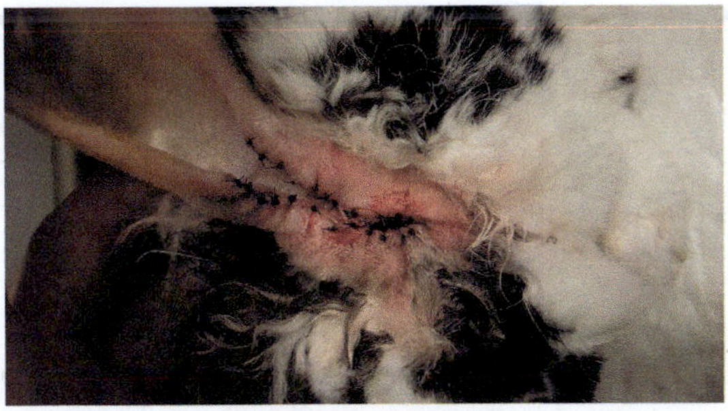

Fig. 12. LECARBOM in a rabbit. Immediate postoperative aspect. (Image Courtesy of EnvT.)

Partial Ear Canal Ablation and Lateral Bulla Osteotomy

Surgical technique

This technique involves a single vertical skin incision over the base of the ear canal. The canal is circumferentially dissected, and the distal vertical portion is transected approximately 1 to 2 cm ventral to the external meatus, preserving the distal healthy section. Dissection continues to the bony acoustic meatus, where a lateral bulla osteotomy is performed using rongeurs and curettes to remove caseous debris and the secretory epithelial lining of the bulla. The cavity is gently lavaged with warm saline and suctioned. From this point, 2 surgical options may be considered with primary closure or marsupialization of surgical site. In the first option, the tissues overlying the bulla are closed with absorbable sutures, the mucosa of the distal canal incision is apposed, and a single horizontal mattress suture is placed across the cut cartilage to close the vertical canal. Subcutaneous tissues and skin are closed in simple interrupted or subcuticular patterns (**Fig. 14**). Unlike marsupialized approaches, the surgical site is completely closed, which improves cosmetic outcomes but requires meticulous removal of all infected and epithelial tissue to prevent recurrence.[16,17] Some surgeon may choose the marsupialization option to allow monitoring for potential recurrence through periodic rechecks, with delayed wound closure performed at a later stage.

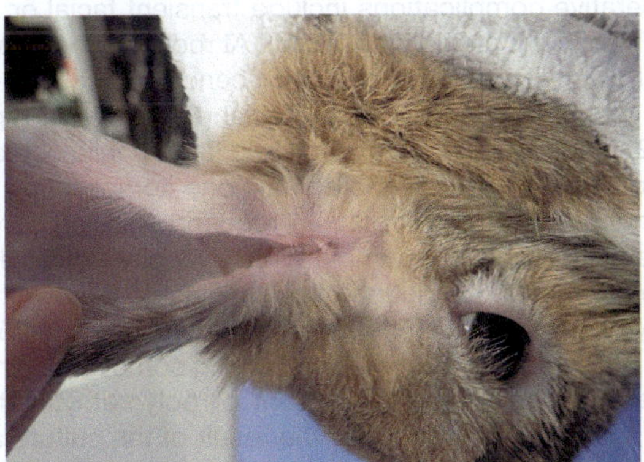

Fig. 13. LECARBOM in a rabbit. Aspect after a complete healing. (Image Courtesy of EnvT.)

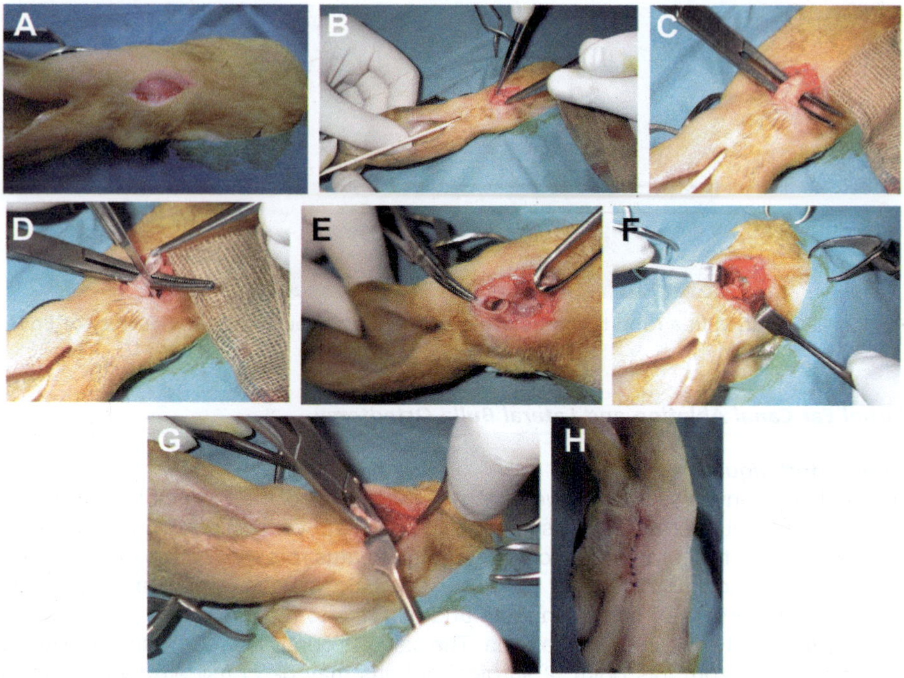

Fig. 14. (*A–H*) Illustration showing all steps of the PECALBO surgery in a rabbit. (*A*) Cutaneous incision over the base of the ear canal. (*B*) Gentle dissection of the subcutaneous tissues to exposed the lateral part of the cartilage of the external ear canal. (*C, D*) The external ear canal is circumferentially dissected, and the distal vertical portion is transected approximately. (*E, F*) Dissection continue to the bony acoustic meatus. (*G*) Lateral bulla osteotomy with rongeur. (*H*) Immediate postoperative appearance of PECALBO after primary closure. (Image Courtesy of Dr José Rosas-Navarro.)

Postoperative care

The rabbit is discharged, with pain medications and antibiotics. As the skin is closed, no daily flushing is performed.

Complications

Immediate postoperative complications include transient facial or palpebral paresis, corneal ulceration, vestibular ataxia, or head tilt. At recheck (median 36 days), complications such as surgical site infection and dehiscence (typically 16–21 days postop), ear base abscess recurrence, and vestibulofacial deficits were reported. In a retrospective study of 27 partial ear canal ablation and lateral bulla osteotomy (PECALBO) procedures, 65% of rabbits experienced at least one complication (most of them minor and self-limiting).[17] Three rabbits (15%) required revision surgery for recurrent abscessation or fistulation due to incomplete removal of epithelial lining. Twelve rabbits (60%) achieved complete resolution of clinical signs, 3 (15%) had minor residual signs (eg, facial asymmetry without functional impairment), and 5 (25%) died of causes possibly related to otitis or surgery. The risk of having some remaining infected tissues is high. Some authors recommend placement of polymethylmethacrylate (PMMA) beads mixed with antibiotics but because the result of the culture and the sensitivity is taking days to be released after the surgery, there is a possibility that bacteria could be resistant to the selected antibiotic.[18]

Total Ear Canal Ablation and Lateral Bulla Osteotomy

Some authors described a total ear canal ablation technique in addition to the lateral bulla osteotomy similar to what was described in dogs and cats.[18–20]

A T-shaped skin incision is made with the horizontal component parallel and ventral to the dorsal edge of the tragus. A vertical incision is made from the midpoint of the horizontal incision extending ventral to the right tympanic bulla. The horizontal incision is extended circumferentially around the opening of the external ear canal. Loose connective tissue is bluntly dissected until the lateral aspect of the vertical canal was exposed. The cartilage of the acoustic meatus and the scutiform cartilage are dissected from surrounding tissues. The canal attachment to the bony acoustic duct is excised, and the entire external ear canal with cartilage plates is removed. Soft tissues are bluntly dissected and elevated from the tympanic bulla. Lempert rongeurs are used to remove the lateral aspect of the bony acoustic duct and to perform an osteotomy at the lateral aspect of the bulla. Cotton-tipped applicators and a curette are used to remove the caseous debris and epithelial lining within the bulla. The subcutaneous and subcuticular layers are closed with monofilament absorbable suture material in a simple continuous pattern.

This technique is more invasive than the previous ones, which leads to the risk of more trauma to the surrounding tissues such as blood vessels and nerves. It also increases the difficulty of managing pain medically. In non-lop breeds, the total ablation of the ear canal could also induce a bending ear after the surgery. Another main difference between TECALBO and lateral ear canal resection and bulla osteotomy with marsupialization (LECARBOM) is that the surgical wound is closed at the end of the surgery with the same limitation as discussed previously.

Partial Ear Canal Ablation Without Bulla Osteotomy

A recent less invasive technique is described for surgical management of otitis media in rabbits. In this technique, the acoustic meatus is preserved and only a flush or superficial curettage of the tympanic bulla is performed, which spares most or all of the tympanic epithelium.[21]

Indications

Partial ear canal ablation without bulla osteotomy (PECAWBO) is indicated for rabbits with CT-confirmed otitis media (including cases presenting with vestibular signs, facial paresis, or auricular canal stenosis) when disease control is unlikely with medical therapy alone and when no lesions of osteomyelitis are present. It is particularly relevant for lop-eared rabbits with conformational stenosis and poor bulla ventilation. PECAWBO aims to restore aeration and drainage by creating a wide lateral opening while avoiding bulla osteotomy, thereby limiting surgical invasiveness and anesthetic time. Preoperative CT (with Richardson grading) guides case selection and prognostic.[7]

Surgical technique

Under general anesthesia in lateral recumbency, the periaural region is clipped and aseptically prepared (temporary tarsorrhaphy to protect the cornea). Two parallel skin incisions are made along the external canal toward the base; dissection continues to expose the lateral canal wall. The lateral wall is incised and resected to the level of the annular cartilage and the ostium of the tympanic bulla, leaving 1 to 2 mm of annular cartilage on bone to anchor closure. The canal is copiously irrigated with warm sterile saline; if the tympanic membrane is intact, perform a myringotomy to access the bulla. Superficial, targeted curettage may be performed through the natural ostium when feasible (no ostectomy). Bulla contents are collected for culture. Closure creates a wide otostomy by placing simple interrupted sutures every 2 mm between the canal epithelium, annular cartilage, and skin; distally, 2 continuous intradermal lines complete marsupialization (**Fig. 15**). Hemorrhage is controlled with pressure and bipolar cautery as needed.

Postoperative care

Hospitalize for monitoring and supportive care: IV fluids (then subcutaneous [SC] boluses), multimodal analgesia (eg, fentanyl–lidocaine–ketamine constant rate infusion [CRI] transitioning to opioids and meloxicam), and empirical antibiotics pending culture, then targeted therapy for 6 to 8 weeks where indicated. Daily local care (gentle cleansing; povidone-iodine as used in the study protocol) maintains stoma patency. Rechecks at 7 to 15 days (wound assessment, suture removal if healed) and 3 to 4 weeks (evaluate opening caliber and secretion control) are advised, with additional visits if complications arise.

Complications

In this 26 case series, all rabbits survived anesthesia; intraoperative issues were limited to minor bleeding managed with electrocautery.[21] Overall success (resolution of preoperative signs within 2 months) occurred in 24 of 26 (92%); vestibular syndrome

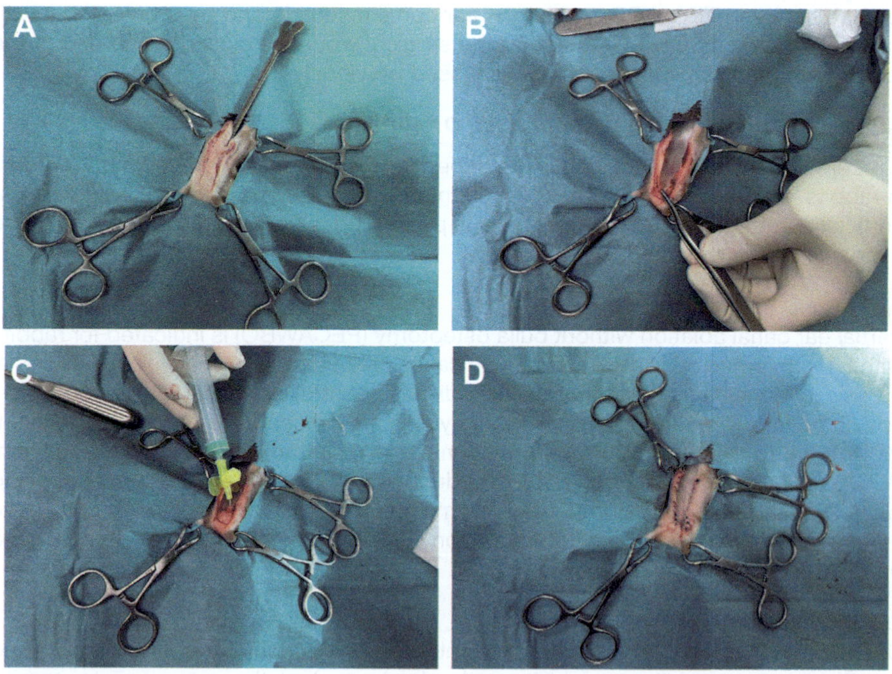

Fig. 15. (*A–D*) Surgical approach to the middle ear by partial ear canal ablation without bullotomy. (*A*) Skin incisions are made along the external auditory canal. (*B*) The lateral wall of the canal is removed up to the level of the annular cartilage, exposing the entrance to the tympanic bulla. (*C*) The canal is flushed using a 24 gauge catheter with warm, sterile 0.9% NaCl solution. (*D*) The incision is closed with simple interrupted sutures, and the pretragic incisure is reconstructed using 2 continuous suture patterns on the external ear canal (4–0 absorbable monofilament). (Image Courtesy of Dr Graham Zoller.)

resolved in 10 of 12 and remained stable in 2. Complications occurred in 9 of 26 (35%): major 2 of 26 (8%) (focal otostomy stenosis requiring revision) and minor 7 of 26 (27%), including focal stenosis not requiring surgery, pretragic dehiscence healing by second intention with local care/antibiotics, and transient rhinitis responsive to doxycycline. One late otitis externa recurrence with para-auricular swelling was noted at 6 months. No deaths were reported.

In case of osseous modification of the tympanic bulla (osteitis or osteolysis) this technique is not recommended.

Ventral Bulla Osteotomy

Indications

The indication for a ventral bulla osteotomy (VBO) is an otitis média without otitis externa, and with no osteolysis of the tympanic bulla.[22]

Surgical technique

A VBO is performed in dorsal recumbency with the neck fully extended. Because of the presence of a prominent semicircular mandibular angle in rabbits, the bulla cannot be directly palpated until the overlying muscles are partially dissected. A 4 to 5 cm skin incision is made parallel and medial to the mandible. The incision is continued through the platysma muscle medial to the mandibular salivary gland. The digastricus muscle is dissected from the hyoglossus and styloglossus muscles taking care to avoid the hypoglossal nerve coursing lateral to the hyoglossus muscle. Lone star retractors are used to provide exposure of underlying tissues throughout the procedure. The bulla is palpated between the jugular process of the skull and mandibular angle. Using a Freer periosteal elevator, blunt dissection is continued until the ventral surface of the bulla is exposed. The bulla is entered on the ventral aspect with a Steinmann pin and hand chuck. The osteotomy is extended circumferentially with rongeurs or a pneumatic burr to allow adequate access and drainage. The bulla is carefully curetted to remove any debris as well as the epithelium lining the middle ear. Samples for culture and susceptibility and histopathology are obtained as necessary and the site lavaged with sterile saline.[23] The surgical site is closed in a routine fashion using 4-0 or smaller absorbable suture material for the muscle and subcutaneous tissue and 4-0 or smaller nonabsorbable monofilament suture material for the skin. An alternative to the use of PMMA is to place an active drain and to rinse the bulla using the drain.[15]

Myringotomy

In case of otitis media without otitis externa (or when the ear canal could be perfectly cleaned under endoscopy), an endoscopic examination of the tympanic bulla could be performed.[24] Depending on the size of the rabbit, a 5 mm otoscope optic, a 2.7 mm 30° or 0° or a 1.9 mm 0° optic with their operating channel sheath could be used. The external ear canal needs to be thoroughly cleaned and flushed with sterile saline. The tympanic membrane is visualized and is perforated with a myringotomy needle. The content is aspirated and sampled to send for a bacterial culture and sensitivity. Then, the tympanic bulla is flushed with sterile saline. A large incision of the tympanic membrane is often necessary, to allow adequate lavage of debris and exudate from the middle ear. As the rabbits' pus often present in the middle ear is thick, it could be challenging to fully clean the tympanic bulla during the first procedure. The author recommends repeating this procedure once a week until the tympanic bulla is perfectly clean.

CLINICS CARE POINTS

- In lop-eared rabbits with severe external ear canal stenosis, LECAR is a recommended surgical procedure, as it restores ventilation and drainage while carrying a lower morbidity than bulla-involving techniques.
- Otitis media is frequently subclinical in rabbits, and a normal neurological examination does not rule out tympanic bulla involvement.
- Once otitis media is confirmed on CT, medical therapy alone is rarely curative, and early surgical management should be considered the treatment of choice.
- During lateral approaches to the tympanic bulla, the facial nerve lies medioventrally to the bulla. Always submit middle ear contents for bacterial culture and susceptibility testing and empirical antibiotic choices should be reassessed once the antibiogram is available, as multidrug-resistant infections have been reported.
- The most common complications are wound dehiscence, delayed healing, transient facial nerve paresis, and possible late recurrence.
- In rabbits with a pre-existing head tilt, warn owners that vestibular signs may persist or only partially resolve despite successful surgical management of the underlying otitis.

DECLARATION OF AI AND AI-ASSISTED TECHNOLOGIES IN THE WRITING PROCESS

During the preparation of this work the authors used Generative AI. After using this tool, the authors reviewed and edited the content as needed and takes full responsibility for the content of the publication.

DISCLOSURE

The authors declare no conflicts of interest, financial or otherwise, related to the content of this article.

REFERENCES

1. O'Malley B. Section four, rabbits. In: O'Malley. Clinical anatomy and physiology of exotic species, structure and function of mammals, birds, reptiles, and amphibians. St Louis (MO): Elsevier et Saunders WB; 2005. p. 163–261.
2. Stott P, Jennings N, Harris S. Is the large size of the pinna of the ear of the European hare (Lepus europaeus) due to its role in thermoregulation or in anterior capital shock absorption? J Morphol 2010;271:674–81.
3. Popesko P, Rajtova V, Jindrich Horak J. A Colour Atlas of Anatomy of small laboratory animals: volume 1 Rabbit, Guinea pig. London: Saunders; 1992.
4. Donnelly TM. Basic anatomy, physiology and husbandry of rabbits (chapter 11). In: Quesenberry KE, Mans C, Orcutt C, editors. Ferrets, rabbits and rodents: clinical medicine and surgery. 4th edition. St Louis (MO): Saunders, Imprint of Elsevier; 2020. p. 131–49.
5. Johnson JC, Burn CC. Lop-eared rabbits have more aural and dental problems than erect-eared rabbits: a rescue population study. Vet Rec 2019;185(24):758.
6. de Matos R, Ruby J, Van Hatten RA, et al. Computed tomographic features of clinical and subclinical middle ear disease in domestic rabbits (Oryctolagus cuniculus): 88 cases (2007-2014). J Am Vet Med Assoc 2015;246(3):336–43.
7. Richardson J, Longo M, Liuti T, et al. Computed tomographic grading of middle ear disease in domestic rabbits (Oryctolagus cuniculi). Vet Rec 2019;184-(22):679.

8. Liatis T, Makri N, Czopowicz M, et al. Otitis media/interna and encephalitozoonosis are the most common causes of head tilt in pet rabbits in the UK: 73 cases (2009–2020). Vet Rec 2024;195(1):e4267.
9. Handerson R, Horne R. Pinna in slatter textbook of small animal surgery section 14: ear. 3rd edition. New York: Saunders; 2002. p. 1737–46.
10. Manjunatha D, Mahesh V, Ranganath L. Surgical management of aural hematoma in Russian grey giant rabbit. Int J Agric Sc Vet Med 2014;2(3):37–8.
11. Krahwinkel D. External ear canal in in slatter texterbook of small animal surgery section 14: ear. 3rd edition. New York: Saunders; 2002. p. p1746–56.
12. Monge E, Donnelly TM, Coutant T, et al. Lateral ear canal resection and bulla osteotomy with marsupialization to treat otitis media in rabbits: forty-eight procedures. Vet Surg 2023;52(8):1100–11.
13. Willems A, Hetterich J, Thöle M, et al. Evaluation of lateral Ear Canal Ablation (LECA) as a surgical treatment option for external ear canal disease in lop-eared pet rabbits (Oryctolagus cuniculus). Animals (Basel) 2025;15(8):1142.
14. Kimmel S, Bakaj M, Di Girolamo N. Progression of otitis media in rabbits after bulla osteotomy or medical management assessed via computed tomography. In: Proceeding of the Exotic365 annual conference;. Seattle; 2025. p. 130.
15. White R. Midle ear in *in* slatter texterbook of small animal surgery section 14: ear. 3rd edition. New York: Saunders; 2002. p. 1757–66.
16. Eatwell K, Mancinelli E, Hedley J, et al. Partial ear canal ablation and lateral bulla osteotomy in rabbits. J Small Anim Pract 2013;54(6):325–30.
17. Dobberstein REA, Brisson BA, McMillan S, et al. Perioperative complications and outcomes following partial ear canal ablation and lateral bulla osteotomy in pet rabbits: 20 cases (2009-2021). J Small Anim Pract 2023;64(5):350–8.
18. Chow EP, Benett RA, Whittington JK. Total ear canal ablation and lateral bulla osteotomy for treatment of otitis externa and media in a rabbit. J Am Vet Med Assoc 2011;239(2):228–32.
19. Smeak D. Management of complications associated with total ear canal ablation and bulla osteotomy in dogs and cats. Vet Clin Small Anim 2011;41:981–94.
20. Chow EP. Surgical management of rabbit ear disease. J Exot Pet Med 2011;20(3): 182–7.
21. Favier S, Rafael P, Zoller G, et al. Surgical management of otitis media in pet rabbits by partial ear canal ablation without bulla osteotomy: a retrospective study of 26 cases. J Am Vet Med Assoc 2025;1–7.
22. Chow EP, Benett RA, Dustin L. Ventral bulla osteotomy for treatment of otitis media in a rabbit. J Exotic Pet Med 2009;18(4):299–305.
23. Csomos R, Bosscher G, Mans C, et al. Surgical management of ear diseases in rabbits. Vet Clin North Am Exot Anim Pract 2016;19(1):189–204.
24. Jekl V, Hauptman K, Knotek Z. Video otoscopy in exotic companion mammals. Vet Clin North Am Exot Anim Pract 2015;18(3):431–45.

Thoracic Surgery in Small Mammals

Mathilde Charrasse, DVM[a,*], Diego Rossetti, DVM, Dipl ECVS[b],
Carlo Paoletti, DVM, Dipl ECZM (Small Mammals); Postgraduate University Diploma in Microsurgical Techniques (Faculty of Medicine, Sorbonne University, Paris)[a],
José Rosas-Navarro, DVM, Dipl ECZM (Small Mammals); Postgraduate University Diploma in Microsurgical Techniques (Faculty of Medicine, Sorbonne University, Paris)[a]

KEYWORDS

• Thymoma • Pulmonary abscess • Thoracotomy • Thoracoscopy • Chest tube

KEY POINTS

- Assisted ventilation is essential in thoracic surgery to ensure lung inflation despite the absence of a pleural vacuum.
- Preserve the last 1 or 2 sternebrae during thoracic surgery to maintain structural stability.
- Identify and protect the phrenic nerves during rabbit thymectomy to avoid diaphragmatic paralysis.
- Apply a hilar clamp immediately during lobectomy for abscesses to prevent intraoperative contamination.
- Reserve chest drains for chylous or purulent effusions or persistent pneumothorax; they are generally unnecessary for iatrogenic pneumothorax.

INTRODUCTION

Advances in imaging, anesthesia, and surgical techniques have made thoracic surgery in small mammals clinically feasible, yet it remains challenging due to their small size, unique physiology, and the anatomic complexity of the thorax. Improvements in computed tomography (CT), endoscopy, and perioperative care now allow safer and more precise diagnosis and treatment, but successful intervention still demands meticulous planning and a thorough understanding of species-specific limitations.

GENERAL CONSIDERATIONS

Anesthetic Concern

A major challenge in thoracic surgery in small mammals is maintaining adequate ventilation once the thoracic cavity is opened. Endotracheal intubation has been described

[a] Exotic Animal Department, Centre Hospitalier Vétérinaire AniCura-ADVETIA, 9 Avenue Louis Breguet, 78140 Vélizy-Villacoublay, France; [b] Department of surgery, Centre Hospitalier Vétérinaire AniCura-ADVETIA, 9 Avenue Louis Breguet, 78140 Vélizy-Villacoublay, France
* Corresponding author.
E-mail address: mathilde.charrasse@gmail.com

Vet Clin Exot Anim 29 (2026) 669–693
https://doi.org/10.1016/j.cvex.2026.04.009 vetexotic.theclinics.com
1094-9194/26/

Abbreviations	
CT	computed tomography
EP	epicardial pacemaker

in guinea pigs, with successful intubation of guinea pigs[1,2] and chinchillas using a 2.0 mm tube via a blind approach or rigid endoscope. When intubation is not feasible due to small size or tracheal diameter, a preoperative tracheostomy can be performed, allowing intubation through the tracheostomy site.

Positive-pressure ventilation is essential,[3,4] with airway pressures kept below 12 cm H_2O. Small mammals have very low tidal volumes, which often necessitates the use of specialized nonrebreathing systems such as T-piece occluders. These pressure-cycled systems deliver small tidal volumes determined by the target airway pressure and the fresh gas flow. However, they become unsuitable during open thoracic surgery, where the loss of the normal thoracic wall constraint alters airway pressures, increasing the risk of volutrauma. In larger species, such as rabbits, mechanical ventilators and rebreathing systems commonly used in cats can be effective. A volume-controlled ventilation mode with a set maximum inspiratory pressure can help limit barotrauma. Using an inspiratory-to-expiratory ratio of 1:2 or 1:3 further helps reduce the cardiovascular impact of mechanical ventilation. An experienced anesthetist should be prepared to adjust mechanical ventilation based on direct visual assessment of lung inflation once the thoracic cavity is opened. Careful recruitment of chronically atelectatic lung tissue may be performed, particularly after the removal of a large thoracic mass. Partially reducing the delivered tidal volume while increasing the respiratory rate can also facilitate optimal visualization and dissection of key thoracic structures for the surgeon.[5]

In larger species (ferrets, rabbits, and guinea pigs), and depending on the surgical approach, unilateral or bilateral intercostal nerve blocks can be performed. An ultrasound-guided serratus plane block can also be used, although this technique has not yet been described in the literature. Different types of local anesthetics can be selected depending on the desired onset and duration of the neural blockade. Bupivacaine and ropivacaine are particularly effective options for providing long-lasting analgesia.[6,7]

Surgical Approach and Thoracic Access

Conventional surgical approach

Compared with dogs and cats, the thoracic cavity is proportionally much smaller relative to the abdominal cavity, which makes surgical interventions particularly challenging.[3] **Table 1** serves to highlight the anatomic characteristics of the different species discussed.

The 3 surgical approaches to the thorax are the intercostal approach, the sternotomy, and the transdiaphragmatic approach. The surgical approaches are summarized for the different procedures in **Table 2**. Due to the narrow width of the sternebrae, longitudinal splitting is generally not feasible; consequently, the term "median sternotomy" is not anatomically accurate for this species. The terms "ventral midline thoracotomy" are then preferred.[6,8]

The equipment required for performing a thoracotomy is shown in **Fig. 1**.

A rotary tool (diamond disc) has been suggested for midline transection of the sternebrae, although a sagittal saw is preferred to minimize the risk of injury to vital structures.[6,8]

Table 1
Comparative anatomy of the thorax of small mammal species

Species	Thymus Involution in Adults?	Notes	Number of Thymus Lobes	Number of Lung Lobes	Number of Thoracic Vertebrae (T)
Ferret	High variability among individuals	Some adults retain an astonishingly large thymus	2 lobes (strictly thoracic)	4 lobes (right) and 2 lobes (left)	14–15
Rabbit	No	The thymus persists into adulthood with minimal involution	3 lobes (1 main left thoracic lobe and the dorsal and ventral right thoracic lobes)	4 lobes (right) and 3 lobes (left, the left cranial lobe is divided in 2 parts)	12
Guinea pig	Sometimes, partial involution	The pattern of atrophy is histologically more similar to humans than many other rodent species	2 lobes (strictly thoracic)	4 lobes (right) and 2 lobes (left)	13
Chinchilla	Yes—documented	Study of chinchillas from 2 wk to 8 y showed that older animals had less actual thymic tissue and lower lymphocyte concentration in medullary centers than younger ones—sign of involution	2 lobes (strictly thoracic)	4 lobes (right) and 2 lobes (left)	13
Degu	Yes	Involution is clearly documented in adults; thymus decreases in size and cellularity with age	2 lobes (strictly thoracic)	4 lobes (right) and 2 lobes (left)	13

(continued on next page)

Table 1
(continued)

Species	Thymus Involution in Adults?	Notes	Number of Thymus Lobes	Number of Lung Lobes	Number of Thoracic Vertebrae (T)
Rat	Yes—classic model species	By 5–12 mo, significant involution observed (loss of thymocytes and stromal changes)	4 lobes (2 cervical + 2 thoracic)	4 lobes (right) and 1 lobe (left)	13
Mouse	Yes—clear, well-documented	Thymus volume peaks ~5–7 wk (or around sexual maturity), then begins involution; by 12 mo cellularity is strongly reduced	4 lobes (2 cervical + 2 thoracic)	4 lobes (right) and 1 lobe (left)	12–14
Gerbil	Does not fully involute	Thymus remains relatively large; involution minimal or delayed	2 lobes (strictly thoracic)	4 lobes (right) and 1 lobes (left)	13
Hamster	Yes	Thymus involution occurs; number of lobes varies among species (2–4)	2–4 lobes depending on species (thoracic, sometimes cervical) lobes of thymus	4 lobes (right), 1 lobe (left)	13

Table 2
Surgical procedures and their access approaches

Surgery	Thymectomy	Lung Lobectomy	Chylothorax	Chest Drain Placement	Epicardial Pacemaker Implantation	Diaphragmatic Hernias
Access	Ventral midline thoracotomy	Intercosta thoracotomy (fourth for the cranial lobe or fifth space for the caudal lobe)	Intercostal thoracotomy (8th–10th space) or diaphragmatic incision	Incision at dorsal aspect of the 10th intercostal space, position the drain by subcutaneous tunneling to the level of the second rib	Transdiaphragmatic access or left eighth intercostal thoracotomy	Ventral midline laparotomy

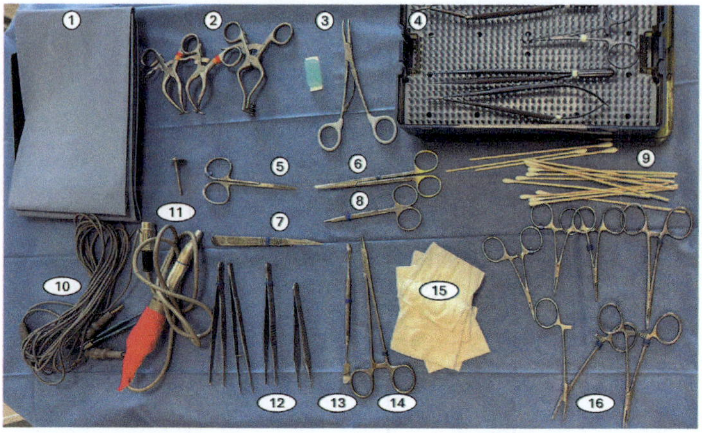

Fig. 1. (1–16) Surgical instruments for a thoracotomy. 1: Sterile drape. 2: Gelpi retractors. 3: Hemoclips. 4: Microsurgery instrument set. 5: Micro-dissecting scissors. 6: Metzenbaum scissors. 7: Scalpel. 8: Stevens scissors. 9: Cotton tips applicators. 10: Bipolar forceps. 11: Dental handpiece with diamond disc. 12: Surgical forceps. 13: Periosteal elevator. 14: Needle holder. 15: Gauzes. 16: Clamps and hemostatic forceps. (Image Courtesy of Dr José Rosas-Navarro.)

Minimally invasive surgery techniques

Currently, diagnostic applications, particularly examination and biopsy of thoracic organs, are the most common uses of these techniques, though therapeutic procedures are rapidly expanding. Endoscopic biopsies generally yield higher quality samples than percutaneous methods due to direct visualization of the target and the ability to obtain larger specimens. The magnification and illumination provided by the endoscope also improve detection of small lesions that may be missed with ultrasonography. Thoracoscopy has been applied across a wide range of surgical procedures in animals, and in small species, the potential for minimally invasive interventions continues to grow, constrained mainly by equipment availability and surgical innovation.[9]

Rigid endoscopes with a diameter of 1.9 or 2.7 mm and 0° or 30° lenses are ideal for use in small mammals. A CO_2 insufflator is generally unnecessary for thoracoscopy in mammals. For biopsy procedures, oval biopsy cup forceps are recommended for sampling pleura, lymph nodes, and masses, while core biopsy needles are preferred for deeper tissues. Additional essential instruments include various grasping forceps, retractors, needle holders, and scissors. Most instruments are equipped with monopolar electrosurgical capability at their tips, allowing both tissue dissection and hemostasis. Proper positioning of the surgical team and equipment is a skill that improves with experience and varies depending on the procedure. Likewise, patient positioning can significantly enhance the operative field by using gravity to aid in the retraction of viscera.[10]

Some studies described the feasibility of a thoracoscopic technique combining an intercostal and a transdiaphragmatic approach in rabbits positioned in dorsal recumbency for lung biopsy collection (**Fig. 2**).[11,12]

SURGERIES BY ANATOMICAL REGION

Mediastinal Surgery

Mediastinal masses in rabbits

Epidemiology, clinical presentation, diagnosis. In rabbits, the thymus persists in adulthood and is easily identified bilaterally, cranial and ventral to the heart. Thymomas

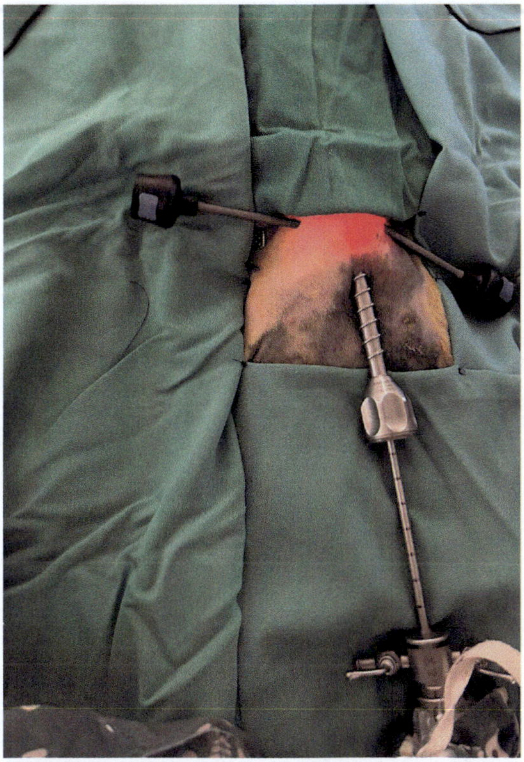

Fig. 2. Thoracoscopy setup. Triangulation involves using a scope portal in the center (through diaphragm) and 2 thoracic ports, one on each side of the scope portal. (Image Courtesy of Dr Laura Vilalta.)

account for 2.1% of all rabbit tumors[13] and arise from thymic epithelial cells, typically containing variable benign lymphocytic infiltration. They are classified based on epithelial characteristics.[14–16] Although histologically benign, their clinical behavior ranges from benign to malignant depending on invasiveness. Thymic lymphoma and thymic carcinoma are rare; metastasis has not been reported for thymoma, but a single case of renal metastasis from a thymic carcinoma exists.[17–19] Thymomas occur most frequently in middle-aged to older rabbits (6–10 years of age), and recent reports suggest that they are relatively common in this species.[14,20,21] A genetic predisposition associated with immunodeficiency and hemolytic anemia has been identified in 3 rabbits.[22]

The most common clinical signs are dyspnea (76.9%) and exercise intolerance (53.9%)[14]; bilateral exophthalmos (**Fig. 3**) and third-eyelid prolapse occur in nearly 50% and 25% of cases, respectively.[15,23–25] Paraneoplastic exfoliative dermatitis (**Fig. 4**) has been described in several species and presumptively in 5 rabbits.[26,27] Hypercalcemia and myasthenia gravis have not been definitively documented in rabbits, though 1 historical case involved suspected concurrent hypercalcemia.[25]

Imaging is essential for evaluating, diagnosing, staging, and planning treatment of mediastinal disease. Thoracic radiographs often reveal mediastinal masses incidentally (**Fig. 5**), and echocardiography may identify them in rabbits with nonspecific thoracic signs while also assessing hemodynamic consequences of intracardiac

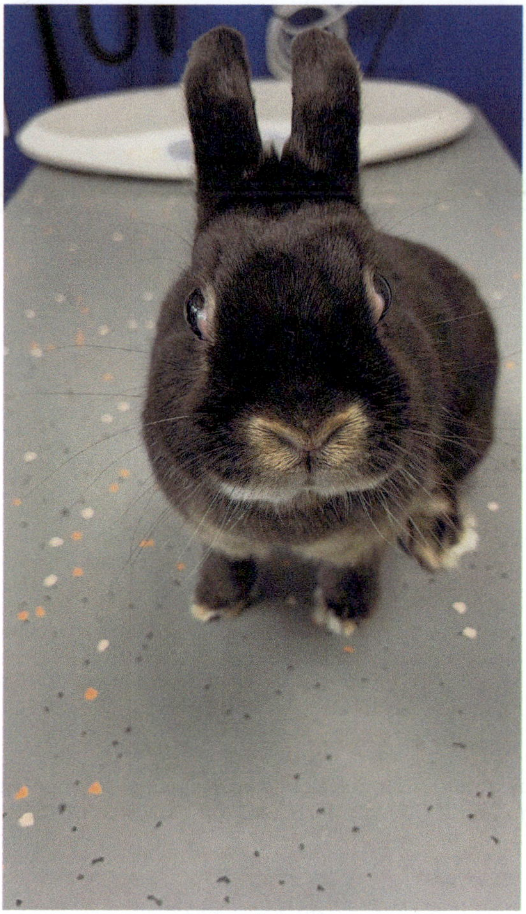

Fig. 3. Bilateral exophthalmos in a rabbit presenting a mediastinal mass (confirmed thymoma). (Image Courtesy of Dr José Rosas-Navarro.)

extension. evaluate internal composition and vascularity, distinguishing solid from cystic structures, identifying fat or calcifications. Postcontrast studies further assess potential involvement of major vessels (**Fig. 6**).[28]

Treatments. Surgical excision, chemotherapy, and radiation therapy have all been reported as treatment options for thymoma in rabbits.[15] Recommendations for surgery or radiation depend on factors such as concurrent diseases (eg, cardiopulmonary conditions), overall clinical status, access to radiation facilities, and owner preference.[14,15]

In a prospective study of 15 rabbits treated with hypofractionated stereotactic volumetric modulated arc radiotherapy, contrast-enhanced CT demonstrated complete tumor elimination for up to 2 years. Ten rabbits remained recurrence-free, 2 died of unrelated causes, and 3 were lost to follow-up. No radiation side effects were observed. The median survival time of the remaining animals (ie, those that survived anesthesia) was 727 days. In contrast, conventional megavoltage radiation was less effective and caused significant complications.[20] Another study reported a median

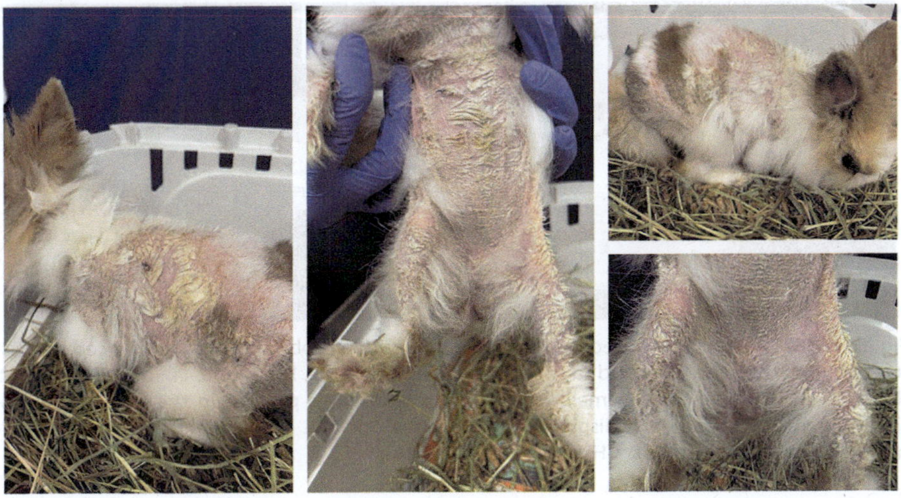

Fig. 4. Exfoliative dermatitis in a rabbit with a concurrent thymoma. (Image Courtesy of Dr José Rosas-Navarro.)

survival time of 213 days with intensity-modulated radiotherapy.[29] Radiation therapy is recommended after incomplete surgical excision or for nonsurgical candidates, although potential complications, including myocardial failure, pneumonitis, pulmonary fibrosis, and thoracic vessel thrombosis, must be considered.

Evidence for chemotherapy is limited, but prednisolone may be used postoperatively, after radiotherapy, or as a sole treatment.[15,29] Glucocorticoid therapy yielded a median survival time of 270 days,[29] though adverse effects such as cheyletiellosis.

Survival time following aspiration of thymic cysts is not well documented; one reported case survived 150 days postaspiration[14] (**Fig. 7**). Clinical experience suggests this procedure improves quality of life and respiratory function, particularly as a preoperative intervention. One study reported a median survival time of 92 days in untreated rabbits.[29]

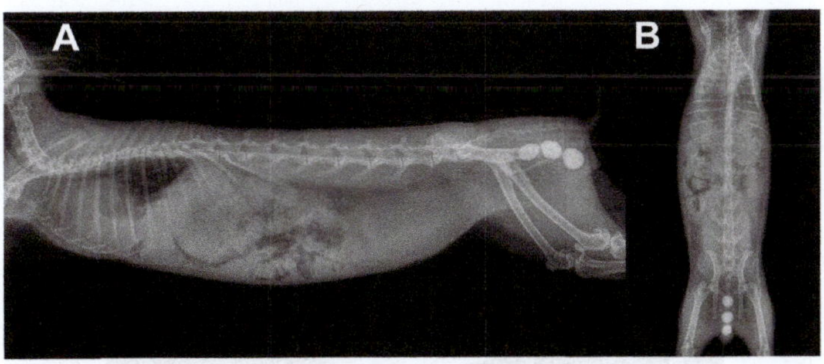

Fig. 5. (*A, B*) Total-body radiographs of a rabbit presented for dysuria. Thoracic findings include dorsal displacement of the trachea, loss of the cardiac silhouette, and pleural effusion, consistent with the presence of a large mediastinal mass. Three urethral calculi and a dilated urinary bladder are also visible. (*A*) Right lateral radiograph. (*B*) Ventrodorsal radiograph. (Image Courtesy of the Exotic Pet Medicine Department, CHV AniCura-ADVETIA.)

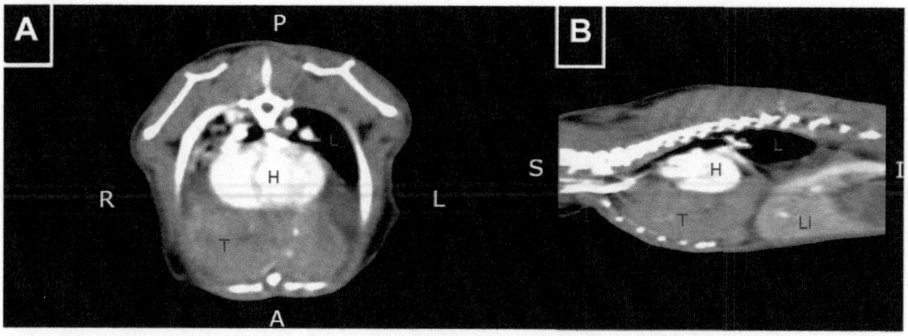

Fig. 6. (*A, B*) Thoracic computed tomography images of a rabbit. Contrast-enhanced soft tissue window: transverse (*A*) and sagittal (*B*) views. H, heart; L, lung lobe; Li, liver; T, enlarged thymus. A soft tissue opacity mass (confirmed thymoma) is present in the cranial mediastinum, ventral to the heart, displacing the trachea dorsally. (Image Courtesy of the Diagnostic Imaging Department, CHV AniCura-ADVETIA.)

Surgery. The first reported thymoma excision in a rabbit (1992)[23] was performed via an intercostal approach; although the tumor was removed, the rabbit died postoperatively, likely due to limited surgical exposure. The first successful long-term postoperative survival was later achieved using a median sternotomy, which provides superior access to the cranial mediastinum and is now the recommended approach.[30]

Although mediastinal masses may recur after surgery, recurrence is not the main cause of mortality.[14] Perioperative deaths are thought to result from pain, stress, anesthetic complications, or incomplete excision.[15] Five rabbits showed pleural and pericardial effusion and chronic epicardial and pericardial inflammation at necropsy, likely contributing to postoperative death. Reported survival after sternotomy ranges widely (0–955 days; median 3 days), largely influenced by selection bias, as only rabbits in sufficiently stable condition undergo invasive surgery.[14] Long-term survival rates vary: one report described 50% long-term survival with most complications occurring within 10 days,[8] while another reported roughly 75% long-term survival, with all fatal events occurring in the first postoperative week (a rate consistent with the present authors' impression of approximately 80%).[5]

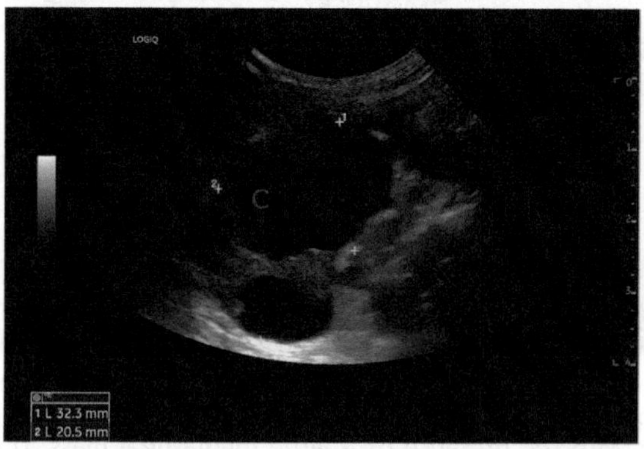

Fig. 7. Thoracic ultrasonography of a polycystic thymoma in a rabbit. C, cyst; M, solid tissue component of the mass. (Image Courtesy of the Diagnostic Imaging Department, CHV AniCura-ADVETIA.)

Key surgical considerations

- The last 1 or 2 sternebrae should remain intact to support thoracic stability during recovery (total of 6 sternebrae in rabbits); if exploring the caudal thorax, the manubrium can be preserved while transecting the last sternebrae (**Fig. 8**).
- The thymic mass is bluntly dissected from surrounding tissues with care to avoid major vessels (cranial vena cava, jugular and subclavian veins, carotid, subclavian arteries, ascending aorta, and pulmonary arteries) and to identify and preserve the phrenic nerves dorsally. Thoracic fat can be abundant. Adhesions, especially to the pericardium, sometimes necessitate pericardiectomy.
- After excision, the thoracic cavity may be rinsed with warm saline to remove blood clots and debris, followed by suction. Careful inspection for hemorrhage and air leaks should be performed prior to closure.

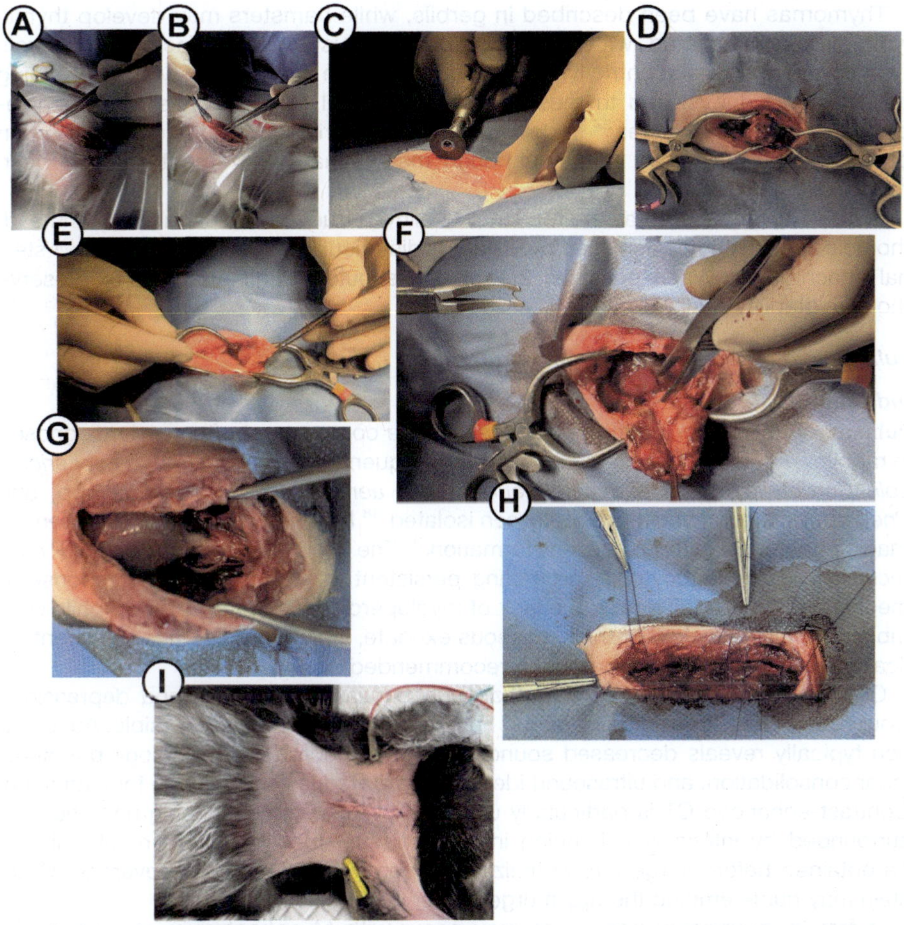

Fig. 8. (*A–I*) Step-by-step ventral midline thoracotomy in a rabbit for thymoma excision. (*A*) Cutaneous incision along the sternum. (*B*) Muscular disinsertion with a periosteal elevator. (*C*) Osseous opening with a diamond disc. (*D*) Placement of Gelpi retractors to expose thoracic cavity. (*E*) Dissection of adhesions around the mass. (*F*) Externalization of the mass. (*G*) Phrenic nerve visualization. (*H*) Closure of the thorax with interrupted cruciate sutures. (*I*) Skin closure. (Image Courtesy of Dr José Rosas-Navarro.)

- Sternebrae are reapposed using preplaced monofilament sutures, applied circumferentially in interrupted manner; rib reattachment is unnecessary. Muscle, subcutaneous tissue, and skin are closed routinely.
- Residual air in the thoracic cavity is evacuated by a chest drain or a simple thoracocentesis.
- The authors note that a chest tube seems unnecessary after thymectomy, as aspiration with needle and syringe during closure is typically sufficient and less inflammatory.

Other species and size concerns

Mediastinal tumors have been reported in several other small mammal species. In rats, exocrine pancreatic adenocarcinomas have been reported, including a case in a 12 month old animal with widespread metastases involving the heart, lungs, mediastinal lymph nodes, liver, spleen, kidneys, adrenal gland, testis, and sternum.[31,32]

Thymomas have been described in gerbils, while hamsters may develop thymic lymphomas associated with hamster polyomavirus; young infected individuals typically develop multicentric lymphoma originating in the mesentery and spreading to the liver, kidneys, and thymus.[32,33] A mediastinal thymoma has also been reported in a Syrian hamster.[34] In degus, a thymoma arising from the cervical portion of the thymus has been noted, although mediastinal involvement has not been reported.[35]

In rodents, the sternebrae are too small to allow a true median sternotomy. Instead, thoracic access can be achieved by unilateral disarticulation of the ribs from their sternal attachments. When possible, 2 to 3 ribs should be left attached to preserve thoracic stability during closure.[36]

Pulmonary Surgery (Pathology and Procedures)

Indications

Pulmonary abscesses. Pulmonary abscesses are common yet often underdiagnosed in rabbits.[5] *Pasteurella multocida* is the most frequent pathogen, although *Escherichia coli*, *Bordetella bronchiseptica*, *Pseudomonas aeruginosa*,[37] *Chlamydia* spp, and *Pneumocystis oryctolagi* have also been isolated.[38] Myxoma virus may cause hemorrhagic pneumonia without abscess formation.[37] The hyaluronic acid capsule of *P multocida* impairs phagocytosis, promoting persistent infection and poor response to medical therapy. Additionally, the lack of myeloperoxidase in rabbit heterophils contributes to the formation of thick, caseous exudate, which further limits treatment efficacy; lobectomy is, therefore, often recommended.[5]

Clinical signs are nonspecific (lethargy, anorexia, weight loss, and depression). Coughing is rare; sneezing may occur. Fever and leukocytosis are possible. Auscultation typically reveals decreased sounds over the affected lobe. Radiographs show lobar consolidation, and ultrasound identifies cavitated lesions suitable for aspiration. Contrast-enhanced CT is particularly useful, showing a nonenhancing necrotic core surrounded by intensely enhancing inflamed tissue. Ideally, culture results should be obtained before surgery to optimize perioperative antimicrobial coverage; Gram stain may guide empiric therapy if urgent intervention is required.

In ferrets, pulmonary abscesses may occur with *Mycobacterium abscessus*, for which surgery may be useful when the pathogen is nonzoonotic.[39] Ferrets may also develop fungal granulomas (*Blastomyces dermatitidis*) that can require lobectomy.[40]

In guinea pigs, bacterial pneumonia—often linked to inadequate husbandry—is common and associated primarily with *B bronchiseptica*, *S pneumoniae*, *Streptococcus equi* subsp *zooepidemicus*, and *P aeruginosa*. *B bronchiseptica* may cause severe purulent bronchopneumonia with pleuritis and systemic complications (otitis media, encephalitis, metritis, abortions, and even death).[41]

Neoplasia. In rabbits, metastatic pulmonary disease is most common and often originates from uterine adenocarcinoma, osteosarcoma, lymphoma, or mammary carcinoma. Primary lung tumors are rare but cases of pulmonary histiocytic sarcoma and acinar adenocarcinoma have been reported (**Fig. 9**).[42–45]

In guinea pigs, lung tumors account for 30% to 35% of all neoplasms in animals aged over 3 years; most are benign bronchogenic adenomas while bronchogenic and alveolar carcinomas have also been described. These tumors typically grow slowly, and clinical signs often remain unnoticed until advanced stages.[32]

In mice, lung tumors are the most common neoplasm (incidence 28%[46]). Other rodents rarely develop primary pulmonary tumors, though chinchillas may present lymphoma or adenocarcinoma of the lung[32] and a rat case of pulmonary squamous cell carcinoma has been reported.[47] In ferrets, the lungs are a frequent site of lymphoma metastasis, whereas primary lung tumors are extremely rare.[48]

Lung lobe torsion. A 360° torsion of the right cranial lung lobe associated with pneumothorax and pleural effusion has been reported in a 3 year old castrated male ferret, constituting the first described case in a small mammal.[49]

Key surgical considerations

- Select the appropriate intercostal space (fourth or fifth) based on the lobe to remove, using the scapular caudo-dorsal border as a landmark (corresponding to the fourth intercostal space; **Fig. 10**).
- Incise the skin parallel to the rib, subcutaneous tissue, and latissimus dorsi, then separate the serratus ventralis and transect the scalenus if needed.
- Incise the intercostal muscles carefully, avoiding the internal thoracic vessels ventrally and the azygos vein dorsally.
- Enter the thoracic cavity and begin assisted ventilation.

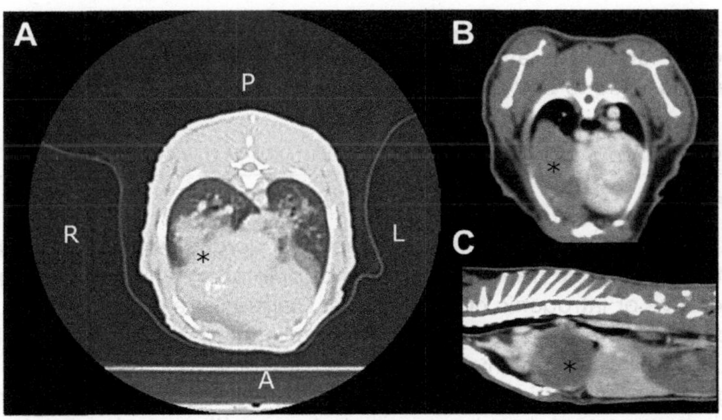

Fig. 9. (*A–C*) Thoracic computed tomography images of a rabbit. Lung window: transversal view (*A*). Contrast-enhanced soft tissue window: transverse (*B*) and sagittal (*C*) views. *: Right caudoventral intrathoracic mass originating from the right caudal lung lobe, histologically identified as a carcinoma associated with an abscess (carcinoma likely metastatic). (Image Courtesy of the Diagnostic Imaging Department, CHV AniCura-ADVETIA.)

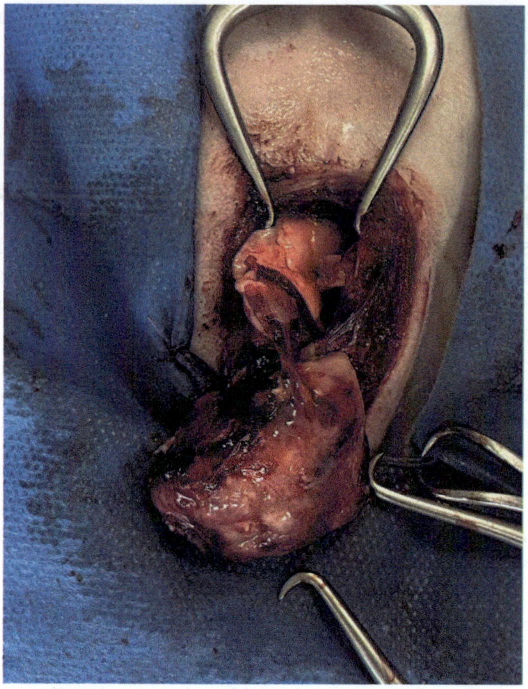

Fig. 10. Externalization of the lung mass described by **Fig. 9**. (Image Courtesy of Dr José Rosas-Navarro.)

- Gently elevate the affected lung lobe and ligate/clip/staple the bronchus and vessels (or perform a partial lobectomy if indicated).
- Check for hemorrhage and air leaks, then place a thoracostomy tube.
- Close the thoracic wall: place and tie rib sutures, then close the scalenus, serratus ventralis, and latissimus dorsi.

Manipulation of infected lung tissue may cause pus to escape from the lobar bronchus into other lobes. The affected lobe should be elevated carefully, and the hilum immediately clamped to prevent contamination.

Pleural Cavity Surgery

Pleural effusion

Pyothorax. Pyothorax is uncommon but reported across small exotic mammals. It may result from thoracic trauma, extension of pulmonary infection, foreign bodies, or postoperative or iatrogenic complications. Diagnosis relies on imaging (**Fig. 11**), cytology demonstrating a neutrophilic/heterophilic exudate with intracellular bacteria, and culture.[50] Treatment involves thoracic drainage (via chest drain or thoracotomy), targeted antimicrobial therapy, and nutritional and fluid support. In a ferret, successful management has been reported using thoracostomy tubes, lavage (5 mL of warm sterile 0.9% saline) every 4 hours for 7 days, and broad-spectrum antibiotics (ceftazidime and clindamycin), with survival beyond 78 days.[51] Reported pathogens in ferrets include *Fusobacterium* spp, *Actinomyces hordeovulneris*, and *Pseudomonas luteola*.[51,52]

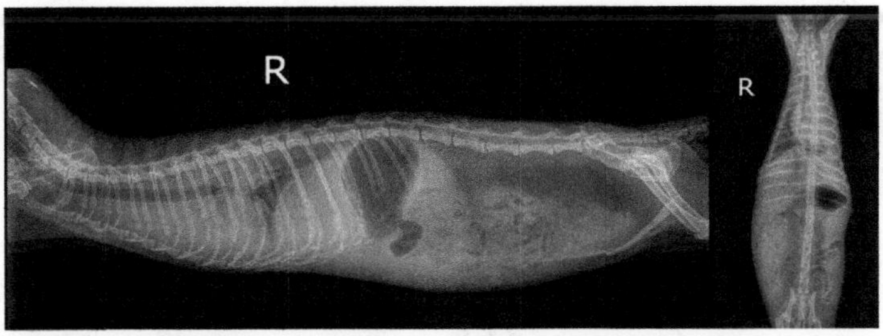

Fig. 11. Total-body radiographs of a ferret presenting a pyothorax. Pleural effusion more pronounced in the left hemithorax. (Image Courtesy of the Exotic Animal Department, CHV AniCura-ADVETIA.)

Guinea pigs are known to develop bronchopneumonia associated with inflammatory and/or septic pleural effusion; however, reported pyothorax cases in the literature involve experimental models. Another study showed a higher virulence of gram-negative bacteria inoculated.[53,54]

Chylothorax. Causes include mediastinal masses, cardiac disease, fungal granulomas, venous thrombi, congenital thoracic duct abnormalities, and peritoneopericardial hernias; in many cases, the etiology remains undetermined. Trauma is an uncommon cause of chylothorax in dogs and cats due to rapid healing of the lymph ducts.[55]

Chylothorax has been reported secondary to thymic lymphoma in rabbits, idiopathically in chinchillas,[18,56] and in ferrets following adrenocortical carcinoma surgery with septic peritonitis.[57] The authors also report a rabbit with chylothorax due to cranial vena cava compression by a thymoma. Prognosis is poor across species.

Respiratory signs predominate, though coughing may be the only sign in ferrets. Diagnosis is based on imaging and thoracocentesis, with confirmation by higher triglyceride concentration in the effusion than in serum.[55]

Advanced imaging includes CT lymphangiography, with species-specific techniques such as testicular contrast injection in rabbits[58,59] or intrametatarsal pad lymphangiography in ferrets as made in cats.[60] Direct lymph node contrast injection yields superior enhancement in mice.[61] The standard technique involves the popliteal lymph node.[55]

Medical treatment includes pharmaceutical treatment, intermittent thoracocentesis and dietary management (mainly applicable to ferrets). Traditional management uses a high-protein, low-fat diet. Although this does not reduce effusion volume, it lowers triglyceride content and may improve fluid reabsorption.[62,63] Octreotide (2 µg/kg, subcutaneous, bid[57]), a synthetic long-acting somatostatin analog, may inhibit the lymph fluid excretion from the lymphatic vessels of the intestinal wall. Rutine (50–100 mg/kg, po, tid[55]), a benzopyrone drug, may act to increase the number and function of macrophages to remove the protein content from the effusion facilitating fluid reabsorption.[57]

Surgery, extrapolated from canine/feline protocols, is reserved for refractory cases and may involve thoracic duct ligation and partial pericardiectomy associated or not with cisterna chyli ablation and omental drainage.[64–67]

Key surgical considerations

- Approach the thoracic duct via intercostal thoracotomy (8th–10th space) or diaphragmatic incision.

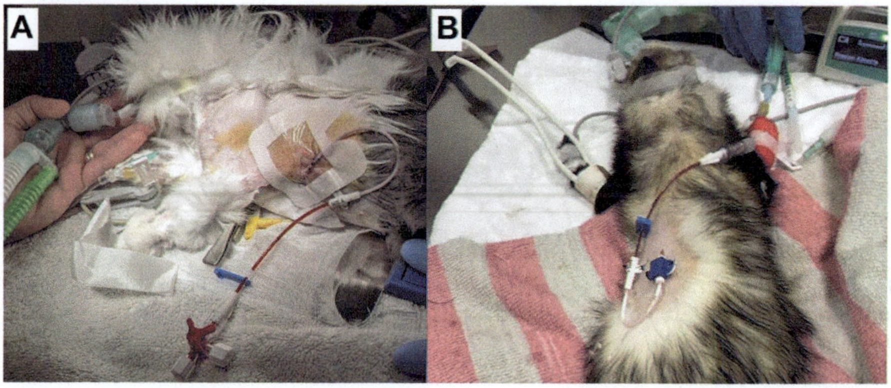

Fig. 12. (*A, B*) Chest drain in a rabbit (*A*) and in a ferret (*B*). (Image Courtesy of Dr Laura Vilalta.)

- Identify and ligate ducts with clips or silk sutures; methylene blue injection enhances visualization.
- Perform subtotal pericardectomy and place a chest drain before closure.

This procedure has also been described under thoracoscopic guidance in dogs and cats.[68,69]

Pneumothorax

Spontaneous pneumothorax has been reported in rabbits due to pulmonary histiocytic sarcoma, emphysematous bullae, cavitary lesions, or neoplasia.[70,71] CT is regarded as the diagnostic imaging modality of choice. Medical management is generally favored when diffuse disease is present. Antibiotic treatment was selected to treat the suspected infectious component. One rabbit underwent doxycycline pleurodesis, which appears more effective than autologous blood or talc. Prognosis is poor, with survival often limited to weeks to months.[71,72]

Iatrogenic tension pneumothorax and oxygen therapy to accelerate pneumothorax resolution have also been described in rabbit models (resolution by 36 hours).[73,74]

In rats, ultrasound has proven useful for diagnosis.[75] While no small-mammal surgical cases are reported, lobectomy may be considered when imaging identifies a discrete bulla and surrounding lung tissue is normal.

Chest drain placement

Chest drains enable continuous evacuation of pleural air or fluid and reduce the need for repeated thoracocentesis (**Fig. 12**).

- A stab incision is made at the dorsal aspect of the 10th intercostal space.
- The drain (usually 2.0 mm internal diameter), mounted on a trocar, advanced cranially through a subcutaneous tunnel to the eighth intercostal space, then gently introduced perpendicular to the thoracic wall while avoiding the caudal rib edge, ensuring minimal penetration to avoid organ injury.
- Position the drain parallel to the thoracic wall to the level of the second rib, withdraw the trocar, and immediately occlude the tube before connecting it to a 3 way stopcock.
- Aspirate excess air gently, close all ports, and secure the drain with a Chinese finger-trap suture, dressing, and bandage.

The presence of a chest tube induces an inflammatory response, resulting in pleural effusion at a rate of approximately 1 to 2 mL/kg/d, with signs of infection (pyothorax) typically observed 4 to 6 days after tube placement.[76]

Cardiac Surgery

Cardiac surgery in small mammals, particularly ferrets, primarily involves epicardial pacemaker implantation for second-degree or third-degree atrioventricular block, with collapse as the main clinical sign. Techniques include transdiaphragmatic access or left eighth intercostal thoracotomy in ferrets aged 4.5 to 7.5 years.[77,78]

Key surgical considerations

- Temporary intraoperative epicardial pacing (EP) of the left ventricle was performed through the pericardiotomy incision to maintain heart rate between 80 and 140 bpm.
- The pacing lead was attached to the left ventricle via the pericardiotomy incision using various fixation techniques (screwing, suturing, or stabbing into the apex), then sutured in place using 4-0 polypropylene.
- The lead exited through the diaphragm or costophrenic junction to connect with a pulse generator placed either in the abdomen or an intermuscular pocket (between the transversus abdominis and internal abdominal oblique muscles for transdiaphragmatic EP, or between the latissimus dorsi and external abdominal oblique muscles for intercostal thoracotomy EP).
- Muscle pockets were closed with absorbable monofilament suture.
- After permanent pacing was initiated (120–160 bpm), the temporary lead was removed.
- Pericardiotomy may be left open or closed; incisions are closed routinely. Pneumothorax is evacuated.[78]

Intraoperative risks include arrhythmia progression, hypotension, low cardiac output, cardiac arrest, and hypoxia. Despite appropriate intervention, some cases progressed to fatal cardiopulmonary arrest. Postoperative complications related to the pacing device included muscle fasciculations caused by unipolar pacing and undersensing of sinus beats, which resolved after adjustment of the pacemaker's refractory period.[78]

Thoracic Wall and Diaphragm Surgery

Thoracic wall neoplasia

Thoracic wall neoplasms can originate from the ribs, thoracic muscles, or pleura. Chondrosarcomas are tumors that arise from cartilage, whereas osteosarcomas arise from bone (**Fig. 13**).

En bloc resection involves wide-margin excision and reconstruction with polypropylene mesh; in dogs and cats, stabilization with spinal plates or rib grafts is recommended if multiple ribs are removed. Muscle or omental flaps may cover the mesh.

Partial sternectomy is reserved for small sternal tumors without intrathoracic invasion; the affected sternebrae and adjacent ribs are excised, preserving or ligating internal thoracic arteries as needed. Closure involves suturing ribs, muscles, and skin layers, minimizing dead space, and placing a thoracostomy tube to evacuate air.

To date, no surgical procedures are reported in small mammal veterinary medicine.

Diaphragm surgery

Diaphragmatic hernias may arise from either congenital or traumatic causes but in rabbits they are most often incidental findings. Congenital diaphragmatic hernias in small

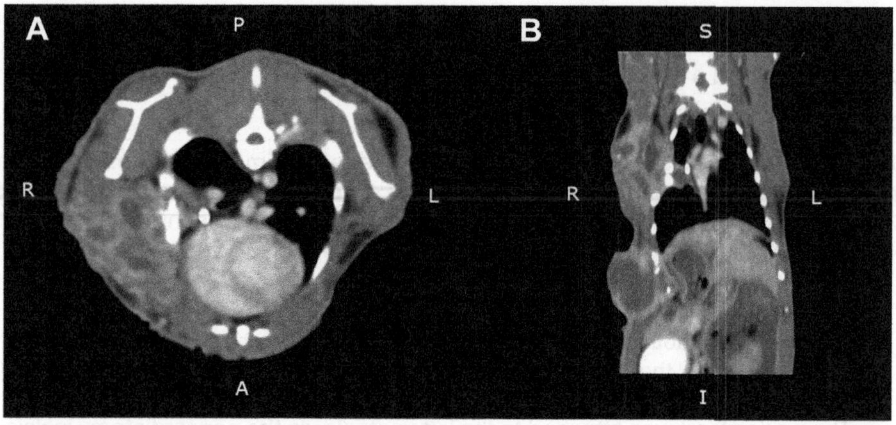

Fig. 13. (*A, B*) Thoracic computed tomography images of a rabbit. Contrast-enhanced soft tissue window: transverse (*A*) and frontal (*B*) views. Two large right thoracic wall masses causing thoracic wall deformation with extensive rib lysis. The cranial mass extends moderately into the thoracic cavity with mass effect and atelectasis, while the caudal mass shows mild intra-abdominal extension displacing the stomach and descending duodenum. (Image Courtesy of the Diagnostic Imaging Department, CHV AniCura-ADVETIA.)

animals are usually considered to be chance embryonic anomalies (5% to 10% in dogs and cats[79]) rather than heritable defects, while traumatic diaphragmatic hernias (77%–85% in dogs and cats[79]) occur due to blunt abdominal traumas, like car accidents, falls, or other traumatic abdominal injuries.[55,80] A previous report on hereditary diaphragmatic hernias showed about 0.8% rabbits suffering perinatal deaths had diaphragmatic hernias. Clinical signs include dyspnea, abdominal organ displacement, and, occasionally, gastrointestinal disturbances. Diagnosis is based on radiography (with or without contrast medium) or ultrasonography, which may reveal loss of the diaphragmatic outline, displacement of lung fields, presence of abdominal organs in the thoracic cavity, gas-filled intestinal loops in the thorax, or pleural effusion.[81]

In a retrospective study, 6 of 16 rabbits underwent hernia repair (mean age 5 years); 2 died within 2 days, and 4 survived to discharge. Long-term follow-up showed survival of 778 and 604 days without hernia recurrence. Four additional rabbits with concurrent conditions (eg, uterine disease) did not undergo repair. Right-sided hernias predominated, with right kidney displacement but no renal dysfunction.[82] A separate case involved a 6 year old neutered male rabbit with right kidney and perirenal fat herniation, successfully corrected surgically by diaphragmatic herniorrhaphy after replacement of the right kidney and the perirenal fat in the retroperitoneal space.[80]

In a chinchilla, a congenital diaphragmatic hernia with bilateral glomerulonephritis displaced half of the stomach into the thorax.[83]

Key surgical considerations

- Perform a ventral midline abdominal incision; extend cranially through the sternum if additional exposure is needed.
- Return abdominal organs to the cavity; enlarge the diaphragmatic defect if necessary.
- Gently dissect adhesions from thoracic structures to avoid pneumothorax or bleeding.

- Close the diaphragmatic defect using a simple continuous suture; incorporate a rib if the diaphragm is avulsed for added strength.
- Evacuate air from the pleural cavity after closure; place a chest tube if persistent pneumothorax or effusion is expected.
- Inspect the abdominal cavity for associated injuries (intestinal, splenic, renal, or bladder) and repair any defects.
- Large defects and chronic hernias can be repaired using muscle flap grafts from the transversus or rectus abdominis muscles, or with synthetic mesh; however, these techniques have not yet been described in small mammals.
- Recommended suture materials include nonabsorbable (polypropylene) or absorbable (polydioxanone and polyglyconate) sutures.[55]

Postoperative pneumothorax is the most common complication, especially if the hernia is chronic and adhesions are present.[55]

Intrathoracic Esophageal Surgery

Esophageal surgery in ferrets addresses foreign bodies and strictures. Diagnosis relies on esophagoscopy and/or iodine-contrast esophagography (radiography or fluoroscopy).[84,85] Foreign bodies are ideally removed endoscopically or surgically by lateral thoracotomy or gastrotomy, while strictures are treated by balloon dilation, occasionally requiring stent placement.[84] Only 1 thoracotomy has been described: a right lateral approach for an esophageal perforation near the heart base, involving surgical debridement and closure, removal of a pleural foreign object, lavage, chest drain placement, and temporary gastrostomy tube.[85]

Intrathoracic Tracheal Surgery

Tracheal tumors are rare in small mammals compared to dogs and cats and may mimic upper airway infections, presenting as progressive dyspnea.

Diagnosis relies on radiographs and CT to detect intraluminal or extraluminal masses. Tracheoscopy is challenging due to small airway diameter but feasible in larger rabbits and ferrets for biopsy or brush cytology.

Reported cases include intraluminal tracheal adenocarcinoma and hemangioma in rabbits, both untreated surgically.[86,87]

No intrathoracic tracheal surgeries have been described in small mammals, and surgical principles are extrapolated from dogs and cats. Rabbits and ferrets are commonly used as an experimental model for the development of tracheal surgery.[88–90] The only reported procedures in rabbits involve surgery or endoscopy of the extrathoracic trachea for tracheal collapse or stenosis.[91,92] One frequent condition of tracheal disease is tracheal strictures secondary to tracheal tube placement for intubation (reported 17–21 days later).[93]

CLINICS CARE POINTS

- During open thoracic surgery, airway pressures should remain below 12 cm H_2O to reduce the risk of barotrauma and volutrauma.
- Mechanical ventilation settings should be adjusted according to direct visualization of lung inflation, with lower tidal volumes and higher respiratory rates improving surgical exposure and limiting cardiopulmonary compromise.
- Careful recruitment of chronically atelectatic lung tissue after thoracic mass removal may improve postoperative pulmonary function while minimizing ventilator-associated lung injury.

- Advanced imaging is essential for diagnosis, staging, and surgical planning of mediastinal disease in rabbits.
- During rabbit sternotomy, preserving 1–2 sternebrae improves postoperative thoracic stability.
- In rabbits and ferrets, multifocal pulmonary lesions should raise suspicion for metastatic or systemic disease.
- Guinea pigs may develop slow-growing pulmonary tumors with minimal clinical signs until advanced stages.
- Pulmonary abscesses are likely underdiagnosed in rabbits.

ACKNOWLEDGMENTS

We warmly thank our team of anesthesia residents, Raphaelle Laffitte and Giacomo Giannettoni, for their daily dedication in the clinic and for their valuable assistance in writing the section on anesthetic management.

DISCLOSURE

The authors have nothing to disclose.

REFERENCES

1. Kramer K, Grimbergen JA, van Iperen DJ, et al. Oral endotrachael intubation of guineapigs. Lab Anim 1998;32:162–4.
2. Turner MA, Thomas P, Sheridan DJ. An improved method for direct laryngeal intubation in the guineapig. Lab Anim 1992;26:25–8.
3. Johnson DH. Endoscopic intubation of exotic companion mammals. Vet Clin Exot Anim Pract 2010;13:273–89.
4. Lennox AM, Capello V. Tracheal intubation in exotic companion mammals. J Exot Pet Med 2008;17:221–7.
5. Bennett RA. Rabbit soft tissue surgery. In: Bennett RA, Pye GW, editors. Surgery of exotic animals. 1st edition. Wiley; 2021. p. 240–76.
6. Szabo Z, Bradley K, Cahalane AK. Rabbit soft tissue surgery. Vet Clin Exot Anim Pract 2016;19:159–88.
7. Aguilar LAB, Portela DA, Moura RA, et al. Ultrasound-guided intercostal nerve injection in rabbit cadavers: technique description and comparison with blind approach. Vet Anaesth Analg 2025;52:228–35.
8. Lewis W. Mediastinal masses and other thoracic surgery. In: Harcourt-Brown Chitty, editor. BSAVA manual of rabbit surgery, dentistry and imaging. British Small Animal Veterinary Association; 2013. p. 257–68.
9. Mehler SJ. Minimally invasive surgery techniques in exotic animals. J Exot Pet Med 2011;20:188–205.
10. Mehler SJ, Bennett RA. Minimally invasive surgery techniques in exotic animals. In: Bennett RA, Pye GW, editors. Surgery of exotic animals. 1st edition. Wiley; 2021. p. 204–26.
11. Wittmaack MCN, Barros FFPC, Silva PES, et al. The feasibility and effectiveness of thoracoscopic transdiaphragmatic approach for lung biopsy in rabbits. A randomized study. Acta Cir Bras 2020;35:e202000501.
12. Wittmaack MCN, Sembenelli G, Conceição MEBAM, et al. Thoracoscopy pulmonary biopsy by two portals with a novel pre-tied loop ligature device in rabbits: an

experimental study. 2022. Available at: http://hdl.handle.net/11449/236892. Accessed November 12, 2025.
13. Bertram CA, Bertram B, Bartel A, et al. Neoplasia and tumor-like lesions in pet rabbits (Oryctolagus cuniculus): a retrospective analysis of cases between 1995 and 2019. Vet Pathol 2021;58:901–11.
14. Künzel F, Hittmair KM, Hassan J, et al. Thymomas in rabbits: clinical evaluation, diagnosis, and treatment. J Am Anim Hosp Assoc 2012;48:97–104.
15. Morrisey J, Mcentee M. Therapeutic options for thymoma in the rabbit. Seminars Avian Exot Pet Med 2005;14:175–81.
16. Robson HR, Yanez RA, Magestro LM, et al. Type A thymoma in a pet rabbit. J Vet Diagn Invest 2022;34:327–30.
17. Huston SM, Ming-Show Lee P, Quesenberry KE, et al. Cardiovascular disease, lymphoproliferative disorders, and thymomas. Ferrets, Rabbits, and Rodents 2012;257–68.
18. Pilny AA, Reavill D. Chylothorax and thymic lymphoma in a pet rabbit (oryctolagus cuniculus). J Exot Pet Med 2008;17:295–9.
19. Wagner F, Beinecke A, Fehr M, et al. Recurrent bilateral exophthalmos associated with metastatic thymic carcinoma in a pet rabbit. J Small Anim Pract 2005;46: 393–7.
20. Andres KM, Kent M, Siedlecki CT, et al. The use of megavoltage radiation therapy in the treatment of thymomas in rabbits: 19 cases. Vet Comp Oncol 2012;10: 82–94.
21. Dolera M, Malfassi L, Mazza G, et al. Feasability for using hypofractionated stereotactic volumetric modulated arc radiotherapy (VMAT) with adaptive planning for treatment of thymoma in rabbits : 15 cases. Vet Radiol Ultrasound 2016;57: 313–20.
22. Weisbroth SH, Flatt RE, Kraus AL. The biology of the laboratory rabbit. Burlington: Elsevier Science; 2013.
23. Kostolich M, Panciera RJ. Thymoma in a domestic rabbit. Cornell Vet 1992;82: 125–9.
24. Pignon C, Jardel N. Bilateral exophthalmos in a rabbit. Diagnosis: thymoma. Lab Anim (NY) 2010;39:262–5.
25. Vernau KM, Grahn BH, Clarke-Scott HA, et al. Thymoma in a geriatric rabbit with hypercalcemia and periodic exophthalmos. J Am Vet Med Assoc 1995;206: 820–2.
26. Florizoone K. Thymoma-associated exfoliative dermatitis in a rabbit. Vet Dermatol 2005;16:281–4.
27. Rostaher PA, Jassies-van der Lee A, Mueller RS, et al. Presumptive paraneoplastic exfoliative dermatitis in four domestic rabbits. Vet Rec 2013;172:155.
28. Ahuja J, Strange CD, Agrawal R, et al. Approach to imaging of mediastinal masses. Diagnostics (Basel) 2023;13:3171.
29. Palmer A, Wu CC, Miwa Y, et al. Outcomes and survival times of client-owned rabbits diagnosed with thymoma and treated with either prednisolone or radiotherapy, or left untreated. J Exot Pet Med 2021;38:35–43.
30. Clippinger TL, Bennett RA, Alleman AR, et al. Removal of a thymoma via median sternotomy in a rabbit with recurrent appendicular neurofibrosarcoma. J Am Vet Med Assoc 1998;213:1140–3, 1131.
31. Benitz KF, Roth RN. A spontaneous metastasizing exocrine adenocarcinoma of the pancreas in the rat. Lab Anim Sci 1980;30:64–6.
32. Greenacre CB. Spontaneous tumors of small mammals. Vet Clin Exot Anim Pract 2004;7:627–51.

33. Simmons JH, Riley LK, Franklin CL, et al. Hamster polyomavirus infection in a pet Syrian hamster (Mesocricetus auratus). Vet Pathol 2001;38:441–6.
34. Rother N, Bertram CA, Klopfleisch R, et al. Tumours in 177 pet hamsters. Vet Rec 2021;188:e14.
35. Okumura N, Kondo H, Suzuki S, et al. Thymoma originating from the cervical component of the thymus in a degu. J Vet Diagn Invest 2022;34:126–9.
36. Bennett RA. Rodent soft tissue surgery. In: Bennett RA, Pye GW, editors. Surgery of exotic animals. 1st edition. Wiley; 2021. p. 297–321.
37. Marlier D, Mainil J, Linde A, et al. Infectious agents associated with rabbit pneumonia: isolation of amyxomatous myxoma virus strains. Vet J 2000;159:171–8.
38. Dei-Cas E, Chabé M, Moukhlis R, et al. Pneumocystis oryctolagi sp. Nov., an uncultured fungus causing pneumonia in rabbits at weaning: review of current knowledge, and description of a new taxon on genotypic, phylogenetic and phenotypic bases. FEMS Microbiol Rev 2006;30:853–71.
39. Lunn JA, Martin P, Zaki S, et al. Pneumonia due to Mycobacterium abscessus in two domestic ferrets (Mustelo putorius furo). Aust Vet J 2005;83:542–6.
40. Darrow BG, Mans C, Drees R, et al. Pulmonary Blastomycosis in a Domestic Ferret (Mustela putorius furo). J Exot Pet Med 2014;23:158–64.
41. Quesenberry KE, Donnelly TM, Mans C. Biology, husbandry, and clinical techniques of Guinea pigs and chinchillas. In: Ferrets, rabbits, and rodents. Elsevier; 2012. p. 279–94.
42. Cooper TK, Griffith JW, Chroneos ZC, et al. Spontaneous Lung Lesions in Aging Laboratory Rabbits (Oryctolagus cuniculus). Vet Pathol 2017;54:178–87.
43. Leissinger M, Brandão J, Wakamatsu N, et al. Pulmonary histiocytic sarcoma in a rabbit. Vet Clin Pathol 2013;42:364–7.
44. Mercado L, Desprez I, Lafuma F, et al. Successful management of acinar adenocarcinoma by pulmonary lobectomy in a pet rabbit (Oryctolagus cuniculus). J Exot Pet Med 2023;47:9–13.
45. Weisbroth SH, Hurvitz A. Spontaneous osteogenic sarcoma in Oryctolagus cuniculus with elevated serum alkaline phosphatase. Lab Anim Care 1969;19:263–5.
46. Prejean JD, Peckham JC, Casey AE, et al. Spontaneous tumors in Sprague-Dawley rats and Swiss mice. Cancer Res 1973;33:2768–73.
47. Chen HC, Liang CT, Hong CC, et al. Spontaneous pulmonary squamous cell carcinoma in an aging CD rat. Vet Pathol 1996;33:228–30.
48. Williams BH, Wyre NR. Neoplasia in Ferrets. Ferrets, Rabbits, and Rodents 2020:92–108.
49. Vuong KS, Fazio C, Greenacre CB, et al. Right cranial lung lobe torsion in a domestic ferret (*Mustela putorius furo*). Vet Radiology Ultrasound 2025;66:e13457.
50. Demetriou JL, Foale RD, Ladlow J, et al. Canine and feline pyothorax: a retrospective study of 50 cases in the UK and Ireland. J Small Anim Pract 2002;43:388–94.
51. Sladakovic I, Brainard BM, Lane SL, et al. Diagnosis and management of pyothorax in a domestic ferret (Mustela putorius furo). J Vet Emerg Crit Care 2017;27:479–85.
52. Martínez J, Martorell J, Abarca ML, et al. Pyogranulomatous Pleuropneumonia and Mediastinitis in Ferrets (Mustela putorius furo) associated with Pseudomonas luteola Infection. J Comp Pathol 2012;146:4–10.
53. Mavroudis C, Ganzel BL, Cox SK, et al. Experimental aerobic-anaerobic thoracic empyema in the Guinea pig. Ann Thorac Surg 1987;43:298–302.

54. Mavroudis C, Katzmark SL, Ganzel BL, et al. Successful treatment of empyema thoracis with polymethylmethacrylate antibiotic-impregnated beads in the Guinea pig. Ann Thorac Surg 1988;46:615–8.
55. Fossum TW. Surgery of the lower respiratory System: pleural cavity and Diaphragm. In: Small animal surgery. 5th Edition. Mosby; 2018. p. 916–57.
56. Ratliff C, Zaffarano B. Generalized edema and chylothorax in a 5-year-old female intact chinchilla (*Chinchilla lanigera*). J Exot Pet Med 2017;26:219–23.
57. Vilalta L, Altuzarra R, Molina J, et al. Chylous Ascites in 2 ferrets. J Exot Pet Med 2017;26:150–5.
58. Iwai T, Sonoda A, Watase S, et al. Thoracic duct lymphangiography via the testicular parenchyma in a rabbit model. J Vasc Interv Radiol 2022;33:1543–7.e1.
59. Tsuruno A, Shibazaki A, Kanda N, et al. Visualization of the thoracic duct with injections of dyes or contrast media into the testicular parenchyma in the rabbit. J Vet Med Sci 2009;71:759–62.
60. Chiang C, Chen K-S, Chiu H-C, et al. Computed tomography lymphangiography via intrametatarsal pad injection is feasible in cats with chylothorax. Am J Vet Res 2021;83:133–9.
61. Sugawara H, Furuta T, Sumiyoshi A, et al. Feasibility study of direct CT lymphangiography in mice: comparison with interstitial CT/MR lymphangiography. Eur Radiol 2023;33:5028–36.
62. Almakdisi T, Massoud S, Makdisi G. Lymphomas and chylous ascites: review of the literature. Oncologist 2005;10:632–5.
63. Al-Busafi SA, Ghali P, Deschênes M, et al. Chylous ascites: evaluation and management. ISRN Hepatol 2014;2014:240473.
64. Reeves LA, Anderson KM, Luther JK, et al. Treatment of idiopathic chylothorax in dogs and cats: a systematic review. Vet Surg 2020;49:70–9.
65. Stockdale SL, Gazzola KM, Strouse JB, et al. Comparison of thoracic duct ligation plus subphrenic pericardiectomy with or without cisterna chyli ablation for treatment of idiopathic chylothorax in cats. J Am Vet Med Assoc 2018;252:976–81.
66. Kanai H, Furuya M, Hagiwara K, et al. Efficacy of en bloc thoracic duct ligation in combination with pericardiectomy by video-assisted thoracoscopic surgery for canine idiopathic chylothorax. Vet Surg 2020;49(Suppl 1):O102–11.
67. Bussadori R, Provera A, Martano M, et al. Pleural omentalisation with en bloc ligation of the thoracic duct and pericardiectomy for idiopathic chylothorax in nine dogs and four cats. Vet J 2011;188:234–6.
68. Haimel G, Liehmann L, Dupré G. Thoracoscopic en bloc thoracic duct sealing and partial pericardectomy for tho treatment of chylothorax in two cats. J Feline Med Surg 2012;14:928–31.
69. Allman DA, Radlinsky MG, Ralph AG, et al. Thoracoscopic thoracic duct ligation and thoracoscopic pericardectomy for treatment of chylothorax in dogs. Vet Surg 2010;39:21–7.
70. Feyer S, Bertram CA, Klopfleisch R, et al. Spontaneous pneumothorax secondary to pulmonary histiocytic sarcoma in two pet rabbits (Oryctolagus cuniculus). J Exot Pet Med 2021;38:48–9.
71. Guillerit F, Gros L, Touzet C, et al. Spontaneous pneumothorax pet rabbits (Oryctolagus cuniculus): four cases (2017–2022). J Exot Pet Med 2023;45:30–7.
72. Mitchem RE, Herndon BL, Fiorella RM, et al. Pleurodesis by autologous blood, doxycycline, and talc in a rabbit model. Ann Thorac Surg 1999;67:917–21.
73. Reuter JD, Fowles KJ, Terwilliger GA, et al. Iatrogenic tension pneumothorax in a rabbit (Oryctolagus cuniculus). Contemp Top Lab Anim Sci 2005;44:22–5.

74. Hill RC, DeCarlo DP, Hill JF, et al. Resolution of experimental pneumothorax in rabbits by oxygen therapy. Ann Thorac Surg 1995;59:825–7 [discussion: 827–828].
75. Piskovská A, Kraszewska K, Hauptman K, et al. RATTUS (Rat Thoracic Ultrasound): diagnosis of pneumothorax in pet rats. Front Vet Sci 2024;11. Available at: https://www.frontiersin.org/journals/veterinary-science/articles/10.3389/fvets.2024.1394291/full. Accessed November 4, 2025.
76. Hung GC, Gaunt MC, Rubin JE, et al. Quantification and characterization of pleural fluid in healthy dogs with thoracostomy tubes. Am J Vet Res 2016;77:1387–91.
77. Sanchez-Migallon Guzman D, Mayer J, Melidone R, et al. Pacemaker implantation in a ferret (Mustela putorius furo) with third-degree atrioventricular block. Vet Clin North Am Exot Anim Pract 2006;9:677–87.
78. Alvarez-Sanchez A, Townsend KL, LeBlanc NL, et al. Epicardial pacemaker implantation and outcome in eight pet ferrets (Mustela putorius furo). J Vet Cardiol 2022;41:44–56.
79. Blake CA. Diaphragmatic Hernia. In: Drobatz KJ, Hopper K, Rozanski E, et al, editors. Textbook of small animal emergency medicine. 1st edition. Wiley; 2018. p. 298–303. Available at: https://onlinelibrary.wiley.com/doi/10.1002/9781119028994.ch47. Accessed November 13, 2025.
80. Wu R-S, Chu C-C, Wang H-C, et al. Clinical diagnosis and surgical management of diaphragmatic retroperitoneal perirenal fat and kidney herniation in a pet rabbit. 2016. Available at: https://avmajournals.avma.org/view/journals/javma/248/12/javma.248.12.1399.xml. Accessed September 15, 2025.
81. Fox RR, Crary DD. Hereditary diaphragmatic hernia in the rabbit. J Hered 1973;64:333–6.
82. Takimoto H, Miwa Y. A retrospective study of diaphragmatic hernia in rabbits (oryctolagus cuniculus): 16 CASES (2009 to 2016). J Exot Pet Med 2019;30:17–21.
83. Vetere A, Bertocchi M, Moggia E, et al. Concomitant Congenital Diaphagmatic Hernia (CDH) and bilateral bacterial glomerulonephritis in a pet chinchilla (Chinchilla lanigera). BMC Vet Res 2021;17:370.
84. Webb J, Graham J, Fordham M, et al. Diagnosis and treatment of esophageal foreign body or stricture in three ferrets (Mustela putorius furo). JAVMA (J Am Vet Med Assoc) 2017;251:451–7.
85. Caligiuri R, Bellah JR, Collins BR, et al. Medical and surgical management of esophageal foreign body in a ferret. 1989. Available at: https://avmajournals.avma.org/view/journals/javma/195/7/javma.1989.195.07.969.xml. Accessed September 15, 2025.
86. Bertram CA, Klopfleisch R, Müller K. Tracheal and laryngeal tumors in two domestic rabbits (Orytolagus cuniculus). J Exot Pet Med 2019;29:142–6.
87. Kandefer-Gola M, Żebrowski K, Ciaputa R, et al. Tracheal hemangioma causing lung emphysema and pneumopericardium in a rabbit—A case report. Animals (Basel) 2022;12:1907.
88. Peleg H, Rao UN, Emrich LJ. The rabbit as an experimental animal for tracheal surgery. J Surg Oncol 1988;37:49–51.
89. Kaye R, Goldstein T, Grande DA, et al. A 3-dimensional bioprinted tracheal segment implant pilot study: rabbit tracheal resection with graft implantation. Int J Pediatr Otorhinolaryngol 2019;117:175–8.
90. Barber HW, Small PA. Construction of an improved tracheal pouch in the ferret. Am Rev Respir Dis 1977;115:165–9.

91. Swisher S, Lennox A, Vecchio N. Tracheal resection and anastomosis for treatment of tracheal collapse in a rabbit. J Exot Pet Med 2020;33:46–9.
92. Ferris RL, Quesenberry KE, Weisse CW. Outcome of intraluminal tracheal stent placement for tracheal stenosis in a rabbit (Oryctolagus cuniculus). J Exot Pet Med 2019;31:23–7.
93. Grint NJ, Sayers IR, Cecchi R, et al. Postanaesthetic tracheal strictures in three rabbits. Lab Anim 2006;40:301–8.

Intestinal Surgery in Rabbits

Nicola Di Girolamo, DVM, PhD, DiplECZM(Herp), DiplACZM, DiplACVPM

KEYWORDS

• Rabbit • Computed tomography • Enterotomy • Enterectomy • Trichobezoar

KEY POINTS

- Advances in rabbit intestinal physiology and diagnostic imaging (especially computed tomography) have clarified when intestinal surgery is needed and improved safety with modern anesthesia and critical care.
- Mechanical obstruction is most commonly due to trichobezoars/phytobezoars; duodenal proximal obstructions often require surgery, while jejunal/ileal obstructions can be managed medically in some cases.
- Preoperative management emphasizes careful fluid therapy, avoidance of prokinetics, and judicious stomach decompression; enterotomy is preferred over resection when feasible.
- Appendiceal disorders may require appendectomy; intestinal biopsies are usually obtained via laparotomy due to risks with endoscopic sampling.
- Post-operative care requires intensive monitoring (72–96 hours), intravenous antibiotics and fluids, and consideration of vasopressors in critical cases; rabbits may have longer GI transit times affecting recovery.

INTRODUCTION

Thanks to a better understanding of rabbit intestinal physiology and advances in diagnostic imaging, indications for intestinal surgery are becoming clearer. Concurrent advances in anesthesia and critical care have made intestinal surgery safer. This review focuses on mechanical obstructions, appendiceal disorders, and intestinal biopsies.

CLINICAL ANATOMY AND PHYSIOLOGY OF THE RABBIT INTESTINAL TRACT

The intestinal tract of rabbits is unique among mammals and has several anatomic features with important clinical implications (**Fig. 1**).[1] Rabbits possess a well-developed lower esophageal sphincter,[2] which prevents vomiting or eructation and predisposes them to gastric distension in case of intestinal obstruction. The stomach is proportionally large and is normally palpable on physical examination. Ingesta are almost always present, even during prolonged anorexia, with approximately half of the gastric

Department of Clinical Sciences, College of Veterinary Medicine, Cornell University, Ithaca, NY, USA
E-mail address: nicoladiggi@gmail.com

Vet Clin Exot Anim 29 (2026) 695–714
https://doi.org/10.1016/j.cvex.2026.04.013 vetexotic.theclinics.com

Abbreviation	
CT	Computed tomography

contents remaining after a 24 hour fast.[3] The small intestine has a relatively narrow luminal diameter, making rabbits particularly susceptible to obstruction by even small foreign bodies. The proximal duodenum, especially its initial cranio-caudal curvature, is a common site for severe, non-transient obstructions.[4] The presence of a functional ileo-colic junction is relevant because that is another location where foreign bodies can result in non-transient obstruction.[4] At this junction lies the sacculus rotundus, a lymphoid structure unique to lagomorphs that marks the transition between small and large intestine and may be mistaken for a pathologic structure on imaging or exploratory laparotomy. The large intestine has a markedly wider diameter, allowing foreign bodies that would be obstructive in the small intestine to pass without complication.[5] The large intestinal tract is characterized by a well-developed vermiform appendix, a feature shared only with a limited number of other mammals (primates, wombat, among others).[6] The appendix of the rabbit has a readily discernible boundary from the body of the cecum, marked by a distinct decrease in the diameter and the lack of sacculations. The appendix is connected to the ileum through the ileocecal

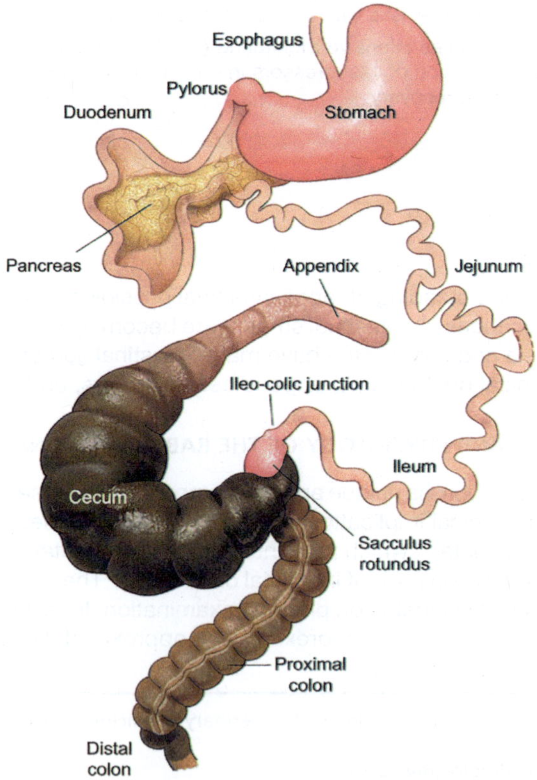

Fig. 1. Anatomical features of primary clinical relevance in the gastro-intestinal tract of rabbits. (*Modified from* Abby Brown, Dissection Lab Guide for Ungulate Anatomy, https://pressbooks.umn.edu/ungulateanatomylabguide/.)

fold, a short mesenteric ligament infiltrated by a number of small, short vessels.[7] The appendix is the part of the gut associated lymphoid tissue that has predominant B cell production, as opposed to the Peyer's patches, ileocecal plaque, and cecal tonsils that have predominantly T-cell production.[8] The vermiform appendix has been proved to be important for the development of the individual's immune function. This function is mostly carried out early after birth, with a 99% reduction of B lymphopoiesis by 16 weeks of age, and no evidence of progenitor B cells in the appendix of adult rabbits.[9] It is unclear whether in the adult rabbit the appendix is involved in any physiologically relevant role. A laboratory study showed that rabbits fed diets high in silicate accumulated sand in the cecal appendix.[10] However, it is unknown whether a similar process of sand accumulation would occur in natural conditions. Finally, the fusus coli represents a physiologically thickened segment of the colon that regulates fecal separation and pellet formation and should not be misinterpreted as an abnormal thickening of the large intestinal tract on diagnostic imaging.

MECHANICAL OBSTRUCTION

Mechanical intestinal obstruction is a common emergency in rabbits.[4,5] For years, intestinal obstructions have been difficult to diagnose due to the generic clinical signs that this condition may present with, and the complex intestinal anatomy of rabbits, which renders diagnostic imaging less clear than in other species. Most commonly, intestinal obstructions of rabbits affect the small intestinal tract and are caused by a trichobezoar, or pellet of compressed hair and fibers (**Fig. 2**). The second most common cause for mechanical obstruction in rabbits are intestinal neoplasms. Occasionally, large intestinal obstructions occur. Small intestinal obstruction typically cause gas build-up orad to them. The esophageal sphincter of rabbits is well developed and does not allow rabbits to eruct or vomit. The modest amount of fermentation that normally occurs in the stomach of rabbits cannot be eliminated through the intestinal tract due to the obstruction, nor it cannot be eructated, and as such accumulates orad to the obstruction. The stomach is gas distended in about 4 out of 5 intestinal obstructions.[4]

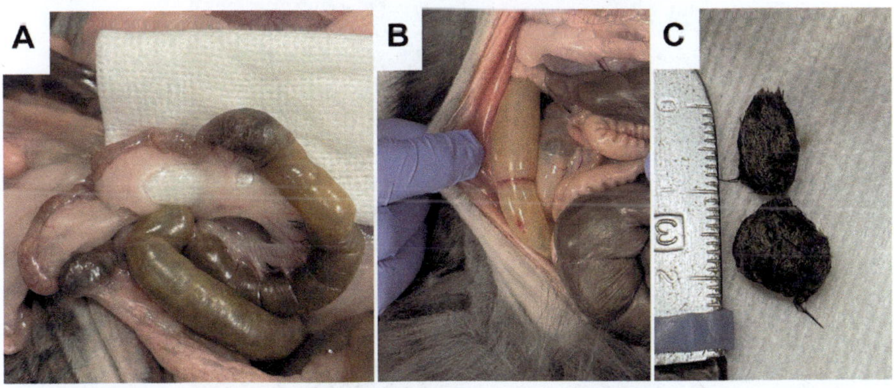

Fig. 2. Mechanical obstruction in rabbits. (*A*) Postmortem image of a rabbit that was dead on arrival after referral for severe gastric distension. A trichobezoar was identified at the level of the jejunum. Notice the typical gas and fluid distension orad to the obstruction, and intestinal emptiness abroad to it. (*B*) Same rabbit as in panel *A*. Notice a circumferential lesion at the level of the duodenum, a finding commonly observed in areas where trichobezoars have remained for prolonged periods during transit. (*C*) Gross aspect of a trichobezoar after section. Trichobezoars are often the same size or just slightly larger than a normal fecal pellet. (Image Courtesy of Dr Nicola Di Girolamo.)

If the small intestinal obstruction is at the level of the ileum, both the stomach and the small intestinal tract will be gas filled, while if the obstruction is at the level of the duodenum, only the stomach is typically gas filled. Based on current knowledge, it is clear that the vast majority (close to 90% of the ones presented in hospital)[11] of the trichobezoars causing small intestinal obstruction will slowly advance through the small intestinal tract until they reach the ileo-colic junction. Once transited through the ileo-colic junction and in the cecum, the trichobezoars are of a size that is not concerning for further obstruction in the large intestine and are eliminated among the rest of the feces. Due to their size and appearance, they are difficult to recognize from normal fecal pellets. In a minority of cases, somehow around 10% of the cases presented to the hospital,[11] the trichobezoar does not progress through the intestinal tract and can cause severe inflammation and perforation of the intestinal tract (**Fig. 3**). These cases require prompt surgical treatment.

Causes

The striking majority of mechanical obstruction events in rabbits are caused by pellets of compressed hair (trichobezoars) similar in size to a large fecal pellet (approximately 1 cm in size) (see **Fig. 2**). Based on 2 studies, trichobezoars account for 76% to 81% of the intestinal obstructions.[4,12] The second most common cause for mechanical obstruction are intestinal neoplasms (5 of 64, 8%),[1] or obstructions caused by synthetic material (5 of 36, 14%), depending on the study.[12]

Presenting Complaints and Physical Examination Findings

Rabbits suffering mechanical obstruction are always anorexic,[5] often dehydrated, and present with an enlarged stomach. Evidence that gastric dilation is a consequence of

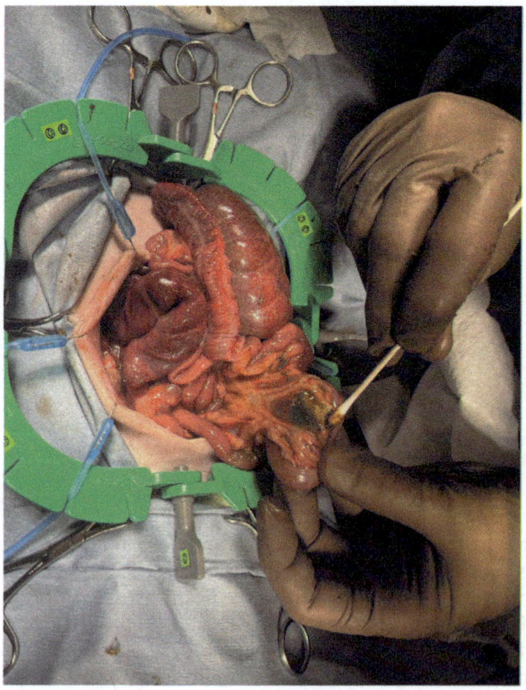

Fig. 3. Intestinal perforation in a rabbit following untreated small intestinal obstruction. (Image Courtesy of Dr Nicola Di Girolamo.)

an intestinal obstruction comes primarily from 2 studies.[4,12] In a case series reporting outcomes of 84 events of gastric dilation in rabbits, at least 64 cases (76%) had an intestinal obstruction.[1] The other 20 cases recovered without surgery or, in 4 cases, were euthanized and the owners declined a postmortem examination.

Diagnostics

Imaging

Historically, radiographs have been used as first line diagnostic in rabbits that presented with generic clinical signs of anorexia and lack of defecation (**Fig. 4**). While radiographs are effective in diagnosing the presence of small intestinal obstructions in rabbits, because they can delineate the presence of gas build-up in the stomach and visualize the increase in size of the stomach, they are not able to locate exactly the obstruction, nor to measure its size.[12] The extensive use of radiography, in combination with the fact that intestinal obstructions are often transient, resulted in the definition of conditions such as "acute gastric distension,"[11] which are likely just the consequence of the pathophysiological process described earlier on, rather than an actual gastric disorder.

The other common imaging modalities used in small animal practice, ultrasound and computed tomography (CT), obviates this issue.[2] CT, including without contrast, allowed visualization of the trichobezoar in all cases in which a trichobezoar was

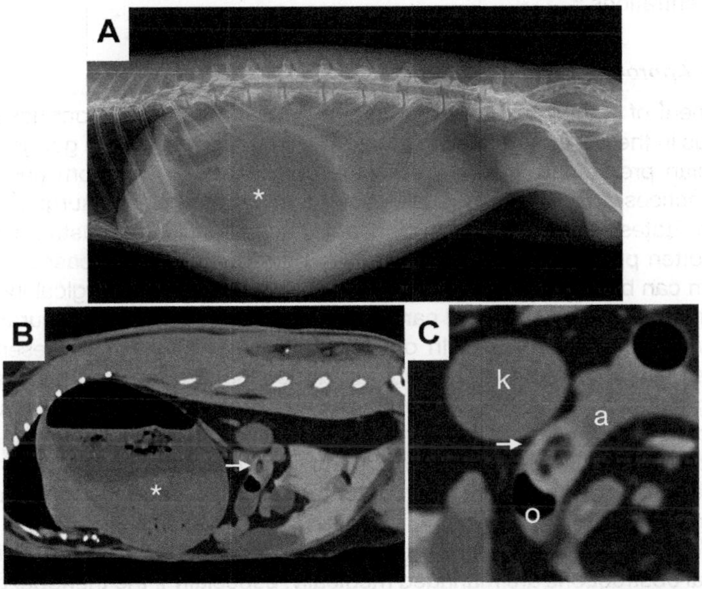

Fig. 4. (*A*) Lateral radiograph of a rabbit with small intestinal obstruction. Notice the marked distension of the stomach (*asterisk*) and gas in the proximal duodenum. (*B*) Computed tomography, parasagittal view, of a rabbit with small intestinal obstruction. The stomach (*asterisk*) is distended, and a trichobezoar is identified in the distal jejunum (*arrow*). (*C*) Close-up view of the trichobezoar (*arrow*) in axial view. On CT, trichobezoars appear as hypoattenuating structures with a hyperattenuating rim and different degrees of internal gas. The intestinal tract orad to the trichobezoar (o) is gas distended, while the intestinal tract aborad to it (a) is empty. The kidney is shown (k). Both location and size of the trichobezoar can be extrapolated from the CT scan. (Image Courtesy of Dr Nicola Di Girolamo.)

present, and allowed determination of its exact location in the intestinal tract and its size (see **Fig. 4**).[5] Following the entire intestinal tract in the CT, allows to identify how far the trichobezoar is from the ileo-cecal junction, which is important to decide on the best treatment course.[5] Ultrasonography, if performed by an experienced operator, it is likely to provide somehow similar indications, albeit limited by intestinal gas.

Blood work

Glucose has been shown to be increased in rabbits with intestinal obstruction.[13] Similar to standard radiographs, the presence of increased glucose is a finding that only suggests the presence of intestinal obstruction, rather than its exact location or size (ie, severity), and as such does not provide further insights on whether a small intestinal obstruction will be able to transit through the intestinal tract or requires surgery.[5] Furthermore, it is not uncommon for small intestinal obstructions to present without elevation of glucose levels.[5] It is particularly important to not use higher glucose levels as the sole indicator for surgery. There have been rabbits with glucose levels over 500 mg/dL that had transient intestinal obstruction medically managed, and rabbits with glucose levels below 200 mg/dL with severe duodenal obstructions and consequent peritonitis.[5] Other common findings in rabbits with intestinal obstruction include indicators of dehydration and/or acute kidney injury, such as increased blood urea nitrogen, creatinine, and packed cell volume, and increase in total magnesium concentrations.[5]

Treatment Approaches

The treatment of small intestinal obstructions caused by trichobezoar has been heterogeneous in the literature and it seems to be highly dependent on geographic location, clinician preference and practice type. In the United Kingdom and Australia, several practices approach most cases of intestinal obstruction surgically.[4,12,14] In the United States, it seems that medical approaches, including gastric decompressions are often prioritized.[15,16] Based on current evidence, some cases of intestinal obstruction can be managed medically, whereas others require surgical intervention; appropriate initial diagnostics and careful follow-up are essential to accurately distinguish between these scenarios. In our hospital, most rabbits that present with an enlarged stomach are advised to undergo abdominal CT, with or without contrast depending on the presence of azotemia, which is common during intestinal obstructions. Since the abdominal CT allows a clear visualization of the obstruction, we can then decide what is the best treatment option based on location and size. Typically, rabbits with proximal duodenal obstruction that have been unwell for several hours are managed surgically because it is unlikely that the trichobezoar will progress through the entire small intestinal tract without consequences. Instead, rabbits with jejunal or ileal obstructions are managed medically, especially if the trichobezoar is relatively small. This approach has significantly reduced the mortality of rabbits presenting for intestinal obstruction caused by trichobezoar, resulting in a small percentage of rabbits undergoing surgery and a large percentage of rabbits managed medically. This approach is not perfect, however, since some trichobezoar (estimated 6%)[5] can get lodged at the level of the ileo-cecal junction. As such, close monitoring of rabbits with foreign body obstruction is required to ensure that the trichobezoar is safely passed into the large intestinal tract. Typically, we advise to repeat imaging techniques adequate to visualize the foreign body (ultrasound or CT), 4 to 8 hours after the initial diagnosis, if there is no clinical improvement.

Medical Treatment

Medical treatment of rabbits with intestinal obstruction should be tailored at reducing discomfort and ensuring that the rabbit is properly hydrated. Prokinetics, assisted feeding and stomach decompression are suggested by some practitioners but the author does not use them for the reasons highlighted below. Anecdotally, rabbits with small intestinal obstructions do not have decreased intestinal motility, but rather the opposite. Hyper-motile intestinal tracts are often visualized through ultrasound. As such, and considering the lack of evidence of their effectiveness, potential risk for intestinal rupture, and indications in other species, prokinetics are not advised in rabbits with intestinal obstruction.[17,18] Assisted feeding, while important when rabbits are unwilling to eat for specific reasons, can result in worsening clinical signs in rabbits with intestinal obstructions. If the trichobezoar is lodged in the duodenum or the ileo-colic junction and does not progress, administration of food is going to increase the size of the stomach, which is going to worsen the clinical signs of the rabbit. Anecdotally, the most severe cases of intestinal obstruction managed by the author are those that have been forced fed before presentation by the owners or other veterinarians. Stomach decompression has become popular in the last decade and a study showed promising results.[15] However, stomach decompression does not remove the cause of the intestinal obstruction. What stomach decompression does is to relieve the clinical signs in rabbits with an enlarged stomach, but since stomach decompression requires general anesthesia or deep sedation to be performed, there is risk associated with it. By reviewing the medical records of Cornell University Hospital for Animals, where stomach decompression was a common practice in the past, several rabbits died during the procedure. Conversely, the author has managed several rabbits with a severely distended stomach that fit the criteria described earlier for medical management without stomach decompression, with resolution. This considered, the author current approach for medical management of rabbits with intestinal obstruction consists in aggressive intravenous fluid therapy (7.5–10 mL/kg/hour for up to 12 hours, in cases with severe azotemia including few hours at 20 mL/kg/hour), intravenous lidocaine (75 mcg/kg/min) and methadone (0.5 mg/kg q6-12h).[5,16] If there is no azotemia, meloxicam (1 mg/kg q12–24h) can be included in the treatment protocol. If arterial pressure can be measured and hypotension is present, vasopressors, particularly norepinephrine (0.2–0.5 mcg/kg/min), should be considered.[19] Rabbits that have a distal small intestinal obstruction that are treated with this approach should improve in the following 4 to 8 hours. If no improvements are observed, additional imaging is important to confirm that the trichobezoar is still transiting.

Surgical Treatment

Perioperative management and stomach decompression

The anesthetic management of patients with potential obstruction is critical. In the author's experience, rabbits suffering mechanical obstruction often have different degrees of metabolic alkalosis, and the anesthetic plan including fluid therapy should be corrected accordingly. The rabbit is pre-medicated, induced and endoscopically intubated. Once the rabbit is stable, the stomach is decompressed. A recent study showed that the enlarged stomach in obstructed rabbits compresses the caudal vena cava, decreasing vascular return.[20] A rubber tube of 18 to 24 French (larger size fitting depending on the size of the rabbit), that has been previously modified by creation of multiple, elliptical (10 mm × 4 mm) holes is passed through the oral cavity into the stomach (**Fig. 5**). The tube is connected to a 60 mL cone syringe in which the cone has been shortened to provide a larger diameter (see **Fig. 5**). This is critical as

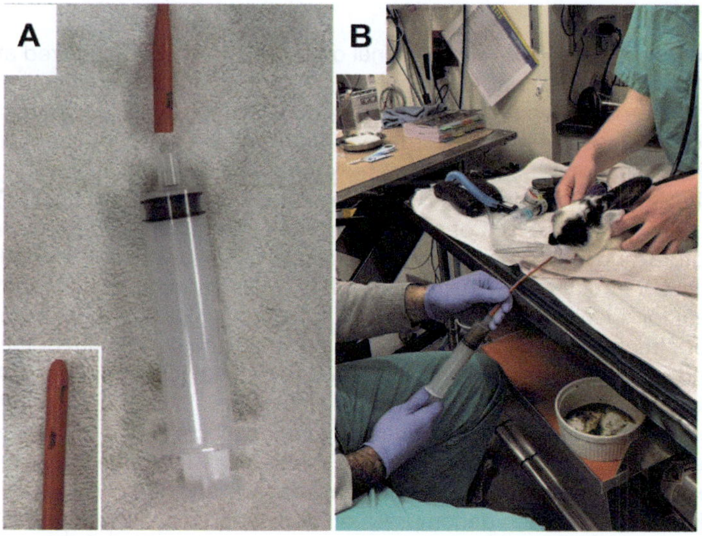

Fig. 5. (*A, B*) Presurgical stomach decompression. (*A*) A 16 to 18 Fr red rubber tube is connected to a 50 to 60 mL catheter-tip syringe. The tip of the syringe is clipped shorter to increase its diameter. Additional holes are pierced on the distal 3 to 4 cm of (*inset*). (*B*) Once the rabbit is under general anesthesia and intubated, the tube is passed orally into the stomach, and gastric contents are aspirated. In addition to decreasing the size of the stomach, and alleviating its compression on the caudal vena cava, this technique often allows the removal of significant quantities of fur. (Image Courtesy of Dr Nicola Di Girolamo.)

the ingesta in the stomach is often mixed with fur/hair that would clog a traditional syringe. Typically, 100 to 300 mL of ingesta mixed with hair can be removed by this method. Once the stomach is decompressed the rabbit is prepared for standard laparotomy.

Surgical technique—laparotomy, detection, and isolation of affected intestinal tract
A 4 to 5 cm midline laparotomy incision is made through the skin and linea alba. The linea alba, incision is performed with forceps rather than scalpel in order to avoid iatrogenic rupture of the GI tract. An auto-static retractor (Lone Star retractor, Cooper Surgical ©) or a circumferential wound protector/retractor (Alexis, Applied Medical ©) is positioned to maximize exposure of the abdomen (**Fig. 6**). Without exteriorizing the entire intestinal tract, the stomach and the duodenum are gently palpated, progressing distally over the small intestine until the site of obstruction is detected. Only the affected intestinal section is then exteriorized. Wet gauze sponges are placed around the isolated intestinal section and either sterile hair clips are placed proximally and distally to the obstruction, or a second surgeon may perform a manual compression. In the authors' experience the use of stay sutures are contraindicated in the intestinal tract of the rabbit due to its fragility. Some authors routinely 'milk' the trichobezoar through the small intestinal tract until it reaches the cecum.[14] This is an acceptable option if the trichobezoar is easily mobile and located distal in the small intestinal tract (ileum/jejunum), but, as mentioned earlier, the author does not approach with surgery cases that have distal intestinal obstructions anymore (**Fig. 7**). If the trichobezoar is in the proximal duodenum and tightly adhered to the intestinal wall, enterotomy or, rarely, enterectomy are indicated.

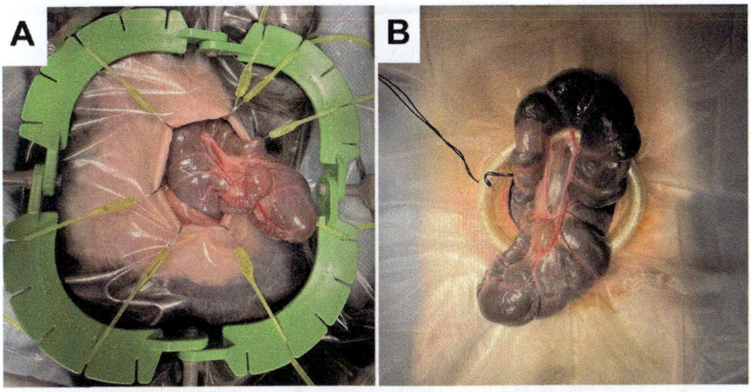

Fig. 6. Options for abdominal wall retraction. (*A*) Use of a self-retaining retractor with elastic stays (Lone Star retractor, Cooper Surgical). The author prefers use of blunt elastic stays for abdominal surgeries in rabbits to prevent iatrogenic damage to the intestinal tract. (*B*) Use of a circumferential wound protector/retractor (Alexis, Applied Medical). The advantage of this retractor is a better distributed pressure on the abdominal wall and additional protection to the abdominal organs if they are exteriorized, preventing their contact with the skin. (Image Courtesy of Dr Nicola Di Girolamo.)

Given that intestinal resection and anastomosis are generally considered higher risk in rabbits than enterotomy, the latter should be preferred whenever feasible. The author frequently observes areas of intestinal damage visible from the serosal surface at sites where foreign bodies have transited. Determining whether such lesions warrant resection and anastomosis can be challenging; however, the rabbit intestinal tract appears capable of healing satisfactorily despite a certain degree of mural damage (**Fig. 8**).

Surgical technique—enterotomy

Once the affected tract is isolated, an incision, usually 4 to 5 mm in length, but dependent on the size of the foreign body, is performed orad to the foreign body, in an area

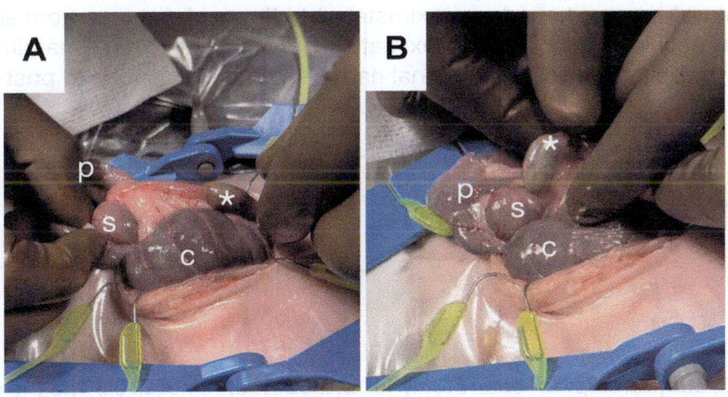

Fig. 7. (*A, B*) Milking of the trichobezoar from the ileum into the large intestinal tract. This rabbit underwent surgery because, even if the trichobezoar was identified on CT scan being close to the ileo-colic junction, it had a size that was concerning for transition. (*A*) The trichobezoar (*asterisk*) is noted to be approximately 4 cm away from the sacculus rotundus (s). The proximal colon (p) and cecum (c) are shown. (*B*) The trichobezoar is milked through the ileo-colic junction, directly into the proximal colon. Saline is injected with a 27 gauge needle in the proximal colon to decrease friction. (Image Courtesy of Dr Nicola Di Girolamo.)

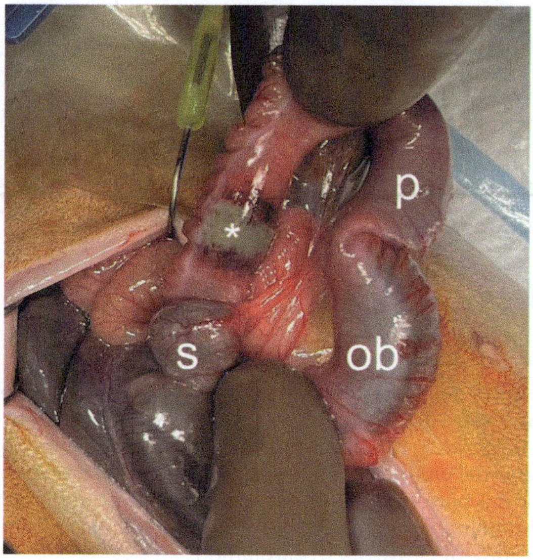

Fig. 8. Damage (*asterisk*) to the proximal colon (p) during a large intestinal obstruction caused by a fecalith (ob). The sacculus rotundus is identified (s). The fecalith was removed with an enterotomy, and a decision was made to not perform a resection and anastomosis of the damaged portion of the intestinal tract. The rabbit recovered and was clinically well at follow-up weeks after the surgery. (Image Courtesy of Dr Nicola Di Girolamo.)

where the tissue is not visibly damaged (**Fig. 9**). While this is in contrast with standard surgical principles in small animals, it is ideal in rabbits since it is challenging to remove the intestinal foreign body from an incision aborad to it. The foreign body is grasped with forceps and removed through the incision (see **Fig. 9**) Care is paid to avoid elongation of the surgical incision of the intestine at the moment of exteriorizing the foreign body. The intestinal tract is sutured with 5-0 PDS, in a simple interrupted pattern (see **Fig. 9**). Sutures are positioned approximately 1 to 2 mm of distance from each other. The sutures should incorporate approximately 1 mm of the intestinal margin; inclusion of excessive tissue may result in luminal narrowing and predispose to post-operative

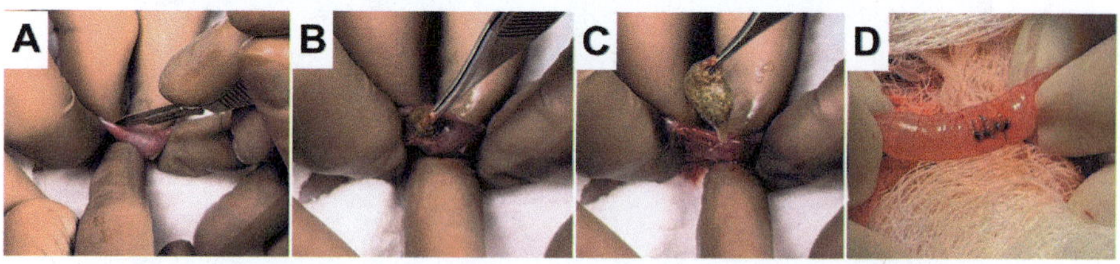

Fig. 9. (*A–D*) Surgical steps for enterotomy for trichobezoar removal. (*A*) The trichobezoar is identified, and the operator occludes the intestinal tract orad and aborad to it. A small incision is made orad to the trichobezoar using a No. 15 blade. (*B*) The trichobezoar is grasped with rat-tooth forceps and gently exteriorized. Note the small size of the incision, which allows tight passage of the trichobezoar. (*C*) The trichobezoar after excision. (*D*) The intestinal incision is closed with simple interrupted sutures using 5-0 absorbable monofilament (eg, polydioxanone, PDS). A leak test is performed to confirm closure integrity. (Image Courtesy of Dr Nicola Di Girolamo.)

stenosis, whereas insufficient tissue purchase may lead to tearing of the intestinal wound edges. A leak test is performed administering 0.5 to 1 mL of saline via a syringe with a 25 gauge needle or smaller (see **Fig. 9**). The intestinal tract is flushed, the surgeons change gloves and surgical instrument pack. The abdomen is explored for further foreign bodies or other abnormalities. The laparotomy incision is closed as per surgeon preference.

Surgical technique—resection and anastomosis

In cases where the intestinal tract is severely damaged or perforated by an untreated foreign body, or of intestinal tract neoplasia or granulomas, resection and anastomosis should be considered. The preparation of the patient is identical to what is described earlier. After visualization of the affected tract, the surgeon needs to evaluate the diameter of the intestinal lumen proximally and distally to the pathologic intestinal section. In the author's experience often rabbits with chronic sub-obstruction such as the one caused by neoplasm, show an abnormal distension of the intestinal tract proximal to the affected section (**Fig. 10**). In these cases, an incision perpendicular to the intestinal length is performed orad to the affected section. An incision at 45° is performed aborad to the affected section (see **Fig. 10**). If the oblique incision is not sufficient in

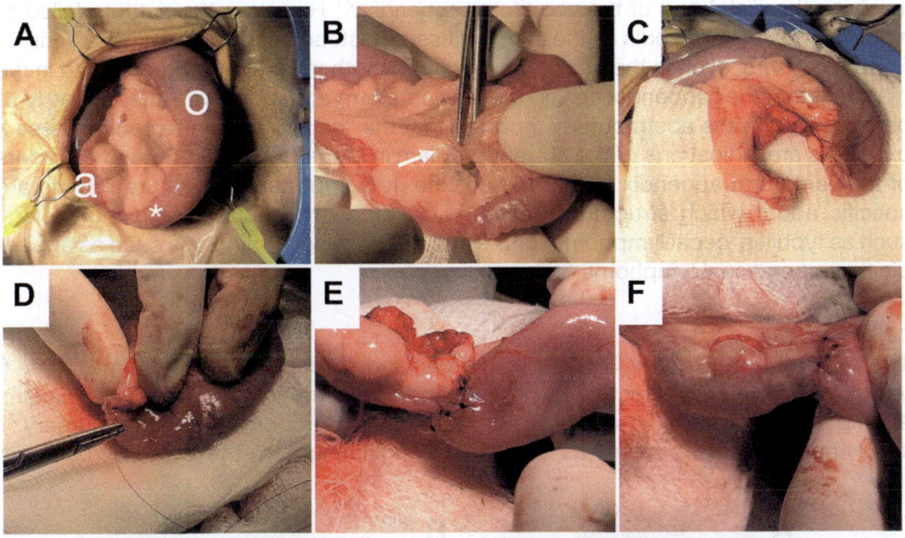

Fig. 10. (*A–F*) Surgical steps for small intestinal resection and anastomosis due to segmental narrowing caused by neoplasm. (*A*) Isolation of the affected area. Notice that the small intestinal tract orad (o) to the neoplasia (*asterisk*) is widely distended due to chronic sub-obstruction, while the small intestinal tract aborad (a) to the neoplasia is normal in diameter. (*B*) Double ligation of the appropriate mesenteric and omental vessels (*arrow*) adjacent to the segment to be resected to provide hemostasis. (*C*) Transection of the affected intestinal segment. The cut angles are planned such that the orad margin is transected at 90° perpendicular to the bowel axis and the aborad margin at 45° relative to the mesenteric border to help match luminal diameters. (*D*) Placement of the initial simple interrupted suture with 5-0 absorbable monofilament (eg, polydioxanone, PDS) at the antimesenteric border, followed by a corresponding suture at the mesenteric border. (*E*) Sequential simple interrupted appositional sutures are placed to approximate the full circumference of the anastomosis. (*F*) The completed anastomosis is leak-tested (eg, saline distention). The previously created omental defect is apposed to restore omental integrity (not shown). (Image Courtesy of Dr Nicola Di Girolamo.)

making intestinal tract of the same lumen diameter, one side of the proximal intestinal end is sutured in order to result in a lumen diameter similar to the one of the distal ends. An end-to-end anastomosis is then performed by placing simple interrupted sutures (PDS 5–0) at 1 to 2 mm of distance from each other around the entire perimeter of the intestinal lumen (see **Fig. 10**). A leak test is performed administering 3 to 5 mL of saline with a syringe with a 25 gauge needle or smaller proximal to the anastomosis and by manipulation of the tract in order to expose any potential leakage (see **Fig. 10**). The intestinal tract is flushed, the surgeons change gloves and the surgical instrument pack. The abdomen is explored for further foreign bodies or other abnormalities. The laparotomy incision is closed as per surgeon preference.

APPENDICEAL DISORDERS

Inflammation, infection, impaction, and neoplasia of the appendix have been described (**Fig. 11**). The inconsistent use of nomenclature for conditions affecting the appendix in the veterinary literature has created confusion in the past. In published case reports, conditions affecting the appendix have been reported affecting the cecum instead, even if the anatomy and function of these 2 contingent tissues are distinct.[21,22] For example, one report had an image showing a neoplasia clearly involving the distal end of the vermiform appendix.[21] However, the authors failed to acknowledge the appendix as the affected tissue, instead defining the tumor as arising from the cecum, even in the title of the article.[21] Another case report mentioned in the main text that the "appendix caecii" (ie, the vermiform appendix) was affected by lymphoma, while in the abstract they reported that the "cecum" was affected.[22] These 2 examples are indications of the current problem in identifying and reporting disorders of the vermiform appendix in rabbit medicine. It is important that future reports are specific about which structure is affected, whether the cecum, using terminology such as typhlitis, cecal lymphoma, or the appendix, using terminology such as appendicitis, appendiceal lymphoma, etc.

Causes

The appendix of the rabbit is a lymphoid organ and susceptible to lymphoma.[21,22] A 6 year old rabbit was affected by an appendiceal lymphoma.[21] The veterinarians attempted removal of the appendiceal mass, but the rabbit died during surgery.[21] The lymphoma in this case was considered originating from the B cells. In another

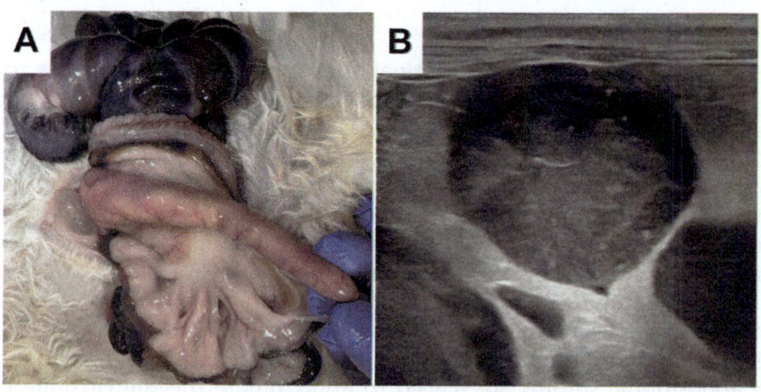

Fig. 11. Appendiceal lymphoma. (*A*) Gross aspect of the appendix upon postmortem. (*B*) Ultrasonographic image of the appendix of the rabbit in panel A, transverse view. Note the thick intestinal wall, loss of wall layering, and lack of normal intestinal content.

report, a 22 month old rabbit suffered a B-cell lymphoma that affected the Harder's gland, mesenteric lymph nodes, and both kidneys, in addition to the appendix.[22] To date there are no reports of successful treatment of appendiceal neoplasia in rabbits. If an actual mass of the appendix is present, excision of the mass in combination with appropriate ancillary oncologic treatments is advised. As such, this article would focus on surgical removal of the appendix during inflammatory conditions.

Although the most obvious explanation for inflammation of the appendix of rabbits may be the invasion of the tissue from bacteria, the process may be more complicated than that. Infiltration with organisms from the lumen, presence of bacteria and debris in the macrophages, and presence of multinucleated giant cells are all typical features of the appendix of clinically healthy rabbits. In humans, there is still controversy over the exact pathophysiology of appendicitis. For example, it is unclear whether bacterial flora within the appendix differs between patients with and without appendicitis.[23] Based on a recent study, the increased diversity of anaerobes and specific anaerobe bacteria may be associated with an increased risk of acute appendicitis, rather than the aerobe bacteria.[24] In rabbits with appendicitis, it is unclear whether bacteria isolated from the appendix are actually responsible for the inflammation, proliferate as a consequence of disrupted activity of the organ, or are normal commensals of the intestinal tract. In a case series of rabbits with appendicitis, 3 out of 5 anaerobic culture grew *Bacteroides fragilis*, and 4 out of 6 aerobic isolates were identified as *Escherichia coli*.[25] In a report including 2 rabbits with appendicitis, both of them grew *Klebsiella variicola*, and one of them grew *Bacteroides sp.*[26] Both *Bacteroides spp.* and *Escherichia* are common inhabitants of the cecum of rabbits.[27,28] In a recent study, epizootic rabbit enteropathy has been induced in rabbits by administration of a low fiber diet.[28] In the rabbits suffering epizootic rabbit enteropathy, the abundance of certain bacteria, including *Escherichia* and *Bacteroides* increased.[28] Perhaps this could predispose rabbits to develop appendicitis. However, none of the rabbits with appendicitis in a case series were fed an improper diet or a diet low in fiber.[25] Other bacteria, cultured from the appendix of rabbits with appendicitis include *Pseudomonas aeruginosa* and *Yersinia pseudotuberculosis*.[25] In some cases of appendicitis, no specific bacteria can be cultured either.[25,29] To further complicate this scenario, a number of potentially pathogenic organisms has been isolated from the appendix of presumed healthy farm rabbits, including *Mycobacterium avium avium*.[30]

Most cases of appendicitis in rabbits occur during summer and fall.[25] Although this trend could merely reflect a higher number of rabbits presented in that period of the year, a previous epidemiologic study on rabbits showed no seasonal variations in number of animals that presented for anorexia and/or lack of defecation to a veterinary clinic.[31] It is possible that exposure to higher environmental temperature during warmer months alters the gastrointestinal microbiota in rabbits and is a concurring factor in the development of acute appendicitis. This hypothesis is supported by the fact that the majority of cases of rabbit appendicitis originates from European countries, where there is a less widespread use of air conditioning as compared with the United States.[32]

Appendicitis seems to be more common in young rabbits, with the median age of affected rabbits being of 2 years of age.[25] This is lower than the median age of presentation of rabbits to primary veterinary care in England (3.2 years)[33] and the mean age of rabbits presented in a different study (3.1 years).[31] It has been observed that appendix size decreases with age both in laboratory and client-owned rabbits.[34,35] Therefore, it is possible that acute appendicitis affects rabbits that still have a well-developed appendix or that are undergoing involution of the organ.

Presenting Complaints and Physical Examination Findings

Almost all rabbits with appendicitis in a case series were anorectic, and over half of them showed a decreased activity or responsiveness.[25] In most rabbits, appendicitis seems to be an acute process, with clinical signs evident for less than 48 hours or no clinical signs at all. However, in some cases appendicitis can be a chronic condition, observed as repeated episodes of anorexia and lack of defecation over time.[25]

More specific findings that could orient the clinician toward appendicitis include elevated temperature, palpation of a tubular abdominal mass, and discomfort on abdominal palpation. In fact, temperature was elevated in over half of the rabbits with appendicitis.[25] The role of fever has been a matter of debate in clinical rabbit medicine, since hyperthermia is rare in hospitalized rabbits, with an estimated prevalence of 1.7% to 2.2% (7 of 316; 2 of 117).[36,37] However, laboratory research has proved that hyperthermia increases the survival rate in rabbits experimentally infected with bacteria.[38] Based on the fact that hyperthermia is uncommon in rabbits, appendicitis should be considered as a differential in rabbits presenting unexplained hyperthermia.

Diagnostics

Blood work

The most characteristic blood work findings in rabbits with appendicitis were hypocalcemia, seen in over two-third of the cases; hypoglycemia, seen in about half of the cases; and anemia, also seen in over half of the cases.[25] Hypoglycemia is an uncommon finding in rabbits, being described in just 1.7% to 4% of rabbits presented to veterinary practices.[13,37] The most likely explanation for hypoglycemia in rabbits with appendicitis is either the consequence of an ineffective colonic fermentation and decreased intestinal absorption, or the development of sepsis. In rabbits with hypoglycemia and hypocalcemia undergoing appendectomy, blood sampling following appendectomy show normalization of these values.[25]

Imaging

Ultrasound and CT can provide an antemortem suspicion of appendiceal disorders in rabbits (see **Fig. 11**).[25,29] The appendix has characteristics ultrasonographic features as compared with the rest of the rabbit gastrointestinal tract. The appendix can be visualized through median and/or left paramedian views in 95.2% (40/42) of the rabbits.[35] The appendix appears as a tubular structure with a multilayered wall, a luminal content with alimentary pattern, and a rounded, closed end. In healthy rabbits, the appendix had no evidence of fluid content, and only in 1 out of 40 healthy rabbits the luminal pattern generated a posterior acoustic shadow that limited visualization of the distal wall of the appendix.[35] Appendiceal disorders should be suspected based on increased thickness of the wall of the appendix, loss of the typical multilayered structure of the appendiceal wall, increase in overall diameter of the appendix, presence of fluid or mucoid content rather than alimentary content in the appendix, or a combination of these factors.[25] Considering that clinical presentations of rabbits with liver lobe torsion are similar to rabbits with appendicitis, inclusion of contrast-enhanced CT or ultrasound in the work-up of rabbits with anorexia is encouraged to rule out both these disorders. It is unknown whether ultrasound or CT can distinguish between inflammation and neoplasia of the appendix.

Treatment Approaches

In humans, treatment of appendicitis depends on several factors.[39–41] In recent years, a non-surgical approach, including administration of antimicrobials, has been proven effective for treatment of uncomplicated appendicitis.[40,41] Cases of complicated appendicitis, such as when there is presence of appendicoliths, perforation, or abscesses of the appendix, typically require surgical treatment. Appendectomy is one of the most common surgical procedures and has been the standard treatment for acute appendicitis for over a century.[39] In rabbits, both medical and surgical treatments have been reported to be effective. A distinction between complicated and uncomplicated appendicitis, similar to that used in human medicine, would likely be beneficial in guiding optimal treatment selection.

Medical Treatment

Medical management of rabbits with appendicitis includes antimicrobial therapy and supportive care. Selection of appropriate antibiotics should take into account the bacteria most commonly involved and their expected antimicrobial susceptibility profiles.[25] Antibiotic coverage for aerobic and anaerobic bacteria should be provided. Based on published susceptibility profiles, fluoroquinolones, particularly marbofloxacin, represent appropriate therapeutic options for treatment of the aerobic bacteria,[25,26] while metronidazole has been used to cover for the anaerobic bacteria.[25,26] However, depending on various factors, including presence of impaction in the appendix, timeliness of the initial medical treatment, medical treatment may be insufficient. In those cases, appendectomy may be required to prevent rupture of the appendix, peritonitis and death. Monitoring should include serial clinical chemistry evaluations, with particular emphasis on glucose and calcium concentrations, as well as point-of-care ultrasonography to assess for signs of peritonitis. Decreases of glucose and calcium levels should be taken as a sign of likely sepsis and treated accordingly.[25]

Surgical Treatment

Surgical technique—appendectomy

Laparotomy is performed as described earlier. When enlarged, the appendix is typically in contact with the ventral abdominal wall and can be easily visualized. In contrast, retrieving a normal-sized appendix requires retraction of the cecum dorsocranially to expose the appendix located dorsal to it (**Fig. 12**). During appendectomy, the ileocecal fold needs to be excised in order to isolate the rabbit appendix from the remainder of the intestinal tract. Considering the large number and small caliber of vessels, as well as the length of the ileocecal fold, radiosurgery is ideal for excision of this ligament (see **Fig. 12**). Cautery should be applied as close to the appendix as possible to minimize the risk of iatrogenic injury to the ileum. After excision of the ileocecal fold, 2 circumferential ligatures are placed at the base of the appendix, followed by placement of an intestinal clamp distal to the sutures and subsequent excision of the appendix (see **Fig. 12**).[25] An alternative technique, analogous to intestinal resection and anastomosis, has also been described, in which the appendix is first resected and the cecum subsequently sutured. Given the thinness of the cecal wall, direct cecal suturing rather than circumferential ligation may be technically more challenging. Notably, both rabbits that underwent this alternative technique died during the post-operative period.[25] Based on these findings, the former technique is recommended.

Intestinal Biopsy

Indications for intestinal biopsy in rabbits include protein-losing enteropathy, intestinal thickening/masses visualized on imaging, or chronic, unresponsive diarrhea. In rabbits, upper gastrointestinal endoscopy and biopsy are not routinely performed. Endoscopic biopsies are difficult to obtain because complete removal of gastric ingesta is

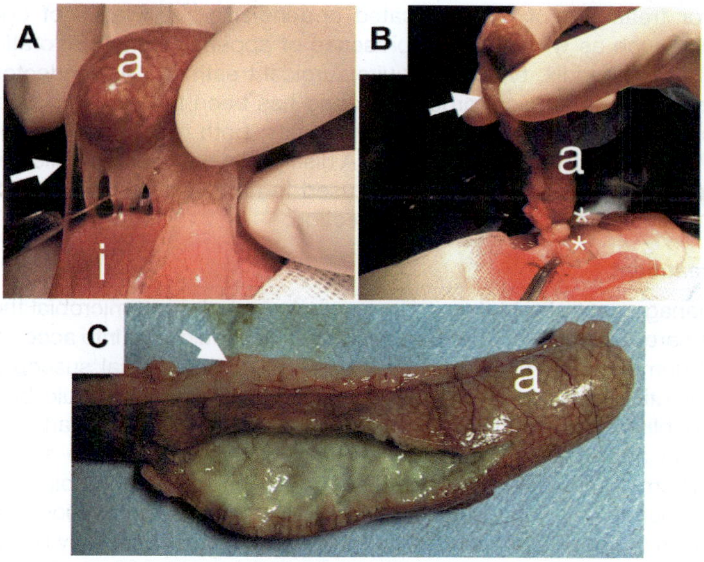

Fig. 12. (*A–C*) Surgical steps for appendectomy in the rabbit. (*A*) Following identification of the appendix (a), the ileocecal ligament (*arrow*) is cauterized using bipolar electrosurgery or ligated and sharply transected as close to the appendix as possible to minimize risk of iatrogenic trauma to the ileum (i). (*B*) After division of the ileocecal ligament (*arrow*), 2 circumferential ligatures using 4-0 absorbable monofilament suture are placed on the proximal appendix approximately 2 to 3 mm distal to the cecal junction (*asterisks*). The appendix is then sharply excised distal to the ligatures. (*C*) Appendix after excision showing purulent content. Samples are collected for aerobic, anaerobic, and fungal culture, and the excised tissue is submitted for histopathologic evaluation. Note the ileocecal ligament (*arrow*). (Image Courtesy of Dr Nicola Di Girolamo.)

technically challenging and carries inherent risks. In addition, the rabbit gastrointestinal tract is fragile, and excessive insufflation or intraluminal pressure may result in rupture. In a pilot study, gastrointestinal endoscopy was attempted in 2 New Zealand white rabbits.[42] One of the 2 rabbits suffered a perforation of the esophagus in the 24 hours following the procedure.[42] As such, in cases in which an intestinal biopsy is indicated, laparotomic, incisional biopsies are typically obtained.

Surgical technique—intestinal biopsies

Laparotomy and isolation of the intestinal tract are performed as previously described. Luminal contents are gently milked away from the biopsy site, which is then isolated using sterile hair clips or manual compression by an assistant. A full-thickness incision is made using a No. 11 or No. 15 scalpel blade, preferably on the antimesenteric border of the intestine, oriented either perpendicular or parallel to the long axis of the intestine. A second incision is then made to obtain an intestinal biopsy measuring approximately 1 to 2 mm in width (**Fig. 13**). The sample is placed in a cassette and immersed in formalin. The enterotomy site is subsequently closed as previously described (see **Fig. 13**).

POSTOPERATIVE CARE

Rabbits undergoing intestinal surgery often require intensive post-operative monitoring. Rabbits should be monitored closely for 72 to 96 hours to detect intestinal dehiscence early. In case of generic intestinal surgery, intravenous antimicrobial

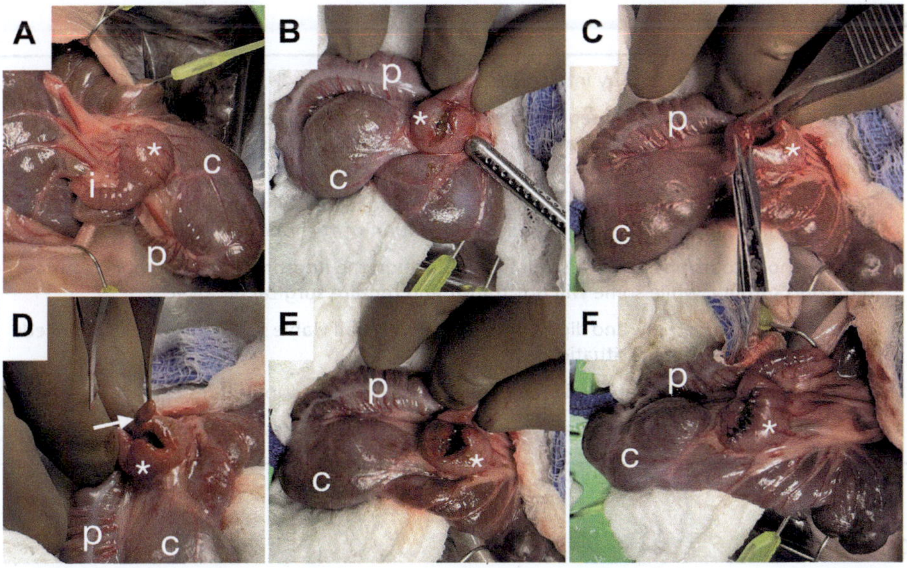

Fig. 13. (*A–F*) Surgical steps for obtainment of an intestinal biopsy from the sacculus rotundus. (*A*) the sacculus rotundus (*asterisk*) is identified, together with its connections with the ileum (i), cecum (c), and proximal colon (p). (*B*) A 4 to 5 mm incision is performed with a blade No. 15 of the center of the sacculus rotundus. Suction is used as needed. (*C*) Tenotomy scissors are used to obtain a full-thickness biopsy, in this instance approximately 2 mm in width. (*D*) Close-up view of the full thickness biopsy (*arrow*). (*E*) Appearance of the sacculus rotundus after obtainment of the biopsy. (*F*) The intestinal tract is apposed with simple interrupted suture with 5-0 absorbable monofilament (eg, polydioxanone, PDS). (Image Courtesy of Dr Nicola Di Girolamo.)

therapy cover typically consists in metronidazole (20 mg/kg, q12 h) and enrofloxacin (7.5 mg/kg q24 h). Fluid therapy (LRS, 5 mL/kg/hour) and lidocaine CRI is typically continued for the following 2 to 3 days. In more critically ill rabbits, vasopressors, particularly norepinephrine (starting from 0.2 mcg/kg/min), have anecdotally appeared to be beneficial during the post-operative period. Antimicrobial therapy is subsequently transitioned to oral administration and continued for approximately 10 days, depending on the individual case.

It is not uncommon for normal defecation to resume 24 to 48 hours following surgery, and this delay is not necessarily indicative of abnormal healing. Rabbits have a significantly longer gastrointestinal transit time compared with carnivorous mammals. Reported transit times in rabbits are approximately 14 hours when fed a high-fiber diet and up to 20 hours when fed a low-fiber diet,[43] assuming a normal caloric intake, which is rarely achieved in the immediate post-operative period.

SUMMARY

Intestinal surgery in rabbits is still poorly described in the scientific literature. Advances in diagnostic imaging, particularly the introduction of abdominal CT scans, now allow more precise diagnosis of intestinal disorders in rabbits. Advances in anesthesia and post-operative care results in improved outcomes. Overall, these medical advances enable veterinarians to offer tailored treatment options to the individual rabbit patient in a similar fashion as it is offered to dogs and cats.

CLINICS CARE POINTS

- Rabbits are often affected by intestinal disorders.
- Intestinal disorders that may require a surgical approach include obstructions caused by trichobezoars/phytobezoars, subobstructions caused by hyperplasia, neoplasia or adhesions, appendiceal inflammation and neoplasia, among others.
- Advanced diagnostic imaging, particularly CT scanning, allows a more precise visualization of the rabbit intestinal tract, including size and location of trichobezoars/phytobezoars.
- Most trichobezoars/phytobezoars will transit through the intestinal tract of rabbits, without requiring surgery, while some will not transit and require surgical removal.
- Enterotomy, enterectomy, and digital manipulation are all viable surgical options, that needs to be applied in different situations.
- The rabbit appendix can be safely removed surgically without long term implications.
- Intestinal biopsies can be obtained for diagnosis of chronic intestinal conditions.

DISCLOSURE

The author would like to thank Dr Paolo Selleri for his early collaboration in the development of the surgical techniques presented here.

REFERENCES

1. Huffman KW. Gross and histological studies of the digestive tract of the rabbit. Thesis. Kansas State University; 1958. Available at: https://krex.k-state.edu/server/api/core/bitstreams/414f5173-8133-464e-a063-25060030732f/content.
2. Botha GM. Histological observations on the gastro-oesophageal junction in the rabbit. J Anat 1958;92(Pt 3):441.
3. Carmichael EB, Strickland JT, Driver RL. The contents of the stomach, small intestine, cecum and colon of normal and fasting rabbits. Am J Physiol 1945;143(4):562–6.
4. Harcourt-Brown FM. Gastric dilation and intestinal obstruction in 76 rabbits. Vet Rec 2007;161(12):409–14.
5. Di Girolamo N, Tollefson C. Computed tomographic diagnosis and clinical outcomes of small intestinal obstruction caused by trichobezoars in client-owned rabbits. Vet Radiol Ultrasound 2024;65(3):264–74.
6. Smith HF, Fisher RE, Everett ML, et al. Comparative anatomy and phylogenetic distribution of the mammalian cecal appendix. J Evol Biol 2009;22(10):1984–99.
7. Barone R, Pavaux C, Blin PC, et al. Atlas d'anatomie du lapin: atlas of rabbit anatomy. Masson & Cie, Soulisse et Cassegrain 1973;pp1–219.
8. Haines RA, Urbiztondo RA, Haynes RA, et al. Characterization of New Zealand white rabbit gut-associated lymphoid tissues and use as viral oncology animal model. ILAR J 2016;57(1):34–43.
9. Jasper PJ, Zhai SK, Kalis SL, et al. B lymphocyte development in rabbit: progenitor B cells and waning of B lymphopoiesis. J Immunol 2003;171(12):6372–80.
10. Winter N, Clauss M, Codron D, et al. Sand accumulation in the digestive tract of rabbits (Oryctolagus cuniculus) and Guinea pigs (Cavia porcellus): the role of the appendix. J Morphol 2022;283(1):5–15.
11. Schuhmann B, Cope I. Medical treatment of 145 cases of gastric dilatation in rabbits. Vet Rec 2014;175(19):484.

12. Debenham JJ, Brinchmann T, Sheen J, et al. Radiographic diagnosis of small intestinal obstruction in pet rabbits (Oryctolagus cuniculus): 63 cases. J Small Anim Pract 2019;60(11):691–6.
13. Harcourt-Brown FM, Harcourt-Brown SF. Clinical value of blood glucose measurement in pet rabbits. Vet Rec 2012;170(26):674.
14. Sheen JC, Sladakovic I, Finch S. Prognostic indicators for survival in surgically managed small intestinal obstruction in pet rabbits: 141 presentations (2011-2021). J Am Vet Med Assoc 2023;261(12):1–10.
15. Steinagel AC, Oglesbee BL. Clinicopathological and radiographic indicators for orogastric decompression in rabbits presenting with intestinal obstruction at a referral hospital (2015-2018). Vet Rec 2023;192(5):e2481.
16. Huckins GL, Tournade C, Patson C, et al. Lidocaine constant rate infusion improves the probability of survival in rabbits with gastrointestinal obstructions: 64 cases (2012-2021). J Am Vet Med Assoc 2023;262(1):61–7.
17. Di Girolamo N, Maranville RE, Pathak D, et al. The 4 prokinetic drugs metoclopramide, cisapride, pyridostigmine, and capromorelin do not increase fecal output or food intake in healthy New Zealand rabbits (Oryctolagus cuniculus). J Am Vet Med Assoc 2025;2:1–7.
18. Husnik R, Gaschen F. Gastric motility disorders in dogs and cats. Vet Clin North Am Small Anim Pract 2021;51(1):43–59. PMID: 33187622.
19. Uccello O, Sanchez A, Valverde A, et al. Cardiovascular effects of increasing dosages of norepinephrine in healthy isoflurane-anesthetized New Zealand white rabbits. Vet Anaesth Analg 2020;47(6):781–8.
20. CVC E365.
21. Ishikawa M, Maeda H, Kondo H, et al. A case of lymphoma developing in the rabbit cecum. J Vet Med Sci 2007;69:1183–5.
22. Volopich S, Gruber A, Hassan J, et al. Malignant b-cell lymphoma of the Harder's gland in a rabbit. Vet Ophthalmol 2005;8:259–63.
23. Flum DR. Clinical practice. Acute appendicitis–appendectomy or the "antibiotics first" strategy. N Engl J Med 2015;372:1937–43.
24. Hattori I, Yuasa N, Ikegami S, et al. Culture-based bacterial evaluation of the appendix lumen in patients with and without acute appendicitis. J Infect Chemother 2019;25:708–13.
25. Di Girolamo N, Petrini D, Szabo Z, et al. Clinical, surgical, and pathological findings in client-owned rabbits with histologically confirmed appendicitis: 19 cases (2015-2019). J Am Vet Med Assoc 2021;260(1):82–93.
26. Jekl V, Piskovska A, Drnkova I, et al. Case report: spontaneous appendicitis with suspected involvement of Klebsiella variicola in two pet rabbits. Front Vet Sci 2021;8:779517.
27. Velasco-Galilea M, Piles M, Viñas M, et al. Rabbit microbiota changes throughout the intestinal tract. Front Microbiol 2018;9:2144.
28. Jin DX, Zou HW, Liu SQ, et al. The underlying microbial mechanism of epizootic rabbit enteropathy triggered by a low fiber diet. Sci Rep 2018;8:12489.
29. Longo M, Thierry F, Eatwell K, et al. Ultrasound and computed tomography of sacculitis and appendicitis in a rabbit. Vet Radiol Ultras 2018;59:E56–60.
30. Arrazuria R, Sevilla IA, Molina E, et al. Detection of Mycobacterium avium subspecies in the gut associated lymphoid tissue of slaughtered rabbits. BMC Vet Res 2015;11:130.
31. Huynh M, Vilmouth S, Gonzalez MS, et al. Retrospective cohort study of gastrointestinal stasis in pet rabbits. Vet Rec 2014;175:225–6.

32. Jakubcionis M, Carlsson J. Estimation of European Union residential sector space cooling potential. Energy Policy 2017;101:225–35.
33. O'Neill DG, Craven HC, Brodbelt DC, et al. Morbidity and mortality of domestic rabbits (*Oryctolagus cuniculus*) under primary veterinary care in England. Vet Rec 2020;186:451.
34. Dasso JF, Obiakor H, Bach H, et al. A morphological and immunohistological study of the human and rabbit appendix for comparison with the avian bursa. Dev Comp Immunol 2000;24:797–814.
35. Nicoletti A, Di Girolamo N, Zeyen U, et al. Ultrasound morphology of cecal appendix in pet rabbits. J Ultrasound 2018;21:287–91.
36. Di Girolamo N, Toth G, Selleri P. Prognostic value of rectal temperature at hospital admission in client-owned rabbits. J Am Vet Med Assoc 2016;248:288–97.
37. Oparil KM, Gladden JN, Babyak JM, et al. Clinical characteristics and short-term outcomes for rabbits with signs of gastrointestinal tract dysfunction: 117 cases (2014-2016). J Am Vet Med Assoc 2019;255:837–45.
38. Kluger MJ, Vaughn LK. Fever and survival in rabbits infected with Pasteurella multocida. J Physiol 1978;282:243–51.
39. McBurney C. Experience with early operative interference in cases of disease of the vermiform appendix. NY Med J 1889;50:676–84.
40. Salminen P, Paajanen H, Rautio T, et al. Antibiotic therapy vs appendectomy for treatment of uncomplicated acute appendicitis: the APPAC randomized clinical trial. JAMA 2015;313:2340–8.
41. Vons C, Barry C, Maitre S, et al. Amoxicillin plus clavulanic acid versus appendicectomy for treatment of acute uncomplicated appendicitis: an open-label, non-inferiority, randomised controlled trial. Lancet 2011;377:1573–9.
42. Pignon C, Crescence L. Upper gastrointestinal flexible endoscopy in rabbits: a pilot study. Exoticscon conference proceedings 2023;443.
43. Gidenne T. Effect of fibre level, particle size and adaptation period on digestibility and rate of passage as measured at the ileum and in the faeces in the adult rabbit. Br J Nutr 1992;67(1):133–46.

Gastrointestinal Surgery in Other Small Mammals

Isabelle Desprez, DVM, Dipl ECZM (SM), Dipl ABVP (ECM)[a,*],
David Guillier, DVM, Dipl ECZM (SM)[b],
Laëtitia Volait-Rosset, DVM, MVS, Dipl ECZM (SM), Dipl ABVP (ECM)[c]

KEYWORDS

- Ferret • Guinea pig • Chinchilla • Rat • African pigmy hedgehog
- Gastrointestinal surgery • Gastrointestinal biopsy • Gastric dilatation and volvulus

KEY POINTS

- Exotic small mammals require species-specific perioperative strategies, with hypothermia, hypoglycemia, and hyperglycemia being key prognostic indicators guiding stabilization and anesthetic planning.
- GI surgery in ferrets, rodents, and hedgehogs has evolved toward early intervention and minimally invasive-inspired approaches, with recent case reports demonstrating successful adaptations of stenting, feeding tubes, and refined reconstructive techniques.
- Hindgut fermenters (especially guinea pigs and chinchillas) are uniquely predisposed to postoperative ileus and dysbiosis, making gentle surgical handling, multimodal analgesia, early enteral nutrition, hydration, and prudent antimicrobial use central to outcome.
- Outcome is highly variable and condition-dependent, with guarded prognosis in pathologies like gastric dilatation-volvulus in guinea pigs but excellent recovery potential in focal, well-stabilized surgical cases (eg, foreign bodies in ferrets).

INTRODUCTION

Gastrointestinal (GI) diseases are considered as common in pet ferrets, rodents, and African pygmy hedgehogs (APH), and surgical management may be indicated.[1–6] Many procedures performed in companion exotic mammals are similar to those performed in dogs and cats, the main differences being perioperative management and adjusting to exotic patients' size and specific anatomy.[7] This review aims at providing an overview of the most recent information available on surgical management of GI diseases in pet ferrets, rodents and APH, excluding disorders of the oral cavity.

[a] Department of Small Animal Clinical Sciences, Western College of Veterinary Medicine, Saskatoon, Saskatoon, Canada; [b] Exotic Pet Service, Clinique Vétérinaire Ric et Rac, Le Cannet, France; [c] Rabbit, Exotics & Wildlife Medicine and Surgery, Royal (Dick) School of Veterinary Studies, Easter Bush Campus, Midlothian, UK
* Corresponding author. 52 Campus Drive, Saskatoon, SK S7N 5B4 Canada.
E-mail address: isabelle.desprez@gmail.com

Vet Clin Exot Anim 29 (2026) 715–730
https://doi.org/10.1016/j.cvex.2026.04.014 vetexotic.theclinics.com

Abbreviations	
APH	African pygmy hedgehogs
GDV	gastric dilatation-volvulus
GI	Gastrointestinal
PCV	packed cell volume
POI	postoperative ileus

PRESURGICAL CONSIDERATIONS

Irrespective of the surgical indication, presurgical assessment of the patient is essential to minimize the risk of adverse surgical outcomes. Whenever possible, appropriate triage and stabilization should be performed before anesthesia and surgery.

A thorough physical examination should be conducted, including rectal temperature measurement as part of the triage protocol.[8–11] Hypothermia at presentation has been associated with increased mortality in several species. In ferrets, hypothermia (<37.8°C) was associated with 3.72 times the odds of death compared with normothermia.[12] A similar association has been reported in guinea pigs (<37.9°C), where hypothermic individuals had nearly 3 times the odds of death.[13] Hyperthermia was less frequently observed and did not appear associated with outcome in these studies. Therefore, identification of hypothermia is important for prognostic assessment and perioperative management.

While complete blood count and serum biochemistry are part of a suitable initial database for general health status assessment, it may not be realistic in all patients, especially if unstable or very small in size.[7] Collection of a small amount of blood may, however, still be beneficial to help determine prognosis. A drop of blood allows for immediate blood glucose measurement, and marked hyperglycemia has been associated with less favorable outcomes in several species. Ferrets that were presented with a blood glucose over 152 mg/dL (8.64 mmol/L) had 2.61 times the odds of dying compared to normoglycemic ferrets[12] while in APH, severe hyperglycemia (≥180 mg/dL or 10 mmol/L) on presentation was associated with increased mortality.[14] In hyperglycemic APH, mortality also increased with increasing degree of anorexia, reaching 82% in APH that were simultaneously severely hyperglycemic and completely anorectic.[14] Determining packed cell volume (PCV) is also relevant to assess a patient's general condition and prognosis. A study conducted in ferrets showed that ferrets presented with a PCV lower than 33% had 4.74 times the odds of dying compared to ferrets that did not have anemia on presentation. These elements, along with physical examination and history collection, allow for estimation of the overall anesthetic and surgical risk, and give an opportunity for better preparation.

ANESTHESIA AND ANALGESIA CONSIDERATIONS

Recommended preoperative fasting times are generally short for rodents as they are unable to vomit and have fast metabolic rate, predisposing them to possible complications following prolonged fast, such as hypoglycemia.[7,15] The main goal of fasting rodents is to allow for them to swallow their oral cavity content and prevent aspiration of that content during anesthesia. Depending on patient age, health status, and size, fasting times of 0 to 3 hours are typically sufficient for pet rodents.[15] While ferrets can vomit, they also have a short GI transit time and are prone to insulinomas, which predispose them to hypoglycemia. Prolonged fasting is therefore not recommended, and 1 to 4 hours is usually deemed sufficient.[7,15] Conflicting information is found on preanesthetic fasting in APH, some sources stating that APH should be fasted for 4 to 6 hours before anesthesia, especially if the procedure is anticipated to last more than 20 minutes,[16,17] while other sources state that fasting is not recommended due to the small body size, small glucose reserves, and high metabolic rates.[18,19] In a study investigating the postanesthetic effects of two durations of isoflurane anesthesia in APH, the animals were fasted for a minimum of 80 minutes before being masked down with isoflurane and maintained under anesthesia for either 15 or 45 minutes.[20] No GI adverse effects, such as vomiting or regurgitations, were observed during that study, and the authors therefore suspect that prolonged preanesthetic fasting time may not be necessary in that species.[20]

While ferrets are easily intubated, rodents may pose more of a challenge and may require the use of an endoscope. An alternative to endotracheal intubation for pet rodents is to use a tight-fitting facemask. This does not protect the airway, but allows for delivery of oxygen and inhalant anesthesia and some degree of manual ventilation if needed.[15] As the airway remains unprotected, rinsing the oral cavity before anesthesia is advisable. The successful use of a rabbit supraglottic airway device has been reported in an APH, which offers another option for airway control in that species.[21] A complete review of anesthesia protocols is beyond the scope of this review, but the anesthesia protocol should be tailored to each individual patient, taking into account the overall health status, procedure planned, and anticipated risks. Various resources can be consulted to optimize the choice for anesthesia protocol.[15,22–24] Monitoring during anesthesia is essential, as ferrets, rodents and APH are small size patients, all prompt to hypothermia, hypoventilation, and hypotension under anesthesia, and the clinical status can change quickly.[15] Supportive care, such as active warming or fluids, should be provided as needed, but also preemptively if possible, to reduce the intensity of changes that may occur during anesthesia and surgery. Analgesia should also be provided preemptively to minimize the risk for central sensitization, which may lead to increased postoperative pain.[25]

SURGICAL PREPARATION

Surgeon's aseptic preparation for GI surgeries in exotic companion mammals is similar to that for canine or feline patients. For patient preparation, care must be taken not to damage the skin during clipping or aseptic preparation.[7] This can be achieved by being very delicate while shaving, and using very fine clipper blades. The action of scrubbing may also lead to skin lesions that are detrimental to prevention of infection. Application of chlorhexidine gluconate 4% solution for 225 seconds was shown to be equally as effective as mechanical scrubbing of the surgical area with the same solution in horses.[26] This represents a suitable alternative to mechanical scrubbing, which is more likely to damage the skin in exotic companion mammals. Another concern about surgical aseptic preparation is the potential for hypothermia caused by the surgical scrub. A study conducted on mice compared the effects of rinsing with 70% isopropyl alcohol to rinsing with saline, either room temperature or warmed to 37°C (98.6°F). These various options were used alone or following surgical preparation with povidone-iodine.[27] The study showed that all scrubbing regimens significantly decreased body temperature at the time of application. Treatments including povidone-iodine decreased core temperature the most and for the longest and rinsing it with warm saline rather than room-temperature saline did not improve heat loss. Interestingly, isopropyl alcohol triggered the most intense cooling, but also a rebound effect, leading to body temperature returning to the level of control animals within minutes of application.[27] The conclusion of the study was that while isopropyl alcohol is not a suitable scrubbing regimen as a standalone, using it to rinse instead of saline should be encouraged as it appears to cause less hypothermia.[7,27] Alcohol-based antiseptic solution also appears to evaporate faster and cause less prolonged hypothermia, and is suitable for surgical preparation.[7]

Proper draping is indicated and should follow the same principles as for canine or feline patients. Using clear plastic drapes is beneficial in small patients to allow for breathing monitoring visually, should other equipment fail.[7] The drapes can be secured in various ways. Sticky drapes are available, with the limitation that some do not seem to be sticky enough to stay in place, while some others stick too much and can cause skin damage upon removal. If surgical drape forceps are deemed too traumatic for smaller patients, the drapes can be sutured or stapled to the patient.

Appropriate surgical instruments and magnification should be used. A wide array of microsurgical tools are available and can be used for smaller patients. Additionally, surgical tools can be repurposed as needed. For example, blepharostats can be used as abdominal retractors in smaller patients, and sterilized bobby pins can be used *in lieu* of Doyen intestinal forceps. Retractors with elastic stays are also popular for various purposes in exotic pet medicine, as well as sterile cotton tip applicators, which can be used to aid in blunt dissection, tissue handling, and hemostasis. As any blood loss will matter for a small-sized patient, magnification (eg, surgical loupes or surgical microscope) should be used to detect and manage any bleeding as early as possible but also visualize smaller vessels and preemptively control bleeding. Various hemostasis techniques should be considered, such as hemostatic clips, which come in a range of sizes and are easier and faster to place than ligatures, absorbable gelatin sponges, and electrocautery or vessel sealing devices.[7]

The overall surgical technique should be as fast as possible while being gentle as in smaller patients, tissues can be more fragile.

SURGICAL TECHNIQUES BY REGION

This review focuses on the major advancements in GI surgery over the last decade. Rather than revisiting long-established procedures such as standard enterotomy or simple gastrotomy, this section highlights modern adaptations, novel case reports, and species-specific refinements that have emerged in the recent literature. Exotic mammal GI surgery now prioritizes minimally invasive approaches when possible, early intervention based on improved diagnostic capabilities, and advanced reconstruction techniques once considered too risky for small patients.

ESOPHAGUS

Esophageal disease remains relatively uncommon in ferrets and is even less frequently reported in rodents and APH. However, recent case reports have demonstrated successful management of esophageal foreign bodies in ferrets using minimally invasive techniques, including endoscopic retrieval, balloon dilation, and in one case esophageal stenting.[28] Treatment included endoscopic retrieval, balloon dilation, and in one case esophageal stenting. Outcomes were generally favorable, with most patients able to return to a normal diet and high owner satisfaction reported.

In APH, placement of an esophagostomy tube following traumatic subtotal glossectomy has been demonstrated to be feasible with species-specific modifications, using an 8 Fr red rubber catheter.[29] Secure dorsal fixation methods allowed hedgehog to maintain natural rolling behaviors without risking tube displacement. These innovations illustrate how techniques traditionally reserved for dogs and cats have been successfully adapted to small exotic mammals.

STOMACH

Gastric Dilatation-Volvulus

Gastric dilatation-volvulus (GDV) has become increasingly recognized in guinea pigs, but still carries a poor prognosis. In a recent review of eight cases of GDV diagnosed on pet guinea pigs, only 2 animals survived surgical correction.[30]

The etiology of GDV in guinea pigs is likely multifactorial, and a combination of intrinsic and extrinsic factors may contribute to the development of GDV in this species. In this case series, postmortem examinations failed to determine a definitive underlying cause in any case. Diagnosis is based on orthogonal radiographic projections with the stomach conspicuously displaced to the right side of the abdomen in cases involving a 180° torsion (**Fig. 1**). Common other radiographic findings include a markedly dilated, gas-filled stomach, with small intestinal loops displaced cranially.

As in dogs, treatment is surgical. Exploratory laparotomy is performed through a ventral midline incision (**Fig. 2**). After identification of the stomach, ventral gastrotomy is performed between the greater and lesser curvatures to evacuate gastric contents. The stomach is lavaged and closed in 2 inverting seromuscular layers. The small intestines are repositioned anatomically, and the stomach returned to its normal orientation. The abdomen is lavaged with sterile saline and closed routinely in 3 layers. Gastropexy was attempted in some cases, although notably, both survivors did not undergo gastropexy.

GDV has been recently described in a 7 month old neutered male pet rat that presented for acute onset of pica, regurgitation, anorexia, and lethargy.[31] The rat exhibited marked pain responses upon cranial abdominal palpation, including vocalization. Whole-body radiographs of the anesthetized patient revealed a severely gas-dilated stomach containing soft tissue material. Based on the history of foreign material ingestion and persistent regurgitation, gastric dilatation secondary to foreign-body obstruction was suspected, and exploratory laparotomy was elected. Celiotomy revealed a small volume of serosanguinous fluid and a markedly distended stomach rotated approximately 180° clockwise, confirming GDV. Gentle derotation with moistened cotton applicators resulted in spontaneous gastric decompression without the

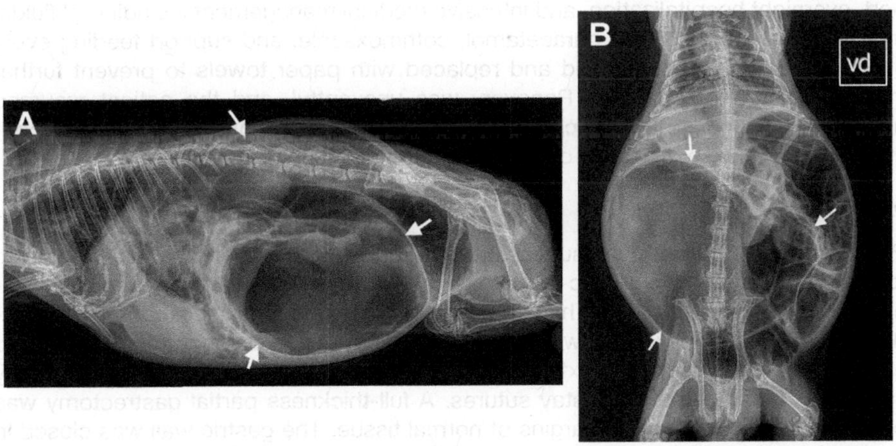

Fig. 1. (*A, B*) Radiography of a guinea pig with GDV. (*A*) Right latero-lateral view, (*B*) Ventro-dorsal view. The stomach (*white arrows*) is severely dilated, displaced in the right part of the abdomen, and filled with gas. (Image Courtesy of Dr José Rosas-Navarro.)

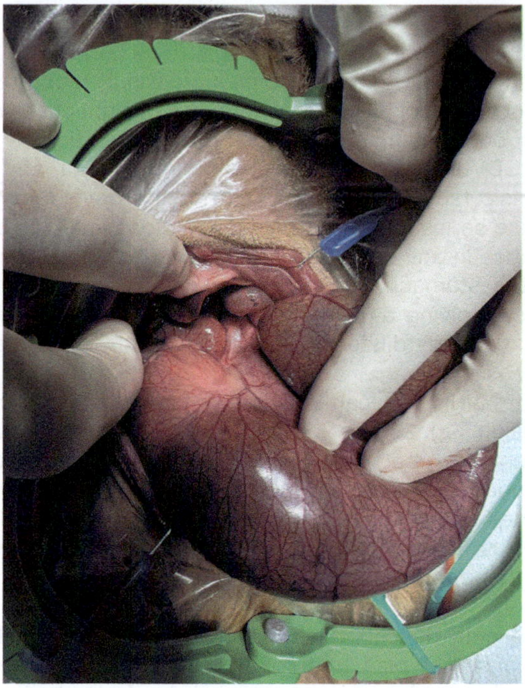

Fig. 2. Intraoperative view showing the torsion of the stomach. (Image Courtesy of Dr José Rosas-Navarro.)

need for trocarization or orogastric tubing. The stomach was exteriorized and isolated with saline-moistened swabs. A full thickness gastrotomy was performed in the fundus and extended approximately 2 cm. Large quantities of blue bedding material were removed. The gastrotomy was closed in 2 layers. Abdominal exploration revealed no additional GI pathology. The abdomen was lavaged with warm sterile saline and closed routinely. Postoperative care consisted of supplemental oxygen, thermal support, overnight hospitalization, and intensive medical management including IV fluids, maropitant, buprenorphine, paracetamol, cotrimoxazole, and support feeding every 4 hours. Bedding was withheld and replaced with paper towels to prevent further ingestion of foreign material. Recovery was uneventful, and the patient resumed normal activity and appetite. Pica and foreign-material ingestion were suspected contributors in this case, although causation could not be definitively established.

Partial Gastrectomy

Partial gastrectomy has been successfully performed in a 4 year old male guinea pig for the management of a gastric leiomyoma.[32] The animal presented for a routine wellness examination was found to have a small, firm mass in the cranial abdomen. A standard ventral midline celiotomy was performed, and a self-retaining retractor facilitated exposure. The stomach was exteriorized, isolated with saline-moistened laparotomy sponges, and stabilized with stay sutures. A full-thickness partial gastrectomy was performed with 1 cm gross margins of normal tissue. The gastric wall was closed in a full-thickness continuous pattern oriented transversally to the long axis of the stomach to maintain luminal diameter and minimize postoperative functional narrowing. A leak test with sterile saline delivered through a 27 gauge needle confirmed an intact closure. Recovery from anesthesia was uneventful, and abdominal ultrasonography performed 19 months later showed no evidence of recurrence.

Gastrotomy and Jejunostomy Tube Placement

Combined gastrostomy and jejunostomy tube placement can be an effective surgical strategy for managing severe idiopathic gastric distention and ensuring enteral support in ferrets, particularly when conventional correction of pyloric outflow obstruction is not feasible.

To manage a severe gastric stasis and provide enteral nutrition, both a gastrostomy tube and jejunostomy tube were placed in 8 month old spayed female ferret which developed recurrent, severe gastric distention after gastrotomy for foreign-body removal.[33] An 8 Fr jejunostomy tube was introduced through a left abdominal incision and advanced 5 cm into the duodenum via the pylorus, while a 14 Fr gastrostomy tube was placed directly into the left gastric fundus via a reopened gastrotomy. Each tube was secured to the gastric wall with a purse-string pattern, and the skin was anchored using a finger-trap suture. A fundic gastropexy was performed to prevent rotation or displacement of the gastrostomy site. Postoperatively, the feeding tubes allowed gastric decompression, bypass feeding, and intensive medical management. The ferret tolerated both tubes without complications and made a full recovery.

SMALL INTESTINE

Gastrointestinal Biopsies

In ferrets and other small mammals with chronic diarrhea unresponsive to empirical therapy, standard first-line diagnostics (eg, fecal testing, bloodwork, imaging, and fine-needle aspiration) can fail to identify an underlying cause. Because ultrasonographic changes in intestinal thickness or layering may be subtle or entirely absent, and cytology lacks sensitivity for most of lesions, early exploratory laparotomy with full-thickness biopsies should be considered. Comprehensive surgical biopsies of the mesenteric lymph node, stomach, duodenum, jejunum, ileum, liver, and pancreas have been shown to provide the diagnostic clarity needed in ferrets, including confirmation of conditions such as epitheliotropic GI T-cell lymphoma that would otherwise be missed with less invasive methods.[34] Consequently, laparotomy with systematic biopsies remains the most reliable diagnostic approach in ferrets with persistent, unexplained GI disease.

Exploratory laparotomy with targeted gastric and intestinal biopsies has been performed in a 2 month old intact female APH with unexplained vomiting for 1 week.[35] A ventral midline celiotomy was performed and showed mild pyloric wall thickening and moderate gastric gas distension, but no foreign body or mechanical obstruction. Laparotomy allowed a full-thickness gastric biopsy by gastrotomy and enterotomy biopsy, both closed with simple interrupted sutures. Histopathology revealed eosinophilic gastroenteritis. Medical management was instituted following diagnosis, and the patient showed clinical improvement.

Intussusception

Intussusception must be considered a surgical differential in small mammals presenting with gastric dilatation, acute abdominal signs, or a palpable abdominal mass. Obstructive ileus can progress rapidly and requires early exploratory laparotomy for definitive diagnosis and potential surgical correction before irreversible decompensation occurs.

Although intestinal intussusception is considered uncommon in pet guinea pigs, several cases have been reported. These include an ileocolic intussusception in a young female,[36] a case in a 3 day old guinea pig with a congenital imperforate anus and bowel rupture,[37] and a larger case series documenting 49 spontaneous small-intestinal intussusceptions in young guinea pigs within a closed breeding colony, though the specific intestinal locations were not described.[38]

In a recent case report, postmortem examination revealed a jejuno-jejunal intussusception causing mechanical GI obstruction and secondary ileus in a guinea pig presented with hyporexia, painful defecation, and intermittent rolling behavior.[39] Abdominal palpation and imaging identified a firm caudal abdominal mass and a gastric dilatation without volvulus. The patient deteriorated rapidly, developing severe gastric reflux of foul-smelling fluid, and euthanasia was elected due to the grave prognosis.

COLON AND ANUS

Colonic Obstructive Foreign Bodies

A case series describes 7 chinchillas diagnosed with colonic obstructive foreign bodies between 2017 and 2020, all presenting with a complete absence of fecal output.[40] Ultrasonography proved highly informative, revealing a hyperechoic intraluminal structure with marked acoustic shadowing in 86% of cases, while plain abdominal radiographs demonstrated variable degrees of gas or fluid distension. Positive-contrast barium studies further supported the diagnosis by showing markedly prolonged GI transit. Obstruction sites were located in the distal ansa of the ascending colon (3 cases), the descending colon (3 cases), and the mid-ascending colon (1 case), suggesting that foreign bodies may preferentially lodge near the distal ansa, possibly migrating distally during prolonged medical management. All chinchillas underwent exploratory laparotomy with colotomy for foreign body extraction, making surgical intervention central to case management when medical therapy proved ineffective. The perioperative survival rate was 71%, with 2 postoperative deaths attributed to hypoalbuminemia, highlighting albumin as a valuable prognostic and perioperative risk indicator. Hyperglycemia was the most common biochemical abnormality and was likely associated with pain.

Colonic Resection and Anastomosis

Colonic masses and neoplasia are rarely reported in small mammals. Surgical treatment is often mandatory but challenging regarding the size and fragility of colonic tissue.

Colonic resection and anastomosis has been successfully performed in a 9 month old female rat with colonic adenocarcinoma without vascular invasion.[41] The rat presented with history of obstipation and exploratory laparotomy revealed a 5 cm colonic mass spanning the transverse to terminal colon with a marked proximal colonic dilation. A 7 cm colonic segment (tumor plus 1 cm margins) was resected using radiosurgical hemostasis. The distal colon was cut obliquely (45°) to better match the enlarged proximal colon. Anastomosis was completed in 2 hemicircumferential simple continuous patterns. A leak test was performed by injecting sterile saline through the antimesenteric border, confirming lumen patency and watertight closure. The mesentery was reapposed, and routine abdominal closure followed. Remarkably, the rat survived 2 years postoperatively with no recurrence or metastasis and was ultimately euthanized for unrelated reasons.

Congenital Fistula

A spayed 3 year old female ferret was diagnosed with a rectovaginal fistula, a rare congenital communication between the rectum and vagina causing fecal passage through the vulva. Physical examination, ultrasound, contrast radiography, and computed tomography scan confirmed a 1 cm fistulous tract, with a normal anus indicating an isolated anorectal defect.[42] Surgical correction was performed via a vertical midline perineal incision. After standard preparation, tissue tension was maintained with stay sutures placed on each side of the perineum. Blunt dissection was carried cranially to locate the fistula, aided by the placement of a 1.7 mm polypropylene catheter in the rectum to identify the rectal lumen during dissection. Because the rectal and vaginal tissues were extremely thin and could not be safely separated, each lumen was closed from the inside, without further dissection. The ventral rectal wall was sutured with a continuous inverting pattern from within the rectum, and the dorsal vaginal wall was similarly closed from the vaginal lumen. The surgical field was flushed, and closure was completed in 3 layers. Postoperative recovery was uneventful, and no complications such as constipation, fecal incontinence, or perineal soiling, which are commonly reported in dogs and cats, were observed at 7 and 15 day follow-up.

A 6 month old female guinea pig with type II atresia ani and a rectocutaneous fistula was presented for painful defecation through a small abnormal perineal opening. Physical examination confirmed an imperforate anus with a ventral fistulous tract that allowed only minimal fecal passage. Given the congenital obstruction and functional fistula, a rectal pull-through procedure was selected to create a functional, ectopic anal opening. The patient was placed in sternal recumbency with the pelvis elevated, and the perineum was prepared aseptically. Four stay sutures were placed circumferentially around the fistula to improve exposure. The fistulous tract was carefully dissected circumferentially ventral to the rectum until the colon was identified. After debridement of the distal rectum, caudal traction on the stay sutures enabled mobilization and externalization of the rectum through the dermis. The dorsal aspect of the fistula was incised to expose the rectal mucosa. The fistula and 2 to 3 mm of adjacent mucosa were excised, and the rectal mucosa was sutured directly to the surrounding skin using simple interrupted sutures to create a nonpainful, permanent neoanus. The procedure successfully restored comfortable defecation.[43]

Rectal Prolapse

Rectal prolapse in hamsters may occur secondary to severe diarrhea, prolonged tenesmus, or underlying GI disease, including proliferative ileitis. When the prolapse is limited to the rectum, conservative management may be attempted. The prolapsed tissue should be gently cleansed and lubricated, and a small, well-lubricated cotton-tipped applicator can be used to carefully reposition the tissue back into the rectum. Following successful reduction, placement of a temporary purse-string suture is recommended to minimize the risk of recurrence. Patency of the anal opening must be verified to ensure the hamster is able to defecate normally. Sutures are typically removed after 3 to 7 days, depending on clinical progress. The prognosis is more favorable in cases of mild rectal prolapse that are identified early and promptly corrected.

Common etiologies of diarrhea in hamsters that may predispose to rectal prolapse include *Lawsonia intracellularis* (proliferative ileitis), *Clostridium difficile*, *Clostridium piliforme* (Tyzzer disease), GI parasitism (including *Hymenolepis nana* and other helminths), poor environmental hygiene, and sudden dietary changes, particularly abrupt increases in moisture or fermentable carbohydrates. Identification and correction of the underlying cause are essential to reduce recurrence and improve overall outcome.

Helicobacter spp. are among the bacterial organisms most frequently isolated from pet mice. Infected individuals are typically asymptomatic; however, when mice present with rectal prolapse, *Helicobacter* infection should be considered a primary differential diagnosis. Owing to the fastidious nature of this organism and the difficulty associated with routine culture, polymerase chain reaction testing of fecal samples is the diagnostic method of choice.

Recommended treatment consists of triple antimicrobial therapy, including amoxicillin (1.5 mg/30 g mouse), metronidazole (0.69 mg/30 g), and bismuth (0.185 mg/30 g), administered orally every 8 hours for a duration of 14 days. This protocol has been shown to be effective in the eradication of *Helicobacter* species in laboratory mice and is extrapolated for use in pet mice.[44]

POSTSURGICAL CONSIDERATIONS

Analgesia and Sedation

Proactive and multimodal analgesic plan and vigilant recovery monitoring are mandatory across the entire perioperative continuum. Effective multimodal analgesia reduces stress, improves gut motility, and shortens hospitalization. Core principles include pre-emptive analgesia, scheduled dosing for the first 24 to 48 hours, and the use of validated or emerging pain-assessment tools.

Opioids (eg, fentanyl, methadone, morphine, hydromorphone, buprenorphine) remain first line for acute visceral pain management following GI surgery across species. Nonsteroidal anti-inflammatory drugs can be considered on a case-by-case basis once perfusion and renal status are stable; avoid or use extreme caution in compromised herbivores and in any dehydrated patient.[45,46]

Pain scoring

Objective tools to improve detection of undertreated pain. Species-specific behavior-based composite scores and/or grimace scales have been historically and intensively developed for research in rats[47,48] and mice,[49] and more recently ferrets.[50] A clinical pain scale was recently validated for guinea pigs, although its use cannot be recommended in a clinical context.[51] In Syrian hamsters, pain-related behaviors and grimace scores had high specificity; overall none of the tested methods were sufficiently sensitive or reliable to serve as effective pain assessment tools in this species.[52] At present, there is no validated pain assessment tool available for chinchillas.

Antimicrobials

Antibiotic therapy is commonly indicated during and after GI procedures because of the high risk of bacterial contamination and peritonitis. There are no species-specific studies or recommendations addressing antimicrobial prophylaxis for long-duration, contaminated, or clean-contaminated surgeries in ferrets and rodents; current guidance is limited to consensus statements from the research field.[53] Even in dogs and cats, high-quality evidence supporting or refining surgical antimicrobial prophylaxis remains remarkably limited. Most available studies focus on orthopedic procedures in dogs—particularly stifle surgeries such as tibial plateau leveling osteotomy or tibial tuberosity advancement—while only a minority address soft-tissue operations.[54] When antimicrobial use is indicated, agents with low dysbiosis potential and adequate anaerobic coverage should be selected according to species-specific sensitivities and toxicities. Trimethoprim–sulfonamides and metronidazole are considered appropriate first-line choices in herbivorous species when clinically indicated.[55] It should however be noted that metronidazole may have the side effect of significantly reducing appetite during treatment in certain species, such as the chinchilla, regardless of the formulation used.[56] In carnivorous species and in certain rodent species such as rats and mice, amoxicillin can be used.[55]

Thermoregulation, Fluid Therapy, and Oxygen Supplementation

Rectal temperature should be monitored following recovery from anesthesia to ensure the patient remains normothermic. Active warming (forced-air blankets, incubators) should be used as indicated, and temperature reassessed frequently, especially in very small patients. Continue crystalloid fluid support based on ongoing losses and perfusion parameters. Supplemental oxygen is beneficial for any patient with anemia, hypoventilation, or postoperative pain-related hypoventilation.

Nutritional Support and Gastrointestinal Motility

Early, careful enteral nutrition improves outcomes in all species. Syringe feeding with species-appropriate recovery diets should begin as soon as swallowing is safe. Postoperative ileus (POI) can be a clinically significant complication following GI surgery, especially in herbivorous patients. POI risk is peaking at 24 hours postsurgery and can last for 48 to 72 hours and can lead to deadly complications in hindgut fermenters species. It results from a combination of tissue manipulation, intestinal inflammation, increased paracellular permeability, electrolyte imbalance, anesthetic effects, opioid administration, and sympathetic inhibition of enteric activity.[57,58] Laparotomy combined with gentle manipulation of the small intestine and cecum is a well-established method to experimentally induce transient GI hypomotility in laboratory rodents.[57–60]

The consensus across veterinary anesthesia and critical-care literature emphasizes that prevention—through atraumatic surgical handling, adequate analgesia, maintenance of hydration and normothermia, and early enteral feeding—is more effective than pharmacologic intervention alone.[61] Current recommendations advocate for a multimodal, individualized approach, where prokinetics serve as supportive—not curative—agents. Among available drugs, metoclopramide remains the most widely—and empirically—used agent in small mammal medicine. However, experimental studies in rodents highlight potential interest in newer molecules such as itopride, which accelerates colonic transit in a dose-dependent manner in guinea pigs and rats at 10 mg/kg orally,[62] and prucalopride, which restores both upper and lower GI transit after experimental laparotomy in guinea pigs at the same oral dose.[63] Contrary to rats, mosapride (10 mg/kg orally) does not have prokinetic effect on the colon of guinea pigs,[62] but is a promising drug to reduce the inflammation and intestinal permeability involved in the pathogenesis of POI.[58]

Wound Protection and Husbandry

Soft Elizabethan collars or protective garments may be required in small rodents to prevent wound complications, but they are generally unnecessary in guinea pigs, chinchillas, and ferrets, which seldom interfere with their surgical sites. In social species, short-term separation may be warranted to prevent overgrooming or chewing of incisions by cage mates. Postoperatively, patients should be housed on deep, clean bedding with easy access to food and water, and handled in a calm, low-stress manner to support recovery.

Monitoring and Inhospital Recheck

A structured recovery checklist adapted to each species for the first 12 to 24 hours should include:

- Heart/respiratory rate and quality, mucous membranes, temperature (q2–4 hours)
- Pain score using species-appropriate tools (q4–6 hours)

- Hydration/perfusion markers (capillary refill time, lactate if available), the latter extrapolated from small-animal critical care; rising lactate or persistent elevation warrants escalation.
- GI parameters: borborygmi, fecal output/character, appetite, abdominal comfort (q4–6 hours)

Owner follow-up schedule: phone recheck at 24 to 48 hours; in-person examination and weight check at 3 to 5 days; suture removal at 10 to 14 days; additional recheck if anorexia, abdominal distension, diarrhea, or incision changes occur.

PROGNOSIS AND OUTCOME

Prognosis depends on species, primary pathology, extent of contamination or devitalization, time to surgery, and perioperative stabilization quality. Herbivorous hindgut fermenters (guinea pigs, chinchillas) are disproportionately susceptible to POI and dysbiosis, which can lead to less favorable outcomes if analgesia, nutrition, and antibiotic selection are suboptimal.

Published outcome data remain sparse and often limited to case series or single-case reports. For example, GDV in guinea pigs carries a guarded to poor prognosis: a small series reported 2 survivors among 7 surgically treated animals, emphasizing the need for rapid recognition and aggressive perioperative care.[30] Conversely, ferrets undergoing surgery for focal GI disease (eg, foreign bodies) often recover uneventfully when stabilization and analgesia are optimized.[64]

In dogs and cats, the risk of intestinal anastomosis dehiscence peaks during the lag phase of healing, typically 3 to 5 days postoperatively, after which it declines. Applying this window to small mammals is prudent, and discharge instructions should highlight clinical signs to be looking for (eg, acute anorexia, abdominal distension/pain, incisional discharge, dyschezia/diarrhea) and that should warrant prompt reassessment.[65]

FUTURE DIRECTIONS

1. Evidence-based postoperative protocols for small mammals. Adapt and prospectively test dog/cat anesthesia-recovery bundles (standardized pain scoring, hypothermia prevention, early enteral nutrition, manipulation-sparing techniques) to quantify effects on POI, hospitalization duration, and readmission rate.
2. Validated pain-assessment tools across species. Expand grimace/composite scales; validate inter-observer reliability and clinical responsiveness in clinical (not just laboratory) settings, and integrate into discharge instructions for owners (eg, simple behavior checklists).
3. POI mitigation strategies. Translate experimental findings from laboratory POI models (reduced ileus with promotility agents or microbiome-directed interventions) into controlled clinical trials, including standardized endpoints (time to first feces, appetite score, readmission).
4. Antibiotic stewardship in hindgut fermenters. Develop consensus guidelines on perioperative antimicrobial indications, spectra, routes, and treatment durations that minimize dysbiosis while covering realistic contaminants—analogous to small-animal antimicrobial stewardship efforts.
5. Registries and multicenter retrospective studies. Establish species-specific GI surgery registries to capture indications, techniques, complications, and outcomes (short and long term), enabling risk-adjusted benchmarking similar to canine/feline surgical literature.

CLINICS CARE POINTS

- All aspects of perioperative management should be considered and planned for as they are crucial for positive outcomes in small mammals.
- Recent reports focus on minimally invasive techniques and adjustments of exisitng techniques for small mammals.

DECLARATION OF AI AND AI-ASSISTED TECHNOLOGIES IN THE WRITING PROCESS

During the preparation of this work the authors used Generative AI. After using this tool, the authors reviewed and edited the content as needed and takes full responsibility for the content of the publication.

DISCLOSURE

The authors have nothing to disclose.

REFERENCES

1. DeCubellis J, Graham J. Gastrointestinal disease in Guinea pigs and rabbits. Vet Clin North Am Exot Anim Pract 2013;16(2):421–35.
2. Hoefer HL. 3 - gastrointestinal diseases of ferrets. In: Quesenberry KE, Orcutt CJ, Mans C, et al, editors. Ferrets, rabbits, and rodents. 4th edition. Philadelphia (PA): W.B. Saunders; 2020. p. 27–38.
3. Minarikova A, Hauptman K, Jeklova E, et al. Diseases in pet Guinea pigs: a retrospective study in 1000 animals. Vet Rec 2015;177(8):200.
4. Halck ML, van Zeeland YRA, Schoemaker NJ. Ferret gastroenterology. Veterinary Clinics: Exotic Animal Practice 2025;28(2):227–61.
5. Jekl V, Modry D. Gastroenterology in rodents. Veterinary Clinics: Exotic Animal Practice 2025;28(2):263–94.
6. Okada K, Kondo H, Sumi A, et al. A retrospective study of disease incidence in African pygmy hedgehogs (*Atelerix albiventris*). J Vet Med Sci 2018;80(10): 1504–10.
7. Bennett RA. General principles, instruments, and equipment. Surgery of Exotic Animals 2021;1–10.
8. Aguilar LAB, Chávez JO, Watty AD. Comparison of body temperature acquired via auricular and rectal methods in ferrets. J Exot Pet Med 2019;28:148–53.
9. Hepps Keeney CM, Hung CS, Harrison TM. Comparison of body temperature using digital, infrared, and tympanic thermometry in healthy ferrets (Mustela putorius furo). J Exot Pet Med 2021;36:16–21.
10. Levy I, Allender MC, Keller KA. Comparison of axillary and inguinal body temperature to rectal temperature in healthy Guinea pigs (Cavia porcellus). J Exot Pet Med 2020;34:1–5.
11. Ozawa S, Mans C, Beaufrere H. Comparison of rectal and tympanic thermometry in chinchillas (Chinchilla lanigera). J Am Vet Med Assoc 2017;251(5):552–8.
12. Stratton HS, Rao S, Sadar MJ. Hypothermia, anemia, hyperglycemia, and severe hypoglycemia are significant prognostic indicators of death in client-owned ferrets (Mustela putorius furo). Am J Vet Res 2024;85(4). https://doi.org/10.2460/ajvr.23.10.0244. ajvr.23.10.0244.
13. Levy IH, Di Girolamo N, Keller KA. Rectal temperature is a prognostic indicator in client-owned Guinea pigs. J Small Anim Pract 2021;62(10):861–5.

14. Kwak D-H, Kim M-C, Song W-J, et al. Hyperglycemia in pet African pygmy hedgehogs (Atelerix albiventris): prevalence, clinical characteristics, and prognostic indicators of severe hyperglycemia. Animals 2025;15(10):1455.
15. Trenholme HN. Sedation and anesthesia in exotic animal critical care. Vet Clin Exot Anim Pract 2023;26(3):591–622.
16. Doss GA, Carpenter JW. 28 - African pygmy hedgehogs. In: Quesenberry KE, Orcutt CJ, Mans C, et al, editors. Ferrets, rabbits, and rodents. 4th edition. Philadelphia (PA): W.B. Saunders; 2020. p. 401–15.
17. Heatley JJ. Chapter 16 - hedgehogs. In: Mitchell MA, Tully TN, editors. Manual of exotic pet practice. Saint Louis (MO): W.B. Saunders; 2009. p. 433–55.
18. Heard D, Insectivores (Hedgehogs, Moles, and Tenrecs). Zoo animal and wildlife immobilization and anesthesia 2014. p. 529–31.
19. D'Agostino J. Chapter 34 - insectivores (Insectivora, Macroscelidea, Scandentia). In: Miller RE, Fowler ME, editors. Fowler's zoo and wild animal medicine, vol. 8. Saint Louis (MO): W.B. Saunders; 2015. p. 275–81.
20. Hawkins SJ, Doss GA, Mans C. Postanesthetic effects of two durations of isoflurane anesthesia in African pygmy hedgehogs (Atelerix albiventris). J Exot Pet Med 2020;32:27–30.
21. Baldo CF, Boelke R. Rabbit supraglottic airway device (V-GEL) for successful airway control in a hedgehog (Atelerix albiventris). Vet Anaesth Analg 2020; 47(1):141–3.
22. Avelino JA, Walsh CA, Wharton KN, et al. A comparison of three anesthetic drug combinations for use in inducing surgical anesthesia in female Guinea pigs (Cavia porcellus). JAALAS 2024;63(2):182–9.
23. Balko JA, Chinnadurai SK. Advancements in evidence-based anesthesia of exotic animals. Vet Clin Exot Anim Pract 2017;20(3):917–28.
24. van Zeeland YRA, Schoemaker NJ. Analgesia, anesthesia, and monitoring. Exotic Animal Emergency and Critical Care Medicine 2021;95–108.
25. d'Ovidio D, Adami C. Pain management for gastrointestinal conditions in exotic animals. Veterinary Clinics: Exotic Animal Practice 2025;28(2):347–63.
26. Davids BI, Davidson MJ, TenBroeck SH, et al. Efficacy of mechanical versus non-mechanical sterile preoperative skin preparation with chlorhexidine gluconate 4% solution. Vet Surg 2015;44(5):648–52.
27. Skorupski AM, Zhang J, Ferguson D, et al. Quantification of induced hypothermia from aseptic scrub applications during rodent surgery preparation. J Am Assoc Lab Anim Sci 2017;56(5):562–9.
28. Webb J, Graham J, Fordham M, et al. Diagnosis and treatment of esophageal foreign body or stricture in three ferrets (Mustela putorius furo). J Am Vet Med Assoc 2017 2017;251(4):451–7.
29. Adamovicz L, Bullen L, Saker K, et al. Use of an esophagostomy tube for management of traumatic subtotal glossectomy in an African pygmy hedgehog (Atelerix albiventris). J Exot Pet Med 2016;25(3):231–6.
30. Nógrádi AL, Cope I, Balogh M, et al. Review of gastric torsion in eight Guinea pigs (Cavia porcellus). Acta Vet Hung 2017;65(4):487–99.
31. Woodhall H, Barrow K, Brown S, et al. Successful surgical treatment of gastric dilatation and volvulus in a pet domestic rat (Rattus norvegicus). J Exot Pet Med 2024;51:9–12.
32. Gardhouse SM, Sanchez-Migallon Guzman D, Sadar MJ, et al. Partial gastrectomy for resection of a gastric leiomyoma in a Guinea pig (Cavia porcellus). J Am Vet Med Assoc 2016 2016;249(12):1415–20.

33. Adamovicz L, Applegate J, Harris J, et al. Use of a gastrotomy and jejunostomy tube for management of gastric distension following pyloric outflow obstruction in a ferret (Mustela putorius furo). J Exot Pet Med 2019;28:105–10.
34. Sinclair KM, Eckstrand C, Moore PF, et al. Epitheliotropic gastrointestinal T-Cell lymphoma with concurrent insulinoma and adrenocortical carcinoma in a domestic ferret (Mustela putorius furo). J Exot Pet Med 2016;25(1):34–43.
35. Hrysyzen TMS, Malmberg JL, Johnston MS. Diagnosis and clinical management of eosinophilic gastroenteritis in an African pygmy hedgehog (Atelerix albiventris). J Exot Pet Med 2019;30:88–91.
36. Pellaz V, Pellaz U, Müller K. Ileocaecal intussusception in a young Guinea pig - a case report. Kleintierpraxis 2012;57(4):192–5.
37. Rowles TK, Keith JC Jr, Warwick KE, et al. Imperforate anus, colo-colic intussusception, and bowel rupture in a neonatal Guinea pig. Lab Anim Sci 1993;43(3): 255–7.
38. Schoenbaum M, Klopfer U, Egyed MN. Spontaneous intussusception of the small intestine in guinea-pigs. Lab Anim 1972;6(3):327–30.
39. Fetzer TJ, Mans C. Jejuno-jejunal intussusception in a Guinea pig (Cavia porcellus). Open Vet J 2017;7(3):286–9.
40. Koizumi I. Diagnosis and surgical treatment of colonic obstructive foreign bodies in chinchillas (*chinchilla lanigera*): a case series (2017–2020). J Vet Med Sci 2022;84(8):1121–7.
41. Applegate JR, Troan BV, Chen LR, et al. Surgical management of colonic adenocarcinoma in a rat (Rattus norvegicus). J Exot Pet Med 2017;26(1):47–52.
42. Schlax K, Quiévreux L, Mélin M, et al. A rectovaginal fistula in a ferret (Mustela putorius furo) with a normal anus: a case report. J Exot Pet Med 2020;35:20–2.
43. Ribas Jiménez R, Valls Badia X, Moya Clivillé A, et al. Surgical treatment of rectocutaneous fistula in a juvenile Guinea pig (Cavia porcellus) using a rectal pull-through technique. J Exot Pet Med 2020;35:44–7.
44. Foltz CJ, Fox JG, Yan L, et al. Evaluation of antibiotic therapies for eradication of Helicobacter hepaticus. Antimicrob Agents Chemother 1995;39(6):1292–4.
45. Oates R, Tarbort DK. Treatment of pain in rats, mice, and prairie dogs. Vet Clin North Am Exot Anim Pract 2023;26(1):151–74.
46. Petritz OA, de Matos R. Treatment of pain in ferrets. Vet Clin North Am Exot Anim Pract 2023;26(1):245–55.
47. Roughan JV, Flecknell PA. Evaluation of a short duration behaviour-based post-operative pain scoring system in rats. Eur J Pain 2003;7(5):397–406.
48. Sotocinal SG, Sorge RE, Zaloum A, et al. The rat grimace scale: a partially automated method for quantifying pain in the laboratory rat via facial expressions. Mol Pain 2011;7:55.
49. Langford DJ, Bailey AL, Chanda ML, et al. Coding of facial expressions of pain in the laboratory mouse. Nat Methods 2010;7(6):447–9.
50. Reijgwart ML, Schoemaker NJ, Pascuzzo R, et al. The composition and initial evaluation of a grimace scale in ferrets after surgical implantation of a telemetry probe. PLoS One 2017;12(11):e0187986.
51. Benedetti F, Pignon C, Muffat-es-Jacques P, et al. Development and validation of a pain scale in Guinea pig (Cavia porcellus). J Exot Pet Med 2024;50:36–41.
52. Edmunson AM, Duke Boynton FD, Rendahl AK, et al. Indicators of postoperative pain in Syrian hamsters (Mesocricetus auratus). Comp Med 2021;71(1):76–85.
53. ACLAM position statement on rodent surgery. J Am Assoc Lab Anim Sci 2016; 55(6):822–3.

54. Sørensen TM, Scahill K, Ruperez JE, et al. Antimicrobial prophylaxis in companion animal surgery: a scoping review for european network for optimization of antimicrobial therapy (ENOVAT) guidelines. Vet J 2024;304:106101.
55. Broens EM, van Geijlswijk IM. Prudent use of antimicrobials in exotic animal medicine. Vet Clin Exot Anim Pract 2018/05/01/2018;21(2):341–53.
56. Mans C, Fink D. Effects of commercial metronidazole and metronidazole benzoate suspensions on food intake in chinchillas. J Small Anim Pract 2021;62(3):174–7.
57. Lee YJ, Hussain Z, Huh CW, et al. Inflammation, impaired motility, and permeability in a Guinea pig model of postoperative ileus. J Neurogastroenterol Motil 2018;24(1):147–58.
58. Kim YM, Hussain Z, Lee YJ, et al. Altered intestinal permeability and drug repositioning in a post-operative ileus Guinea pig model. J Neurogastroenterol Motil 2021;27(4):639–49.
59. Firpo MA, Rollins MD, Szabo A, et al. A conscious mouse model of gastric ileus using clinically relevant endpoints. BMC Gastroenterol 2005;5(1):18.
60. Mueller MH, Karpitschka M, Gao Z, et al. Vagal innervation and early postoperative ileus in mice. J Gastrointest Surg 2011;15(6):891–901.
61. Hellstrom EA, Ziegler AL, Blikslager AT. Postoperative ileus: comparative pathophysiology and future therapies. Mini review. Front Vet Sci 2021;8:2021.
62. Tsubouchi T, Saito T, Mizutani F, et al. Stimulatory action of itopride hydrochloride on colonic motor activity in vitro and in vivo. J Pharmacol Exp Therapeut 2003;306(2):787–93.
63. Park SJ, Choi EJ, Yoon YH, et al. The effects of prucalopride on postoperative ileus in Guinea pigs. Yonsei Med J 2013;54(4):845–53.
64. Jekl V, Casale S. 31 - soft tissue surgery: ferrets. In: Quesenberry KE, Orcutt CJ, Mans C, et al, editors. Ferrets, rabbits, and rodents. 4th edition. Philadelphia (PA): W.B. Saunders; 2020. p. 432–45.
65. Ralphs SC, Jessen CR, Lipowitz AJ. Risk factors for leakage following intestinal anastomosis in dogs and cats: 115 cases (1991-2000). J Am Vet Med Assoc 2003;223(1):73–7.

Hepatobiliary Surgical Diseases in Small Exotic Mammals

Indications, Techniques, and Outcomes

Minh Huynh, DVM, MRCVS, DECZM (Avian), DACZM[a,*],
Albert Phouratsamay, DVM, DECZM (Small Mammals)[a,b],
Diego Rossetti, DVM, Dipl ECVS[c]

KEYWORDS

• Liver lobe torsion • Extrahepatic biliary obstruction • Cholecystectomy
• Cholecystoduodenostomy • Choledochal stent • Liver biopsy

KEY POINTS

- Hepatobiliary disease in exotic small mammals is increasingly manageable thanks to advances in diagnostic imaging, anesthesia, and microsurgical techniques, with liver lobe torsion (LLT) in rabbits and extrahepatic biliary obstruction (EHBO) in ferrets as key surgical focuses.
- Anatomic and physiologic differences (fragile parenchyma, variable biliary anatomy) require meticulous preoperative assessment (biochemistry, coagulation, albumin, and bilirubin) and careful anesthetic planning.
- Core surgical options include liver biopsy (open, laparoscopic, or percutaneous) and liver lobectomy, plus extrahepatic biliary procedures such as cholecystectomy, choledochotomy, cholecystoduodenostomy, and biliary stenting.
- Portosystemic shunts are rare in exotic mammals; prognosis after EHBO is generally favorable in ferrets, while LLT outcomes in rabbits are relatively good with surgery.
- Postoperative care is critical and includes antibiotics, hepatoprotectants, early nutrition, and regular imaging to monitor for complications (hemorrhage, bile leakage, infection).

[a] Department of Exotic Pet Medicine, Clinique vétérinaire Sevetys Crozatier, 61 Rue Crozatier, 75012 Paris, France; [b] Department of Exotic Pet Medicine, Centre Hospitalier Vétérinaire AniCura ADVETIA, 9 Avenue Louis Breguet, 78140 Vélizy-Villacoublay, France; [c] Department of Surgery, Centre Hospitalier Vétérinaire AniCura ADVETIA, 9 Avenue Louis Breguet, 78140 Vélizy-Villacoublay, France
* Corresponding author.
E-mail address: nacologie@gmail.com

Vet Clin Exot Anim 29 (2026) 731–747
https://doi.org/10.1016/j.cvex.2026.04.015 vetexotic.theclinics.com
1094-9194/26/

Abbreviations	
ALP	alkaline phosphatase
ALT	alanine aminotransferase
AST	aspartate aminotransferase
BUN	blood urea nitrogen
EHBO	extrahepatic biliary obstruction
GGT	gamma-glutamyltransferase
LLT	liver lobe torsion
PSS	portosystemic shunt

INTRODUCTION

Hepatobiliary disease in exotic mammals is a relatively underexplored field compared with that of dogs and cats. However, recent advances in diagnostic imaging, anesthesia, and microsurgical techniques have expanded the range of feasible interventions for species such as rabbits, ferrets, guinea pigs, and other small mammals. Although hepatobiliary disorders remain uncommon in these species, they are often associated with high morbidity and mortality when surgical intervention is delayed or misapplied.

In exotic small mammals, small organ size, friable parenchyma, and species-specific biliary anatomy significantly increase the technical difficulty and risk of surgical procedures. Moreover, limited published data and a lack of standardized surgical protocols contribute to variability in clinical outcomes. For these reasons, most surgical approaches in exotics are still extrapolated from canine and feline literature, then adapted based on the surgeon's experience and the anatomic constraints of each species.

Among exotic mammals, rabbits appear to be the most commonly affected by hepatobiliary pathology, with hepatic lobe torsion representing the predominant surgical indication. In contrast, ferrets more frequently present with cholangiohepatitis or cholecystitis. This review will mainly focus on those 2 conditions and integrates the existing exotic animal literature with well-established principles from canine and feline hepatobiliary surgery.

Anatomic Consideration

The liver of rabbits is divided into 5 lobes. It comprises a left lateral lobe, a left medial lobe, a right lobe, a quadrate lobe, and a caudate lobe. The number of liver lobes is also described as 6 according to other literature sources, with a right lateral lobe and a right medial lobe, which causes confusion.[1,2] Rabbits have a particularly well-developed and partially pedunculated caudate lobe, predisposing them to lobe torsion[1,3] (**Fig. 1**).

Rodents have a more compact liver anatomy, consisting of 6 tightly arranged lobes for guinea pigs, or 4 lobes for rats and chinchillas. Rats do not have a gallbladder.[3] Ferrets exhibit a liver configuration closer to that of carnivores, including a well-defined gallbladder.[4]

The liver receives a dual blood supply from the portal vein and the hepatic artery. Rabbit models have been thoroughly studied, and several arterial and portal variants have been reported.[5,6] The common hepatic artery divides into the gastroduodenal artery and the proper hepatic artery, which further branches into the right hepatic artery and the left hepatic artery (medial and lateral branches). Importantly, the caudate lobe is consistently supplied by a single caudate portal vein, whereas the left portal vein may show a trifurcation or even a quadrifurcation.[6]

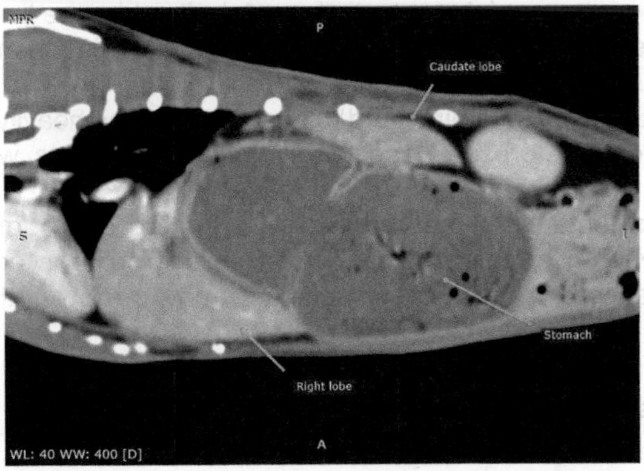

Fig. 1. Postcontrast computed tomography images of a healthy rabbit, showing the anatomic topography and aspects of liver lobes, particularly the caudate liver lobe which is well developed and partially pedunculated. (Image Courtesy of Dr Minh Huynh.)

Preoperative Consideration

Biochemical assessment

A thorough biochemical assessment is recommended before undergoing hepatic surgery. Several risk factors need to be addressed specifically (beyond traditional parameters considered for general anesthesia including alanine aminotransferase [ALT], aspartate aminotransferase [AST], and alkaline phosphatase [ALP]).

- *Hemoglobin:* Anemia is frequently observed in hepatic disease and is particularly common in cases of liver lobe torsion in rabbits. Preoperative blood collection should be considered so that a transfusion is available in the event of significant intraoperative hemorrhage.
- *Coagulation panel:* In severe hepatic dysfunction, coagulation parameters may be altered. Reference ranges for coagulation tests have been established in rabbits and ferrets.[7,8] However, a major limitation is the relatively large blood volume required, which can be counterproductive in unstable patients or those with suspected coagulopathies. Vitamin K may be administered preoperatively because biliary dysfunction can reduce its intestinal absorption and increase the risk of deficiency.
- *Albumin:* Hypoalbuminemia commonly accompanies liver disease, leading to reduced oncotic pressure and decreased tolerance of fluid therapy. Albumin levels also affect drug protein-binding, particularly for anesthetic agents, making accurate dosing more challenging.
- *Bilirubin:* Elevated bilirubin concentrations may influence arterial blood pressure by helping maintain renal perfusion and reducing renal vascular resistance. Consequently, rapid correction or normalization of bilirubin levels could theoretically exacerbate pre-existing hypotension.

Anesthetic consideration

Most anesthetic agents undergo significant hepatic metabolism, which can complicate their use in patients with liver failure (although true hepatic failure remains uncommon). Inhalant anesthetics such as isoflurane and sevoflurane are eliminated primarily via the lungs and therefore represent the safest maintenance option in these cases.

Both alfaxalone and propofol are partially metabolized by the liver but also rely on substantial extrahepatic clearance (lungs and kidneys), making them suitable choices for anesthetic induction.

In contrast, α_2-agonists, ketamine, and midazolam depend heavily on hepatic metabolism and should therefore be used with caution in patients with impaired liver function.

Opioids such as fentanyl or methadone are preferred over morphine, which depends more heavily on hepatic metabolism. Buprenorphine is an acceptable and safe alternative, although its analgesic efficacy may be lower than that of other opioids.

Surgical Techniques in Hepatobiliary Disease

Liver biopsy

Liver biopsy is a fundamental diagnostic and, in selected cases, therapeutic tool in the evaluation of hepatobiliary disease across all small mammals.

Indications include evaluation of diffuse hepatopathies, diagnosing and staging of neoplastic disease, characterization of focal lesions, and confirmation of infectious or inflammatory processes. Specifically in ferrets, liver biopsy can be used for quantification of hepatic copper concentration, which may be of importance in case of hepatobiliary disease.[9]

Three major approaches are adapted from canine and feline surgery:

- *Open wedge or guillotine biopsy* allows for controlled visualization and hemostasis, suitable for larger patients such as rabbits and ferrets.
- *Minimally invasive (laparoscopic) biopsy.* Rabbits are used as a laboratory model for laparoscopic techniques for liver surgery.[10] Whether the technique can be transposed to clinical cases in pet rabbits and be clinically beneficial remains to be determined. A study comparing fine needle aspiration, 1.7 and 3.0 mm biopsy forceps in rabbits showed that the latter has greater diagnostic value.[11] Some sampling artifacts were observed but the 3.0 mm biopsies had a mean of 4.0 portal triads and 4.14 central veins per biopsy. Regarding diagnostic adequacy and portal triad counts in canine medicine, an average of 2.9 or greater portal triads per sample is suggested for an adequate diagnostic yield (versus earlier recommendations of 4–6 triads).[12,13] In a cadaveric canine study, 3 and 5 mm laparoscopic cup biopsies showed no significant difference in diagnostic agreement for key histologic features.[14] These data support the feasibility of 3 mm cup instruments for small exotic mammals.
- *Percutaneous ultrasound-guided biopsy* retains the advantages of minimal invasiveness and brief anesthesia but carries nonnegligible hemorrhagic risk. Pre-biopsy coagulation screening and post-biopsy monitoring of packed cell volume and abdominal effusion are strongly recommended.

Hemorrhage remains the principal intraoperative and postoperative complication in all species. Because hepatic vessels in exotics are fragile and the parenchyma is friable, meticulous hemostasis is essential. Application of absorbable gelatin sponge, digital pressure, and bipolar vessel-sealing devices can help minimize blood loss.

Liver lobectomy

Liver lobectomy is a major surgical procedure indicated for focal, potentially resectable hepatic diseases, including lobe torsion, abscess, cyst, and primary (biliary cystadenoma or carcinoma) or metastatic neoplasia. In exotic mammals, it is most frequently performed in rabbits for torsion and, less commonly, in ferrets and guinea pigs for tumors or abscesses.

Surgical approach is typically via a ventral midline celiotomy, allowing access to the entire liver and gallbladder. For lobectomy, the vascular pedicle of the affected lobe is carefully isolated and ligated. Ligation can be achieved using absorbable monofilament suture (3-0 to 5-0), hemostatic clips, instrument ligation tools (eg, SurgiTie, Surg-I-Loop), metal clips, or a vessel-sealing device (eg, LigaSure). In smaller species, hand ligation or transfixation remains the preferred method (**Fig. 2**).

Partial versus complete lobectomy depends on lesion size, vascular involvement, and species tolerance to blood loss. Because hepatic regeneration potential in exotic mammals is unknown, conservative resections are favored whenever margins are histologically clean.

Extrahepatic biliary surgery

Cholecystectomy. Cholecystectomy is an uncommon but essential surgical procedure in exotic mammals, indicated for primary gallbladder diseases such as cholecystitis, cholelithiasis, mucocele, infarction, or neoplasia. Although the gallbladder is a small and delicate organ in species such as the ferret, its removal may be curative in selected cases when performed before rupture or systemic compromise occurs.[15] Cholecystectomy has been described as a treatment of cholelithiasis in a guinea pig.[16]

Before performing the procedure, patency of the extrahepatic biliary tract must be verified, as cholecystectomy in the presence of obstruction is contraindicated and may be fatal. Patency can be evaluated intraoperatively through anterograde flushing of the common bile duct after gallbladder removal, or retrograde catheterization via duodenotomy. If patency cannot be demonstrated, biliary rerouting (eg, cholecystoduodenostomy) must be considered instead.

Two main dissection strategies are described in both domestic and exotic species. In the classic technique, dissection begins by identifying and isolating the cystic duct and artery before detaching the gallbladder from its hepatic fossa. Alternatively, some surgeons prefer to first separate the gallbladder from the hepatic parenchyma before vascular control. Dissection is performed sharply or bluntly using fine Metzenbaum scissors, electrocautery, or bipolar energy. Gentle traction is essential to avoid parenchymal tearing (**Fig. 3**). Bleeding from the hepatic fossa can be controlled with direct pressure, hemostatic agents (eg, Gelfoam, Surgicel), or low-temperature electrocautery.

Extrahepatic biliary obstruction. Extrahepatic biliary obstruction (EHBO) encompasses mechanical or functional impairment of bile flow due to cholelithiasis, cholangitis, pancreatitis, or neoplasia. While well characterized in dogs and cats, its occurrence in exotic mammals has been rarely documented. In ferrets, reported

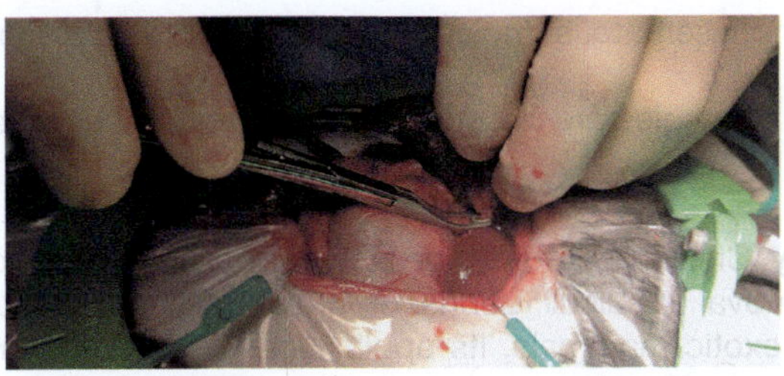

Fig. 2. Ligation of a torsed liver lobe achieved using a metal clip in a rabbit. (Image Courtesy of Dr Carlo Paoletti.)

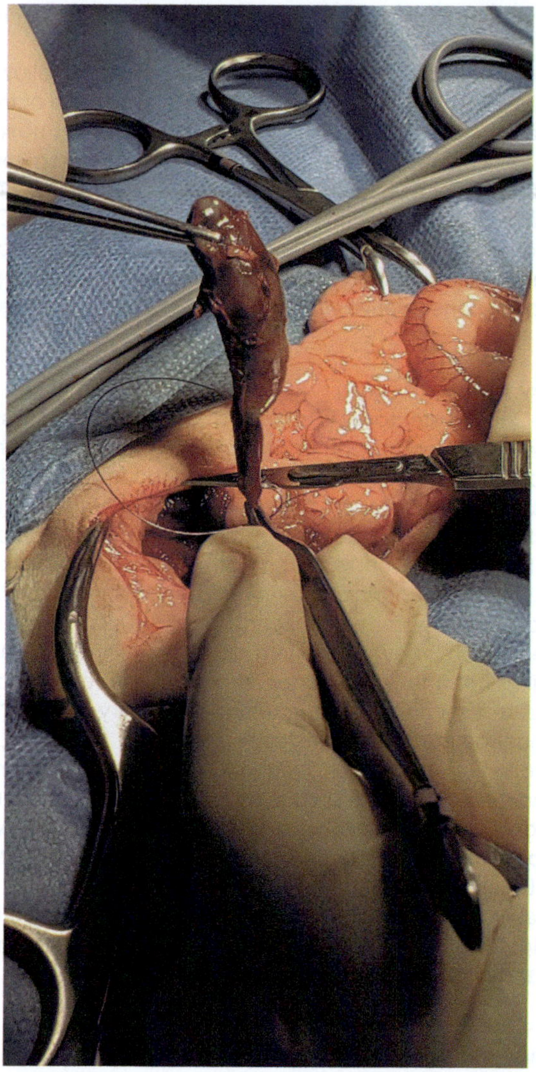

Fig. 3. Cholecystectomy in a ferret. The gallbladder is gently dissected and detached from the hepatic fossa. The ligation and excision are performed on the cystic duct area. (Image Courtesy of Dr Carlo Paoletti.)

causes include emphysematous cholecystitis with rupture, gallstones, and bile duct strictures.[17,18]

Several surgical strategies are described depending on the site and reversibility of obstruction.

Choledochotomy Choledochotomy, the surgical incision into the common bile duct, is indicated for removal of calculi, debris, or intraluminal masses, or for obtaining biopsy samples. In exotic mammals, its application is limited to larger species such as rabbits or ferrets due to the narrow duct diameter. A longitudinal incision is made on the ventral aspect of the common bile duct, with minimal traction applied to surrounding tissues. The choledochotomy is performed directly over, or just proximal to, the site of obstruction. Closure is performed with simple interrupted or continuous 6-0 to 7-0 monofilament absorbable sutures, ensuring watertight apposition. Leakage or stricture formation is the most feared complications; therefore, intraoperative duct flushing and postoperative imaging are recommended.

Choledochal stenting Choledochal stenting can provide temporary drainage across an obstructed or traumatized duct. In veterinary medicine, this technique has been successfully used in dogs and cats for reversible obstruction due to pancreatitis or cholangitis.[19] Although it has also been successfully used in a ferret.[20]

The stent, often a segment of red rubber catheter (3.5–5 Fr in cats), is inserted through a duodenotomy at the major papilla and advanced into the bile duct across the obstruction (**Fig. 4**). Care is taken to ensure that the stent does not completely occlude the ductal lumen, thereby preserving bile flow and minimizing the risk of pressure necrosis. The duodenal end is secured to the duodenal mucosa and submucosa using a 4 or 5-0 absorbable monofilament suture. As the suture material undergoes resorption, the stent is expected to dislodge spontaneously and pass through the gastrointestinal tract within the following weeks. Follow-up ultrasonography is recommended 3 to 4 weeks after stent placement to confirm spontaneous expulsion.

Cholecystoenterostomy When obstruction is permanent or nonreversible, a biliary–enteric anastomosis such as cholecystoenterostomy becomes the treatment of choice. Indications include bile duct neoplasia, strictures, or duodenal obstruction preventing normal bile flow. In these cases, the gallbladder must be viable and its vascular supply preserved.

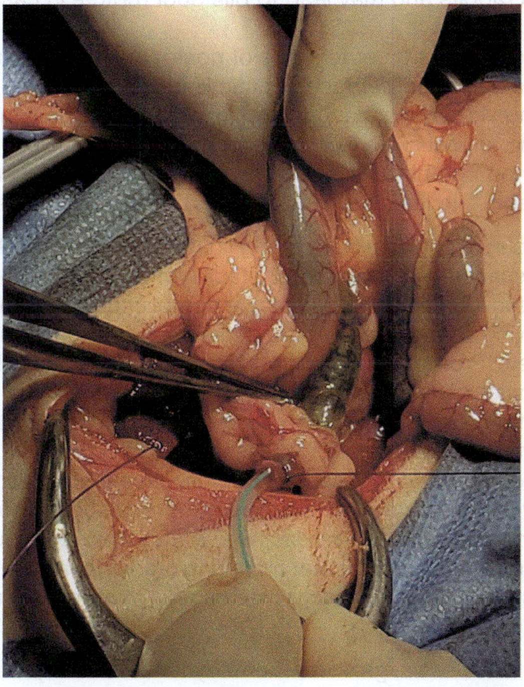

Fig. 4. Placement of a choledochal stenting in a ferret. (Image Courtesy of Dr Carlo Paoletti.)

Among surgical options, cholecystoduodenostomy and cholecystojejunostomy are the most practical. The mucosa-to-mucosa appositional technique described in dogs remains the gold standard and is readily adaptable to exotics with meticulous microsurgical technique.[21] A stoma of at least 2.5 cm (scaled appropriately for body size) is recommended to prevent reflux cholangitis due to inadequate drainage.

Cholecystoduodenostomy has been reported successfully in a ferret.[20] The primary limitations are anatomic—narrow cystic ducts, short mesenteric attachments, and the risk of bile leakage.

Portosystemic shunts

Portosystemic shunts (PSS) are vascular anomalies that permit portal blood to bypass hepatic sinusoids. While well characterized in dogs and cats, congenital PSS are rarely reported in exotic mammals, with only one documented case in a ferret.[22] Surgical techniques are numerous and will not be developed further given the rarity of this condition in small exotic mammals.

Postoperative Care

Postoperative management plays a pivotal role in the outcome of hepatobiliary surgery across all species.

Antibiotic therapy is indicated for all hepatobiliary surgeries due to the high risk of bacterial contamination from bile and the gastrointestinal tract. Broad-spectrum coverage targeting *Escherichia coli*, *Enterococcus*, and anaerobes is advised. Culture of bile or hepatic tissue during surgery can guide postoperative adjustments.

Hepatoprotective medications, such as S-adenosylmethionine and vitamin E, are extrapolated from canine and feline protocols and may support recovery by promoting bile flow and reducing oxidative injury. Ursodeoxycholic acid is used with caution as it is reported toxic in rabbits and may lead to bile duct rupture in case of obstruction in other species.[23]

Early nutritional support is a cornerstone of postoperative care in exotic mammals. Prolonged anorexia can rapidly induce hepatic lipidosis, especially in rabbits and ferrets. Enteral feeding via syringe, nasogastric, or esophagostomy tube should be initiated as soon as the animal is alert and normothermic.

The most common complications following hepatobiliary surgery in exotic mammals are hemorrhage, bile leakage, infection, and hepatic insufficiency.

- *Hemorrhage* can occur from inadequate ligation or coagulopathy. Re-exploration may be necessary if hemodynamic instability persists despite transfusion.
- *Bile peritonitis* is a severe but preventable complication; it should be suspected in animals showing fever, icterus, and abdominal effusion within 48 to 72 hours postoperatively. Prompt diagnostic abdominocentesis and culture are essential.
- *Sepsis* is a major cause of death in small exotic species due to rapid systemic decompensation. Early institution of intravenous fluids, antibiotics, and nutritional support can be lifesaving.
- *Iatrogenic pneumothorax* is a serious complication that should be considered in any patient with peroperative or postoperative respiratory distress. The shape of the diaphragm in rabbits and ferrets, which attaches very caudally on the sternum, predisposes to tear or laceration during cranial laparotomy. The diaphragm should be inspected closely before closure and any breach should be corrected promptly.

Close attention should be given to hemodynamic stability and signs of intra-abdominal bleeding, which include pallor, tachycardia, weak pulses, and abdominal distension. Measurement of packed cell volume and total solids every 4 to 6 hours during the first 24 hours can aid in detecting occult hemorrhage. Ultrasound assessment is a minimally invasive and valuable method for identifying free fluid or bile leakage.

Assessment of hepatic recovery involves serial measurement of serum bile acids, bilirubin, ALT, and ALP. Increases in these parameters may reflect transient postoperative hepatocellular injury, while persistent elevation suggests ongoing cholestasis or hepatic insufficiency. In ferrets and rabbits, mild hyperbilirubinemia can persist for several days without clinical consequence if appetite and activity are maintained.

Ultrasonography is recommended within 5 to 7 days after surgery to confirm the integrity of biliary anastomoses or ligations and to evaluate for effusion and patency of the duct.

Liver Lobe Torsion in Rabbits

The first descriptions of liver lobe torsion (LLT) in rabbits date back to the end of the 20th century in laboratory breeds.[24–26] Over the past 2 decades, there has been an increasing number of published papers on LLT in pet rabbits, totaling 211 cases.[27–39]

Several hypotheses have been proposed to explain why rabbits are prone to liver lobe torsion. The specific anatomy of the caudate liver lobe makes it more likely to twist.[1,3] Other hypotheses—traumatic event, congenital absence or laxity of hepatic ligaments, abdominal organ dilation, bacterial or parasitic hepatitis, or neoplasia—have been proposed in dogs and cats and could contribute to LLT.[40]

Epidemiology

A retrospective study from 4 North American veterinary institutions covering 82 cases found the prevalence of LLT to be 0.7% in pet rabbits.[36] In laboratory rabbits, the prevalence was estimated at 0.3%.[24] Rabbits affected by LLT are typically middle-aged, with median ages ranging from 3 to 5.15 years.[32,35–37,39]

The youngest reported case was 6 month old and the oldest 10 year old.[36]

Lop breeds and castrated males appeared overrepresented, although no statistical confirmation exists.[27–39]

Of the 211 published cases in pet rabbits, the torsed lobe was specified in 200 cases. The caudate lobe was most commonly involved (82.5%), followed by the right (13%), left lateral (3%), quadrate (1%), and left medial (0.5%) lobes. Some rabbits had simultaneous torsion of two lobes.[32,36,37]

Clinical presentation

The progression of clinical signs is generally acute, with most rabbits presented within 48 hours.[32,36,37] Chronic LLT has also been described as an incidental necropsy finding in laboratory rabbits with some individuals surviving untreated.[24]

Clinical signs are nonspecific. The most common include reduced appetite or anorexia (92.7%–100%), lethargy (56%–80%), and decreased fecal production (38%–46.3%).[32,36,37] Common physical findings include abdominal pain, tachypnea, dull mentation, gastric distension, and pale mucous membranes.

Palpation of a cranial abdominal mass effect or pale mucous membranes should strongly raise suspicion for LLT.[32,37]

Ancillary tests

Bloodwork abnormalities are frequent but nonspecific. Marked increases in ALT, AST, and ALP are common.[32,36,37] A small proportion of rabbits (6.3%) show no enzyme elevation.[36]

Azotemia, hyperglycemia, elevated creatinine, hypoproteinemia, hypercholesterolemia, electrolyte abnormalities, and anemia (59.5%–76.9%) are often reported.[32,36,37]

Thrombocytopenia is also common.[32,36] Leukopenia or leukocytosis occurs less frequently.[30,32,36]

Imaging is essential. Radiographs are nonspecific, but ultrasonography is diagnostic in nearly all cases.[32,36] Findings include an enlarged, rounded, hypoechoic lobe, absent Doppler flow, and inconsistent effusion[30,32,36,38,39] (**Fig. 5**).

Contrast-enhanced computed tomography is highly accurate,[34,35,37] revealing a hypoattenuating, poorly enhancing torsed lobe (**Fig. 6**). Torsed caudate lobe position relative to the pylorus can help with surgical planning.[37]

Surgical indication

Historically, lobectomy was the only treatment.[27–31] Recently, successful medical management has been reported.[32,36,37] Whole blood transfusion is recommended in rabbits with hematocrit less than 20%.[37]

Surgical techniques

Detorsion should not be performed to avoid reperfusion injury.[30] Most surgeries use a ventral midline approach[27–30,32,36,37] (**Fig. 7**). A paracostal approach for caudate lobectomy (**Fig. 8**) provides reduced gastrointestinal manipulation and faster recovery, it is especially advised in case of gastric dilation because it provides a better access to the caudate lobe.[35]

Outcome and prognosis

Post-lobectomy survival ranges from 77.3% to 100%.[30,32,35–37] Medical management alone yields 43% to 80% survival.[32,36,37] Overall survival is 61% to 75% with no significant difference between treatments.[36–38]

Median survival is longer with surgery (1452 versus 530 days).[36] Perioperative mortality is estimated at 17%.[36] Rabbits surviving medical treatment frequently experience recurrent gastrointestinal stasis in the first 2 months but not LLT recurrence.[32]

Risk factors for poor outcome include moderate to severe anemia, tachycardia, prolonged absence of defecation, and right lobe torsion.[36] Each 1% decrease in hematocrit increases the odds of poor outcome by 12%, and each unit increase in blood urea nitrogen (BUN) by 13%.[37] In one study, tramadol administration was associated with higher survival but this finding was unexpected and should be interpreted with

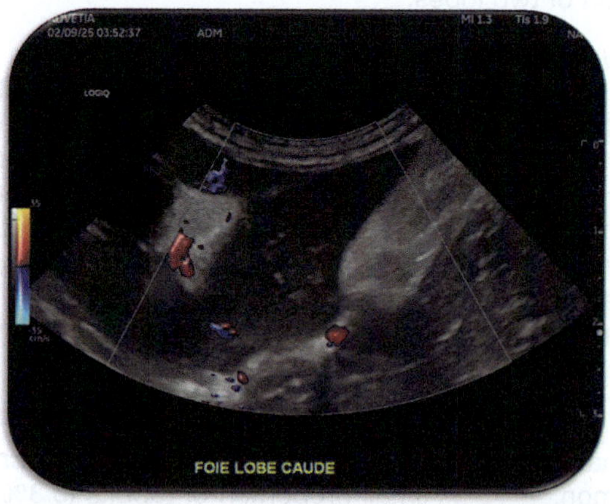

Fig. 5. Abdominal ultrasound demonstrating minimal to absent blood flow within the torsed caudate liver lobe on directional Power Doppler. (Image Courtesy of Dr José Rosas-Navarro.)

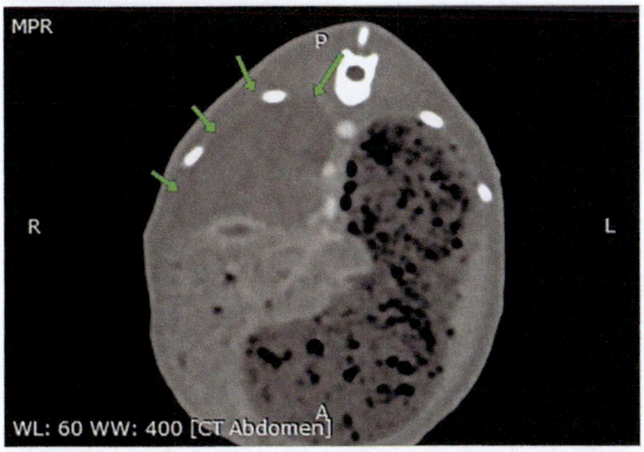

Fig. 6. Postcontrast computed tomography images of a rabbit with torsion of the caudate liver lobe, which is enlarged, rounded, hypoattenuating, and minimally contrast enhancing (*green arrow*) (Image Courtesy of Dr Minh Huynh.)

caution, as the analgesic efficacy of tramadol in rabbits remains controversial and the association may have been confounded by case selection (outpatients were more likely to receive tramadol and were potentially more stable).[36]

Histopathology typically reveals necrosis, congestion, thrombosis, and hemorrhage.[27,28,30,36,37] Bacterial culture is infrequently positive.[30,32,37]

Liver lobe torsion in other species

LLT is rarely reported in other exotic mammals, with isolated cases in a ferret[41] and a guinea pig,[42] both involving the left lateral lobe.

Biliary Tract Disease in Ferrets

Epidemiologic data

Liver and biliary diseases are relatively well described in domestic ferrets, including cholangiohepatitis, hepatic steatosis, and infectious or inflammatory biliary

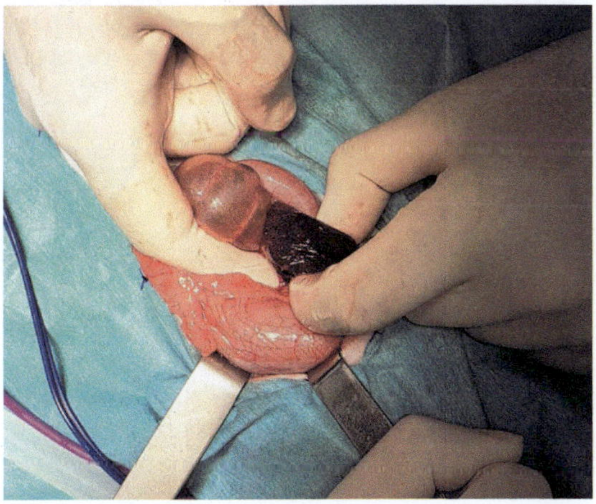

Fig. 7. Macroscopic aspect of a torsed caudate liver lobe in a rabbit during surgery, access through a ventral midline approach. The torsed lobe is dark, firm, and friable. (Image Courtesy of Dr Minh Huynh.)

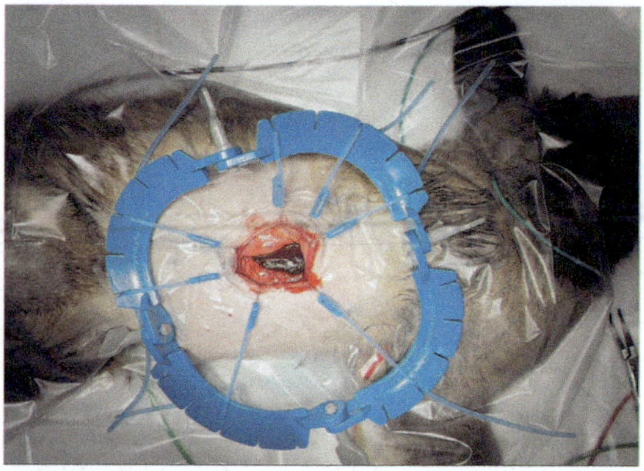

Fig. 8. Macroscopic aspect of a torsed caudate liver lobe in a rabbit during surgery, access through a right paracostal approach. (Image Courtesy of Dr Carlo Paoletti.)

disorders.[4,43] One of the most important conditions requiring prompt surgical intervention is EHBO (**Fig. 9**).

Early literature consisted of isolated case reports, including 2 cases of obstruction due to inspissated bile,[17] 1 case of gallbladder rupture associated with bacterial cholecystitis,[15] and a case of cholestasis related to biliary sediment without clinical signs.[18] A multicenter retrospective series including 17 ferrets affected with EHBO showed that this condition appears predominantly in adult and older animals

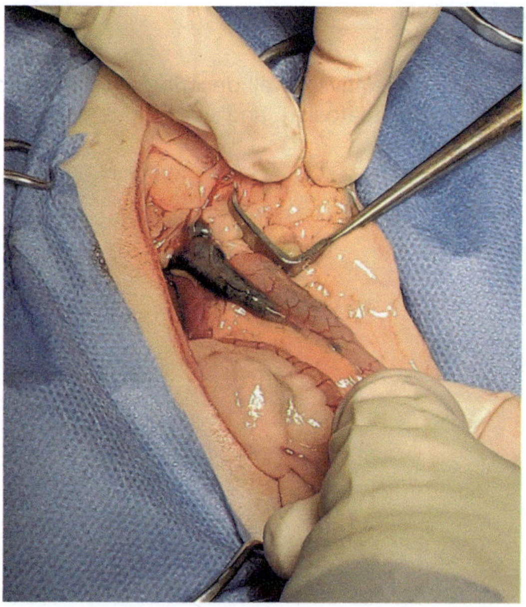

Fig. 9. Macroscopic aspect of an extrahepatic bile duct obstruction in a ferret during surgery, access through a ventral midline approach. The common bile duct is severely distended. (Image Courtesy of Dr Carlo Paoletti.)

(3–8 years old) and is associated mainly with chronic inflammatory biliary disease rather than acute, isolated obstructive lesions.[20]

Clinical data

Ferrets with EHBO demonstrate a range of nonspecific clinical presentations, including anorexia, hyporexia, lethargy, weakness, dehydration, and weight loss (cases reported in[15,17,18,20]). Acute abdominal pain is an important clinical indicator that should prompt further investigation, particularly to identify potential bile peritonitis.

Icterus is relatively uncommon in ferrets due to rapid renal excretion of bilirubin.[4] When present, it represents a very significant clinical sign consistent with biliary dysfunction. It was reported in 3 of 11 cases of cholecystitis and 6 of 17 cases of EHBO.[20,43]

Clinicopathologic data

Ferrets with EHBO display a characteristic biochemical profile consistent with cholestasis and hepatocellular injury. Common abnormalities include

- Marked ALT elevation, often greater than 500 IU/L
- Increased ALP and gamma glutamyl-transferase (GGT), though less consistently than ALT
- Hyperbilirubinemia in most reported cases
- Neutrophilic leukocytosis, especially in infectious or perforation cases[15]
- Evidence of dehydration and mild electrolyte disturbances

Because ferrets have an efficient bilirubin metabolic pathway, bilirubin rarely increases in early liver disease. When hyperbilirubinemia occurs, it is typically marked and reflects advanced choledochal obstruction. In case of bile duct rupture, the ALP and bilirubin may decrease, masking the initial biochemical alteration.

Bile bacteriology is informative and may reveal *E. coli* in many cases, although bile may also be sterile.[17,18]

It is suggested that ascending opportunistic bacterial infections may cause or worsen EHBO.

Preoperative liver cytology may help in ruling out potential neoplastic infiltration (hepatic lymphoma), which may account for severe postoperative comorbidities.

Diagnostic

Abdominal ultrasonography is the gold standard for diagnosis.[43] Typical ultrasonographic findings include dilation of the common bile duct, thickened ductal or gallbladder walls, intrabiliary debris or inspissated material, and hyperechoic peribiliary fat indicating inflammation. Free abdominal fluid can be seen in case of biliary tract rupture.

Cholelithiasis is very rarely observed in ferrets; obstruction is more commonly caused by inspissated biliary material associated with ductal dilatation.

Surgical indication

Several clinical parameters are taken into account for surgical decision. Acute pain, icterus, and hyperbilirubinemia should be considered strong indicators for rapid surgical intervention.

However, surgery may have to be deferred in case of severe hypoalbuminemia (<20 g/L), which is relatively common with hepatic conditions. A plasma transfusion can be indicated.

Whenever surgery cannot be performed, ferrets may survive for several days with an EHBO but may eventually die if the obstruction is not relieved.[20]

Surgical interventions

Because EHBO represents mechanical obstruction, surgery is the treatment of choice. Several techniques are described. In the cohort of 17 cases, 10 cholecystectomies, 1 choledochotomy, 2 cholecystoduodenostomies, and 2 choledochal stentings were reported.[20] One case consisted only of manual pressure evacuation of ductal content, allowing successful restoration of duct patency. Most cases were successful except 2 undergoing cholecystectomy. Cholecystectomy was systematically combined with manual bile duct patency restoration in order to perform histologic and bacterial analysis.

Prognostic data

Ferrets appear to tolerate biliary surgery exceptionally well compared to cats and dogs, even with severe biochemical abnormalities.[20]

In small animals overall, EHBO carries a guarded prognosis. Combined data from canine and feline studies report survival rates of 66% in dogs and 65% in cats following surgery.[44,45] Pancreatitis may occur as a consequence of excessive traction or manipulation of the pancreas during surgery, leading to iatrogenic damage of the pancreatic tissue, ducts, or vascular supply. The pancreas is also highly susceptible to ischemic injury secondary to systemic conditions such as shock or sepsis. Therefore, postoperative pancreatitis can develop even in the absence of direct pancreatic handling.

In all individual case reports found in the literature, the ferrets survived the surgery. In the retrospective cohort, 15/17 ferrets survived the surgery, with 75% 1 year survival and 44% 2 year survival.[20]

Normalization of liver enzymes is expected within 5 days after surgery.[18] The generally good prognosis may be related to factors such as the low incidence of pancreatitis in ferrets.

However, among the different underlying causes, neoplastic disease (hepatic lymphoma) is most strongly associated with reduced survival in ferrets.

SUMMARY

As microsurgical and anesthetic techniques advance, the feasibility of complex hepatobiliary surgery in small exotic mammals continues to expand. For LLT in rabbits and EHBO in ferrets, prognosis seem to be fair to good which should encourage prompt recognition of those condition and surgical intervention whenever possible.

Future research should focus on evaluating long-term outcomes of liver surgeries through multicenter prospective studies and the importance of oncologic liver surgery in exotic pet species.

CLINICS CARE POINTS

- In rabbit liver lobe torsion, the caudate lobe is most commonly involved.
- Elevated ALT, AST and ALP, coupled with anemia is strongly suggestive.
- Liver lobectomy has a good prognosis in rabbit.
- Ferret with EHBO are often presented with ALT values higher than 500 IU/L and elevated bilirubinemia.
- Bile duct surgery has a good prognosis in ferret.

DECLARATION OF AI AND AI-ASSISTED TECHNOLOGIES IN THE WRITING PROCESS

During the preparation of this work the authors used Generative AI. After using this tool, the authors reviewed and edited the content as needed and takes full responsibility for the content of the publication.

DISCLOSURE

The authors declare no conflicts of interest related to this work. No external funding was received for this study.

REFERENCES

1. Donnelly TM, Vella D. Basic anatomy, physiology, and husbandry of rabbits. In: Ferrets, rabbits, and rodents: clinical medicine and surgery. 4th edition. Elsevier; 2020. p. 131–49.
2. Popesko P, Rajtová V, Horák J. A colour atlas of anatomy of small laboratory animals. Wolfe Publishing; 1992.
3. Stan FG. Comparative study of the liver anatomy in the rat, rabbit, Guinea pig and chinchilla. Bull Univ Agric Sci Vet Med Cluj-Napoca 2018;75:33–40.
4. Huynh M, Laloi F. Diagnosis of liver disease in domestic ferrets. Vet Clin North Am Exot Anim Pract 2013;16:121–44.
5. Tam AL, Melancon MP, Ensor J, et al. Rabbit hepatic arterial anatomy variations: implications on experimental design. Acta Radiol 2014;55(10):1226–33.
6. Páramo M, García-Barquin P, Santa María E, et al. Evaluation of the rabbit liver by direct portography and contrast-enhanced computed tomography: anatomical variations of the portal system and hepatic volume quantification. Eur Radiol Exp 2017;1:7.
7. Mentré V, Bulliot C, Linsart A, et al. Reference intervals for coagulation times using two point-of-care analysers in healthy pet rabbits (*Oryctolagus cuniculus*). Vet Rec 2014;174:658.
8. Bernhard C, Linsart A, Larrat S, et al. Use of two point-of-care analyzers provides reference intervals of prothrombin time and activated partial prothrombin time in nonanesthetized healthy ferrets (*Mustela putorius furo*). J Am Vet Med Assoc 2023;261(5):713–7.
9. Richard JN, Graham JE, Center SA, et al. Hepatic copper accumulates in ferrets with and without hepatobiliary disease. Am J Vet Res 2022;83:371–80.
10. Wittmaack MCN, Conceição MFBAM, Vera MCM, et al. Comparative evaluation of three laparoscopic cholecystectomy techniques in rabbit's model. Acta Cir Bras 2023;38:e383523.
11. Proença LM, Camus M, Nemeth N, et al. Diagnostic quality of percutaneous fine-needle aspirates and laparoscopic biopsy specimens of the liver in rabbits (*Oryctolagus cuniculus*). J Am Vet Med Assoc 2015;246:313–20.
12. Kemp SD, Zimmerman KL, Panciera DL, et al. A comparison of liver sampling techniques in dogs. J Vet Intern Med 2015;29:51–7.
13. Cole TL, Center SA, Flood SN, et al. Diagnostic comparison of needle and wedge biopsy specimens of the liver in dogs and cats. J Am Vet Med Assoc 2002;220:1483–90.
14. Kimbrell TL, Milovancev M, Olsen R, et al. Comparison of diagnostic accuracy of laparoscopic 3 mm and 5 mm cup biopsies to wedge biopsies of canine livers. J Vet Intern Med 2018;32:701–6.

15. Huynh M, Guillaumot P, Hernandez J, et al. Gall bladder rupture associated with cholecystitis in a domestic ferret (*Mustela putorius*). J Small Anim Pract 2014;55: 479–82.
16. Bochmann M, Knell S, Dennler M, et al. Clinical presentation, diagnosis, and treatment of cholelithiasis in a pet Guinea pig (*Cavia porcellus*). J Exotic Pet Med 2016;25(4):327–31.
17. Hauptman K, Jekl V, Knotek Z. Extrahepatic biliary tract obstruction in two ferrets (*Mustela putorius furo*). J Small Anim Pract 2011;52:371–5.
18. Hall BA, Ketz-Riley CJ. Cholestasis and cholelithiasis in a domestic ferret (*Mustela putorius furo*). J Vet Diagn Invest 2011;23:836–9.
19. Mayhew PD. Choledochal stenting in small animals. Adv Small Anim Med Surg 2009;22(9):1–3.
20. Huynh M, Di Girolamo N, Modesto F, et al. Biliary tract disease in ferrets: 17 cases. In: Proceedings of ICARE; 2017.
21. Tangner CH. Cholecystoduodenostomy in the dog comparison of two techniques. Vet Surg 1984;13:155–61.
22. Visser J, Schoemaker NJ, van Zeeland YRA, et al. Diagnosis and treatment of a congenital portosystemic shunt in a ferret (*Mustela putorius furo*). J Small Anim Pract 2024;65:75–8.
23. Miyai K, Javitt NB, Gochman N, et al. Hepatotoxicity of bile acids in rabbits: ursodeoxycholic acid is less toxic than chenodeoxycholic acid. Lab Invest 1982;46: 428–37.
24. Weisbroth SH. Torsion of the caudate lobe of the liver in the domestic rabbit (*Oryctolagus*). Vet Pathol 1975;12:13–5.
25. Wilson RB, Holscher MA, Sly DL. Liver lobe torsion in a rabbit. Lab Anim Sci 1987; 37:506–7.
26. Fitzgerald AL, Fitzgerald SD. Hepatic lobe torsion in a New Zealand white rabbit. Canine Pract 1992;17:16–9.
27. Taylor HR, Staff CD. Clinical techniques: successful management of liver lobe torsion in a domestic rabbit (*Oryctolagus cuniculus*) by surgical lobectomy. J Exotic Pet Med 2007;16:175–8.
28. Wenger S, Barrett EL, Pearson GR, et al. Liver lobe torsion in three adult rabbits. J Small Anim Pract 2009;50:301–5.
29. Saunders R, Redrobe S, Barr F, et al. Liver lobe torsion in rabbits. J Small Anim Pract 2009;50:562.
30. Stanke NJ, Graham JE, Orcutt CJ, et al. Successful outcome of hepatectomy as treatment for liver lobe torsion in four domestic rabbits. J Am Vet Med Assoc 2011;238:1176–83.
31. Pignon C, Donnelly TM, Mayer J. Hepatic lobe torsion in a rabbit (*Oryctolagus cuniculus*). Prat Med Chir Anim 2013;48:91–8.
32. Graham JE, Orcutt CJ, Casale SA, et al. Liver lobe torsion in rabbits: 16 cases (2007–2012). J Exotic Pet Med 2014;23:258–65.
33. Stock E, Vanderperren K, Moeremans I, et al. Use of contrast-enhanced ultrasonography in the diagnosis of a liver lobe torsion in a rabbit (*Oryctolagus cuniculus*). Vet Radiol Ultrasound 2020;61:31–5.
34. Daggett A, Loeber S, Le Roux AB, et al. Computed tomography with hounsfield unit assessment is useful in the diagnosis of liver lobe torsion in pet rabbits (*Oryctolagus cuniculus*). Vet Radiol Ultrasound 2021;62:210–7.
35. Leonard KC, Zhao Q, Taber RH, et al. Paracostal versus ventral midline approach for caudate liver lobectomy in the rabbit. Vet Surg 2022;51:920–8.

36. Ozawa SM, Graham JE, Guzman DS, et al. Clinicopathological findings in and prognostic factors for domestic rabbits with liver lobe torsion: 82 cases (2010–2020). J Am Vet Med Assoc 2022;260:1334–42.
37. Sheen JC, Vella D, Hung L. Retrospective analysis of liver lobe torsion in pet rabbits: 40 cases (2016–2021). Vet Rec 2022;191:e1971.
38. Chapple AR, Mikoni NA, Dutton CJ, et al. Left medial liver lobe torsion and post-operative acute gastric rupture in a 2.5 year old male-castrated Flemish giant rabbit (*Oryctolagus cuniculus*). Vet Radiol Ultrasound 2024;65:14–8.
39. Louvard C, Mathieu L. Clinical study on 30 cases of hepatic lobe torsion in rabbits (*Oryctolagus cuniculus*) between January 2021 and February 2024 clinical study on 30 cases of hepatic lobe torsion in rabbits (*Oryctolagus cuniculus*) between January 2021 and February 2024. Rev Vet Clin 2025;60:115–7.
40. Swann HM, Brown DC. Hepatic lobe torsion in 3 dogs and a cat. Vet Surg 2001; 30:482–6.
41. Vilalta L, Espada Y, Majó N, et al. Liver lobe torsion in a domestic ferret (*Mustela putorius furo*). J Exotic Pet Med 2016;25:321–6.
42. Waugh S, Andrie KM, Johnson V, et al. Liver lobe torsion in a Guinea pig (*Cavia porcellus*). Top Companion Anim Me 2021;43:100517.
43. Basse CV, Ruel Y, Agoulon A, et al. Domestic ferrets (*Mustela putorius furo*) with cholecystitis commonly show hyperbilirubinemia and common bile duct dilation, gallbladder sludge, and gallbladder wall thickening on ultrasound. Am J Vet Res 2024;86(1). ajvr.24.07.0191.
44. Amsellem PM, Seim HB 3rd, MacPhail CM, et al. Long-term survival and risk factors associated with biliary surgery in dogs: 34 cases (1994–2004). J Am Vet Med Assoc 2006;229(9):1451–7.
45. Speelman JP, Hui KL, Woodbridge NT, et al. Prognostic factors in 26 cats undergoing surgery for extra-hepatic biliary obstruction. Vet Sci 2024;11(12):610.

Reproductive Surgery in Rabbits, Rodents, and Ferrets

Sheyla Dominguez, DVM, DECZM (Small Mammal)[a],
Vicente Soler, DVM, DECZM (Small Mammal)[b],
Laura Vilalta, DVM, PhD, DECZM (Small Mammal)[c,*]

KEYWORDS

- Small mammals • Ovariohysterectomy • Ovariectomy • Orchiectomy
- Accessory glands • Mastectomy

KEY POINTS

- Reproductive anatomy differs substantially among rabbits, rodents and ferrets, requiring species-specific surgical planning and techniques to minimize complications.
- Selecting the neutering approach should be guided by the indication and patient-specific disease prevalence, and individual patient factors, rather than surgeon preference alone.
- The optimal timing of elective neutering for disease prevention varies among species and target conditions; in some species like ferrets, elective surgical neutering is not routinely recommended.
- Surgical management of accessory sexual gland disease requires precise anatomic knowledge to guide approach selection and minimize iatrogenic injury.
- Gentle tissue handling, meticulous hemostasis, and effective analgesia are critical to minimize complications such as gastrointestinal stasis, self-mutilation, wound infection, and scrotal or abdominal herniation.

INTRODUCTION

Reproductive surgery is commonly performed in small mammal practice. Different surgical approaches can be used for the same procedure, depending on species, patient size, and whether the surgery is elective or therapeutic. Approach must be tailored to each case due to anatomic variations among small mammals (**Tables 1** and **2**).

[a] Department of Exotic Animal, Exovet - Exotic Veterinary Hospital, Ngau Tau Kok, Hong Kong; [b] Department of Exotic Animal, Tai Wai Small Animal and Exotic Hospital, New Territories, Hong Kong; [c] Department of Exotic Animal, Hospital Veterinari Canis, Girona, Spain
* Corresponding author.
E-mail address: lauravilalta84@hotmail.com

Vet Clin Exot Anim 29 (2026) 749–780
https://doi.org/10.1016/j.cvex.2026.04.016 vetexotic.theclinics.com
1094-9194/26/

Abbreviations	
AGD	adrenal gland disease
VMA	ventral midline approach
VSD	vessel-sealing device

This article provides an overview of reproductive procedures in rabbits, rodents, and ferrets, highlighting the principal surgical approaches used for prophylactic gonadectomy and for the management of reproductive disorders.

PATIENT PREPARATION

Following patient induction, positioning, and surgical preparation, performing a local anesthetic block is advised (**Fig. 1**).

Antimicrobial prophylaxis is indicated when the risk of contamination or infection is high.[1] In such cases, presurgical intravenous administration is recommended. Routine sterile procedures like gonadectomy do not require perioperative antibiotics. Postoperative incision evaluation at 3 and 7 days is advised to identify early complications, and antimicrobial therapy should be initiated only after culture and sensitivity testing.

OVARIAN AND UTERINE SURGERY

Indications: Prevent unwanted pregnancies and pseudopregnancies, reduce hormonal-driven behavioral disorders, prevent or treat reproductive tract disease, and decrease the incidence of mammary gland disease.[8] The optimal age for spaying differs among species and is influenced by factors such as sexual maturity and species-specific disease risk.

A reduced incidence of mammary neoplasia after ovariectomy has been reported in rats, in which both early (3 months)[9] and late (5–7 months)[8] ovariectomy significantly decrease the incidence of mammary tumors.

In ferrets, elective neutering is not routinely recommended, as it may be a contributing factor in the development of adrenal gland disease (AGD).[10] When performed therapeutically, the authors recommend concurrent deslorelin acetate implantation.

Ovariectomy

Ovariectomy is technically simpler, faster, with lower risk of complications than ovariohysterectomy. However, it is contraindicated when uterine pathology is present.[11–15] It is commonly performed in rabbits up to 6 to 9 months of age.[13,14,16] Following ovariectomy, the uterus normally atrophies, and subsequent uterine disease is rarely observed. Rabbits present a high incidence of uterine disease, particularly malignant neoplasia,[14,17] specially in females older than 3 years, although uterine tumors have been reported in rabbits as young as 5 to 6 months old.[14,17] Papillary adenocarcinomas, the most common uterine adenocarcinoma subtype in rabbits, are frequently negative for estrogen receptor-α and progesterone receptors, suggesting that hormonal stimulation may not be essential for tumor progression.[18] Protective effect of ovariectomy against these tumors remains uncertain. In rats, a few cases of uterine pathology have been reported following elective ovariectomy, with or without partial hysterectomy, suggesting a potential risk of leaving residual reproductive tissue.[19]

Macroscopic uterine evaluation before ovariectomy has been recommended; however, gross inspection alone may fail to detect occult pathology, without

Table 1
Anatomic reproductive features of rabbits, rodents, and ferrets

Species	Female Reproductive Tract	Male Reproductive Tract	Mammary Glands
Rabbit	Uterus duplex bicollis Vagina simplex Vagina is long, flaccid, and fills with urine during micturition	No os penis Two hemiscrotal sacs Testes located cranial to the penis Open inguinal canal communicating with the abdominal cavity Accessory sexual glands (ASG)*: Vesicular (bilobed or paired glands), proprostate, prostate, paraprostate, and bulbourethral	Four to five pairs
Chinchilla	Uterus duplex bicollis Vagina simplex Vagina and urethral orifice are separated	Os penis S-shaped penis Two external opening in the glans (intromittent sac ventral to urethral opening) Not well-developed scrotum (scrotal pouches) Open inguinal canal communicating with the abdominal cavity ASG*: Vesicular, prostate, and bulbourethral	Three pairs
Guinea pig	Uterus duplex bicollis* Vagina simplex Vagina and urethral orifice are separated	Os penis Two external opening in the glans (intromittent sac caudoventral to urethral opening) Not well-developed scrotum (scrotal pouches) Open inguinal canal communicating with the abdominal cavity ASG*: Vesicular, prostate, bulbourethral, coagulating, ampullary, and preputial. The vesicular glands are blind-ending tubular sacs, up to 10 cm in length	One pair
Degu	Bicornuate uterus* Vagina and urethral orifice are separated	Os penis Two external opening in the glans (intromittent sac ventral to urethral opening) Not true scrotum (scrotal pouches) Open inguinal canal communicating with the abdominal cavity ASG*: Vesicular, prostate, and bulbourethral	Three to four pairs

(continued on next page)

Table 1
(*continued*)

Species	Female Reproductive Tract	Male Reproductive Tract	Mammary Glands
Rat	Uterus duplex bicollis Vagina simplex Vagina and urethral orifice are separated	Os penis Scrotum Open inguinal canal communicating with the abdominal cavity ASG*: Vesicular, prostate, bulbourethral, coagulating, ampullary, and preputial	Six pairs
Mouse	Uterus duplex bicollis* Vagina simplex Vagina and urethral orifice are separated	Os penis Scrotum Open inguinal canal communicating with the abdominal cavity ASG*: Vesicular, prostate, bulbourethral, and ampullary	Five pairs
Hamster	Uterus duplex bicollis* Vagina simplex Vagina and urethral orifice are separated	Os penis Scrotum Open inguinal canal communicating with the abdominal cavity ASG*: Vesicular, prostate, bulbourethral, coagulating, and ampullary	Six to seven pairs
Gerbil	Uterus duplex bicollis* Vagina simplex Vagina and urethral orifice are separated	Os penis Scrotum Open inguinal canal communicating with the abdominal cavity ASG*: Vesicular, prostate, bulbourethral, and coagulating	Four pairs
Ferret	Bicornuate uterus Vagina simplex	J-shaped os penis Scrotum ASG*: Prostate and preputial	Three to five pairs

Asterisk denotes inconsistent terminology in the literature; terms were chosen based on the most anatomically supported and recent references.

Data from Refs.[1,2–7]

histopathological examination.[20] Authors recommend careful case selection considering uterine disease prevalence in each species and performing preoperative radiographic and ultrasonographic assessment to help exclude uterine pathology.[21,22]

Surgical techniques

Ventral midline approach

- Make a 2 cm incision midway between the umbilicus and pubis. When incising the linea alba, gently elevate the muscular layer to avoid traumatizing the bladder and, in hindgut fermenters, the cecum.[23]

Table 2
Uterine types and principal anatomic characteristics

Uterine Type	Anatomic Illustration	Characteristics
Duplex bicollis	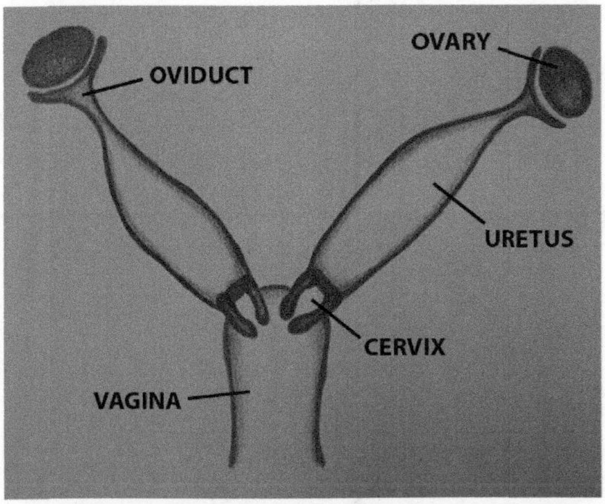	Two uteri and 2 cervices, eg.,: rabbits
Bicornuate	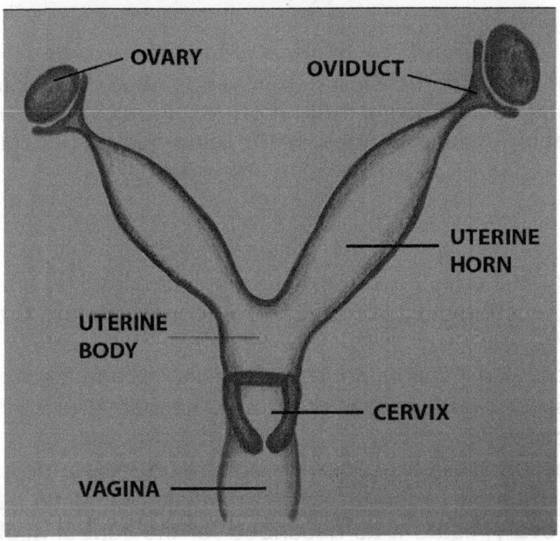	Two uterine horns (Y-shaped) separated medially but fused distally, where they form a common chamber, the uterine body. Uterine body opens into the vagina through a single cervix, eg, ferrets

Data from Refs.[4–7]

- Use a finger to exteriorize an ovary.[1,24] The weak suspensory ligament can be gently transected to allow further ovarian exteriorization. Place a clamp across the ovarian vessels. Use a ligature, hemostatic clip, vessel-sealing device (VSD), or bipolar electrocautery (for vessels 1–2 mm in diameter) at the ovarian pedicle and remove the ovary.[1,13,24] Suture materials and patterns used in the described techniques are summarized in **Table 3**
- Repeat the procedure on the contralateral ovary.
- Close the abdominal wall routinely.

Comments: Approach most commonly performed in rabbits.

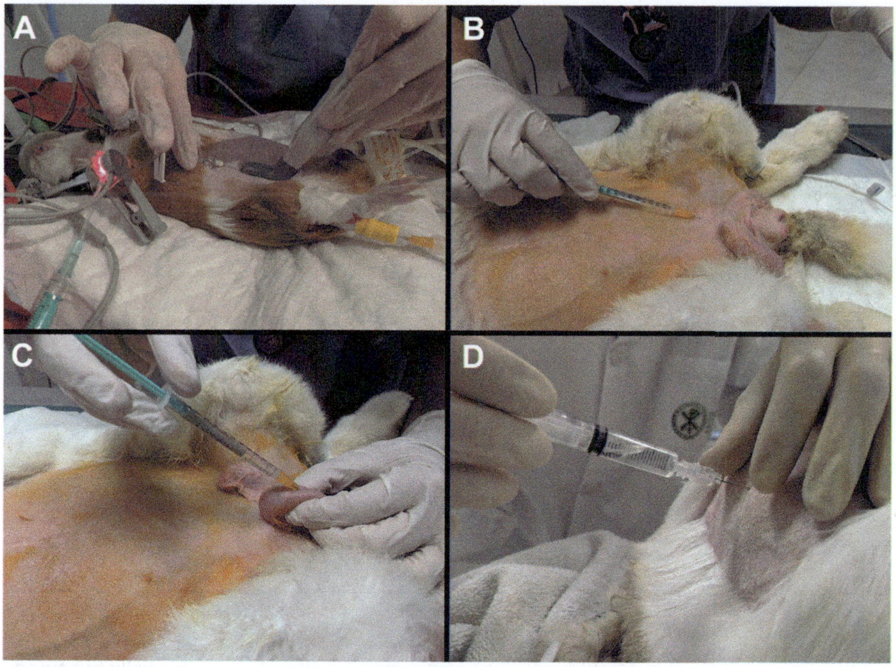

Fig. 1. (*A–D*) Locoregional anesthetic blocks: transversus abdominis plane block in a guinea pig (*A*), prescrotal subcutaneous infiltration (*B*), intratesticular infiltration (*C*), and epidural (*D*) in a rabbit. (Image Courtesy of Dr Laura Vilalta, DECZM and Dr Elena Ríos, DECVAA.)

Lateral approach

- Position the patient in sternal (myomorph rodents) or lateral recumbency (hystricomorph rodents, rotating the patient during surgery to access the contralateral ovary) (**Fig. 2**).[15,26]
- Perform a 1 to 2 cm skin incision, caudal to the last rib and approximately 1 cm ventral to the dorsal spinous process of the third lumbar vertebra in an oblique[27] or horizontal direction.[15]
- Dissect bluntly the abdominal oblique muscles and incise the peritoneum to expose the adipose tissue of the broad ligament. Apply gentle lateral pressure to exteriorize the ovary, ligate it as described for the ventral midline approach (VMA) and transect it. Confirm complete ovary removal.[15,26]
- Repeat the procedure on the contralateral ovary.
- Close the abdomen routinely.

Comments: This approach allows a smaller incision, easier access to the ovary, and reduces the risk of evisceration or incision contamination.[28] In rats, a comparison between VMA and flank approaches detected no differences in complication rates.[19] In guinea pigs with cystic ovaries, ovariohysterectomy remains the preferred treatment as concurrent uterine pathology is frequently present.[28]

Laparoscopic approach. Laparoscopic techniques are similar to those used in dogs and cats, with adjustments for anatomic and size differences.[16] Described laparoscopic techniques and complications are summarized in **Table 4**.

Table 3
Characteristics of suture materials and suture patterns used for the surgical techniques described in this article

SUTURE TYPES							
Brand name	Composition	Tensile strength over time	Tissue reactivity	Handling	Relative knot security	Approximate absorption	Suture sizes and needle types
Absorbable multifilament sutures							*Suture sizes:* should be adjusted to patient size and tissue characteristics. As a general guideline, suture sizes of 6-0 to 4-0 are used in myomorph rodents; 4-0 to 3-0 in hystricomorph rodents, rabbits and ferrets. *Needles types:* - Blunt point. Uses: friable tissues. - Taper point. Uses: delicate tissues such as reproductive tissue and muscle, especially in situations in which the size of the needle hole must be kept as small as possible. - Cutting point. Tapercut needles are a combination of taper and cutting needles. Standard cutting needles are triangular with the cutting surface on the concave surface of the needle. Reverse-cutting needles have the cutting surface on the convex surface having less risk of inadvertent needle hole elongation during needle passage and consequently less risk of suture pull-through. Uses: skin (dermal and intradermal) and muscle. The authors prefer the use of minimally traumatic taper-point needles and monofilament suture material for reproductive tissue and abdominal wall closures. Rapidly absorbable sutures are reserved for the subcutaneous tissue and skin, whereas slowly absorbable sutures for the musculature. Nonabsorbable sutures are reserved for skin closure.
Vicryl	Polyglactin 910	+++ (50% at 2-3 weeks)	+	++++	++	Predictable 56-70 days	
Vicryl Rapide	Polyglactin 910	+ (0% at 2-3 weeks)	+	++++	++	Predictable 42 days	
Monosyn Dexon	Polyglycolic acid	+++ (50% at 2-3 weeks)	+	++	+++	Predictable 90 days	
Absorbable monofilament sutures							
Monocryl	Poliglecaprone 25	+++ (50% at 1-2 weeks)	+	+++	++	Predictable 119 days	
Biosyn	Glycomer 631	+++ (50% at 2-3 weeks)	+	+++	++	Predictable 90-110 days	
PDS II	Polydioxanona	+++ (50% at 5-6 weeks)	+	+++	++	Predictable 180 days	
Maxon	Polyglyconate	+++ (50% at 4-5 weeks)	+	+++	+++	Predictable 180 days	
Non absorbable monofilament sutures							
Nylon, Supramid	Polyamide	460-710 MPa	Low	++	+		
Prolene	Polypropylene	410-460 Mpa	Low	+	+		
Novafil	Polyester	510-1060 Mpa	Moderate	++	++		

SUTURE PATTERNS					
	Advantages	Disadvantages	Patterns used	Uses	Comments
Interrupted pattern	Every suture has a knot associated with it. More precise wound margins apposition (selective adjustments can be made). Provides greater security than a continuous pattern.	More time is needed to close a wound. Common errors include excessive tightening and insufficient space between the knot and the skin.	Simple interrupted, modified Gambee, and four mattress patterns (horizontal, vertical, cruciate and Lembert).	Variety of tissues: viscera, body wall, subcutaneous, and skin.	Cruciate, simple, interrupted, or simple continuous patterns may be used for the abdominal muscle. Subcutaneous tissues are apposed with a simple continuous pattern, and the skin with an intradermal suture secured with an Aberdeen Knot. The numbers of throws appropriate to use in a surgical knot is influenced by suture material characteristics and the type of pattern used. In general, at least four throws are appropriate for surgical knots, with the five-throw square knot considered as the gold standard in conventional surgery. Ending knots of continuous patterns require two to three additional throws because such knots are composed of three suture strands (single strand and suture loop).
Continuous patterns	Quicker and easy to perform. Tension distribution along the entire length of the wound. For abdominal wall closure, it provides similar strength and complication rates to simple interrupted sutures.	Usually reserved for noncutaneous locations because of the risk of suture line compromise by self-inflicted trauma.	Simple continuous, continuous lock, horizontal mattress, purse-string, Cushing, Connell, and continuous Lembert patterns. Intradermal pattern (variation of horizontal mattress pattern).	Common locations for use: intradermal sites, subcutaneous tissue, body wall, and viscera; temporarily orifice closure (purse-string pattern, a circular variation of continuous Lembert).	

Rapidly absorbable synthetic sutures (blue); slowly absorbable synthetic sutures (green). +: poor, ++: fair, +++: good, ++++: very good.
Data from Refs.[25]

Ovariohysterectomy

Technique of choice when uterine pathology is present. In rabbits, surgery is easier after puberty (6–9 months), when the uterus enlarges and the ligaments become slightly looser, and before significant fat accumulation occurs.[11,20]

Surgical techniques

Ventral midline approach

- Position the patient in dorsal recumbency (**Fig. 3**). Make a 2 to 3 cm skin incision midway between the umbilicus and pubis. In gerbils and dwarf hamsters, make a paramedian incision to avoid the midventral sebaceous gland. Celiotomy is performed as described for ovariectomy.[11,19,24,28] Carefully exteriorize the uterus, ovaries, fallopian tube, and associated fat pads using a finger or blunt

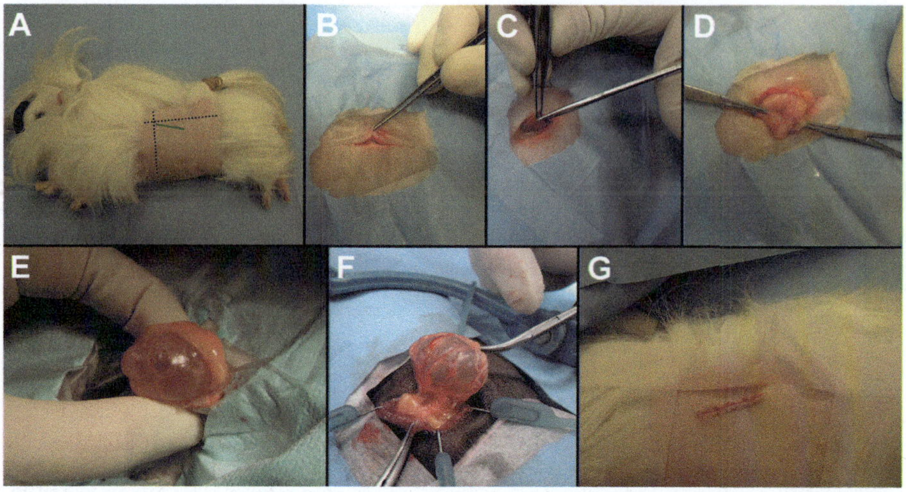

Fig. 2. (*A–G*) Bilateral flank ovariectomy in a guinea pig. Determination of the incision start point (*black dashed lines*) and incision orientation (*green line*) (*A*). Skin incision (*B*). Abdominal muscle dissection (*C*). Identification of the broad ligament adipose tissue (*D*). Gentle lateral pressure facilitates ovarian exteriorization, particularly in patients with ovarian cysts (*E, F*). Abdominal closure (*G*). (Image Courtesy of Dr Laura Vilalta.)

instrument.[1,23] Transect the ovarian ligament to facilitate exposure. Double ligate the ovarian vascular pedicle after creating a small fenestration through the mesometrium, using the standard two-clamp technique, or with vascular clips, VSD or bipolar electrocautery.[11,23,36] Transect the pedicle above the second ligature, confirm hemostasis, and return it to the abdomen. Confirm complete ovary removal and repeat the procedure on the opposite side.[23,36]

- Identify the uterine vessels within the mesometrium. In rabbits, they lie farther from the cervices and vagina than in ferrets, dogs, or cats and fat may hinder their visualization. Some authors ligate the vessels separately on each side, whereas others prefer a transfixing ligature.
- In rabbits, opinions differ regarding whether the cervices should be removed during ovariohysterectomy.[12] Vaginectomy and hysterectomy techniques, along with their respective advantages and disadvantages, are described in **Table 5**. In other species, hysterectomy is routinely performed.

The use of VSDs for occlusion of uterine tissue has shown promising results in dogs and was effective in sealing the uterus in rabbits; however, it failed to achieve a reliable seal at the vagina.[37,38] This difference is likely anatomic, as vaginal, uterine, or cervical tissue differ in elastin-to-collagen ratio,[37] with organ size potentially contributing as well. Despite this limitation, the use of VSDs for vascular occlusion significantly reduces surgical and anesthetic times compared to conventional ligation.[38,39]

- Close the abdomen routinely.

Comments: The authors routinely perform vaginectomy to ensure complete removal of uterine tissue in rabbits, with no major complications. A literature review did not reveal reports of uroabdomen or septic peritonitis following vaginectomy.[24] Postoperative adhesions may develop after ovariohysterectomy, particularly in rabbits;

Table 4
Laparoscopy gonadectomy techniques in small mammals

Surgery	Technique	Description
Ovariectomy	Two ports	• Place the patient in dorsal recumbency (reverse Trendelenburg position). Make a small midline incision (1–2 cm caudal to the umbilicus) to expose and incise the linea alba, elevating the body wall to avoid visceral trauma. • Insert the sheathed telescope as the first portal and secure it with a mattress suture to obtain an airtight seal. Initiate CO_2 insufflation and examine the abdominal viscera for abnormalities. Insert an additional cannula on the midline, 2–3 cm cranial to the first portal, under direct camera visualization to prevent abdominal organ injury. • Rotate the patient approximately 30°–45° laterally in rabbits or 90° in guinea pigs down on the surgeon's side, to displace the voluminous gastrointestinal tract away from the surgical area and allow visualization of the contralateral ovary. Grasp the ovary with forceps inserted through the cranial portal, elevate and tack it to the body wall using a transabdominal suspension suture. Replace the forceps with the preferred ligating device (endoscopic clips, suture ligatures, electrosurgery, or a tissue-sealing device) and dissect free the ovarian pedicle, proper ligament and mesovarium. After ensuring hemostasis, leave the ovary tacked to the body wall using a hemostat on the skin for later retrieval. • Rotate the patient to the opposite side and dissect the contralateral ovary as described above. Remove both ovaries though the cranial cannula. Remove the instruments, evacuate the insufflating gas by manual expression, and close routinely. Comments: A 2.7 mm telescope and 3 mm instruments are preferred. For larger animals, 5 mm instrumentation can be used, with the main advantage being the time-saving use of a combined sealing and cutting device (eg, LigaSure Atlas, Covidien) instead of separate bipolar forceps and scissors. This technique is limited for elective ovariectomy in simple monogastric species, as visualization of the ovaries may be challenging in species with voluminous gastrointestinal tract.
	Three ports	• Make a 3–10 mm skin incision through or caudal to the umbilicus and place the first cannula as described in the technique above. • Insert 2 additional instrument cannulae cranial and caudal to the first port through the linea alba. Use the telescope to visualize the entry of each cannula. • Insert grasping forceps through a cannula and grasp the ovary. Gentle manipulation of intestinal structures may be required to reveal the ovary. As the ovary is elevated, the vascular supply is exposed.

(*continued on next page*)

Table 4
(*continued*)

Surgery	Technique	Description
		• Insert the preferred ligating device through the right cannula to ligate or coagulate the vasculature and transect the ovary. • Once the ovary is free, remove the cannula and the ovary through the port site and confirm hemostasis. • Place the patient on the opposite side and repeat the procedure from the other side of the table. • Conventional closure. Comments: Most common approach in hindgut fermenters, as it allows the use of additional instrumentation to retract the gastrointestinal tract and facilitate ovarian identification and manipulation.
Ovariohysterectomy	Two-three ports	• Perform the preferred ovariectomy as described above. After ovarian resection, perform the hysterectomy. Hysterectomy can be accomplished using a pre-tied ligature loop introduced into the abdomen through one of the cannulae. Pull the ovaries and uterus through the suture loop and tighten it at the level of the cervix or vagina, then transect the uterus cranial to the loop. • Control hemostasis and remove the ovaries and uterus through an instrument portal, enlarging the portal, if needed. • Close the incisions routinely.
	Scope assisted	• Alternatively, a laparoscopic-assisted ovariohysterectomy can be performed following laparoscopic ovarian resection, by enlarging the caudal opening enough to exteriorize the uterus and ovaries. Once exteriorized, ligate the vessels and the reproductive tissue as in an open procedure (see ovariohysterecteomy section). • A single-incision laparoscopic surgery (SILS) technique using only one port containing multiple lumens for cannulae has been described in rabbits. This SILS port allows easy transition of instruments, telescope, and bipolar electrocautery devices between cannulae, improving triangulation and reducing surgical time and complications. The system consists of a foam port with 3 cannula openings (2 5 mm cannulae and a 12 mm cannula), and a small opening for the insufflator tubing. A 2–3 cm ventral midline incision is made approximately 1 cm caudal to the umbilicus. Before insertion, the intra-abdominal portion of the port is occluded with Carmalt forceps to protect the viscera, as the insufflator tubing contains a firm plastic component that protrudes slightly from the concave surface. Use a Gelpi retractor to elevate the body wall and facilitate port insertion. The ovaries are approached as in standard techniques, introducing the telescope

(*continued on next page*)

Table 4
(continued)

Surgery	Technique	Description
		through 1 cannula and instruments through the remaining 2. After resection of the second ovary, and while is grasped, insufflation is discontinued and the remaining instruments are removed. The foam SILS port is gently removed from the abdomen with the grasper in place, holding the reproductive tract. Once exteriorized, hysterectomy or vaginectomy is performed (see ovariohysterectomy section).
Orchiectomy	One or two ports	• Place the patient in reverse Trendelenburg dorsal recumbency to move the viscera cranially. • Position the telescope cannula cranial to the umbilicus, then place 1 or 2 instrument cannulae as described for ovariohysterectomy. • Identify the ductus deferens dorsal to neck of the urinary bladder and ventral to the colon. Grasp it and apply gentle traction to locate the testicle. • Ligate the spermatic cord with vascular clips, pre-tied suture loops, or a tissue-sealing device, and transect distal to the ligature. This leaves the testicle unattached within the abdomen. Often, a cryptorchid testicle is small enough to be removed through the cannula, enlarge the instrument port incision as needed for retrieval. • Repeat the procedure on the contralateral testicle. Remove the instruments, evacuate the insufflation gas and close routinely.
	Scope assisted	• Only 2 portals are required: a midline umbilical telescope portal and one instrument portal. • Identify and grasp the testicle as described above, then enlarge the midline portal incision to expose it. • Apply a conventional open technique to ligate and transect the spermatic cord. • Repeat the procedure on the contralateral testicle and complete the procedure as described for the technique above.
Complications	Complications such as intestinal trauma, hemorrhage, and prolonged surgical and anesthetic times are primarily linked to operator inexperience and tend to decrease with training. In rabbits, a study comparing laparoscopic ovariectomy with open ovariectomy found no reduction in pain or recovery time; laparoscopic ovariectomy required twice the surgical time, and one rabbit sustained an intestinal perforation requiring euthanasia. Insufflation-related complications include impaired ventilation, acidosis, reduced venous return, and postoperative discomfort. In guinea pigs, although increased working space was achieved at intraabdominal pressures of 6 and 8 mm Hg compared to 4 mm Hg, further research is needed due to associated negative cardiovascular effects. In rabbits, 8 mm Hg provided adequate working space with fewer cardiorespiratory changes than 12 mm Hg. Isobaric abdominal lifting technique is a feasible alternative to insufflation in rabbits and requires less specialized equipment.	

Data from Refs.[13,16,29–35]

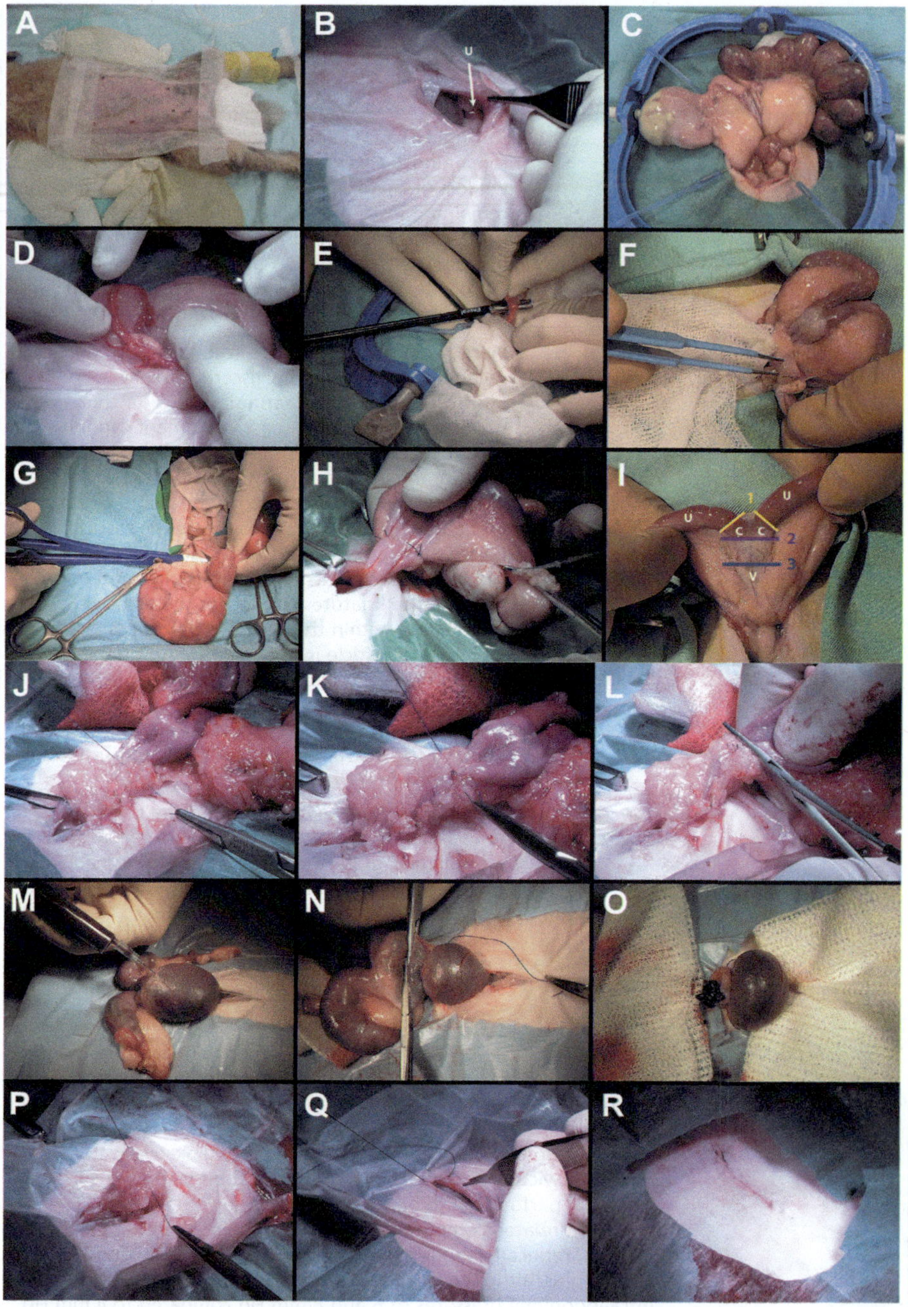

Fig. 3. (*A–I*) Ventral midline ovariohysterectomy in a rabbit: part 1. Patient preparation; clipping can be minimized by securing surrounding hair with adhesive tape (*A*) (Image Courtesy of Dr Laura Vilalta and Dr Sheyla Dominguez). Abdominal wall incision, and uterus and associated fat pad visualization (*arrow*) (*B*) (Image Courtesy of Dr Laura Vilalta.). Exteriorization of the reproductive tract (*C*). Inspection of the ovary; note the fallopian tube forming a semicircle around it (*D*).

therefore, intrabdominal tissues should be handled gently, and devitalized tissue within the abdomen minimized to reduce this risk.[36] When uterine pathology is present, histopathological examination is recommended.

Lateral approach

Unilateral

- Place the patient in lateral recumbency (**Fig. 4**). In young and clinically healthy guinea pigs, either flank can be used. However, in those with ovarian cysts, position the smaller ovary uppermost to facilitate its localization and access.[15]
- Abdominal access and ovarian pedicle ligation are performed as described for flank ovariectomy. Ligate the mesometrium and expose the uterus and uterine bifurcation. Place a transfixing ligature and transect the cervix. Locate the contralateral ovary and repeat the process.[15,28]
- Close the abdomen routinely.

Comments: Approach primarily described in guinea pigs, with a reported 93% success rate.[15] Compared with VMA, it carries a lower risk of complications and mortality due to the deep ovarian location, short suspensory ligaments, and cecum handling; it also shortens surgery time, minimizes visceral manipulation (reducing the risk of gastrointestinal stasis and adhesions), wound contamination and dehiscence.[15,27,28] It has also been successfully performed in rats.[19] Both flanks and ventral abdomen should be prepared in case conversion to a bilateral or VMA is required due to complications or unexpected uterine pathology.[28]

Bilateral

- Position the patient in left lateral recumbency, and make the incision as described earlier. Ligate and dissect the right ovary and uterus, then either transect and remove them, or replace them within the abdomen before routine closure. Reposition the patient and prepare aseptically the opposite flank. Make the second incision slightly more caudal to facilitate access to the left ovary and uterus and repeat the procedure.[28,36]

Comments: Preferred approach in large guinea pigs with abundant abdominal fat or reproductive pathology to allow a complete reproductive tract removal.[28,36]

Laparoscopic approach. Described laparoscopic techniques and complications are summarized in **Table 4**.

Hysterotomy

Indications: Dystocia.

Ovarian vascular pedicle ligation using a vessel-sealing device (VSD) or bipolar electrocautery (*E, F*). Uterine vessels identification and ligation using a VSD or a transfixing ligature (*G, H*). Potential ligation sites for hysterectomy or vaginectomy include uterine bifurcation (1), cervices (2), or vaginal body (3) (*I*). U: uterus, C: cervices, V: vagina. (*J–R*) Ventral midline ovariohysterectomy in a rabbit: part 2. Vaginectomy (*J–P*). A transfixing ligature is placed through the vaginal vestibule below cervices (*J–L*). In cases of aneurysm, fine-needle aspiration of vaginal fluid reduces its size, facilitating ligatures placement (*M, N*). Transection above the ligature and closure of the vaginal lumen (*O, P*). Abdominal closure (*Q, R*). (*Image Courtesy* This image is the courtesy of Laura Vilalta and Sheyla Dominguez, DECZM.)

Table 5
Comparison of hysterectomy and vaginectomy techniques

	Surgical Approach	Advantages	Disadvantages
Vaginectomy	Recommended only in rabbits. Place a transfixing ligature through the vaginal vestibule below the cervices. Transect the tissue above the ligature. As the vagina is nonsterile and may contain urine, close its lumen, using a continuous Lembert suture pattern.	Quick and simple. Treatment of choice when reproductive pathology exists, allowing complete removal of reproductive tissue.	If the cervices are removed, urine leakage into the abdomen may occur unless the vaginal stump is effectively repaired or ligated. The friable nature of the vaginal tissue can make oversewing difficult, as the suture material may tear through it. The uterine artery lies in close proximity to the cervices and vaginal wall, and a transfixing suture can easily penetrate it.
Histerectomy	In rabbits, 2 different techniques have been reported. • Clamp and double ligate the cervices with 3–0 or 4–0 absorbable suture material and transect above the second ligature (at least one of the ligatures must be transfixing). • Ligate each uterus individually at the bifurcation with the same suture, then encircle the cervices; cut the suture only after securing the cervical ligature. Remove the uterus and transect the mesometrium and the cervical stump. Confirm hemostasis before replacement into the abdomen. In other species, the uterus and uterine vessels are ligated along the cervix or distal uterine body using a transfixing ligature.	Quick and simple. The ligature sits securely in the cervical tissue, which is much firmer than the flaccid vaginal tissue. Remaining cervical tissue serves as an effective seal against infection or urine leakage. Transfixing suture is unnecessary, eliminating the risk of hemorrhage. The ligature is not close to the ureters, bladder or rectum, minimizing the risk of postoperative adhesions to these organs.	Residual uterine tissue left behind; this is clinically insignificant unless neoplastic or abnormal. Primarily indicated in very young animals, as reproductive pathology is common. Preoperative diagnostic imaging is recommended to rule out reproductive disease. This technique should only be performed when no uterine pathology is present.

Data from Refs.[8,11,19,24,28,40,41]

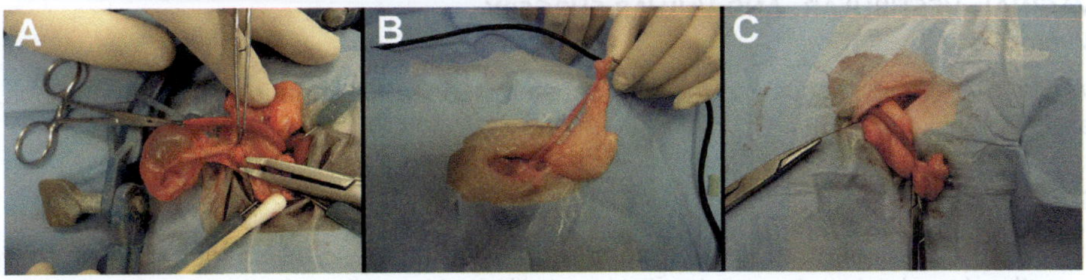

Fig. 4. (*A–C*) Bilateral flank ovariohysterectomy in a guinea pig. Ovary and uterus exteriorization. Ligation of the ovarian pedicle (*A*). Mesometrium exposition and uterus ligation (*B*, *C*). (Image Courtesy of Dr Laura Vilalta.)

Surgical technique

- Perform a midline incision as described for the VMA ovariohysterectomy. Avoid traumatizing the uterus when incising the linea alba.
- Exteriorize and isolate the uterus with moist sponges. Make a longitudinal incision on the ventral surface of the uterus or bilateral incisions on each uterine horn (depending on species-specific anatomy and fetal distribution). In ferrets, grasp the fetus, apply gentle traction until the endotheliochorial placenta detaches,[42] and transfer them to an assistant. If the placenta is firmly attached to the uterus, as occurs in rabbits and rodents due to their deeply invasive hemochorial placenta,[42] clamp the umbilical cord, avoiding placental traction. If placental removal is not possible without causing excessive hemorrhage or endometrial trauma, leave them to pass naturally. Lavage any lochia from the uterus and incision site, minimizing abdominal contamination. Close the uterus using a simple continuous appositional inner layer and continuous inverting outer layer. Suture material should engage the submucosa but not penetrate the uterine lumen.[28,43]
- Close the abdomen routinely.

Comments: Dystocia is relatively common in guinea pigs and chinchillas and can be managed by performing either an ovariohysterectomy or a cesarean section (hysterotomy). Cesarean section is preferred in breeding or anemic animals, followed by oxytocin administration to induce uterine involution and minimize blood loss. In nonbreeding animals, en bloc resection of the uterus and enclosed fetuses provides simultaneous ovariohysterectomy and dystocia treatment without a significant increase in neonatal mortality rate. Ligate the ovarian vessels first to maintain fetal oxygenation. Fetuses should be removed within 60 seconds of clamping uterine blood supply to minimize hypoxemia.[28,43,44]

Uterine Prolapse

Surgical technique

- Position the patient in dorsal recumbency. Clean and lubricate the prolapsed uterus. If the tissue is viable, attempt replacement using gentle compression. Success is uncommon and recurrence frequent.[44]

If replacement is unsuccessful, perform laparotomy. Apply simultaneous external pressure (use multiple cotton-tipped applicators to increase surface area, avoiding vaginal perforation) and internal traction to aid prolapse reduction.[45] Once the uterus is repositioned, perform an ovariohysterectomy.

VAGINAL, VESTIBULAR, AND VULVAR SURGERY

Vulvoplasty

Indications: Vulvar tissue overgrowth causing perineal dermatitis, vulvar lacerations, and neoplasia (**Fig. 5**).

Surgical technique

- Place the patient in dorsal recumbency. Make a crescent-shaped incision from the dorsal vulvar area, extending ventrally and laterally to both sides of the vulva. Carefully estimate the amount of skin resection required. Use bipolar electrocautery to achieve hemostasis and close the subcutaneous tissue and skin with interrupted sutures to prevent dog-ear formation.[24,46,40]

Vaginal Prolapse

Surgical technique

- Position the patient in dorsal recumbency. Clean and lubricate the prolapsed vagina. Resect the affected portion of the vagina if nonviable tissue is observed. Manually reduce the vagina and decrease the vaginal lumen using a purse-string suture.[11,24,44]

Comments: Vaginal prolapse is distinguished by the "doughnut-shaped" protrusion of the entire vaginal circumference and lumen. Ovariohysterectomy is recommended in cases of recurrence.[11,24,44]

Rectovaginal Fistula Repair

Indications: rare congenital disorder reported in ferrets[47,48] and rabbits.[49] May occur with or without imperforate anus. Fecal contamination of the vagina results in vaginitis, vulvitis, and associated dermatitis.

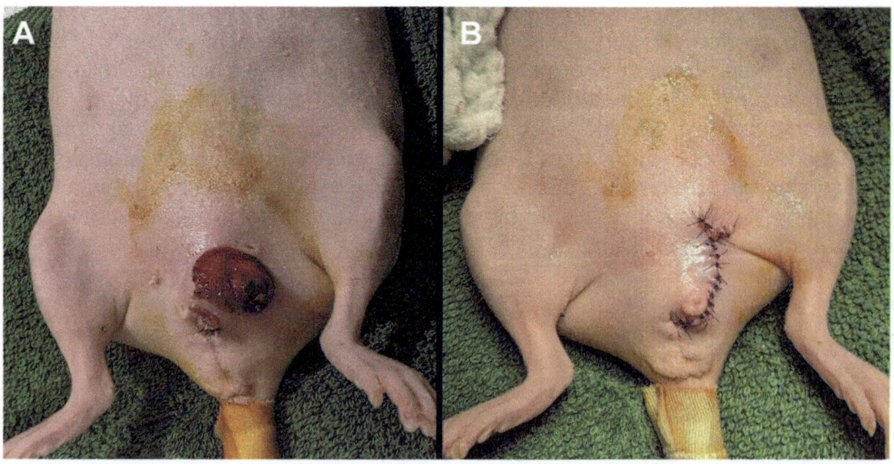

Fig. 5. (*A, B*) Vulvoplasty in a rat. Preoperative image of a perivulvar squamous cell carcinoma (*A*). The mass was in close contact with the urethra and involved the ventral aspect of the vagina, causing ventrolateral displacement. Postoperative image following mass excision and vulvar reconstruction (*B*). (Image Courtesy of Dr Laura Vilalta.)

Surgical techniques

- Make a vertical perineal incision and locate the fistula opening. Insert a catheter into the rectum to identify the rectal lumen and close the rectal and vaginal defects separately. Close the musculature, subcutaneous, and skin routinely.[47]
- Isolate and repair the fistula via horizontal incision between the anus and vagina. In cases of imperforate anus, incise the anal button, locate the rectal stump, and suture the terminal part to the anus.[48]

Comments: Reported complications include fecal incontinence, obstipation, tenesmus, constipation, anal gland odor, anal edema, rectal prolapse, urinary incontinence, anal stenosis, and wound dehiscence.[47,48]

TESTICULAR, AND SCROTAL SURGERY

Orchiectomy

Indications: Prevent breeding, reduce sexually driven behaviors (urine marking and aggression),[50] and manage or prevent testicular and prostatic disorders (tumors, infections, torsions, or cryptorchidism). Orchiectomy can be performed once the testicles descend to the scrotal area. Elective orchiectomy in ferrets is not recommended, due to its potential association with AGD.[10]

Surgical techniques

Three surgical approaches have been described for castration in rabbits and rodents: scrotal, prescrotal, and abdominal.[28,51] As rabbits and rodents have a permanently open inguinal canal, its closure and preservation of epididymal fat are recommended to reduce the risk of postoperative herniation.[1,50,52]

Scrotal approach

- Place the patient in dorsal recumbency. If the testicles are intra-abdominal, apply gentle manual pressure on the caudal abdomen to return them to the scrotal area.
- Make a 0.5 to 1 cm longitudinal incision through the scrotal skin. Bluntly dissect the subcutaneous tissue to expose the vaginal tunica. Gentle back-and-forth movement of the testicles may facilitate its identification.[11]
- Once the vaginal tunica is identified, proceed according to the selected technique (**Table 6**), depending on whether the vaginal tunica and inguinal canal are managed using a closed (**Fig. 6**), open–closed, or open technique (**Fig. 7**).
- Because rabbit and ferret scrotal skin is very thin, it is preferable to seal the incision with surgical adhesive or allow healing by second intention.[23] In rodents, intradermal suture is recommended as they are prone to scrotal abscessation and wound infection.[36,53]
- Repeat the procedure on the contralateral side.

Comments: Although technically simpler, this approach has been associated with longer anesthetic times in rabbits and degus,[50,54] higher rates of postoperative self-trauma in rabbits,[50] and a higher incidence of postoperative infection in guinea pigs.[53] When testicular pathology is present, histopathological examination is recommended.

Prescrotal approach

- Make a single 1 to 2 cm midline prescrotal incision to access both testicles (**Fig. 8**). Bluntly dissect the subcutaneous tissue to expose the vaginal tunica.
- Follow the instructions described earlier for the scrotal technique.

Table 6
Surgical orchiectomy techniques according to inguinal canal management

Technique	Description	Comments
Closed	• Expose the vaginal tunica and dissect it from the internal wall of the scrotum. • Exteriorize the vaginal tunica containing the spermatic cord and testicle. Separate it from the scrotal sac using a sterile gauze. • Clamp, ligate, and transect the spermatic cord covered by the vaginal tunica. • Remove the testicle and confirm hemostasis. In rabbits, use a hemostat to replace the inverted scrotal sac.	Technique recommended in rabbits and rodents to prevent herniation of the intestine or urinary bladder through the open inguinal canals.
Open closed	• Isolate the vaginal tunica and place a circumferential ligature around it using curved hemostatic forceps; this ligature will later be used to close the inguinal canal once the testicle is excised. • Incise the vaginal tunica and exteriorize the testicle, everting the scrotal sac. • Separate the attachment between the tail of the epididymis and the scrotal sac, then return the inverted scrotal sac to its anatomic position. • Clamp and ligate the ductus deferens and testicular vessels, in large rabbits they may be ligated separately. • Resect the testicle and if hemostasis is adequate, return the spermatic cord stump into the inguinal canal with a sterile cotton swab. • Use the initial circumferential ligature around the vaginal tunica to close the inguinal canal and resect the tunic distal to the ligation.	Technique recommended in rabbits and rodents to prevent herniation of the intestine or urinary bladder through the open inguinal canals.
Open	• Incise the vaginal tunica to exteriorize the testicle. • Proceed as described for the open-closed technique until excising the testicle and returning the spermatic cord stump into the inguinal canal. • Suture the vaginal tunica with a cruciate pattern.	Since the inguinal canal remains open in this approach, closure of the tunica is mandatory.

Data from Refs.[1,23,28,51]

- Repeat the procedure on the contralateral side and close the incision with an intradermal suture.

Comments: Preferred approach for rabbits, as it reduces anesthetic time and is associated with less postoperative scrotal edema compared with the scrotal

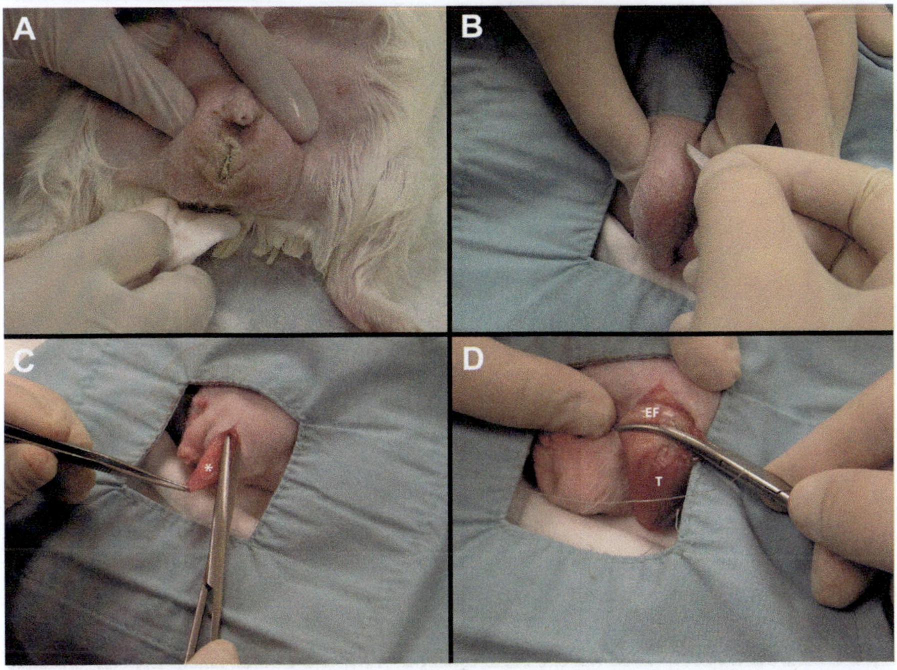

Fig. 6. (*A–D*) Scrotal closed orchiectomy in a guinea pig. Preoperative perineal sac cleaning is recommended to minimize surgical contamination (*A*). Scrotal incision (*B*). Vaginal tunica dissection (*C*). Clamping and ligation of the intact vaginal tunica (*D*). Asterisk: vaginal tunica, T: testicle, EF: epididymal fat. (Image Courtesy of Dr Laura Vilalta.)

technique.[50] Similarly, in degus is faster and requires less anesthetic time.[54] In rodents, particularly hystricomorphs, make a single skin incision cranial to the prepuce or 2 craniolateral incisions, avoiding the penis,[28,52] as postoperative penile complications (prolapse attributable to nerve trauma or displacement related to preputial damage) have been reported.[28,55]

When therapeutic orchiectomy is indicated in ferrets, both prescrotal and scrotal approaches may be used.[41] Their inguinal canal is closed; therefore, vaginal tunica closure is unnecessary. The spermatic cord can be ligated using a "self-tie" technique, tying the ductus deferens to the testicular vessels, or absorbable suture material.[41]

Abdominal approach

- Empty the urinary bladder before surgery and gently reduce the testicles into the abdominal cavity by pressing on the scrotum (**Fig. 9**).
- Make a 2 to 3 cm caudal abdominal celiotomy.
- Identify the testicles craniolateral to the bladder and exteriorize them.
- Dissect the tail of the epididymis free from the scrotal sac, ligate the spermatic cord near the inguinal canal, and remove the testicle.
- Repeat the procedure on the contralateral testicle and close the abdomen routinely.

Comments: Preferred approach for guinea pigs as it is associated with lower postoperative infection rates and shorter anesthetic times.[53] Technique of choice for cryptorchidism and inguinal or hemiscrotal hernia repair in rabbits.[1,11] Advantages include a

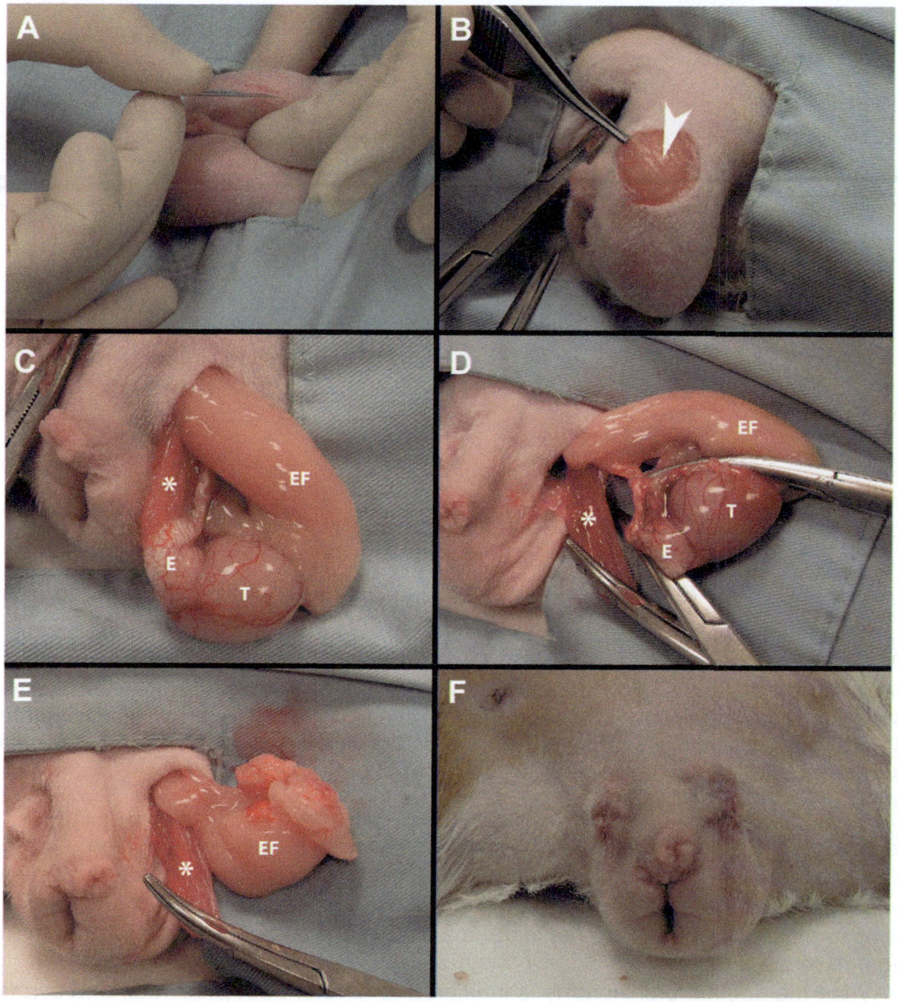

Fig. 7. (*A–F*) Scrotal open orchiectomy in a guinea pig. Scrotal incision (*A*). Exposure and incision of the vaginal tunica with testicular exteriorization (*B, C*). Detachment of the ligament between epididymis and everted vaginal tunica (*D*). Testicle resection preserving epididymal fat (*E*). Final bilateral scrotal wounds (*F*). Arrowhead: vaginal tunica, T: testicle, E: epididymis, EF: epididymal fat, asterisk: everted vaginal tunica. (Image Courtesy of Dr Laura Vilalta.)

single incision that is less likely to become contaminated by substrate and preservation of epididymal fat.[36]

Laparoscopic approach. Described laparoscopic techniques and complications are summarized in **Table 4**.

Scrotal Ablation

Indications: Testicular or scrotal tumors, scrotal trauma, and large pendulous scrotum, causing perineal dermatitis.[40]

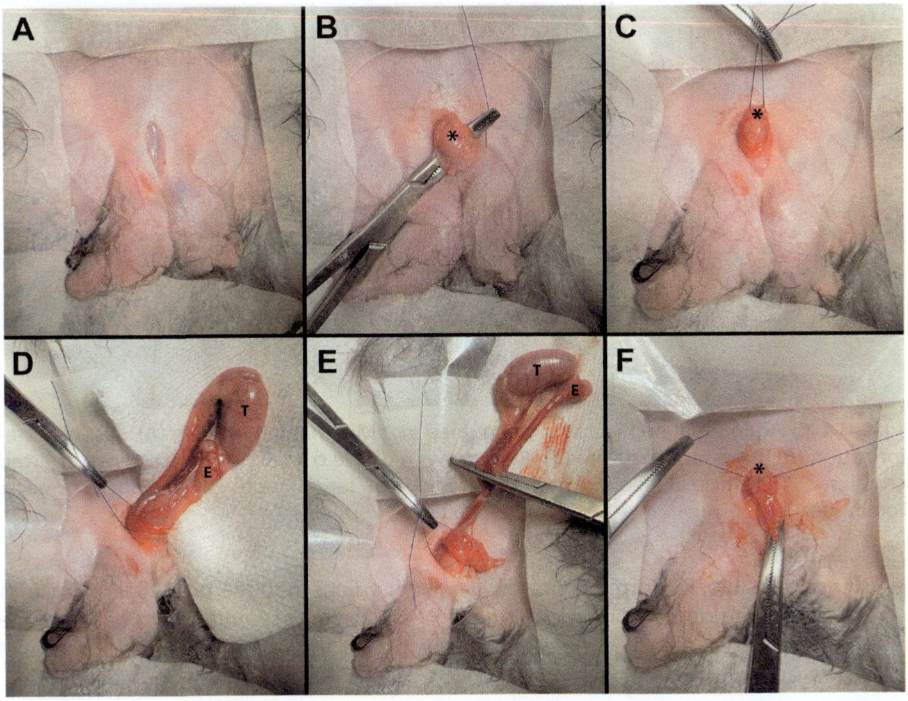

Fig. 8. (*A–F*) Prescrotal open-closed orchiectomy in a rabbit. Prescrotal incision (*A*). Vaginal tunica isolation (*B*). Placement of circumferential ligature around the vaginal tunica (*C*). Vaginal tunica incision, testicular exteriorization, and cord ligation (*D, E*). Tightening of the circumferential ligature to close the inguinal canal (*F*). Asterisk: vaginal tunica, T: testicle, E: epididymis. (Image Courtesy of Dr Sheyla Dominguez.)

Surgical technique

- Place the patient in dorsal recumbency. Make a crescent-shaped incision along the base of the scrotal area. In rabbits requiring scent glands excision extend the incision over the inguinal pouches, dissect the skin, and remove the glands (**Fig. 10**).
- Assess carefully the amount of skin to be excised. Insufficient removal may lead to recurrence, whereas excessive removal may expose the genital orifice, causing urethral mucosal eversion, urethritis, or altered urine flow.
- Once the scrotal skin is excised, perform an open-closed or closed castration. Close the skin routinely.[46,40]

PENILE AND PREPUTIAL SURGERY

Phimosis

Indications: Incapability of protruding the penis, abnormal urination, preputial swelling, preputial dermatitis, or inability to breed.

Surgical technique

- Under anesthesia, examine the prepuce, break down any adhesion between the prepuce and penis, and attempt to exteriorize the penis.

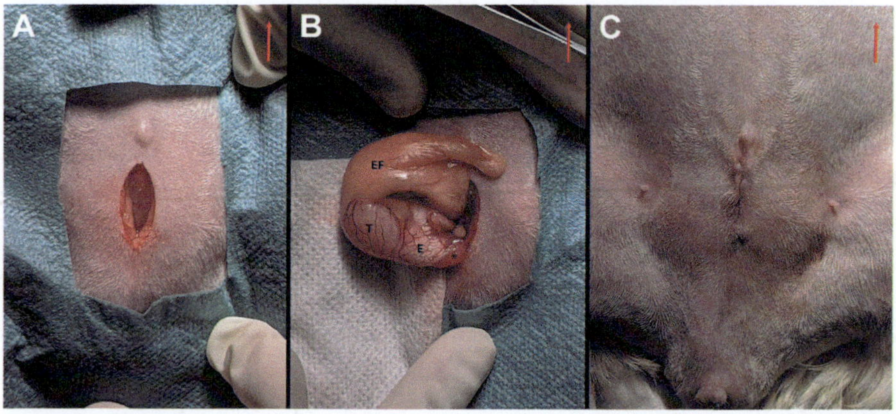

Fig. 9. (*A–C*) Abdominal orchiectomy in a guinea pig. Midline skin incision (*A*). Testicle exteriorization (*B*). Intradermal suture (*C*). Red arrows indicate cranial position; asterisk: everted scrotal sac, T: testicle; E: epididymis, EF: epididymal fat. (Image Courtesy of Dr Sheyla Dominguez.)

- If not possible, perform a semi-oval incision adjacent to the preputial orifice and excise a wedge of skin, subcutaneous tissue, and preputial mucosa. Remove enough tissue to allow exposure of the penile tip while maintaining preputial coverage.

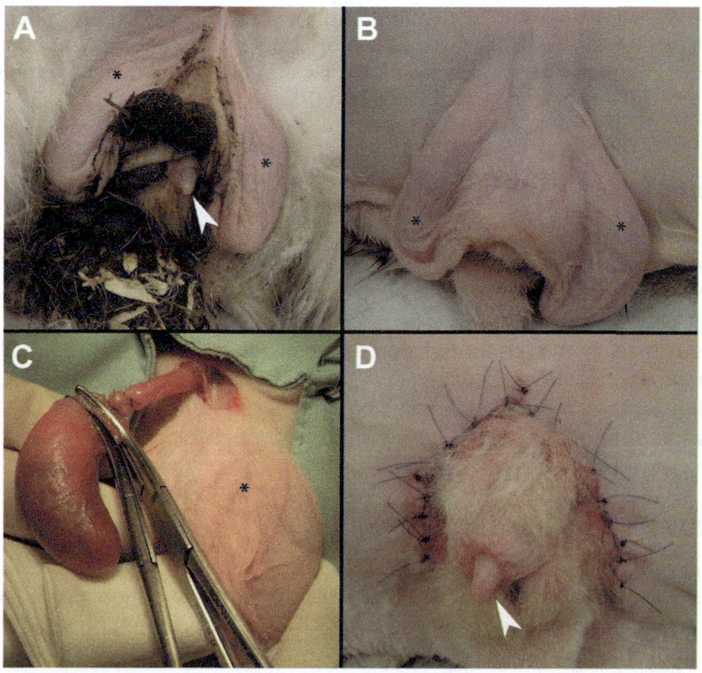

Fig. 10. (*A–D*) Pendulous hemiscrotal sacs in a rabbit before (*A*) and after (*B*) aseptic preparation. Prescrotal closed orchiectomy (*C*) followed by scrotal ablation (*D*). Asterisk: hemiscrotal sacs, arrowhead: protruded penis. (Image Courtesy of Dr Laura Vilalta.)

- Ligate or cauterize bleeding vessels and suture preputial mucosa to the skin with simple interrupted sutures.[56,57]

Comments: Phimosis has been described in ferrets and chinchillas.[56,57] It may be congenital (penile deviation) or acquired (scarring secondary to preputial trauma or neoplasia). Surgical treatment and correction of the primary condition usually resolve clinical signs; however, excessive tissue removal, particularly on the ventral aspect, can result in paraphimosis.[56]

Paraphimosis

Indications: Incapability to retract the penis, abnormal urination, preputial dermatitis, or inability to breed.

Surgical technique

- Mild paraphimosis may be resolved conservatively using lubricants, hyperosmolar solutions, and local temperature therapy (heat or cold). If manual reduction is unsuccessful, surgical enlargement of the preputial orifice may be required (*see phimosis section*).
- Alternatively, a phallopexy, with or without preputial advancement, may be performed. A full-thickness incision is made into the preputial cavity, and strips of preputial and penile epithelium are excised and sutured together. A urethral catheter should be placed to avoid inadvertent urethral injury.[58]
- Penile amputation is indicated in case of necrosis (see article "Urinary Surgery in Small Mammals" by Bernhard and Chassang of this issue for technique).[44,56,59]

Comments: Paraphimosis has been described in ferrets and hystricomorph rodents.[56,59,60] May have congenital (narrowed preputial orifice, or abnormally shortened prepuce) or acquired causes (fur rings, trauma, infection, or priapism).[56,59,60]

Apocrine Gland Adenocarcinomas

These aggressive tumors typically affect ferrets and involve the preputial area, penis, or vulva. Surgical treatment is required, including preputial excision, penile amputation or vulvoplasty, regional lymphadenectomy, and urethrostomy (see article 'Urinary Surgery in Small Mammals' by Bernhard and Chassang of this issue for penile amputation and urethrostomy techniques).[41]

ACCESSORY SEXUAL GLAND SURGERY

Prostate

Prostatic abscesses

Surgical techniques

- Position the patient in dorsal recumbency and place a urethral catheter. The prostate is generally approached through a caudal celiotomy, although a perineal approach may be required for lesions like cysts or abscesses.
- Retract the pubic brim to expose the prostate and carefully remove periprostatic fat for visualization.
- Isolate the prostate with moist sponges and elevate it using Penrose drains.
- Avoid dissecting along the dorsal surface of the prostate to prevent damaging major vessels and the hypogastric and pelvic nerves.
- Make lateral stab incisions and aspirate purulent material from abscess cavities to prevent abdominal contamination.

- Incise the prostatic capsule and control hemostasis using electrocautery. Digitally break down abscess walls and loculations within the parenchyma to create a single communicating cavity. Identify and protect the urethra by palpating the catheter, then irrigate the unified cavity thoroughly to remove residual debris.
- Available surgical options to complete the treatment are summarized in **Table 7**.[61]

Comments: Male ferrets may develop prostatic hyperplasia, cystic prostatic disease, or prostatic abscesses, commonly secondary to AGD.[62] Omentalization and ultrasound-guided drainage are preferred in ferrets to reduce prostatic trauma and postoperative complications. Broad-spectrum perioperative antibiotics are advised, as prostatic surgery, particularly those for cystic or septic conditions, poses a significant risk of intraoperative contamination.[62]

Prostatic cysts
Prostatic cysts can be managed with several techniques; in selected cases, ultrasound-guided drainage offers a minimally invasive alternative to surgery.

Surgical techniques
- Perform a caudal celiotomy to identify and exteriorize the cyst.
- After isolating it with moist sponges, make a single stab through the cyst wall, and aspirate the contents.
- Complete resection is recommended for small or paraprostatic cysts with limited capsular attachment. Partial resection and omentalization are suitable for larger cysts in ferrets.[61]

Table 7
Surgical options for management of prostatic abscesses in small mammals

Surgical Procedure	Technique Description
Marsupialization	Creation of a prostatocutaneous stoma to allow continuous drainage. The prostatic capsule is sutured to a parapenile stoma site. Daily irrigation with povidone-iodine is required to maintain patency and promote abscess resolution. Infrequently used surgery.
Ventral drainage	Passive drainage by using Penrose drains placed through the abscess cavities and exiting via the prostatic capsule and ventral abdominal wall on both sides of the prepuce.
Omentalization	Use the natural drainage properties of the omentum. Lateral capsular incisions are made to access the abscess cavity. The omentum is packed into the cavity and secured with mattress sutures. In cases with multiple abscesses, the omentum must be passed through all communicating cavities. In ferrets, this technique has been reported to be consistently more successful than other drainage techniques. However, due to the small size of the omentum in rabbits, omentalization is generally not possible in this species.
Partial prostatectomy	Two parallel midline incisions are made to expose the abscessed prostatic parenchyma which is debrided by digital disruption and aspiration. Avoid damage to the dorsal neurovascular plexus. The ventral prostatic capsule may be left open, closed, or packed with omentum before tension-free closure

Data from Refs.[11,61,62]

Vesicular Glands—Seminal Vesiculectomy

Indications: Vesiculitis, vesicular gland neoplasia, or lithiasis.

Surgical technique

- Place the patient in dorsal recumbency and perform a caudal midline celiotomy.
- Identify and isolate the affected vesicular glands using cotton-tipped applicators. Manipulate the tissue gently, as the glandular wall is thin and fragile (**Fig. 11**), particularly in hamsters.[63]
- If the glands are distended, aspirate seminal fluid to decompress them and obtain a sample for culture and sensitivity.
- Place transfixing ligatures or hemoclips at the base of each gland before excision.
- Lavage the abdomen thoroughly and close routinely.

Comments: Seminal vesiculectomy has been described in rabbits, guinea pigs, and hamsters.[63–66] Abdominal orchiectomy is frequently performed concurrently, although its effectiveness preventing or treating vesicular disorders is unknown.[64] Submission of samples for histopathology, bacterial culture, and sensitivity is advised.

MAMMARY GLAND SURGERY

Mastectomy

Indications: Mammary gland tumors, abscesses, and chronic mastitis with necrotic tissue.

Surgical techniques

- For benign lesions, marginal excision is indicated, removing the entire affected gland including the areola. Partial mastectomy (**Fig. 12**) may be performed, particularly in rats and mice, as total mastectomy is impractical due to the extensive mammary tissue distribution.[24,28,36]

Make a skin incision at the base of the lesion, extending sufficiently to allow a tension-free closure. Dissect the lesion from the mammary gland without entering it, to avoid hemorrhage or tumor seeding. Blunt dissection is performed, using electrosurgery or VSD to ligate any supplying vessels. For larger lesions, ligate arteries before veins to allow venous drainage from the mass. Replace tumor-contaminated gloves and instruments before closure. To minimize dead space,

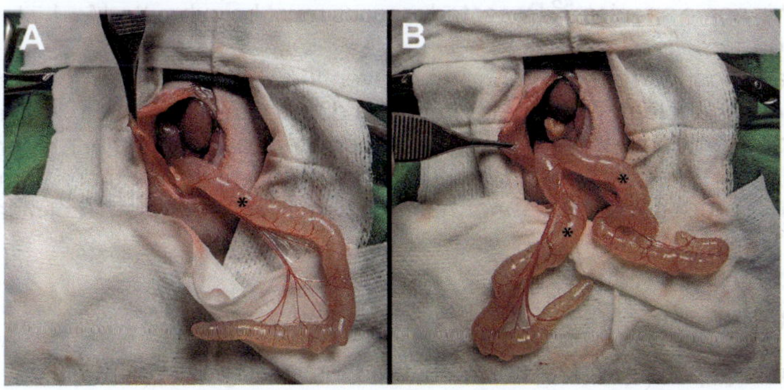

Fig. 11. (*A, B*) Normal appearance of vesicular glands (*asterisk*) in a male guinea pig. (Image Courtesy of Dr Laura Vilalta.)

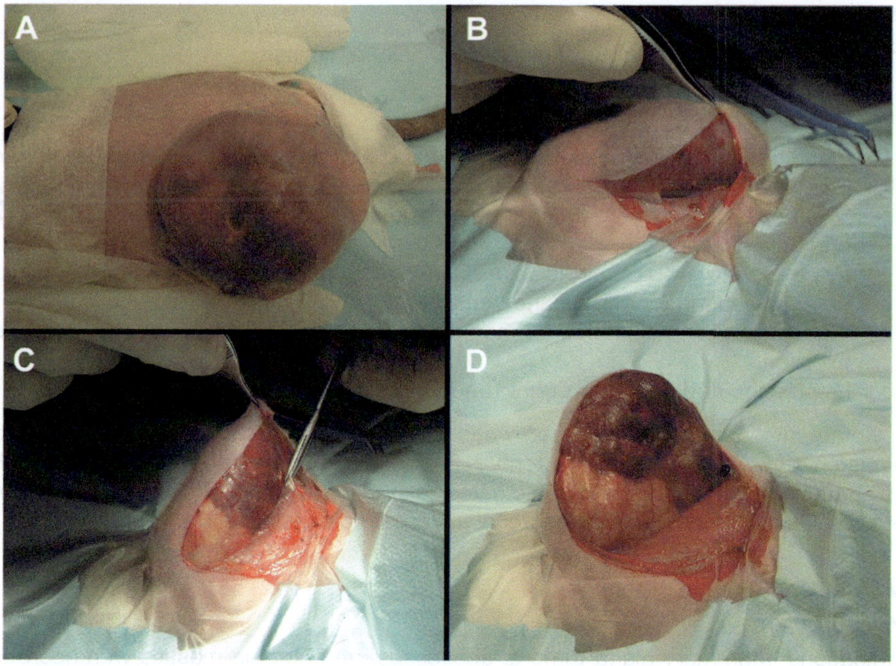

Fig. 12. (*A–D*) Sequence of surgical images depicting a mastectomy in a female rat. (Image Courtesy of Dr Laura Vilalta.)

tack the skin and subcutaneous tissue to the body wall. Close the subcutaneous tissue and skin in 2 layers.[24,28,36]

- For malignant tumors, a fusiform wide excision with 0.5 to 1 cm margins (depending on patient size) is recommended. Remove the overlying skin and the external rectus fascia beneath the mass. Preoperative planning is essential, as available tissue in this area is limited. If there is muscle invasion, excise the affected portion of abdominal wall.

Perform regional lymphadenectomy for histopathologic evaluation and staging. Close the rectus abdominis fascia, subcutaneous, and skin in layers.[24,28,36]

Comments: Fine-needle biopsy should be performed before surgery to determine the biological nature of the lesion, although self-trauma or hematoma-like lesions may occur in some species.[52] Resected masses must be submitted for histopathologic evaluation.[24,28,36,52,67]

The role of concurrent neutering in preventing recurrence or additional tumor development is unclear. No benefit has been demonstrated in mice, in which mammary tumor development is largely virus associated; and results in rats are controversial. However, as approximately 40% of rats with mammary tumors have concurrent reproductive tract abnormalities, neutering is advised in clinically stable patients.[24,28,36,52,67]

POSTOPERATIVE CARE

Postoperatively, patients should be monitored for vital signs, appetite, fecal, and urine output.[23] Nutritional support should begin once the patient is alert and ambulatory, since anorexia is common in rabbits and hystricomorph rodents. Adequate analgesia,

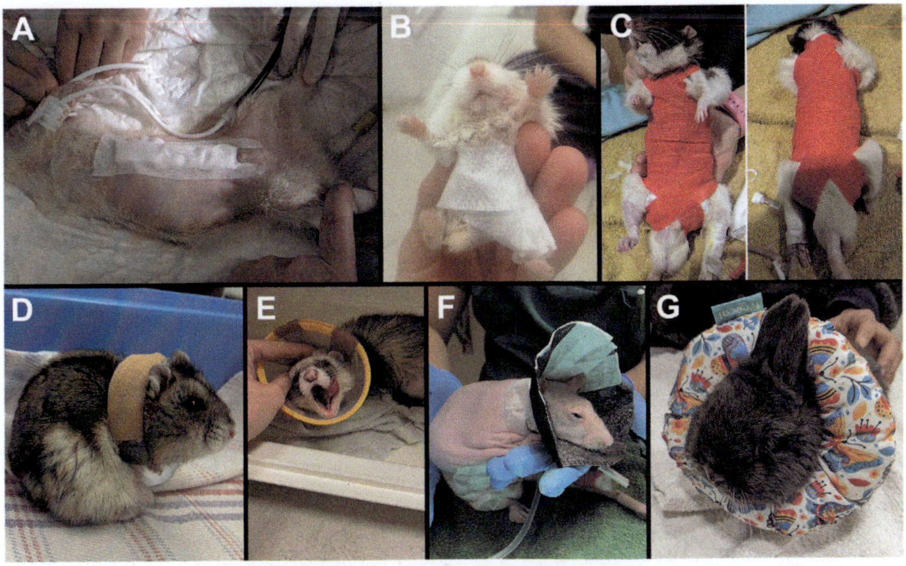

Fig. 13. (*A–G*) Self-mutilation preventive methods. Soft adhesive bandage applied to a ferret (*A*) and hamster (*B*). Ventral and dorsal views of a body wrap in a rat, using Vetrap arranged in an X-pattern over the shoulders and pelvis (*C*). Different types of collars for small mammals (*D–G*): polyethylene pipe-insulation material as a collar in a hamster (*D*); trimmed feline Elizabethan collar adapted for a ferret (*E*); collar made from an FFP2 mask in a rat (*F*); commercial soft feline collar (size XS) used in a rabbit (*G*). (Image Courtesy of Dr Laura Vilalta and Dr Sheyla Dominguez.)

hydration, and nutrition are essential to maintain gastrointestinal motility.[1,28] Postoperative analgesia should include opioids and/or nonsteroidal anti-inflammatory drugs, depending on the procedure invasiveness.[1] For more invasive surgeries, overnight hospitalization is recommended to avoid any major complication related to the surgical procedure.

Close inspection of the incision is essential. In nonhystricomorph rodents, Vetrap bandages or Elizabethan collars help prevent self-mutilation and infection (**Fig. 13**). Rabbits, however, rarely chew their sutures, and adhesive bandages can irritate their skin.[1] Soft adhesive dressings can be used if needed. If rabbits attempt to traumatize the wound, soft collars may be applied, ensuring they do not interfere with feeding or cecotrophy. Substrate should be kept clean and changed frequently to reduce infection risk.

POSTOPERATIVE COMPLICATIONS

Common early complications include gastrointestinal stasis in rabbits and hystricomorph species, wound infection, dehiscence, edema, hematoma, inflammation, and self-inflicted trauma (**Fig. 14**).[1,11]

Following ovariohysterectomy, adhesion involving intestinal or urinary organs may develop.[38,40,68,69] Prevention includes minimizing tissue desiccation, gentle tissue handling, appropriate hemostasis, precise suture placement, removal of debris, and thorough lavage.[68] Other reported complications include fat necrosis, which may calcify and local peritonitis secondary to urine leakage after inadequate vaginal stump ligation.[1,23]

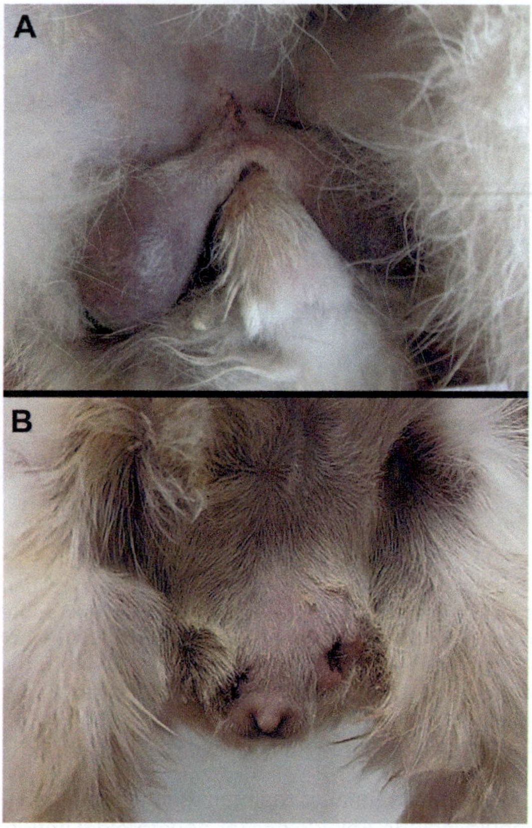

Fig. 14. (*A, B*) Orchiectomy complications. Scrotal edema following prescrotal castration in a rabbit (*A*) and unilateral wound infection, inflammation, and dehiscence following scrotal castration in a guinea pig (*B*). (Image Courtesy of Dr Laura Vilalta and Dr Sheyla Dominguez.)

Scrotal herniation can occur after orchiectomy if the inguinal ring is not adequately closed.[1] Males may remain hormonally active and potentially fertile for 4 to 8 weeks postorchiectomy.[1,11]

Reported complications following prostatic surgery include urinary incontinence, urinary leakage, and sepsis,[61,62,70] In vesicular gland procedures, sepsis secondary to intraperitoneal leakage of glandular contents has been described.[64,66]

CLINICS CARE POINTS

- Rabbits and rodents should not be fasted before surgery because prolonged fasting may predispose to gastrointestinal stasis.
- Ovariectomy is faster and less invasive than ovariohysterectomy but should not be performed when uterine disease is suspected, and its protective effect against uterine disease remains uncertain.
- In rabbits and rodents, closure of the inguinal canal during orchiectomy helps reduce the risk of postoperative herniation.

- Elective neutering is not routinely recommended in ferrets because of its association with adrenal gland disease.
- Scrotal orchiectomy in guinea pigs is associated with higher postoperative infection risk compared with the abdominal approach.
- Gentle tissue handling, meticulous hemostasis, and minimization of tissue desiccation are essential to reduce postoperative adhesions and gastrointestinal complications in rabbits and hystricomorph rodents.
- Postoperative anorexia in rabbits and hystricomorph rodents should be prevented with multimodal analgesia, hydration, and early nutritional support.

DISCLOSURES

The authors declare no commercial or financial conflicts of interest in the preparation of this article.

REFERENCES

1. Pignon C. Rabbit basic surgery. In: Smith MV, editor. Textbook of rabbit medicine. 3rd edition. St Louis (MO): Elsevier; 2023. p. 401–11.
2. Wong AD, Keller KA, Cerreta AJ, et al. Visualization of radiographic mineral opacities in Guinea pigs in the location of the bulbourethral glands may be underdiagnosed. J Exot Pet Med 2024;48:25–30.
3. Călămar CD, Pătruică S, Dumitrescu G, et al. Morpho-histological studies on the male genital apparatus of *Chinchilla laniger*. Sci Pap Anim Sci Biotechnol 2014;47(1):275.
4. Quesenberry KE, Orcutt CJ, Mans C, et al, editors. Ferrets, rabbits, and rodents: clinical medicine and surgery. 4th edition. St Louis (MO): Elsevier; 2021.
5. Barthold SW, Griffey SM, Percy DH. Pathology of laboratory rodents and rabbits. 4th edition. John Wiley & Sons; 2016.
6. Jarrett CL, Jarrett TR, Harvey SB, et al. The uterus duplex Bicollis, vagina simplex of female chinchillas. J Am Assoc Lab Anim Sci 2016;55(2):155–60.
7. Bertram CA, Klopfleisch R, Erickson NA, et al. Uterus duplex bicollis, vagina simplex in laboratory Guinea pigs (*Cavia porcellus*), rats (*Rattus norvegicus forma domestica*) and mice (*Mus musculus forma domestica*). Anat Histol Embryol 2019;48(4):388–93.
8. Planas-Silva MD, Rutherford TM, Stone MC. Prevention of age-related spontaneous mammary tumors in outbred rats by late ovariectomy. Cancer Detect Prev 2008;32(1):65–71.
9. Hotchkiss CE. Effect of surgical removal of subcutaneous tumors on survival or rats. J Am Vet Med Assoc 1995;206(10):1575–9.
10. Schoemaker NJ, Schuurmans M, Moorman H, et al. Correlation between age at neutering and age at onset of hyperadrenocorticism in ferrets. J Am Vet Med Assoc 2000;216:195–7.
11. Guzman DS, Szabo Z, Steffey MA. Soft tissue surgery: rabbits. In: Quesenberry KE, Orcutt CJ, Mans C, et al, editors. Ferrets, rabbits, and rodents: clinical medicine and surgery. 4th edition. St Louis (MO): Elsevier; 2021. p. 446–66.
12. Harcourt-Brown FM. Disorders of the reproductive tract of rabbits. Vet Clin North Am Exot Anim Pract 2017;20(2):555–87.

13. Kabakchiev C, Singh A, Dobson S, et al. Comparison of intra- and postoperative variables between laparoscopic and open ovariectomy in rabbits (*Oryctolagus cuniculus*). Am J Vet Res 2021;82(3):237–48.
14. Settai K, Kondo H, Shibuya H. Assessment of reported uterine lesions diagnosed histologically after ovariohysterectomy in 1,928 pet rabbits (*Oryctolagus cuniculus*). J Am Vet Med Assoc 2020;257(10):1045–50.
15. Rozanska D, Rozanski P, Orzelski M, et al. Unilateral flank ovariohysterectomy in Guinea pigs (*Cavia porcellus*). N Z Vet J 2016;64(6):360–3.
16. Sladakovic I, Divers SJ. Exotic mammal laparoscopy. Vet Clin North Am Exot Anim Pract 2016;19(1):269–86.
17. Bertram CA, Müller K, Klopfleisch R. Genital tract pathology in female pet rabbits (*Oryctolagus cuniculus*): a retrospective study of 854 necropsy examinations and 152 biopsy samples. J Comp Pathol 2018;164:17–26.
18. Asakawa MG, Goldschmidth MH, Une Y, et al. The immunohistochemical evaluation of estrogen Receptor-a and progesterone receptors of normal, hyperplastic, and neoplastic endometrium in 88 pet rabbits. Vet Pathol 2008;45(2):217–25.
19. Frerichs K, Lennox AM, Bocchine A. Comparison of post-surgical complication rates and potential confounding factors in two common approaches for elective altering in female rats (*Rattus norvegicus*). J Exot Pet Med 2022;43:11–8.
20. Mäkitaipale J, Airas N, Engblom S, et al. Prospective survey of neoplastic and non-neoplastic uterine disorders in 116 domestic rabbits (*Oryctolagus cuniculus*). J Exot Pet Med 2022;41:3–8.
21. Lazard M, Muller V, Manon S, et al. Ultrasonographic appearance and histopathological findings of the genital tract in healthy nulliparous female rabbits (*Oryctolagus cuniculus*). J Exot Pet Med 2020;33:1–8.
22. Lübke VC, Fehr M, Köstlinger S. Validation of whole-body radiographs for examining uterine disorders in sexually intact female rabbits. Tierarztl Prax Ausg K Kleintiere Heimtiere 2019;47(1). 14-4.
23. Szabo Z, Bradley K, Cahalane AK. Rabbit soft tissue surgery. Vet Clin North Am Exot Anim Pract 2016;19(1):159–88.
24. Bennett RA. Rabbit soft tissue surgery. In: Bennett RA, Pye GW, editors. Surgery of exotic animals. 1st edition. Hoboken (NJ): Wiley-Blackwell; 2022. p. 240–76.
25. Schmiedt CW. Suture material, tissue staplers, ligation devices, and closure methods. In: Johnston SA, Tobias KM, editors. Veterinary surgery: small animal. 2nd edition. St Louis (MO): Elsevier; 2018. p. 210–24.
26. Steele MS, Bennett RA. Clinical technique: dorsal ovariectomy in rodents. J Exot Pet Med 2011;20(3):222–6.
27. Capello V. Common surgical procedures in pet rodents. J Exot Pet Med 2011; 20(4):294–307.
28. Szabo Z. Soft tissue surgery: rodents. In: Quesenberry KE, Orcutt CJ, Mans C, et al, editors. Ferrets, rabbits, and rodents: clinical medicine and surgery. 4th edition. St Louis (MO): Elsevier; 2021. p. 467–82.
29. Divers SJ. Endoscopic ovariectomy of exotic mammals using a three-port approach. Vet Clin North Am Exot Anim Pract 2015;18(3):401–15.
30. Proença LM. Two-portal access laparoscopic ovariectomy using LigaSure atlas in exotic companion mammals. Vet Clin North Am Exot Anim Pract 2015;18(3): 587–96.
31. McCready J, Beaufrère H, Singh A, et al. Laparoscopic ovariectomy in Guinea pigs: a pilot study. Vet Surg 2020;49:131–7.

32. Mehler SJ, Bennett RA. Minimally invasive surgery techniques in exotic animals. In: Bennett RA, Pye GW, editors. Surgery of exotic animals. 1st edition. Hoboken (NJ): Wiley-Blackwell; 2022. p. 204–26.
33. Coleman KA, Monnet E, Johnston MS. Single-port laparoscopic-assisted ovariohysterectomy in three rabbits. J Exot Pet Med 2018;27:21–4.
34. McCready JE, Gozzard H, Tisotti T, et al. Effect of pneumoperitoneum on gastrointestinal motility, pain behaviors, and stress biomarkers in Guinea pigs (*Cavia porcellus*). Am J Vet Res 2022;83(8).
35. McCracken BD, Beths T, Herbert S, et al. Comparison of isobaric and insufflated laparoscopy-assisted ovariohysterectomy in the common rabbit (*Oryctolagus cuniculus*). J Exot Pet Med 2019;28:193–204.
36. Bennett RA. Rodent soft tissue surgery. In: Bennett RA, Pye GW, editors. Surgery of exotic animals. 1st edition. Hoboken (NJ): Wiley-Blackwell; 2022. p. 297–321.
37. McLean EJ, Woodward AP, Ryan SD. Comparison of the use of a vessel-sealing device versus ligatures for occlusion of uterine tissues during ovariohysterectomy or ovariectomy in rabbits (*Oryctolagus cuniculus*). Am J Vet Res 2020;81(9): 755–9.
38. d'Ovidio D, Adami C. Comparison of two haemostasis techniques on procedural duration, postoperative pain and gastrointestinal function in pet rabbits undergoing ovariohysterectomy. Top Companion Anim Med 2024;62:100906.
39. Dumartinet C, Matres-Lorenzo L, Linsart A, et al. Comparison of conventional ligatures and a vessel sealing device for haemostasis during open ovariohysterectomy in rabbits. N Z Vet J 2022;70(5):256–62.
40. Harcourt-Brown F. Neutering. In: Harcourt-Brown F, Chitty J, editors. Manual of rabbit surgery, dentistry and imaging. 1st edition. Gloucester, UK: British Small Animal Veterinary Association; 2013. p. 138–56.
41. Jekl V. Soft tissue surgery: ferrets. In: Quesenberry KE, Orcutt CJ, Mans C, et al, editors. Ferrets, rabbits, and rodents: clinical medicine and surgery. 4th edition. St Louis (MO): Elsevier; 2021. p. 432–45.
42. Hafez S. Comparative placental anatomy: divergent structures serving a common purpose. Prog Mol Biol Transl Sci 2017;145:1–28.
43. Fransson BA. Ovaries and uterus. In: Johnston SA, Tobias KM, editors. Veterinary surgery: small animal. 2nd edition. St Louis (MO): Elsevier; 2018. p. 2109–30.
44. Kondert L, Mayer J. Reproductive medicine in Guinea pigs, Chinchillas and degus. Vet Clin North Am Exot Anim Pract 2017;20(2):609–28.
45. Di Girolamo N, D'Ovidio D, Del Duca V, et al. Surgical resolution of uterine prolapse in three pet rabbits. J Small Anim Pract 2021;62(3):229–32.
46. Smith MV. Skin disease. In: Smith MV, editor. Textbook of rabbit medicine. 3rd edition. St Louis (MO): Elsevier; 2023. p. 242–67.
47. Schlax K, Quiévreux L, Mélin M, et al. A rectovaginal fistula in a ferret (*Mustela putorius furo*) with a normal anus: a case report. J Exot Pet Med 2020;35(C):20–2.
48. Rectovaginal fistula with atresia ani in a ferret (*Mustela putorius furo*). ICARE 2024. Belgium: Ghent; 2024.
49. Hotchkiss CE, Collins BR. Imperforate anus with rectovaginal fistula in a dwarf rabbit. Lab Anim Sci 1994;44(2):184–5.
50. Duhamelle A, Tessier E, Larrat S. Comparative study of scrotal and prescrotal castration in pet rabbits (*Oryctolagus cuniculus*). J Exot Pet Med 2018;27(3): 15–21.
51. Capello V. Surgical techniques for orchiectomy of the pet rabbit. Exot Dvm 2005; 7(5):23–32.

52. Miwa Y, Sladky KK. Small mammals: common surgical procedures of rodents, ferrets, hedgehogs, and sugar gliders. Vet Clin North Am Exot Anim Pract 2016; 19(1):205–44.
53. Guilmette J, Langlois I, Hélie P, et al. Comparative study of 2 surgical techniques for castration of Guinea pigs (*Cavia porcellus*). Can J Vet Res 2015;79(4):323–8.
54. Malbrue RA, Arsuaga-Zorrilla CB, Bidot W, et al. Evaluation of orchiectomy and ovariectomy surgical techniques in degus (*Octodon degus*). J Exot Pet Med 2019;30:22–8.
55. Powers MY, Campbell BG, Finch NP. Preputial damage and lateral penile displacement during castration in a degu. J Am Vet Med Assoc 2008;232(7): 1013–5.
56. Bulliot C, Flenghi L, Levrier C. Phimosis and paraphimosis in two ferrets (*Mustela putorius furo*). J Exot Pet Med 2021;39(2):59–63.
57. Martel-Arquette A, Mans C. Management of phimosis and balanoposthitis in a pet chinchilla (*Chinchilla lanigera*). J Exot Pet Med 2016;25(1):60–4.
58. Boothe HW. Penis and prepuce. In: Johnston SA, Tobias KM, editors. Veterinary surgery: small animal. 2nd edition. St Louis (MO): Elsevier; 2018. p. 2158–67.
59. Lavallée J. Subtotal penile amputation and preputial urethrostomy in a degu (*Octodon degus).* Can Vet J 2023;64(7):650–3.
60. Calvo Carrasco D, Abou-Zahr T. Surgical narrowing of the preputial orifice for treatment of recurrent penile prolapse in a degu (*Octodon degus*). Vet Rec Case Rep 2015;3(1):e000223.
61. White RAS. Prostate. In: Johnston SA, Tobias KM, editors. Veterinary surgery: small animal. 2nd edition. St Louis (MO): Elsevier; 2018. p. 2168–83.
62. Powers LV, Winkler K, Garner MM, et al. Omentalization of prostatic abscesses and large cysts in ferrets (*Mustela putorius furo*). J Exot Pet Med 2007;16(3): 186–94.
63. Chan SC, Kiupel M. Seminal vesiculitis in golden hamsters (*Mesocricetus auratus*): two cases (2022). J Exot Pet Med 2024;49:58–63.
64. Ardiaca M, Bonvehi C, Cuesta M, et al. Seminal vesiculitis in three pet rabbits (*Oryctolagus cuniculus*). J Am Anim Hosp Assoc 2016;52(5):335–40.
65. de Souza MG, Sueiro FAR, Batalha LFB, et al. Radiographic and ultrasonographic findings of seminal vesiculitis with nonmineral stones in a Guinea pig: case report. Vet Radiol Ultrasound 2025;66(1):e13458.
66. Picazo L, Del Romero A, Rosell J, et al. Vesicular gland infection caused by *Pseudomonas aeruginosa* with secondary prostatitis in a Guinea pig (*Cavia porcellus*). J Exot Pet Med 2024;48:20–4.
67. Vergneau-Grosset C, Keel MK, Goldsmith D, et al. Description of the prevalence, histologic characteristics, concomitant abnormalities, and outcomes of mammary gland tumors in companion rats (*Rattus norvegicus*): 100 cases (1990-2015). J Am Vet Med Assoc 2016;249(10):1170–9.
68. Guzman DS, Graham JE, Keller K, et al. Colonic obstruction following ovariohysterectomy in rabbits: 3 cases. J Exot Pet Med 2015;24(1):112–9.
69. Duhamelle A, Tessier E, Larrat S. Ureteral stenosis following ovariohysterectomy in a rabbit (*Oryctolagus cuniculus*). J Exot Pet Med 2021;35:77–81.
70. Castellier A, Vinomack C, Girard-Luc A, et al. Surgical treatment with adjunctive metronomic chemotherapy of a prostatic adenocarcinoma in a rabbit (*Oryctolagus cuniculus*). J Exot Pet Med 2025;55:11–8.

Urinary Surgery in Small Mammals

Cécile Bernhard, DVM, DECZM (Small Mammals)[a,*],
Lucile Chassang, DVM, DECZM (Small Mammals)[b]

KEYWORDS

• Surgery • Small mammals • Urinary • Soft tissue

KEY POINTS

- Urinary surgery in small mammals applies principles from cats and dogs but requires species-specific adaptation in anatomy knowledge, patient preparation, and instrumentation.
- Urinary surgery requires precise dissection, perfect hemostasis, and strict contamination control.
- Species-specific physiology, such as rabbits' unique calcium metabolism, influences surgical planning and technique selection.
- Minimally invasive techniques are preferred, and handling of tissues should be kept to a minimum to reduce postoperative complications.

INTRODUCTION

Urinary surgery in small mammals follows surgical principles established in domestic carnivores. However, their small size and unique urinary anatomy demand precise planning, careful perioperative care, and suitable instruments. Minimally invasive, tissue-sparing techniques reduce morbidity and improve recovery. As urolithiasis is common and diet contributing to its development, discussing nutrition with the owner is essential for treatment, prevention, and to reduce recurrence.

PRE-, PERI-, AND POSTOPERATIVE CONSIDERATIONS

Each patient requires a thorough history and clinical examination. Bloodwork (biochemistry and complete blood count (CBC), urinalysis, bacterial culture, and imaging are often indicated. Preoperative stabilization typically includes fluids, analgesia, and nutritional support. Aggressive fluids are usually avoided until urinary patency is

[a] Veterinary Clinic l'Arche Des NAC, 20 rue Lavoisier, 95300 Pontoise, France; [b] Eläinsairaala Evidensia Tammisto Animal Hospital, Tammiston kauppatie 29, 01510 Vantaa, Finland
* Corresponding author.
E-mail address: bernhard.ccile@gmail.com

Vet Clin Exot Anim 29 (2026) 781–804
https://doi.org/10.1016/j.cvex.2026.04.010 **vetexotic.theclinics.com**
1094-9194/26/

Abbreviation	
SUB	subcutaneous ureteral bypass

restored. In cases of urolithiasis, radiographs should be performed immediately before surgery to confirm the location of the stone(s). In particular, benzodiazepines, when used as premedication, provide effective muscle relaxation and may allow spontaneous expulsion of large calculi from the bladder via the urethra.[1]

Perioperative care focuses on preventing hypothermia, ensuring intravenous access and intubation, and minimizing tissue trauma. Fine monofilament absorbable sutures are recommended—poliglecaprone 25 for the urinary tract, polydioxanone for the abdominal wall and skin. Poliglecaprone or Glycomer 631 is preferred for faster healing and reduced stone recurrence risk.[2,3] However, an experimental rat study found no stone formation with polydioxanone on bladder wall.[4] The abdominal wall and skin are closed in a routine manner, and the abdomen is lavaged before closure.

Postoperatively, urine output and hydration must be monitored, diuresis ensured, and antibiotics used if needed.[5–7] Dietary management plays a key role in urinary diseases in small mammals, where urolithiasis is a common clinical presentation, particularly in species such as rabbits and guinea pigs.[1] Due to their unique calcium physiology and naturally high urinary calcium excretion, they are especially predisposed to developing urinary calculi. Therefore, limiting dietary calcium intake—along with ensuring adequate hydration—is recommended both for preventing and for reducing the risk of recurrence.

SURGICAL TECHNIQUES

Surgery of the Kidney

Surgical approach of the kidney

Lateral flank approach minimizes visceral manipulation and postoperative pain and is often preferred in herbivorous species such as rabbits and guinea pigs, whereas ventral midline approach is preferred for bilateral exploration.[5,8]

Midline celiotomy

- The animal is placed in dorsal recumbency and surgically prepared from sternum to pelvic inlet.[9]
- A ventral midline incision is performed from the xiphoid process to midway between the umbilicus and pubis.[5,10]
- Self-retaining retractors can be used for better visualization (**Fig. 1**D). Intestines and caecum are exteriorized and protected with moistened gauzes.[5]
- Both kidneys are inspected and sampled if bilateral disease is suspected.[9]
- The kidney is freed from the peritoneum by a caudal incision with Metzenbaum scissors and by dissecting remaining attachments digitally or with cotton swabs (**Fig. 2**A).[10]

Lateral/paralumbar approach

- The animal is placed in right or left lateral recumbency and surgically prepared.
- A horizontal incision is performed caudal to the last rib, over the affected kidney.[5,8,9]

Renal biopsy (wedge or core needle)

Renal biopsy can be performed via open laparotomy (wedge or needle), laparoscopic, or ultrasound-guided percutaneous approaches.[5,9,10] Open surgery generally

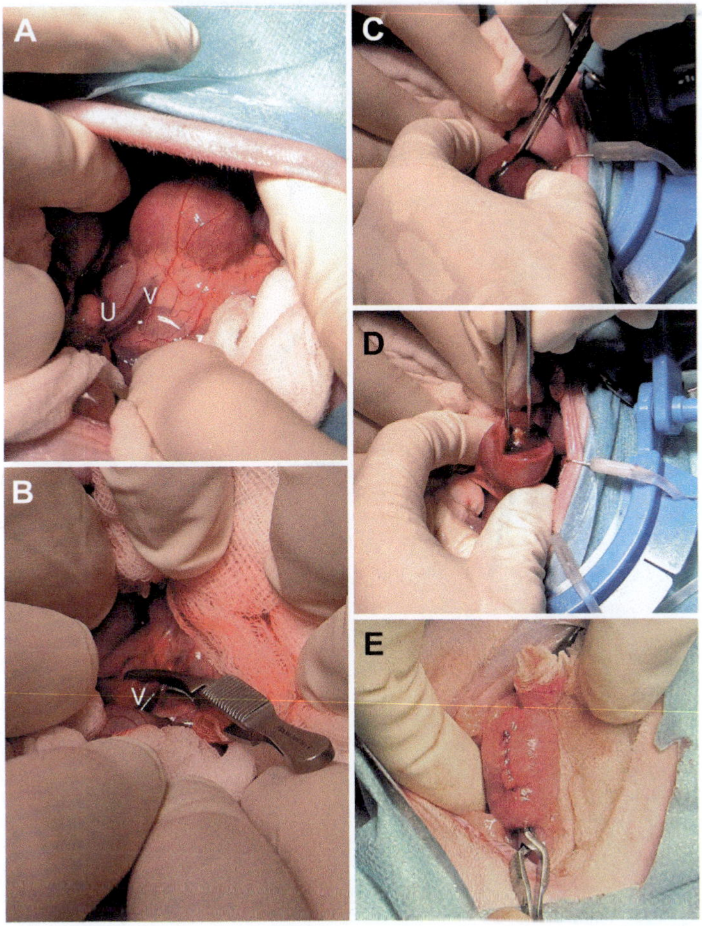

Fig. 1. Nephrotomy in a rabbit (*Oryctolagus cuniculus*). (*A*) Exposure of renal vessels (V) and ureter (U). (*B*) Vascular clamp placement over renal artery/vein (V). (*C*) Midline incision over the renal cortex to expose the pelvis. (*D*) Removal of a calculus. (*E*) Renal capsule closure using continuous sutures with monofilament absorbable material. (Image Courtesy of Dr Cécile Bernhard.)

yields higher quality samples with fewer complications.[10] Wedge biopsies provide superior tissue quality, though needle biopsies usually offer sufficient diagnostic value.[10]

Indications. To confirm diagnosis and prognosis in cases of unexplained renal insufficiency, focal masses, suspected neoplasia, unexplained proteinuria or hematuria, and nephropathies such as glomerulonephritis, vasculitis, interstitial nephritis, or amyloidosis.[5,9,10]

Contraindications. Moderate-to-severe thrombocytopenia or coagulopathy, uncontrolled hypertension, severe azotemia, large renal cysts, severe hydronephrosis, extensive pyelonephritis, perirenal abscess, or obstructive uropathy.[5,9,10] Biopsy may further compromise renal function.[10]

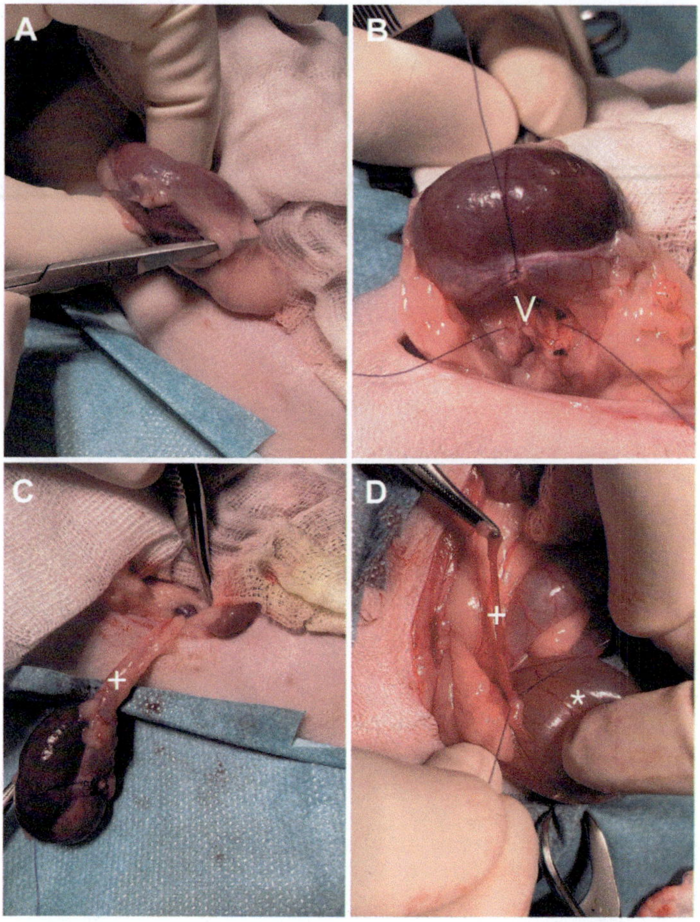

Fig. 2. Nephrectomy in a ferret (*Mustela putorius furo*). (*A*) Dissection of the peritoneum caudal to the kidney. (*B*) Isolation of the renal artery and vein to be double ligated (V). (*C*) Dissection of the ureter (+) along its entire length to the bladder neck. (*D*) Encircling ligature around the ureter (+) close to the bladder (*asterisk*). (Image Courtesy of Dr Véronique Mentré.)

Surgical steps

Wedge biopsy technique:

- The kidney is reflected ventromedially to expose the renal vessels.[10]
- The renal artery is occluded manually by an assistant or with a vascular clamp (**Fig. 1**B) for a maximum of 20 minutes, causing the kidney to get darker and softer. Some oozing of dark blood will still occur upon incision of the parenchyma (**Fig. 1**C).[10]
- The kidney is elevated with laparotomy sponges, and 2 cortical incisions at approximately 60° angle are made on the greater curvature with a scalpel blade. A small wedge, no more than 5 mm long and 5 mm deep, is excised from the outer third of the kidney. The exact depth depends on cortical thickness and species size. The incision is made parallel to the kidney's long axis, and the wedge is removed either by gently elevating it with a blade or by grasping the edge of the renal capsule with forceps.[5,9]

- Thumb forceps are avoided on the parenchyma. Hemostasis is achieved by digital pressure or sterile swabs.[5,9]
- The renal capsule is closed with interrupted sutures.[10] The superficial parenchyma is usually included in the suture, as the capsule is thin. The suture must be passed gently through the tissues. If the needle is lifted during insertion or the suture tied too tightly, the parenchyma may tear.[5,9,10]
- Vascular clamps are removed, and hemostasis reassessed.[10]

Core needle biopsy:

- Manual (eg, Tru-Cut biopsy instrument [Merit Medical Systems, South Jordan, UT, USA]) or spring-loaded biopsy needles (16–18 G) can be used, and at least 2 cores longer than 1 cm should be collected.[9]
- The kidney is stabilized in situ.[10]
- Depending on the desired sample, the needle is inserted either perpendicular to the kidney's long axis at the cranial or caudal pole or parallel to its convex surface. It is then advanced through the capsule into the cortex. The firing mechanism is activated to sever the renal parenchyma, and the needle withdrawn with the sample.[10]
- Samples are dislodged from the biopsy instrument with sterile saline to avoid crushing it.[10]
- Hemostasis is achieved by digital pressure, sterile swabs and/or interrupted sutures if persistent bleeding.[5,10]

Complications and prognosis. Complications include hemorrhage, hematuria, urine leakage, peritonitis, pain, and renal function deterioration if large samples are removed.[5] Prognosis depends on underlying pathology and presence of bilateral disease.[5,9]

Nephrotomy

Ventral and lateral flank approaches are described in rabbits,[9,11] along with endoscopy-assisted methods.[8,12]

Indications. Removal of renal pelvic calculi, abscesses, or intrapelvic masses, and hemostasis in the renal pelvis when conservative management is ineffective.[5]

Contraindications. Irreversible renal parenchymal loss or advanced hydronephrosis.[5,9] Nephrotomy is known to reduce renal function by approximately 30% to 40% and should be avoided in patients with pre-existing renal failure.[11]

Surgical steps

- The kidney is elevated medially to expose the renal vessels and ureter (**Fig. 1**A).[5,9,13]
- Atraumatic vascular clamps are placed on the renal artery/vein to reduce bleeding during the procedure (see **Fig. 1**B).[5,9] Occlusion should be limited to 20 minutes.[10] The kidney will get darker and softer once the artery occluded.[10] The renal parenchyma will still ooze dark blood when incised.[10]
- A sagittal incision is made along the greater curvature of the kidney, through the renal cortex, to reach the pelvis (see **Fig. 1**C). Calculi, abscesses, or masses are removed (see **Fig. 1**D).[5]
- Samples for culture are collected from the renal pelvis and exposed parenchyma when indicated.[5]
- The renal pelvis and parenchyma are irrigated with warm sterile saline to eliminate debris, blood clots, and sludge.[5,9]

- A 3 Fr catheter is inserted through the pelvis into the ureter to confirm patency.[5,9]
- Renal closure is achieved by apposing the 2 halves of the parenchyma and maintaining gentle pressure for a few seconds. In addition, a single horizontal mattress or cruciate suture may be placed through the cortex.[5] The renal capsule is closed using interrupted or continuous sutures (**Fig. 1**E).
- Vascular clamps are removed, and hemostasis reassessed.[5]

Complications and prognosis. Complications include intrarenal hemorrhage, urine leakage, postoperative renal insufficiency, adhesions, and decreased glomerular filtration rate.[5] In cases of persistent dysfunction or obstruction, nephrectomy may be required. Prognosis depends on initial renal function and disease extent.[5,9]

Pyelolithotomy

Indications. Removal of calculi located in the extrarenal portion of renal pelvis or proximal ureter, especially when these areas are distended due to obstruction.[5] When feasible, pyelolithotomy is preferred over nephrotomy, as it minimizes parenchymal damage and reduces postoperative complications.[5,9]

Contraindications. In rabbits, pyelolithotomy is only technically feasible when renal pelvis is sufficiently dilated; a small or nondistended pelvis may preclude this approach.[9]

Surgical steps

- The kidney is reflected medially to expose the extrarenal pelvis and proximal ureter.[5,9]
- Occlusion of renal vessels is not necessary for pyelolithotomy.[5]
- A longitudinal incision over the distended pelvis is performed directly above the calculus.[5]
- The calculus is removed, and pelvic contents sampled for bacterial culture and sensitivity if indicated.[5]
- The renal pelvis is irrigated with warm saline to remove debris and blood clots.[5,9]
- Ureteral patency is confirmed with a 3 Fr catheter.[5,9]
- Pelvic incision is closed using either an interrupted or continuous pattern. Transverse closure is preferred, when possible, to maintain lumen diameter.

Complications and prognosis. Complications include ureteral stricture, adhesion formation, and residual obstruction from blood clots or debris.[5] Prognosis is favorable when obstruction is successfully relieved and underlying cause managed.[9]

Endoscopy-assisted nephrolithotomy has been described and successfully performed in rabbits, providing minimally invasive access.[12]

Nephrectomy/nephroureterectomy

Indications. For irreversibly damaged kidney due to end-stage hydronephrosis, chronic pyelonephritis, severe nephropathies, primary renal neoplasia, severe renal or ureteral trauma, large renal cysts, renal or perirenal abscesses, congenital abnormalities, ureteral stenosis, or refractory obstruction from calculi.[5,9,11,13–15]

Contraindications. In case of azotemia, as renal function is already reduced by at least 75%.[2,10] Ideally, an excretory pyelogram should be performed prior to surgery to confirm adequate contralateral renal function, while taking into account the potential nephrotoxicity of the contrast media used.[5,16,17]

Surgical steps

- The kidney is reflected ventromedially to expose the renal vessels and ureter from the dorsal surface of kidney.[2,5,10,13,14]

- The renal artery and vein are separately isolated (**Fig. 2**B) and clamped using vascular clamps, then double-ligated or triple-ligated (4-0 to 5-0 suture in rabbits) close to the descending aorta and caudal vena cava, respectively,[2,13,14] or sealed using vascular sealing technology such as LigaSure.[2] The vessels are transected between the clamp and the ligatures.[5,10,14]
- The ureter is dissected along its entire length up to the bladder neck (**Fig. 2**C). Leaving a ureteral stump or intact ureter may predispose to vesicoureteral reflux and recurrent lower urinary tract infections, so placing a clip or an encircling absorbable suture close to the bladder is recommended, taking care not to damage adjacent nerves in the lateral ligament of the bladder (**Fig. 2**D).[2,13]
- The kidney and ureter are removed en bloc, transecting the ureter above the ligature or clip.[2,5]

Complications and prognosis. Complications include intraoperative hemorrhage, bladder injury, urine leakage, infection, postoperative renal insufficiency (if contralateral kidney is compromised), adhesions, and recurrent urinary infections.[2,5] Prognosis is favorable when contralateral renal function is intact. Long-term survival is reported in rabbits and ferrets following nephrectomy for kidney tumors.[2,14,18,19]

Surgery of the Ureter

Ureterotomy

Indications. For removal of ureteroliths when medical management fails.[9]

Contraindications. In cases of markedly dilated ureter or hydronephrosis or high risk of postoperative stricture; nephroureterectomy may be indicated instead.[5] In very small species, surgical manipulation may be technically unfeasible.

Surgical steps

- The ureterolith is palpated and localized (**Fig. 3**A, B). Encircling stay sutures may be placed proximally and distally to isolate the segment and gently elevate it.[5]
- A transverse or longitudinal incision is made over or just proximal to the calculus, allowing its removal (**Fig. 3**C).[5] Samples for bacterial culture can be taken.
- Ureteral patency is verified using a 3 Fr catheter, and the proximal ureter and renal pelvis are gently flushed with sterile saline.[5,9]
- The ureter is closed with simple interrupted sutures (7-0 in rabbits), avoiding tension (**Fig. 3**D). An omental wrap may be applied if feasible (usually not possible in rabbits and smaller species). Longitudinal incisions are closed transversely when possible to widen lumen diameter and limit the risk of stricture.[5]

Complications and prognosis. Complications include ureteral stricture, recurrent obstruction, urine leakage, and peritonitis. Prognosis is guarded and depends on the degree of hydronephrosis and contralateral renal function.[5,9] Recurrence of calculi is common.[5]

Uretero-vesical reimplantation/ureteroneocystostomy

Indications. In cases of congenital ureteral anomalies (eg, circumcaval or retrocaval ureter (**Fig. 4**A), which may lead to hydroureteronephrosis), traumatic avulsion near the bladder, or when distal ureter resection and reimplantation are required to restore urinary drainage (eg, ureterovesical junction stenosis).[20–22]

Species-specific considerations. Ureteroneocystostomy is mainly described in ferrets.[20,21,23]

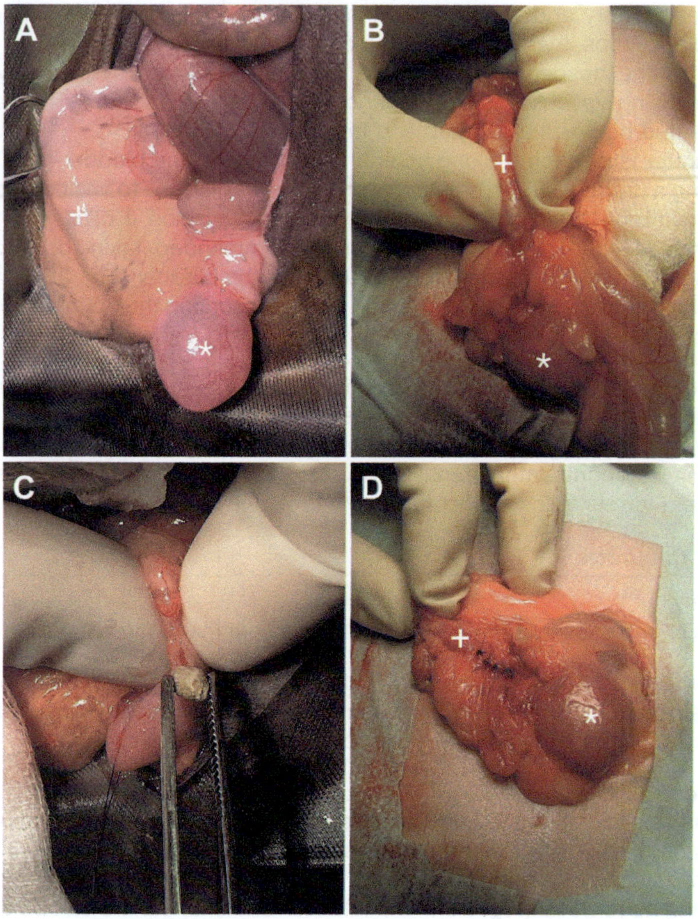

Fig. 3. Ureterotomy in a guinea pig (*Cavia porcellus*). (*A*) Visualization of the ureter (+) and the bladder (*asterisk*). (*B*) Localization of the calculus within the ureter (+). (*C*) Removal of the calculus. (*D*) Longitudinal closure of the ureter (+) using simple interrupted absorbable monofilament suture. (Image Courtesy of Dr Véronique Mentré and Dr Clément Paillusseau.)

Surgical steps

- The bladder is exposed through midline celiotomy and isolated using laparotomy pads.[10] A full-thickness monofilament stay suture is placed at the bladder apex for retraction.[10]
- A cystotomy is performed by making an incision on the ventral surface of the bladder in an avascular area, and urine is suctioned. The ureteral papilla and ureter can then be localized, followed by retrograde ureteral catheterization to confirm patency (**Fig. 4**B).[10,20]
- The ureter is transected close to the bladder, and repositioned in its normal anatomic position if required, as in circumcaval cases.[20]
- The ureter is reimplanted into the bladder mucosa by an end-to-end anastomosis using interrupted sutures (6-0 in ferrets), ensuring mucosa-to-mucosa apposition

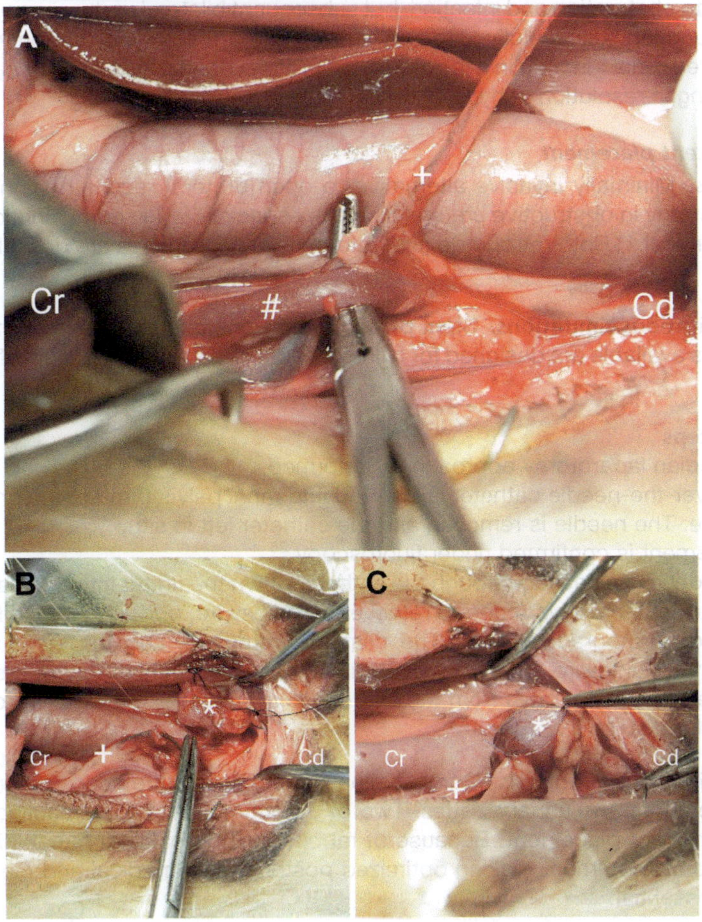

Fig. 4. Ureteroneocystostomy in a ferret with a circumcaval ureter (*M putorius furo*). (*A*) Visualization of the abnormal course of the ureter (+) with a medial and dorsal deviation to the caudal vena cava (#). (*B*) Insertion of a guide into the ureter (+) after its transection close to the bladder (*asterisk*). (*C*) End-to-end anastomosis between the bladder (*asterisk*) and the ureter (+). (*Adapted from* Cécile Bernhard, Adeline Linsart, Véronique Mentré, Circumcaval ureter in two ferrets, Journal of Exotic Pet Medicine, 42, 2022, 42-46, https://doi.org/10.1053/j.jepm.2022.04.006.)

(**Fig. 4**C). Patency is checked by placing a catheter retrogradely through the ureter.[10] A short stent placement is considered if the size permits.[20]

- The bladder is closed in a single-layer with a simple continuous appositional pattern, incorporating the submucosa.[10] An additional Cushing inverting pattern can be added.[10]

Complications and prognosis. Ureteroneocystostomy is technically challenging, and complications include persistent hydronephrosis, anastomotic leak, stricture, or the need for nephrectomy in severe or recurrent cases. Prognosis is variable: in one case of circumcaval ureter in a ferret, a ureterovesical anastomosis was performed, but nephrectomy was ultimately required due to persistent hydronephrosis.[20] In a reported case of bilateral ureterovesical junction stenosis, initial subcutaneous ureteral bypass failed due to obstruction and infection, but subsequent bilateral ureteroneocystostomy restored function successfully.[23] In another report, a ureteroneocystostomy successfully restored renal function in a ferret with left ureteral obstruction caused by urolithiasis, resulting in resolution of hydronephrosis.[21]

Ureteral stent placement

Indications. Minimally invasive alternative to open ureteral reconstruction or nephroureterectomy in obstructive ureteral disease, especially when renal function preservation is critical.[24] Both retrograde and anterograde approaches are described in pet rabbits.[25]

Contraindications/limitations. Stent placement is constrained by animal size. Smallest devices available are designed for feline patients and may be unsuitable for smaller rabbits.[24]

Surgical steps

- A median laparotomy approach is performed.
- An over-the-needle catheter is inserted into renal pelvis through the greater curvature. The needle is removed and the catheter left in situ.[24,25]
- Placement is confirmed under fluoroscopy.[25]
- A guidewire is passed through the catheter down the ureter into the bladder.[24,25]
- A bladder incision is made to retrieve the guidewire, and a ureteral dilator is inserted normograde over it. The dilator is removed, and the stent advanced over the guidewire. The cranial pigtail is positioned within renal pelvis, and the guidewire is withdrawn from the bladder to allow the distal pigtail to curl within the bladder.[24,25]

Complications and prognosis. Complications in rabbits include encrustation, soft tissue proliferation, and urinary issues. Two of 3 documented cases resulted in death within months of placement. Because of rabbits' unique calcium metabolism, stent encrustation is common, making optimized postoperative medical and dietary management essential.[24,25]

Subcutaneous ureteral bypass

Indications. The subcutaneous ureteral bypass (SUB) offers an alternative to open ureteral reconstruction or nephroureterectomy for obstructive ureteral disease, especially when renal function preservation is a priority. This technique avoids the need of ureterotomy, avoids compromising ureterovesical junction and allows postoperative flushing, minimizing encrustation risk.[24]

Contraindications/limitations. Current SUB devices are designed for feline patients and consist of a 6.5 F catheter. Main limitation is renal pelvis size.[24]

Surgical steps

- A median laparotomy is performed.
- An over-the-needle catheter is inserted into the caudal renal pole, midway between dorsal and ventral surfaces, and directed toward renal pelvis. Advancing the nephrostomy catheter down the ureter is generally easier and safer than coiling it within the pelvis.[24]
- Placement is verified under fluoroscopy.[24]
- A 0.035 inch guidewire is inserted through the 18 gauge catheter and coiled in renal pelvis. The catheter is withdrawn over the guidewire.[24]

- A 6.5 F pigtail locking-loop nephrostomy tube is placed over the 1190 Palm and Culp guidewire (Boston Scientific, Marlborough, MA, USA) into the renal pelvis and secured to the renal capsule with tissue adhesive.[24]
- A 6.5 F cystotomy tube is inserted and sutured into the bladder.[24]
- Both tube ends are tunneled through the body wall and connected to a titanium shunting port fixed to the body wall.[24]

Complications and prognosis. In cases reported in rabbits and ferrets, SUB placement lead to urinary tract infection, kinking, or obstruction. Regular port flushing and imaging are essential to maintain function.[24,25]

Surgery of the Bladder

Cystotomy

Indications. For removal of uroliths, initially located in the bladder or retroflushed from the urethra, for repair of bladder rupture, biopsy, removal of intravesical masses and diagnostic exploration of the bladder (eg, cases of chronic cystitis unresponsive to medical treatment).[26]

Surgical steps

- When a cystotomy is performed for the removal of uroliths (vesical and/or urethral), a retrograde urinary catheter is inserted through the external urethral orifice to flush any urethral stones back into the bladder and confirm urethral patency. If retrograde flushing is unsuccessful, urethrostomy may be required.[2,3,26] A Foley catheter can also be used intraoperatively to prevent stone migration.[26]
- A caudal midline laparotomy is performed, ending about 1 cm cranial to the pelvis in rabbits.[3,26] Care is taken to avoid bladder perforation, particularly when the bladder is distended.[26] In male ferrets, the incision is in part parapreputial given the location of the penis and prepuce.[22]
- The bladder is gently exteriorized and isolated with moistened gauze.[2,3] If distended, cystocentesis is performed to minimize contamination of the abdominal cavity with urine.[2]
- Stay sutures are placed cranially and caudally to the bladder incision site (**Fig. 5**A).[2,3]
- The incision is made in an avascular region of the bladder (**Fig. 5**B).[2,3] Bleeding may occur in chronically inflamed bladders.[26]
- Stones are removed using small, dull-edged spoons or forceps, taking care to avoid mucosal injury (**Fig. 5**C).[3] Alternating normograde flushing and retrograde flushing is recommended to ensure complete removal of urethral stones.[3]
- Samples for culture and/or histopathology can be taken. If no preoperative urinary culture was performed, a bladder wall swab can be collected.[2]
- The bladder is flushed with warm sterile saline to remove blood clots and debris.[2]
- Closure is performed using a simple interrupted or continuous full-thickness patterns (4-0 to 6-0 resorbable monofilament; **Fig. 5**D).[2,3] Ideally, sutures should avoid entering bladder lumen to limit the risk of recurrence due to suture material forming a nidus.[2] However, distinguishing submucosa from mucosa is difficult, so full-thickness sutures are often recommended.[3]
- Bladder integrity is tested by filling it with sterile saline via fine needle or catheter; additional simple interrupted or continuous inverting sutures are placed if leakage is detected (**Fig. 5**E).[2,3]

Complications and prognosis. Complications include intraoperative bladder rupture or perforation, ureteral injury, postoperative incisional dehiscence, and uroabdomen.

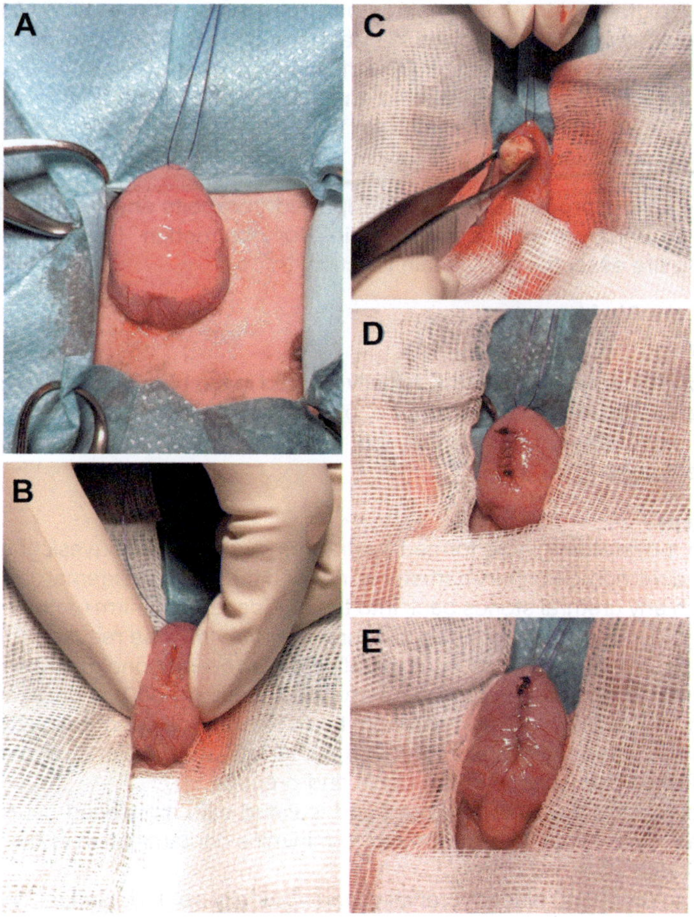

Fig. 5. Cystotomy in a guinea pig (*Cavia porcellus*) with a urolith. (*A*) Placement of a stay suture cranial to bladder incision. Note the markedly thickened bladder wall. (*B*) Incision made in an avascular ventral region of the bladder. (*C*) Removal of the urolith. (*D*) Bladder closure using continuous full-thickness pattern. (*E*) A cushing inverting pattern can be added if necessary. (Image Courtesy of Dr Cécile Bernhard.)

Adhesions can form with intestines or uterus, especially in cases of pre-existing chronic cystitis. Postoperative challenges include persistent hematuria, urinary obstruction from clots, missed uroliths, and straining due to inflammation.[2]

Survival and recurrence have been reported in guinea pigs and chinchillas. In a retrospective study of 25 guinea pigs, 60% survived to discharge, but only 48%- survived the first postoperative month.[27] Prognosis was better in animals exhibiting preoperative signs of discomfort, whereas urethral stones were associated with higher mortality. Surgery failed in 1 patient due to inability to dislodge a urethral stone.[27] In chinchillas, cystotomy was successful in 10 cases. Half experienced recurrence within 19 to 400 days, and most died between 74 and 1074 days postoperatively. Animals without recurrence had a median follow-up of 2204 days.[28]

Bladder biopsy. The technique follows the same principles as cystotomy. Unless full-thickness biopsies are needed, biopsies may be obtained via cystoscopy for a less-invasive approach.[5]

Cystectomy

Indications. In case of bladder tumors, inflammatory polyps, necrotized or traumatic lesions.[2,3,5] In general, up to two-thirds of bladder wall can be resected without impairing function, provided the trigone and ureters are not damaged.[2,3] Anecdotal reports describe successful removal of vesical soft tissue sarcomas in 2 guinea pigs and transitional cell carcinoma in a rabbit.[29,30]

Surgical steps

- The procedure follows the same steps as cystotomy (see earlier discussion).
- The bladder is palpated prior to incision to locate masses, leaving a 1 to 2 cm margin from the mass.[5]
- Stay sutures may assist in mass removal and bladder closure.[5]
- Use of a composite membrane for full-thickness bladder defects is described, but if the trigone remains intact, remaining bladder typically expands postoperatively.[5]
- A urethral catheter can be left in place for 1 to 2 days to allow a fibrin seal to form, especially when a large part of the bladder is resected.[3]

Cystopexy

Indications. In cases of bladder eversion, most commonly reported in postpartum multiparous female rabbits. Prognosis is generally poor, especially if the bladder is severely damaged.[3,5]

Surgical steps

- A midline laparotomy is performed, following the same approach as for cystotomy.
- After thoroughly rinsing the prolapsed bladder, it is gently repositioned through the urethra and grasped with atraumatic forceps through the laparotomy incision.[3,5]
- Once repositioned into the abdomen, partial cystectomy is performed if necrotic lesions are present.[3,5]
- The bladder is sutured to the abdominal wall during closure. Scarification of ventral bladder serosa and internal abdominal oblique muscle is described to promote permanent cystopexy.[3,5]

Tube cystotomy (temporary and long term)

Indications. Temporary tube cystotomy is indicated in ferrets and rabbits with urethral obstruction when catheterization fails, particularly for prostatic or paraurethral cysts in ferrets (**Fig. 6**A). Long-term cystotomy tubes may be considered for permanent damage, such as bladder atony or following penile amputation.[1,9]

Surgical steps

- Midline approach is commonly used, with incision at the bladder midpoint.[1,9] Alternatively, a 2 to 3 cm oblique inguinal incision directly over the bladder is performed.[9]
- Stay sutures and a purse string suture are placed at the intended catheter entry site.[9]
- A separate abdominal wall incision is made to pass a 5 to 8 Fr Foley catheter.[1,9] The bladder is incised within the purse-string suture, emptied, and the Foley

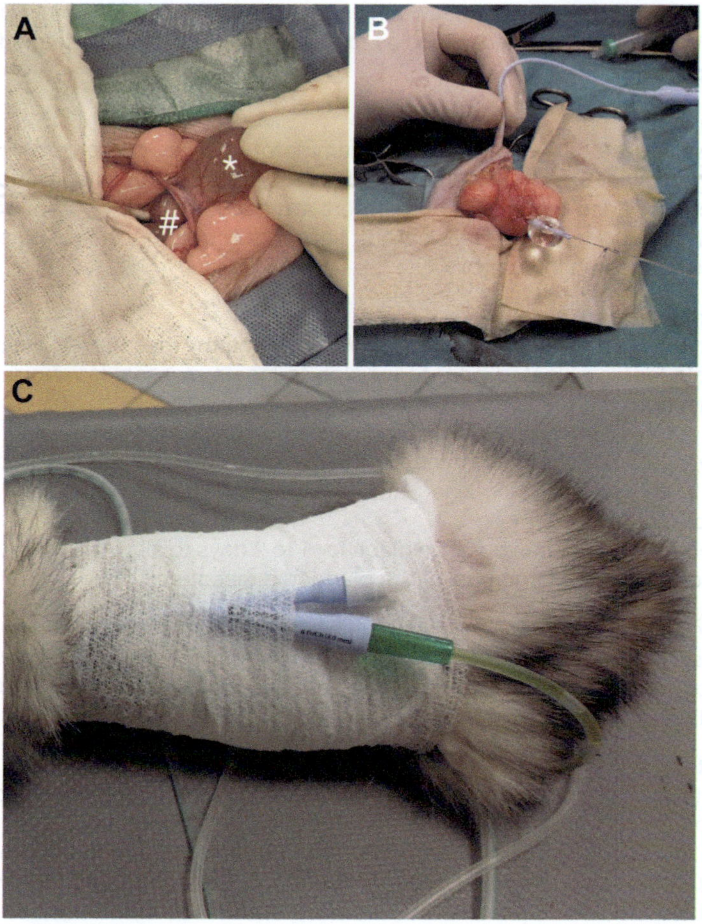

Fig. 6. Management of paraprostatic abscesses in 2 ferrets (*M putorius furo*). (*A*) Identification of the single paraprostatic abscess (#) and bladder (*asterisk*) in ferret 1. (*B*) Placement of a Foley catheter during surgery in ferret 2. (*C*) Foley catheter in place postsurgery. (Image Courtesy of Dr Lucile Chassang.)

catheter inserted through the incision (**Fig. 6**B).[1,3,9] The balloon is inflated with saline and secured by tightening the purse-string suture.

- The bladder is sutured to the body wall with interrupted absorbable sutures. The initial incision is closed routinely and the catheter secured to the skin with a finger-trap suture.[3,9]
- Catheters can be left in place for 1 to 5 days (**Fig. 6**C).[1]

Alternative techniques. Low-profile silicone gastrostomy tubes have been used as long-term cystotomy devices. A Foley catheter is placed for 1 to 2 weeks to create a continuous ostium, after which the low-profile tube is inserted and secured with a purse-string suture. Daily tube care and frequent urine cultures are necessary due to risk of secondary urinary tract infections (UTIs). Documented complications include mechanical cystitis, dislodgement or leakage, urinary tract infection, and septicemia.[1] Percutaneous fluoroscopy-guided cystotomy tube placement has also been described.[3]

Bladder herniation

Indications. Inguinal or scrotal bladder herniation is described in intact male and female rabbits.[7,31,32] Perineal herniation of the bladder is reported in a rabbit and a chinchilla, and midline inguinal wall herniation in rabbits.[33–35]

Surgical steps

Inguinal/scrotal hernia

- A urethral catheter is passed retrogradely to drain urine; alternatively, cystocentesis can be performed.[2,7,32] Urine samples should be collected for urinalysis and bacterial culture.[2]
- An incision is made over the inguinal hernia sac, taking care to avoid damaging herniated structures.[7,32]
- The inguinal ring is often enlarged to allow bladder replacement into the abdomen. In males, open castration is recommended, as the spermatic cord can impede proper closure of inguinal ring.[7,31,32]
- The external inguinal ring is closed with slowly absorbable monofilament suture, taking care to preserve the external pudendal vessels passing through the inguinal canal.[7,31,32,36]
- This approach can be combined with an abdominal approach and excision of the hernia sac or total scrotal ablation.[2,31,32,36]

Abdominal approach

- A caudal midline incision is performed to expose the internal inguinal ring.
- The bladder is gently repositioned into the abdomen using traction and external pressure. Cystopexy can be performed.
- The internal inguinal canal is closed with simple interrupted or horizontal mattress sutures.[2,7]

Perineal and inguinal midline body wall hernias Transposition of the internal obturator muscle was successfully performed in 1 female rabbit and 1 male chinchilla with perineal herniation.[34,35]

For midline abdominal wall herniation in rabbits, surgery consisted in incising the skin at the level of the hernia, dissecting the hernia sac, replacing the organs in their normal anatomic position, followed by excision of the line of contact on the body wall and closure of the fascia (**Fig. 7**A, B).[33]

Complications. Recurrence is fairly common, occurring in 2 of 6 rabbits with inguinal hernia in 1 retrospective study.[32] Other complications include hematoma, seroma, infection, and repair rupture.[2]

Surgery of the Urethra

Urethrotomy

Indications. To remove urethral calculi. In female guinea pigs, large stones may get stuck at urethral papilla. In rabbits, stones often obstruct the urethral opening, the narrowest point in both sexes.[3]

If feasible, stones can be retrogradely flushed into the bladder, which is preferred to reduce risk of postoperative stricture. Chronic, adherent, or very large stones may prevent hydroretropulsion.[2,3,9] Urethral calculi located within the intrapelvic urethra are the most challenging situation because of limited surgical access. When retrograde hydroretropulsion is unsuccessful, a pubiotomy (pubic osteotomy) or symphysiotomy may be required to approach the pelvic urethra.

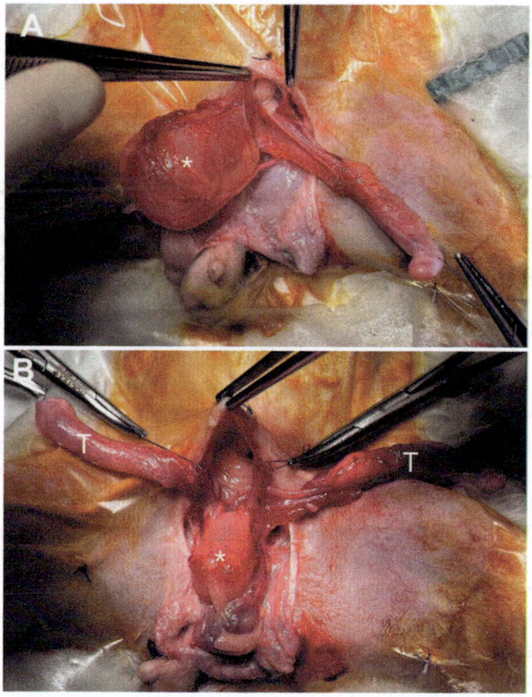

Fig. 7. Inguinal midline body wall hernia in an intact male rabbit (*O cuniculus*) involving the urinary bladder. (*A*) Visualization of the urinary bladder (*asterisk*) within the hernial sac. (*B*) Appearance of the urinary bladder (*asterisk*) after careful dissection of the hernial sac. Testicles (T) are visible prior to castration. (Image Courtesy of Dr José Rosas-Navarro.)

Surgical steps

Distal urethrotomy

Female distal urethrotomy

- The stone is stabilized using fingers, and a sufficiently large incision is made through the skin, urethra, and vagina (in rabbits) to remove it (**Fig. 8**A, B).[3]
- The urethra, vagina, and skin can be sutured close or left to heal by second intention.[3]

In one guinea pig, a urethral diverticulum caused stone recurrence. Urethrostomy including the diverticulum was performed and allowed to create a larger urethral opening.[37]

Penile urethrotomy:

This technique is described in male rabbits.[2]

- The pubic area and scrotum are aseptically prepared, keeping inguinal skin folds lateral to the prepuce draped outside surgery field.[2,5]
- A longitudinal incision is made on ventral or lateral side of the penis skin (**Fig. 9**A), and subcutaneous tissues are dissected onto the palpated stone (**Fig. 9**B). The urolith is localized by palpation or by measuring a urinary catheter inserted to the stone.[2]
- The stone is stabilized between 2 fingers before incising the urethra longitudinally over it (**Fig. 9**C).[2]

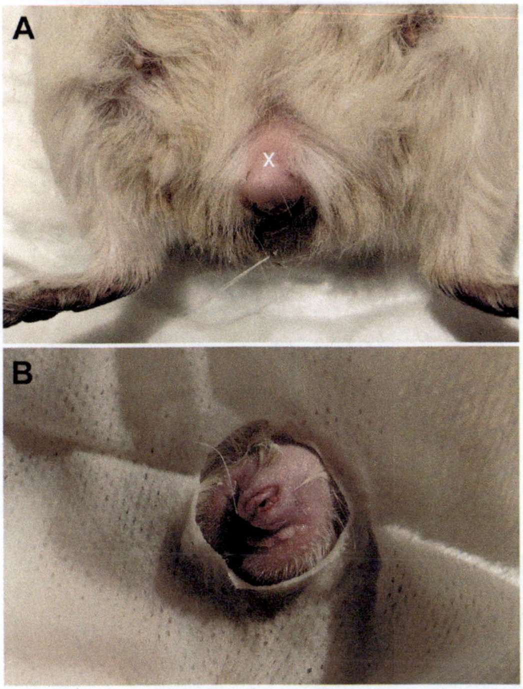

Fig. 8. Distal urethrotomy in a female guinea pig (*Cavia porcellus*). (*A*) Visualization of the urolith in distal urethra (x). (*B*) Incision through skin and urethra. (Image Courtesy of Dr Lucile Chassang.)

- After removal of the stone, urethral patency is confirmed with a urinary catheter before closure with a continuous 5-0 suture. The skin is closed routinely.[2]
- The urinary catheter may be left in place for 24 to 48 hours to decrease the risk of postoperative obstruction.[2]

Intrapelvic urethrotomy (pubiotomy/symphysiotomy approach) Intrapelvic urethrotomy has not been reported in exotic small mammals. The following description is based on surgical techniques described in domestic carnivores.[38]

- A ventral midline incision is performed over the ischium to expose the pubic symphysis.
- A symphysiotomy or partial pubiotomy is performed using an oscillating saw or osteotome regarding the pubis and ischium. The intrapelvic urethra is carefully isolated and incised longitudinally over the stone, which is then removed.
- Urethral patency is confirmed with a urinary catheter before closure of the urethra with simple continuous or interrupted pattern.
- The pubic bones are apposed using orthopedic wire or suture, and routine closure of the abdominal wall and skin is performed.[38]

Complications and prognosis. Postoperative complications include urethral obstruction secondary to swelling, fibrosis, or necrosis. Maintaining a urinary catheter for 24 to 48 hours after surgery helps reduce this risk. Urine leakage into the subcutis may also occur, as well as stricture formation.[2]

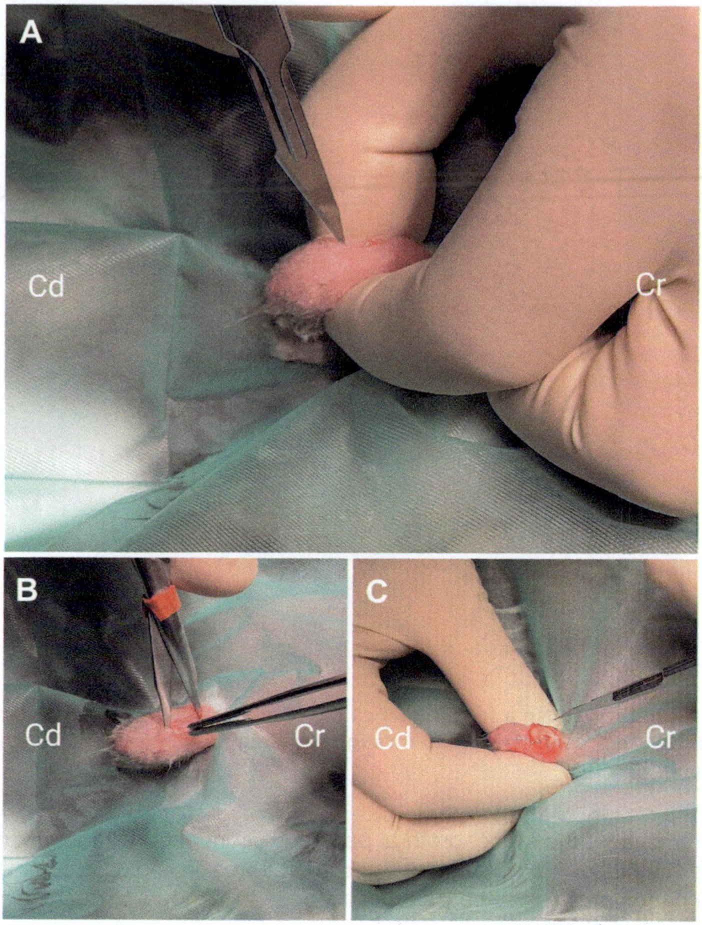

Fig. 9. Distal urethrotomy in a male rabbit (*O cuniculus*). (*A*) Ventral incision on the penis skin. (*B*) Careful dissection of subcutaneous tissues onto the palpated urethral stone. (*C*) Stabilization of the urethral stone between 2 fingers before incision of the urethra. (Image Courtesy of Dr Carlo Paoletti.)

Urethrostomy

Indications. For distal urethral strictures, trauma, neoplasia, or urethral calculi.[3,22,39]

Perineal urethrostomy in ferrets. Penile anatomy is similar to that of dogs. Urethrostomy is performed caudal to the os penis, proximal to the obstruction, and 1 to 2 cm ventral to the anus, where the urethra is wide and superficial.[3,22,40,41] The penis does not require resection.[13]

- The ferret is placed either in dorsal recumbency with the pelvic area elevated or in ventral recumbency with a perineal stand.[22]
- Caudal abdomen and perineal region are aseptically prepared, and a purse-string suture is placed on the anus.[22,40] A urinary catheter is placed retrogradely if possible.[22]
- A vertical skin incision is made 1 to 2 cm ventral to the anus to expose the base of the penis (**Fig. 10**A), then a 1 to 1.5 cm incision is made along ventral penile

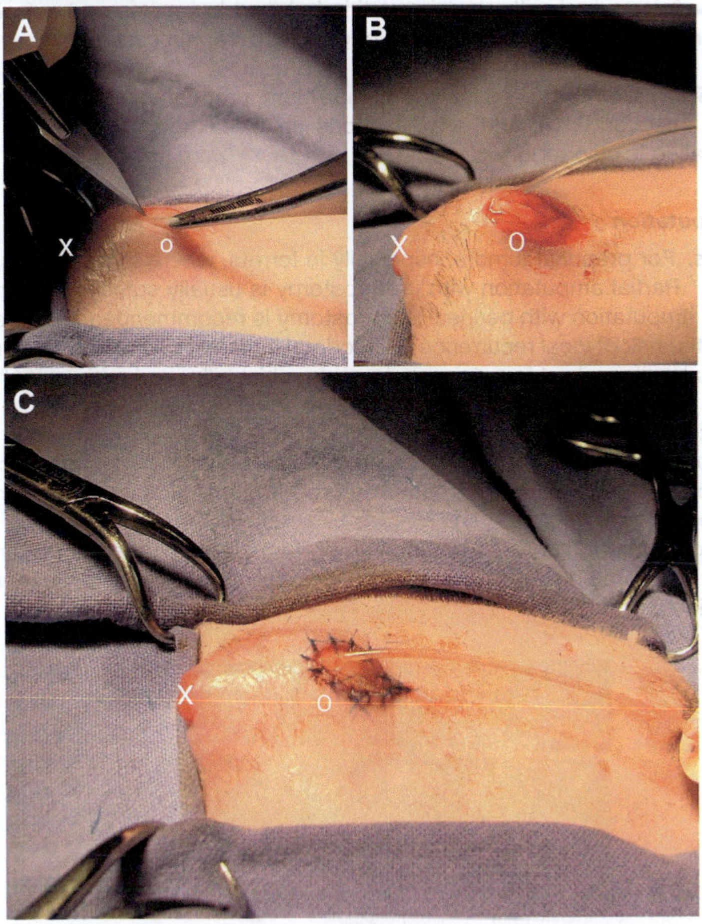

Fig. 10. Urethrostomy in a ferret (*M putorius furo*). (*A*) Vertical skin incision 2 cm ventral to the anus (x) to expose the base of the penis (o). (*B*) Placement of a urinary catheter through the incision. (*C*) Urethral mucosa sutured to skin edges with nonabsorbable simple interrupted sutures. (Image Courtesy of Dr Véronique Mentré.)

urethra. Placement of a urinary catheter facilitates the procedure (**Fig. 10**B). Care is required to avoid the cavernous tissue on both side of the urethra.[22,40] Damage to cavernous tissue can cause bleeding lasting 2 to 4 weeks.[3]

- A larger catheter is placed in proximal urethra, and the bladder emptied if needed.[22,40]
- The urethral mucosa is sutured to skin edges using 5-0 or 6-0 absorbable or nonabsorbable simple interrupted sutures (**Fig. 10**C).[22,40] Stoma should be at least 1 cm long, and sutures removed after 10 to 14 days.[22,40]

Urethrostomy in other species. In other small mammals, urethrostomy is only reported anecdotally. Perineal urethrostomy was described in a rabbit with a urethral stricture.[39] In a guinea pig, prescrotal urethrostomy was performed at the same time as penile amputation for the management of balanoposthitis and urethritis leading to adhesions, mineralizations, and fibrosis.[42] Scrotal urethrostomy was reported in an Eastern fox squirrel with chronic cystitis-induced lower urinary tract obstruction while a scrotal approach was used in a degu with paraphimosis.[43,44]

Complications. Complications include hemorrhage, urethral stricture, urine scald, urinary tract infection (UTI), and subcutaneous urine leakage.[3] Dehiscence and prolonged healing is also reported.[42]

Penile amputation

Indications. For preputial tumors, especially in ferrets, where these tumors are often malignant.[7] Partial amputation with urethrostomy is usually sufficient in most cases, while total amputation with perineal urethrostomy is recommended for larger masses to reduce the risk of local recurrence.[7] Anecdotal cases of partial or total penis amputation are also described in a degu, guinea pig, chinchilla, and rabbit.[39,42,44,45]

Surgical steps

- For partial amputation, after removing distal penis, a 3 Fr urethral catheter is placed and the urethral mucosa is sutured to penile surface using simple interrupted sutures (**Fig. 11**A, B).[7]
- For total amputation, urethrostomy is performed simultaneously at amputation site or more proximally (perineal, scrotal, and so forth) depending on species.[7,39,42,44,45]

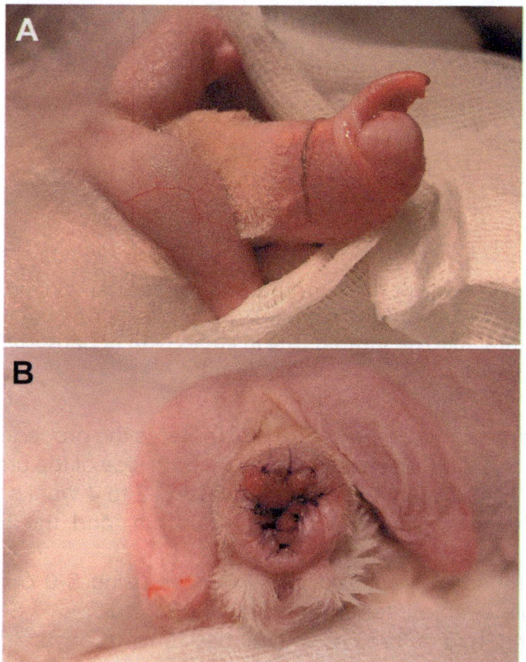

Fig. 11. Partial penile amputation in a rabbit (*O cuniculus*) following a bite wound injury. (*A*) Preoperative appearance of the penis showing stenosis of the distal portion secondary to a bite wound, with proximal urethral distension caused by urine retention. (*B*) Postoperative appearance after partial penile amputation, with urethral mucosa sutured to skin using interrupted sutures. (Image Courtesy of Dr Cécile Bernhard.)

Minimally Invasive Approaches

Alternative to cystotomy and urethrotomy should be considered whenever possible, as minimally invasive options are reported in rabbits, ferrets, and guinea pigs.

Percutaneous cystolithotomy

Percutaneous cystolithotomy is described in ferrets and rabbits, offering a lower complication rate than cystotomy, and a reduced risk of incomplete stone removal when combined with endoscopy. The bladder incision is smaller and manipulation of the viscera is minimal.[3,46]

In rabbits, it is described for single and small bladder calculi. The bladder is filled with saline using a urethral catheter to allow easy palpation, and the cecum and intestine are displaced laterally. A 2 cm abdominal incision is made over the palpable bladder, which is then partially exteriorized and secured to the abdominal wall with stay sutures. A 1 to 2 cm cystotomy is performed to retrieve the stone. When multiple stones are present, endoscopy and normograde or retrograde flushing are used to ensure complete removal. The bladder is closed, fixation sutures are removed, and the abdominal wall is closed routinely.[3]

In ferrets, percutaneous cystolithotomy with endoscopy allows visualization of the urethra up to distal part of ischiatic curve in males. Distal urethral stones can be flushed retrogradely or normogradely using a urinary catheter. Main limitations are the need for specialized equipment and trained operators, high cost, and long procedure time (65–170 minutes in reported cases).[46]

Nonsurgical techniques

In selected cases, urethral or small bladder uroliths may be managed using nonsurgical minimally invasive techniques. In female guinea pigs, transurethral cystoscopy allows removal of stones up to 5 mm in diameter using small rigid endoscopes and grasping forceps or retrieval baskets, avoiding cystotomy.[47,48] Cystoscopy-guided laser lithotripsy has also been reported to fragment larger stones prior to removal.[49] Additionally, extraction of distal urethral uroliths using elastic-band retractors placed along the mucosa at the urethral opening has been described in female guinea pigs and in 1 male rabbit.[50,51] Reported complications of these techniques include mild urethral or bladder trauma, hematuria, overdistension-related bladder injury, and retrograde infection, but overall morbidity appears limited in appropriately selected cases.[47,48,50,51]

CLINICS CARE POINTS

- Obtain radiographs immediately before surgery for urolithiasis, to confirm exact location of the stone(s).
- Active warming should begin before induction and continue throughout recovery, as small mammals are highly prone to perioperative hypothermia during urinary surgery.
- Lateral flank approach of the kidney minimizes visceral manipulation and postoperative pain, ventral midline approach is preferred for bilateral exploration.
- Renal vascular occlusion during renal biopsy or nephrotomy should be limited to less than 20 minutes to minimize ischemic renal injury.
- Always confirm ureteral patency intraoperatively with flushing and/or catheterization after ureterotomy or ureteral reimplantation procedures.
- Full-thickness bladder closure is often technically easier in small mammals because distinguishing the submucosa from the mucosa can be difficult.

- Whenever possible, urethral calculi should be retroflushed into the bladder before urethrotomy to reduce the risk of postoperative urethral stricture and urine leakage.
- Monofilament absorbable sutures with rapid absorption profiles are preferred in the urinary tract to reduce the risk of mineral deposition and recurrent urolith formation.
- Long-term dietary management and optimization of hydration are essential after urinary surgery in rabbits and guinea pigs because recurrence of urolithiasis is common.

DISCLOSURE

The authors have nothing to disclose.

REFERENCES

1. Di Girolamo N, Selleri P. Disorders of the urinary and reproductive systems. In: Quesenberry KE, Orcutt CJ, Mans C, editors. Rabbits, and rodents. 4th edition. St. Louis (MO): W.B. Saunders; 2020. p. 201–19.
2. Sanchez-Migallon Guzman D, Szabo Z, Steffey MA. Soft tissue surgery: rabbits. In: Quesenberry KE, Orcutt CJ, Mans C, et al, editors. Rodents. 4th edition. St. Louis (MO): W.B. Saunders; 2020. p. 446–66.
3. Bennett RA, Pye GW. In: Bennett RA, Pye GW, editors. Surgery of exotic animals. Hoboken (NJ): Wiley; 2022.
4. Kosan M, Gonulalan U, Ozturk B, et al. Tissue reactions of suture materials (polyglactine 910, chromed catgut and polydioxanone) on rat bladder wall and their role in bladder stone formation. Urol Res 2008;36(1):43–9.
5. Keeble E, Benato L. Urinary tract surgery. In: Harcourt-Brown F, Chitty J, editors. BSAVA manual of rabbit surgery, dentistry and imaging. British Sm; 2013. p. 190–211.
6. Varga M. General surgical principles and neutering. In: Varga MBT-T of RM. 2nd edition. Edinburgh: Butterworth-Heinemann; 2014. p. 425–34.
7. Bennett RA. General principles of surgical techniques. In: Quesenberry KE, Orcutt CJ, Mans C, editors. Rabbits, and rodents. 4th edition. St. Louis (MO): W.B. Saunders; 2020. p. 426–31.
8. Martorell J, Bailon D, Majó N, et al. Lateral approach to nephrotomy in the management of unilateral renal calculi in a rabbit (Oryctolagus cuniculus). J Am Vet Med Assoc 2012;240(7):863–8.
9. Szabo Z, Bradley K, Cahalane AK. Rabbit soft tissue surgery. Vet Clin North Am - Exot Anim Pract 2016;19(1):159–88.
10. Tobias KM. Surgery of the urinary tract. In: Tobias KM, editor. Manual of small animal soft tissue surgery. Ames (IA): Wiley-Blackwell; 2010. p. 275–327.
11. Varga M. Urogenital diseases. In: Varga MBT-T of RM. 2nd edition. Edinburgh: Butterworth-Heinemann; 2014. p. 405–24.
12. Greci V, Stefanello D, Di Giancamillo M, et al. The use of endoscopy-assisted nephrolithotomy for unilateral nephrolith removal in a rabbit (Oryctolagus cuniculus). Can Vet J 2009;50(11):1191–4.
13. Mehler SJ. Surgery. In: Fox JG, Marini RP, editors. Biology and diseases of the ferret. 3rd edition. Ames (IA): Wiley-Blackwell; 2014. p. 285–310.
14. Chitty JR, Johnson-Delaney CA. Common surgical procedures. In: Johnson-Delaney CA, editor. Ferret medicine and surgery. Boca Raton (FL): CRC Press; 2016. p. 389–420.

15. Duhamelle A, Tessier E, Larrat S. Ureteral stenosis following ovariohysterectomy in a rabbit (Oryctolagus cuniculus). J Exot Pet Med 2017;26(2):132–6.
16. Goic JB, Koenigshof AM, McGuire LD, et al. A retrospective evaluation of contrast-induced kidney injury in dogs (2006-2012). J Vet Emerg Crit Care 2016;26(5):713–9.
17. Mamoulakis C, Fragkiadoulaki I, Karkala P, et al. Contrast-induced nephropathy in an animal model: evaluation of novel biomarkers in blood and tissue samples. Toxicol reports 2019;6:395–400.
18. Hassan J, Katic N, Klang A, et al. Treatment of nephroblastoma with polycythaemia by nephrectomy in a rabbit. Vet Rec 2012;170(18):465.
19. Wong AD, Laniesse D, Zur Linden A, et al. Development of renal adenocarcinoma in a ferret with renal cortical cysts (Mustela putorius furo). JAVMA 2021;259(12).
20. Bernhard C, Linsart A, Mentré V. Circumcaval ureter in two ferrets (Mustela putorius furo). J Exot Pet Med 2022;42:42–6.
21. Laminette PJ, Trout NJ, Noonan B, et al. Ureteroneocystostomy for treatment of struvite urolithiasis in a ferret. J Am Vet Med Assoc 2023;261(9):1–4.
22. Jekl V, Casale S. Soft tissue surgery: ferrets. In: Quesenberry KE, Orcutt CJ, Mans C, editors. Rabbits, and rodents. 4th edition. St. Louis (MO): W.B Saunders; 2020. p. 432–45.
23. Vilalta L, Dominguez E, Altuzarra R, et al. Imaging diagnosis—radiography and ultrasonography of bilateral congenital ureterovesical junction stenosis causing hydronephrosis and hydroureter in a ferret (Mustela Putorius Furo). Vet Radiol Ultrasound 2017;58(3):E31–6.
24. Huynh M. Permanent implantable medical devices in exotic pet medicine. Vet Clin North Am - Exot Anim Pract 2019;22(3):521–38.
25. Rembeaux H, Langlois I, Burdick S, et al. Placement of ureteral stents in three rabbits for the treatment of obstructive ureterolithiasis. J Small Anim Pract 2021;62(6):489–95.
26. Szabo Z. Soft tissue surgery: rodents. In: Quesenberry KE, Orcutt CJ, Mans C, editors. Rabbits, and rodents. 4th edition. St. Louis (MO): W.B. Saunders; 2021. p. 467–82.
27. Behrens KN, Cray MT, Noonan B. Risk factors, complications, and outcomes of cystotomy in guinea pigs: 25 cases (2010-2023). J Am Vet Med Assoc 2025; 263(2):178–83.
28. Martel-Arquette A, Mans C. Urolithiasis in chinchillas: 15 cases (2007 to 2011). J Small Anim Pract 2016;57(5):260–4.
29. Nógrádi AI , Cope I, Arany-Toth A, et al. Primary urinary bladder tumors in three Guinea pigs (Cavia Porcellus). Top Companion Anim Med 2023;56–7.
30. Cikanek S, Eshar D, Nau M, et al. Diagnosis and surgical treatment of A transitional cell carcinoma in the bladder apex of A pet rabbit (Oryctolagus cuniculus). J Exot Pet Med 2018;27. https://doi.org/10.1053/j.jepm.2018.02.004.
31. Petritz OA, Guzman DS-M, Gandolfi RC, et al. Inguinal-scrotal urinary bladder hernia in an intact Male domestic rabbit (Oryctolagus cuniculus). J Exot Pet Med 2012;21(3):248–54.
32. Thas I, Harcourt-Brown F. Six cases of inguinal urinary bladder herniation in entire male domestic rabbits. J Small Anim Pract 2013;54(12):662–6.
33. Crocker K, Kline S, d'Ovidio D, et al. Diagnosis and treatment of inguinal midline abdominal wall herniation of the urinary bladder in three domestic rabbits (Oryctolagus cuniculus). Top Companion Anim Med 2025;69:101019.
34. Thöle M, Schuhmann B, Köstlinger S, et al. Treatment of unilateral perineal hernias in 2 Male chinchillas (Chinchilla Lanigera). J Exot Pet Med 2018;27(3):43–9.

35. Berk B, Böttcher A, Nagel S, et al. Rabbits: unilateral perineal-urinary bladder hernia in a high-grade cachectic intact female domestic rabbit (Oryctolagus cuniculus). Vet Rec 2017;5. https://doi.org/10.1136/vetreccr-2016-000420.
36. Grunkemeyer VL, Sura PA, Baron ML, et al. Surgical repair of an inguinal herniation of the urinary bladder in an intact female domestic rabbit (Oryctolagus cuniculus). J Exot Pet Med 2010;19(3):249–54.
37. Parkinson LAB, Hausmann JC, Hardie RJ, et al. Urethral diverticulum and urolithiasis in a female Guinea pig (Cavia porcellus). J Am Vet Med Assoc 2017;251(11):1313–7.
38. Fossum TW. Surgery of the bladder and urethra. In: Fossum T, editor. Small animal surgery. 2nd edition. St. Louis (MO): Mosby; 2002. p. 586–607.
39. Lamb S. Perineal urethrostomy in a castrated male pet rabbit (Oryctolagus cuniculus) after development of a urethral stricture. J Exot Pet Med 2024;49:18–22.
40. Mullen HS, Beeber NL. Miscellaneous surgeries in ferrets. Vet Clin North Am Exot Anim Pract 2000;3(3):663–71, vi.
41. Kokkinos P, Carasco D, Shimizu N. Perineal urethrostomy in a ferret (Mustela putorius furo) to treat iatrogenic urethral stricture after orchiectomy. Vet Rec Case Reports 2023;11. https://doi.org/10.1002/vrc2.658.
42. Doneley R. Penile amputation and pre-scrotal urethrostomy in a male Guinea pig (Cavia porcellus). Aust Vet J 2021;99(3):89–92.
43. Kleinschmidt L, Stickney M, Hoppes S. Treatment of lower urinary tract obstruction via scrotal urethrostomy in an Eastern fox squirrel (Sciurus niger). J Exot Pet Med 2016;25(4):314–20.
44. Lavallée J. Subtotal penile amputation and preputial urethrostomy in a degu (Octodon degus). Can Vet J = La Rev Vet Can 2023;64(7):650–3.
45. Grubb R. From abscess to amputation - case example of chinchilla penile surgery. Peterborough, UK: Vet Times; 2008.
46. Branquart M, Langlois I, Vachon C, et al. Removal of lower urinary tract stones by percutaneous cystolithotomy in domestic male ferrets (Mustela putorius furo): four cases (2017–2020). J Exot Pet Med 2023;45:38–44.
47. Wenger S, Hatt J-M. Transurethral cystoscopy and endoscopic Urolith removal in female Guinea pigs (Cavia porcellus). Vet Clin North Am Exot Anim Pract 2015;18(3):359–67.
48. Pizzi R. Cystoscopic removal of a urolith from a pet Guinea pig. Vet Rec 2009;165(5):148–9.
49. Coutant T, Dunn M, Langlois I, et al. Cystoscopic-guided lithotripsy for the removal of a urethral stone in a Guinea pig. J Exot Pet Med 2018;28. https://doi.org/10.1053/j.jepm.2018.02.042.
50. Lewis TT, Lennox AM. Nonsurgical removal of urethral uroliths using a self-retaining retractor with elastic stays in female Guinea pigs (Cavia porcellus): 16 cases (2006–2019). J Exot Pet Med 2021;36:11–5.
51. Lempert M. Urethrolith removal using an elastic band retractor in a male rabbit. J Exot Pet Med 2020;35:112–3.

9780443473166